Atlas of Laparoscopic and Robotic Urologic Surgery

Atlas of Laparoscopic and Robotic Urologic Surgery

THIRD EDITION

Editors

Jay T. Bishoff, MD

Director
The Intermountain Urological Institute
Adjunct Professor of Surgery
University of Utah
Salt Lake City, Utah

Louis R. Kavoussi, MD, MBA

Waldbaum-Gardner Professor and Chairman of Urology
The Arthur Smith Institute for Urology
Hofstra Northwell School of Medicine
Hempstead, New York

Associate Editor

David A. Leavitt, MD

Vattikuti Urology Institute
Henry Ford Health System
Detroit, Michigan

ELSEVIER

ELSEVIER

1600 John F. Kennedy Blvd.
Ste 1800
Philadelphia, PA 19103-2899

Previous edition copyrighted 2007.

Library of Congress Cataloging-in-Publication Data
Names: Bishoff, Jay T., editor. | Kavoussi, Louis R., editor.
Title: Atlas of laparoscopic and robotic urologic surgery / [edited by] Jay
   T. Bishoff, Louis R. Kavoussi.
Other titles: Atlas of laparoscopic urologic surgery (Bishoff)
Description: Third edition. | Philadelphia, PA : Elsevier, [2017] | Preceded
   by: Atlas of laparoscopic urologic surgery / [edited by] Jay T. Bishoff,
   Louis R. Kavoussi. c2007. | Includes bibliographical references and index.
Identifiers: LCCN 2016030629 | ISBN 9780323393263 (hardcover : alk. paper)
Subjects: | MESH: Urologic Surgical Procedures—methods |
   Laparoscopy—methods | Robotic Surgical Procedures—methods | Atlases
Classification: LCC RD572 | NLM WJ 17 | DDC 617.4/60597—dc23 LC record available at
   https://lccn.loc.gov/2016030629

Senior Content Strategist: Charlotta Kryhl
Senior Content Development Specialist: Ann R. Anderson
Publishing Services Manager: Patricia Tannian
Senior Project Manager: Claire Kramer
Design Direction: Christian Bilbow

Printed in China.

Last digit is the print number: 9 8 7 6 5 4 3 2 1

This opus is dedicated to the courageous giants who took the risks that advanced our craft and created time to be incredible mentors and inspiration: Arthur Smith, Ralph Clayman, and Patrick Walsh.

Contributors

Steven F. Abboud, MD
Urologic Oncology Branch
National Cancer Institute
National Institutes of Health
Bethesda, Maryland
Laparoscopic Partial Nephrectomy

Vineet Agrawal, MD, FRCSEd (Uro.), FEBU
Attending Urological Surgeon
The Guthrie Clinic
Sayre, Pennsylvania
Preperitoneal Robotic-Assisted Radical Prostatectomy

Rajesh Ahlawat, MBBS, MS, MNAMS, MCh
Chairman, Division of Urology and Renal Transplantation
Medanta Kidney and Urology Institute
Medanta Hospital
Gurgaon, India
Minimally Invasive Renal Recipient Surgery

Haris S. Ahmed, MD
Urology Resident
The Arthur Smith Institute for Urology
Hofstra Northwell School of Medicine
Hempstead, New York
Laparoscopic Varicocelectomy

Mohamad E. Allaf, MD
Associate Professor of Urology, Oncology, and Biomedical Engineering
Director of Minimally Invasive and Robotic Surgery
Brady Urological Institute
Department of Urology
Johns Hopkins University School of Medicine
Baltimore, Maryland
The da Vinci Surgical System

Tareq Al-Tartir, MD, FRCSC
Department of Urology
Roswell Park Cancer Institute
Buffalo, New York
Robotic-Assisted Intracorporeal Ileal Conduit

Kyle Anderson, MD
Department of Urology
University of Minnesota
Minneapolis, Minnesota
Basic Instrumentation

Sero Andonian, MD, MSc, FRCS(C), FACS
Associate Professor
Division of Urology
McGill University Health Centre
Montreal, Quebec, Canada
Laparoscopic/Robotic Camera and Lens Systems

Judith Aronsohn, MD
Assistant Professor
Anesthesiology
Hofstra Northwell School of Medicine
Hempstead, New York
Anesthetic Considerations for Laparoscopic/Robotic Surgery

Mohamed A. Atalla, MD
Chief of Urology
Department of Urology
Mid-Atlantic Permanente Medical Group
Largo, Maryland
Ports and Establishing Access into the Peritoneal Cavity

Timothy D. Averch, MD
Professor and Vice Chair for Quality
Department of Urology
University of Pittsburgh Medical Center
Pittsburgh, Pennsylvania
Laparoscopic Simple Nephrectomy

Jathin Bandari, MD
University of Pittsburgh
Pittsburgh, Pennsylvania
Laparoscopic Renal Biopsy

Mahendra Bhandari, MD
Director, Robotic Surgery Education and Research
Vattikuti Urology Institute
Henry Ford Hospital
Detroit, Michigan
Minimally Invasive Renal Recipient Surgery

Sam B. Bhayani, MD, MS
Holekamp Family Endowed Chair in Urology
Professor, Urologic Surgery
Chief Medical Officer, Faculty Practice Plan
Co-Director of Robotic Surgery
Washington University Institute for Minimally Invasive Surgery
Division of Urologic Surgery
Department of Surgery
Washington University School of Medicine
St. Louis, Missouri
Laparoscopic Pyeloplasty

Giampaolo Bianchi, MD
Full Professor of Urology
Department of Urology
University of Modena and Reggio Emilia, Italy
Laparoscopic Denervation for Chronic Testicular Pain

Jay T. Bishoff, MD
Director
The Intermountain Urological Institute
Adjunct Professor of Surgery
University of Utah
Salt Lake City, Utah
Endoscopic Subcutaneous Modified Inguinal Lymph Node Dissection for Squamous Cell Carcinoma of the Penis

Sam J. Brancato, MD
Clinical Fellow
Urologic Oncology Branch
National Cancer Institute
Bethesda, Maryland
Laparoscopic Partial Nephrectomy

Jeffrey A. Cadeddu, MD
Professor of Urology and Radiology
Department of Urology
University of Texas Southwestern Medical Center
Dallas, Texas
Laparoscopic Radical Nephrectomy

Peter A. Caputo, MD
Glickman Urologic and Kidney Institute
Cleveland Clinic
Cleveland, Ohio
Retroperitoneal Access

George K. Chow, MD
Consultant
Department of Urology
Mayo Clinic
Rochester, Minnesota
Laparoscopic Adrenalectomy

Daniela Colleselli, MD
Department of Urology and Andrology
Paracelsus Medical University
Salzburg, Austria
Partial Adrenalectomy

Daoud Dajani, MD, MSc
Robotic Surgery and Advanced Laparoscopy Fellow
Department of Urology
University of Southern California
Los Angeles, California
Ports and Establishing Access into the Peritoneal Cavity

Brian D. Duty, MD
Assistant Professor
Department of Urology
Oregon Health and Science University
Portland, Oregon
  *Laparoscopic Appendiceal Onlay Flap
  and Bowel Reconfiguration for Complex
  Ureteral Stricture Reconstruction*

Sammy E. Elsamra, MD
Assistant Professor of Surgery (Urology)
Department of Surgery
Division of Urology
Rutgers Robert Wood Johnson Medical
  School
New Brunswick, New Jersey
  Insufflators and the Pneumoperitoneum

Justin I. Friedlander, MD
Assistant Professor of Urology
Department of Urology
Einstein Healthcare Network
Philadelphia, Pennsylvania
  Pyelolithotomy and Ureterolithotomy

Matthew Gettman, MD
Professor and Vice-Chair
Department of Urology
Mayo Clinic
Rochester, Minnesota
  Laparoscopic Renal Cyst Decortication

Mazyar Ghanaat, MD
Chief Resident
Department of Urology
SUNY Downstate School of Medicine
Great Neck, New York
  Laparoscopic Orchiopexy

Leonard Glickman, MD
Laparoscopic, Robotic, and
  Endourology Fellow
Department of Urology
Hackensack University Medical Center
Hackensack, New Jersey
  *Laparoscopic and Robotic-Assisted
  Laparoscopic Pelvic Lymph Node
  Dissection*

Khurshid A. Guru, MD
Professor of Urologic Oncology
Director of Robotic Surgery
Department of Urology
Roswell Park Cancer Institute
Buffalo, New York
  *Robotic-Assisted Intracorporeal Ileal
  Conduit*

Ashraf S. Haddad, MD
Fellow
Urologic Robotic Surgery
Swedish Medical Center
Seattle, Washington
  *Laparoscopic and Robotic-Assisted
  Retroperitoneal Lymph Node Dissection*

Ashok K. Hemal, MD, MCh, FACS
Professor
Department of Urology and
  Comprehensive Cancer Center,
  Institute for Regenerative Medicine
Wake Forest School of Medicine and
  Baptist Hospital
Winston Salem, North Carolina
  Continent Urinary Diversion

Ahmed A. Hussein, MD, MS, MRCS
Department of Urology
Roswell Park Cancer Institute
Buffalo, New York
  *Robotic-Assisted Intracorporeal Ileal
  Conduit*

James S. Hwong, MD
Harvard Combined Urology Residency
  Program
Boston, Massachusetts
  *Patient Preparation and Positioning for
  Laparoscopic and Robotic Urologic Surgery*

Stephen V. Jackman, MD
Professor
Department of Urology
University of Pittsburgh
Pittsburgh, Pennsylvania
  Laparoscopic Renal Biopsy

Günter Janetschek, MD
Department of Urology and Andrology
Paracelsus Medical University
Salzburg, Austria
  *NOTES-Assisted Laparoscopic
  Transvesical Bladder Diverticulectomy
  Partial Adrenalectomy*

Thomas W. Jarrett, MD
Professor and Chairman
Department of Urology
George Washington University
Washington, District of Columbia
  Nephroureterectomy

Wooju Jeong, MD
Senior Urologist
Vattikuti Urology Institute
Henry Ford Hospital
Detroit, Michigan
  *Minimally Invasive Renal Recipient
  Surgery*

Michael H. Johnson, MD
Assistant Professor of Urology and
  Oncology
Brady Urological Institute
Department of Urology
Johns Hopkins University School of
  Medicine
Baltimore, Maryland
  The da Vinci Surgical System

Jean V. Joseph, MD, MBA
Professor
Department of Urology
University of Rochester Medical Center
Rochester, New York
  *Preperitoneal Robotic-Assisted Radical
  Prostatectomy*

Jin Jung, MD
Resident Physician
Anesthesiology
Northwell Health
Manhasset, New York
  *Anesthetic Considerations for
  Laparoscopic/Robotic Surgery*

Jihad H. Kaouk, MD
Director
Center for Robotics and Minimally
  Invasive Surgery
Glickman Urologic Institute
Cleveland Clinic
Cleveland, Ohio
  Retroperitoneal Access

Louis R. Kavoussi, MD, MBA
Waldbaum-Gardner Professor and
  Chairman of Urology
The Arthur Smith Institute for Urology
Hofstra Northwell School of Medicine
Hempstead, New York
  *Complications of Laparoscopic and
  Robotic-Assisted Surgery*

Nicholas Kavoussi, MD
Department of Urology
University of Texas Southwestern
  Medical Center
Dallas, Texas
  *Laparoscopic and Robotic-Assisted
  Ureteral Reimplantation*

Bohyun Kim, MD, PhD
Professor
Department of Radiology
Mayo Clinic
Rochester, Minnesota
  Laparoscopic Renal Cyst Decortication

Dae Keun Kim, MD
Assistant Professor
Department of Urology
CHA Seoul Station Medical Center
CHA University
CHA Medical School
Seoul, Republic of Korea
  *Laparoscopic/Robotic Boari Flap
  Ureteral Reimplantation*

Jaime Landman, MD
Professor of Urology and Radiology
Chairman, Department of Urology
University of California Irvine
Orange, California
  *Laparoscopic and Percutaneous Delivery
  of Renal Ablative Technology*

Aaron H. Lay, MD
Endourology Fellow
Department of Urology
University of Texas Southwestern
  Medical Center
Dallas, Texas
  Laparoscopic Radical Nephrectomy

David A. Leavitt, MD
Vattikuti Urology Institute
Henry Ford Health System
Detroit, Michigan
  Laparoscopic Varicocelectomy

Ahmed Magdy, MD MSc
Urology and Andrology Department
Faculty of Medicine
Menoufiya University
Menoufiya, Egypt
Department of Urology and Andrology
Paracelsus Medical University
Salzburg, Austria
*NOTES-Assisted Laparoscopic
Transvesical Bladder Diverticulectomy
Partial Adrenalectomy*

Ted B. Manny, MD, MBA
Partner
Alliance Urology Specialists
Greensboro, North Carolina
Continent Urinary Diversion

Sean McAdams, MD
Department of Urology
University of Minnesota
Minneapolis, Minnesota
Basic Instrumentation

Mani Menon, MD
The Raj and Padma Vattikuti
   Distinguished Chair
Vattikuti Urology Institute
Henry Ford Hospital
Detroit, Michigan
*Minimally Invasive Renal Recipient
Surgery*

Salvatore Micali, MD
Associate Professor of Urology
Department of Urology
University of Modena and Reggio
   Emilia, Italy
*Laparoscopic Denervation for Chronic
Testicular Pain*

Debora Moore, MD
Urology Clinic Site Director
Charlotte VA Health Care Center
Charlotte, North Carolina
*Exiting the Abdomen and Closure
Techniques*

Robert Moore, MD
Urology Resident Site Director
Salisbury VA Medical Center
Salisbury, North Carolina
Associate Professor of Urology
Wake Forest Baptist Health–Urology
Winston-Salem, North Carolina
*Exiting the Abdomen and Closure
Techniques*

Monica S.C. Morgan, MD
Department of Urology
Houston Methodist Hospital
Houston, Texas
*Laparoscopic and Robotic-Assisted
Ureteral Reimplantation*

Ravi Munver, MD, FACS
Vice Chairman
Chief of Minimally Invasive and
   Robotic Urologic Surgery
Department of Urology
Hackensack University Medical Center
Hackensack, New Jersey
Associate Professor of Surgery
   (Urology)
Department of Surgery
Division of Urology
Rutgers University–New Jersey Medical
   School
Newark, New Jersey
*Laparoscopic and Robotic-Assisted
Laparoscopic Pelvic Lymph Node
Dissection*

Stephen Y. Nakada, MD, FACS
Professor and Chairman
The David T. Uehling Chair of Urology
Department of Urology
University of Wisconsin School of
   Medicine and Public Health
Professor and Chairman
Department of Urology
University of Wisconsin Hospital and
   Clinics
Madison, Wisconsin
Stapling and Reconstruction

Yasser A. Noureldin, MD, MSc, PhD
Lecturer
Department of Urology
Benha University Hospital
Benha University
Benha, Egypt
*Laparoscopic/Robotic Camera and Lens
Systems*

Michael C. Ost, MD
Associate Professor and Vice Chairman
Department of Urology
University of Pittsburgh Medical Center
Chief of Division
Pediatric Urology
Children's Hospital of Pittsburgh at
   the University of Pittsburgh Medical
   Center
Pittsburgh, Pennsylvania
Ureterolysis

Lane S. Palmer, MD
Professor and Chief
Pediatric Urology
Cohen Children's Medical Center of
   New York
Hofstra Northwell School of Medicine
Hempstead, New York
Laparoscopic Orchiectomy

Jaspreet Singh Parihar, MD
Chief Resident
Department of Surgery
Division of Urology
Rutgers Robert Wood Johnson Medical
   School
New Brunswick, New Jersey
Insufflators and the Pneumoperitoneum

Jeffery E. Piacitelli, PA-C, MS
Robotics and Minimally Invasive
   Surgery–Urology
Intermountain Urological Institute
Intermountain Medical Center–Eccles
   Outpatient Center
Murray, Utah
Considerations for the Assistant

Peter A. Pinto, MD
Head, Prostate Cancer Section
Fellowship Program Director
Urologic Oncology Branch
National Cancer Institute
National Institutes of Health
Bethesda, Maryland
Laparoscopic Partial Nephrectomy

Giacomo Maria Pirola, MD
Urology Resident
Department of Urology
University of Modena and Reggio
   Emilia, Italy
*Laparoscopic Denervation for Chronic
Testicular Pain*

James Porter, MD
Director, Robotic Surgery
Swedish Urology Group
Seattle, Washington
*Laparoscopic and Robotic-Assisted
Retroperitoneal Lymph Node Dissection*

Aaron M. Potretzke, MD
Minimally Invasive/Robotic Surgery
   Fellow
Division of Urologic Surgery
Department of Surgery
Washington University School of
   Medicine
St. Louis, Missouri
Laparoscopic Pyeloplasty

Raj Pruthi, MD
Professor and Chair
Department of Urology
University of North Carolina
Chapel Hill, North Carolina
Robotic-Assisted Radical Cystectomy

**Johar S. Raza, MD, MRCS, FCPS
(urol)**
Department of Urology
Roswell Park Cancer Institute
Buffalo, New York
*Robotic-Assisted Intracorporeal Ileal
Conduit*

Jeremy N. Reese, MD, MPH, MEd
Resident
Department of Urology
University of Pittsburgh Medical Center
Pittsburgh, Pennsylvania
Ureterolysis

Koon Ho Rha, MD, PhD, FACS
Professor
Department of Urology
Urological Science Institute
Yonsei University College of Medicine
Seoul, Republic of Korea
*Laparoscopic/Robotic Boari Flap
Ureteral Reimplantation*

Lee Richstone, MD
System Vice Chairman
The Arthur Smith Institute of Urology
Hofstra Northwell School of Medicine
Hempstead, New York
Chief
Department of Urology
The North Shore University Hospital
Manhasset, New York
*Robotic-Assisted and Laparoscopic
Simple Prostatectomy*

Bijan W. Salari, MD
University of Toledo Medical Center
Toledo, Ohio
*Exiting the Abdomen and Closure
Techniques*

Jason M. Sandberg, MD
Department of Urology
Wake Forest School of Medicine and
Baptist Hospital
Winston-Salem, North Carolina
Continent Urinary Diversion

John Schomburg, MD
Department of Urology
University of Minnesota
Minneapolis, Minnesota
Basic Instrumentation

Michael J. Schwartz, MD
Associate Professor of Urology
The Arthur Smith Institute for Urology
Hofstra Northwell School of Medicine
Hempstead, New York
Laparoscopic Live Donor Nephrectomy

Casey A. Seideman, MD
Pediatric Urology Fellow
Cohen Children's Medical Center of
New York
Hofstra Northwell School of Medicine
Hempstead, New York
Laparoscopic Orchiectomy

Paras H. Shah, MD
The Arthur Smith Institute for Urology
Hofstra Northwell School of Medicine
Hempstead, New York
*Laparoscopic Live Donor Nephrectomy
Robotic-Assisted Laparoscopic Partial
Cystectomy*

Michael Siev, BA
Research Fellow
The Arthur Smith Institute for Urology
Hofstra Northwell School of Medicine
Hempstead, New York
*Complications of Laparoscopic and
Robotic-Assisted Surgery*

Armine K. Smith, MD
Assistant Professor
Brady Urological Institute
Johns Hopkins University
Baltimore, Maryland
Assistant Professor
Department of Urology
George Washington University
Washington, District of Columbia
Nephroureterectomy

Akshay Sood, MD
Resident PGY-1
Vattikuti Urology Institute
Henry Ford Hospital
Detroit, Michigan
*Minimally Invasive Renal Recipient
Surgery*

Arun Srinivasan, MD
Attending Pediatric Urologist
Division of Urology
The Children's Hospital of Philadelphia
Philadelphia, Pennsylvania
Laparoscopic Orchiopexy

Michael D. Stifelman, MD
Chairman
Department of Urology
Hackensack University Medical Group
Hackensack, New Jersey
*Buccal Mucosa Grafts for Ureteral
Strictures*

Necole M. Streeper, MD
Assistant Professor of Surgery
Division of Urology
Penn State Milton S. Hershey Medical
Center
Hershey, Pennsylvania
Stapling and Reconstruction

Li Ming Su, MD
David A. Cofrin Professor of Urology
Associate Chairman of Clinical Affairs
Chief
Division of Robotic and Minimally
Invasive Urologic Surgery
Department of Urology
University of Florida College of
Medicine
Gainesville, Florida
Transperitoneal Technique Prostatectomy

Hassan G. Taan, MD
Clinical Instructor
Department of Urology
University of Pittsburgh Medical Center
Pittsburgh, Pennsylvania
Laparoscopic Simple Nephrectomy

Angelo Territo, MD
Urology Resident
Department of Urology
University of Modena and Reggio
Emilia, Italy
*Laparoscopic Denervation for Chronic
Testicular Pain*

Manish A. Vira, MD
Assistant Professor of Urology
The Arthur Smith Institute for Urology
Hofstra Northwell School of Medicine
Hempstead, New York
*Robotic-Assisted Laparoscopic Partial
Cystectomy*

Andrew A. Wagner, MD
Director of Minimally Invasive
Urologic Surgery
Beth Israel Deaconess Medical Center
Assistant Professor of Surgery and
Urology
Harvard Medical School
Boston, Massachusetts
*Patient Preparation and Positioning for
Laparoscopic and Robotic Urologic Surgery*

Kyle J. Weld, MD
Director of Endourology
Wilford Hall Medical Center
Department of Urology
Lackland Air Force Base
San Antonio, Texas
*Laparoscopic and Percutaneous Delivery
of Renal Ablative Technology*

Mary E. Westerman, MD
Department of Urology
Mayo Clinic
Rochester, Minnesota
Laparoscopic Adrenalectomy

Michael Woods, MD
Associate Professor
Department of Urology
The University of North Carolina
Chapel Hill, North Carolina
Robotic-Assisted Radical Cystectomy

Yuka Yamaguchi, MD
Division of Urology
Department of Surgery
Alameda Health System
Oakland, California
*Buccal Mucosa Graft for Ureteral
Strictures*

Akira Yamamoto, MD
Resident of Urology
Department Urology
University of Florida College of
Medicine
Gainesville, Florida
Transperitoneal Radical Prostatectomy

Ramy Youssef, MD
Assistant Clinical Professor
Department of Urology
University of California Irvine
Orange, California
*Laparoscopic and Percutaneous Delivery
of Renal Ablative Technology*

Lee C. Zhao, MD, MS
Assistant Professor
Department of Urology
New York University School of
    Medicine
New York, New York
    Buccal Mucosa Graft for Ureteral
    Strictures

Philip T. Zhao, MD
Endourology Fellow
The Arthur Smith Institute for Urology
Hofstra Northwell School of Medicine
Hempstead, New York
    Robotic-Assisted and Laparoscopic
    Simple Prostatectomy

Matthew Ziegelmann, MD
Resident Physician
Department of Urology
Mayo Clinic
Rochester, Minnesota
    Laparoscopic Renal Cyst Decortication

Preface

Surgical technique is continuously evolving as physicians remain vigilant in their search for excellence. It has been 10 years since the last edition of this work. Much has changed in these years because of the collective efforts of those surgeons around the globe who are seeking ways to contribute to iterations that progressively make surgery safer, less invasive, and more successful. In addition, modern times have called for a focus on making surgical approaches cost effective. All these were the impetus for us to create a third edition of this text.

The role of minimally invasive surgery has continued to expand over the past decade. This text recognizes this reality through new and updated chapters. Indeed, most extirpative and reconstructive urologic procedures are now performed through keyhole incisions. Facilitating this trend has been the application of da Vinci surgical approaches to surgery. As such, specific sections and chapters have been added in recognition of this phenomenon.

This edition offers an expanded role for illustrative education. Teaching the art of surgery is so much more enhanced through visual lessons. The number of graphics has been increased to help clarify the written word. Moreover, in this edition we have added David Leavitt as the video editor. His guidance has provided for an expanded library that allows enhanced understanding of the nuances of each surgical technique through detailed step-by-step instruction.

We are fortunate to have world experts contributing their experience as authors. This text has both well-recognized pioneers and recent innovators. They have painstakingly updated or added chapters that reflect the most up-to-date minimally invasive techniques to treat urologic disease. These authors selected key technical tips to help readers understand important nuances to successfully undertake described procedures.

Finally, we have to acknowledge the professional staff at Elsevier who truly helped convert our ideas into reality. Lotta Kryhl understood the importance of creating a third edition and demonstrated incredible leadership in helping with organization and crafting the proposal to upper management. Ann Ruzycka Anderson and Claire Kramer did a magnificent job in operationalizing the project and masterfully herding us editors and authors alike.

Contents

Video Contents

Atlas of Laparoscopic and Robotic Urologic Surgery

1

Patient Preparation and Positioning for Laparoscopic and Robotic Urologic Surgery

Andrew A. Wagner, James S. Hwong

"Before anything else, preparation is the key to success."

Alexander Graham Bell

Appropriate patient selection, thorough preparation, and careful patient positioning are essential in achieving a safe and successful outcome in laparoscopic surgery. No matter how prepared a surgeon may be for the technical exercise of laparoscopic surgery, inadequate execution of these important surgical preludes may result in unnecessary complications, extend operative time, and challenge the course of recovery. If the surgeon becomes entangled in a challenging situation, he or she must continuously evaluate for adequate progress to justify continuing laparoscopically versus converting to open surgery. Recognizing these situations during patient selection and proceeding with these cases with a healthy dose of surgical humility is fundamental to avoiding major complications and achieving a successful outcome.

PATIENT SELECTION

Preparation for laparoscopic surgery begins first and foremost with appropriate patient selection. The most experienced laparoscopic surgeons in the world are also experts at patient selection. Each case must be carefully considered prior to the patient reaching the operating room. Several aspects of surgery unique to laparoscopy must be considered before patient selection. The most significant of these include the altered physiology of pneumoperitoneum, the potential for prolonged procedure time during a team's early learning curve, and the dangers of minimally invasive abdominal access.

Pneumoperitoneum of laparoscopy can significantly alter cardiopulmonary physiology, so an experienced anesthesia team is vitally important and should be involved in the preoperative planning of complicated cases. Several medical conditions are worthy of special mention and should prompt a careful review by both surgery and anesthesia teams. These include but are not limited to chronic obstructive pulmonary disease (COPD), restrictive lung disease, active cardiac disease, obesity, glaucoma, and cerebrovascular disease (Table 1-1).

Patients with pulmonary compromise present unique challenges during particularly long surgical cases. Insufflation of the peritoneum with CO_2 can exacerbate hypercarbia in the COPD patient with a severe ventilation-perfusion mismatch. This hypercapnia (arterial CO_2 >60 mm Hg) is cardiodepressive and can lead to acidosis and cardiac arrhythmias if left untreated. The typical treatment for hypercarbia is for the anesthesia team to increase ventilation rate, tidal volume, or both and for the surgical team to reduce intra-abdominal

pressure (IAP). During surgery, the anesthesia team can easily monitor end-tidal CO_2, which is proportional to arterial CO_2. However, in patients with impaired pulmonary gas exchange (e.g., obstructive lung disease, low cardiac output, or pulmonary embolism), arterial CO_2 can be significantly greater than end-tidal CO_2. For these patients, regular measurement of arterial blood gas is recommended for more accurate monitoring. After laparoscopic surgery, patients with pulmonary compromise should be closely monitored for signs of hypercapnia.

Patients with cardiac disease are also at unique risk during laparoscopy. In particular, patients with cardiomyopathy, congestive heart failure, and ischemic heart disease require close monitoring as a result of the altered physiology of pneumoperitoneum. Increased intra-abdominal pressure from insufflation is exerted directly on the vasculature, decreasing venous return and preload, as well as systemic vascular resistance and afterload. These can be further exacerbated by decreased myocardial contractility induced by hypercapnia, ultimately leading to decreased stroke volume and cardiac output. Accordingly, careful fluid resuscitation by the anesthesiologist and attentive control of bleeding by the surgeon are warranted to prevent hypovolemia in these patients.

Other issues that warrant a thoughtful preoperative plan include obesity and central nervous system issues. Prolonged positioning for complex laparoscopy combined with an obese patient may increase the risk of rhabdomyolysis. If positioning is steep Trendelenburg (ST), increased intraocular pressure can lead to ischemic optic neuropathy and postoperative vision loss in the patient with glaucoma. Patients with cerebrovascular disease should be carefully selected because ST positioning can contribute to increased intracranial pressure. The astute urologist should not hesitate to seek specialty evaluation for any of these comorbidities before proceeding with surgery.

Patients with a previous history of abdominal surgery or peritonitis should be carefully considered for laparoscopy. These conditions can result in the formation of a significant amount of adhesions involving intra-abdominal viscera, presenting unique challenges and dangerous pitfalls for trocar placement. In general, for abdominal access, the surgeon should use the technique with which he or she has the most experience. Blind Veress needle placement for insufflation can be used away from the known surgical scars if the surgeon

TABLE 1-1 Comorbidities Exacerbated by Pneumoperitoneum and Robotic Surgery

Comorbidities	Exacerbating Physiology
Coronary artery disease, cardiac disease	Decreased venous return
	Increased systemic vascular resistance
COPD, lung disease	Hypercarbia
	Decreased chest wall compliance
Glaucoma	Increased intraocular pressure
Cerebrovascular disease	Increased intracranial pressure
Kidney or liver disease	Decreased renal and hepatic blood flow
Obesity	Increased venous congestion
	Increased muscle compartment pressures

COPD, chronic obstructive pulmonary disease.

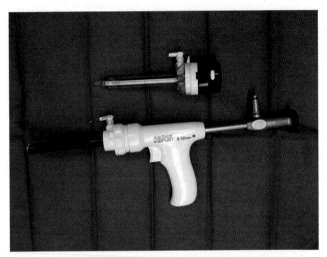

Figure 1-1. Trocars for initial port placement under direct vision. The Visiport Plus and Versaport (Covidien, Norwalk, Connecticut) trocars allow for placement of the initial trocar under direct vision. Both accommodate passage of a 0-degree laparoscope through the body of the trocars, allowing for visualization and identification of abdominal wall tissue through their clear tips during placement. A sharp crescent-shaped blade extends 1 mm through the tip of the Visiport Plus trocar *(bottom)* for sharp tissue dissection with each trigger pull. The sharpened tip of the Versaport trocar *(top)* dissects through the abdominal wall with a twisting motion and firm, steady pressure.

has experience with that technique. If not, then an open Hasson technique should be used for initial access. Regardless of insufflation method, no ports should ever be placed blindly, including the initial abdominal access port. Several varieties of "visual obturator" trocars are available and provide safer options for abdominal access (Fig. 1-1). Moreover, subsequent trocars should always be placed under direct vision after adhesions are cleared from the abdominal wall. Retroperitoneal or preperitoneal access can be considered in patients with a history of multiple complicated surgeries. Experience and additional training with these techniques are recommended. As stated previously, preoperative recognition of challenging situations such as a hostile abdomen is paramount in avoiding complications.

PREPARING THE PATIENT

Before surgery, all patients should be evaluated by the anesthesia team and obtain appropriate specialty clearance. Preoperative testing including electrocardiography, blood work, urinalysis, and cultures should be performed if appropriate. In addition, instructions for stopping anticoagulation

agents and antiplatelet agents should be conveyed to the patient. If an ostomy is planned, the patient should be evaluated by an ostomy nursing team, and potential ostomy sites should be marked bilaterally for placement. Preoperative ostomy education can be reviewed, and supplies such as ostomy pouches, thromboembolism-deterrent (TED) hose, and chlorhexidine body scrubs can be provided at this time.

Prevention of surgical site infections begins preoperatively and includes skin treatment, bowel preparation when necessary, and antibiotic prophylaxis. On the evening before surgery, the patient should shower with a chlorhexidine body scrub and should refrain from waxing, shaving, or trimming the surgical site to prevent microtrauma to the skin. For the same reason, body hair should not be shaved with a blade but rather trimmed with mechanical clippers, which have been demonstrated to decrease the risk of surgical site infection. After the patient has been positioned, abdominal surgical sites should be sterilized with chlorhexidine, and genitalia with povidone-iodine solution.

If the bowel will be manipulated, mechanical bowel preparation with polyethylene glycol or sodium phosphate can be administered the evening before surgery. The constipated patient can be administered enemas or manually disimpacted. The rationale for mechanical bowel preparation includes reduction of fecal flora, easier manipulation of bowel, improved visualization, and easier anastomotic stapling. However, meta-analyses of colorectal surgery have not identified a clear statistical benefit to mechanical bowel preparation. Cochrane reviews were able to demonstrate trends toward decreased rates of anastomotic leakage with mechanical bowel preparation, although these did not reach statistical significance. Maneuvers for aggressive bowel preparation were further detracted by potentially morbid colonic mucosal changes, fluid shifts, and electrolyte derangements. Similar controversy exists surrounding administration of oral antibiotic bowel preparation (OABP) or selective decontamination of the digestive tract (SDD) with regimens such as tobramycin, polymyxin E, and amphotericin B. In general, parenteral antibiotic prophylaxis is used in lieu of these agents.

There is less controversy regarding parenteral antibiotic prophylaxis before incision. For laparoscopic procedures without entry into the digestive or urinary tract, the guidelines of the American Urological Association (AUA) recommend perioperative administration of a first-generation cephalosporin or clindamycin as an alternative in penicillin-allergic patients. If the urinary tract will be entered, a first- or second-generation cephalosporin or aztreonam with metronidazole or clindamycin is recommended. A fluoroquinolone or ampicillin-sulbactam is acceptable as an alternative regimen. For cases involving the intestine, AUA guidelines recommend a second- or third-generation cephalosporin or aztreonam with metronidazole or clindamycin. Fluoroquinolones, ampicillin-sulbactam, ticarcillin and clavulanate potassium (Timentin), and piperacillin and tazobactam (Zosyn) can be used as alternative regimens. At our institution, a third-generation cephalosporin is combined with metronidazole for all cases involving bowel. All antibiotics should be administered 30 to 60 minutes before incision and should be continued for no more than 24 hours if there is no gross contamination during the procedure.

Preoperative preparation should also include measures to prevent venous thromboembolism (VTE), a common cause of preventable death in surgical patients. The American College of Chest Physicians has developed evidence-based clinical guidelines for nonorthopedic surgical patients. Intermittent pneumatic compression (IPC) should be applied to all laparoscopy patients before induction of anesthesia. For patients at moderate and high risk for VTE without high risk of bleeding complications, subcutaneous heparin or low-molecular-weight heparin (LMWH) should be administered. For high-risk cancer patients, extended-duration prophylaxis with LMWH for 4 weeks is recommended. Patients at high risk for bleeding complications can have pharmacologic prophylaxis withheld, although they should have mechanical prophylaxis with IPC preoperatively and pharmacologic prophylaxis should be initiated when the risk of bleeding diminishes. Pharmacologic prophylaxis should be administered 2 hours preoperatively, although LMWH appears to be effective 12 hours preoperatively.

PATIENT POSITIONING: BASIC CONSIDERATIONS

Prevention of positioning-related injuries should be of primary consideration when the anesthetized patient is manipulated. Pharmacologic paralysis required for laparoscopic surgery compounds the risk of injury as a result of decreased muscular tone and prolonged periods of immobility. These injuries can be broadly categorized into peripheral nerve injuries, vascular-mediated injuries, and skin injuries, all of which can result in significant morbidity and mortality to the patient. Recognition of risk factors for positioning-related injuries and diligent prevention is key to avoiding these complications.

Injuries to peripheral nerves are a result of stretch or compression at susceptible nerve segments that can compromise neural blood supply, tear neural tissue, and disrupt axoplasmic flow. When the patient is positioned, care should be taken to ensure adequate padding at the elbow to avoid ulnar nerve compression at the cubital tunnel. If the arms are not tucked at the side, abduction at the shoulder should be limited to less than 90 degrees to prevent stretching of the brachial plexus over the humeral head. In the ST position, shoulder bracing should be avoided to prevent further loading of the brachial plexus. In the full-flank position, an axillary roll should be placed one handbreadth inferior to the axilla to support these important structures. When the patient's lower extremities are positioned, close attention should be directed to the peroneal nerve, which can be compressed at the head of the fibula, and the median nerve, which can be injured at the medial tibial condyle.

Vascular-mediated injuries such as compartment syndrome and rhabdomyolysis are not unique to laparoscopic urology, but their risks may be exacerbated by insufflation, ST positioning, long operative times, and patient factors such as obesity. One possible contributing factor is ST positioning. With the legs elevated in the lithotomy position, perfusion pressure at the calf is reduced, which may increase the risk for compartment syndrome. Insufflation has also been theorized to contribute to decreased lower limb perfusion, and obesity may increase forces exerted at gluteal muscles, back muscles, and lower extremity supports. Long operative times (>4 to 5 hours) have also been associated with the development of rhabdomyolysis. Taken together, prevention of compartment syndrome and rhabdomyolysis should focus on limiting the degree of ST inversion and limiting operative time in morbidly obese patients.

The patient's skin should be closely examined, and any preexisting lesions should be noted. Then all bony protuberances should be comfortably supported to distribute any forces that could lead to skin ischemia during a prolonged case. Similarly, any foreign bodies placed against the patient's skin such as pulse oximeter connectors and intravenous access ports should also be padded. Gel pads, foam pads, egg crate foam, gauze, and towels can all serve in this capacity. For the patient's skin to be protected from electrical burns, the electrocautery grounding pad should be well adhered across its entire surface. If necessary, body hair should be clipped to improve pad adherence. All patient jewelry should be removed, and the

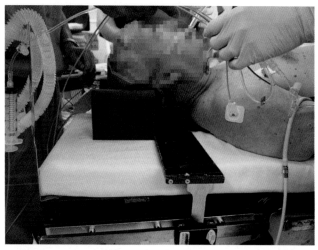

Figure 1-2. TrenGuard device for securing patients in steep Trendelenburg (ST) position. Safely securing a patient in ST position can be achieved with the TrenGuard system from D.A. Medical (Chagrin Falls, Ohio). This system uses a nuchal foam bolster secured to the operating table accessory rails, functioning like chocks for a wheel.

grounding pad should be placed as close to the operative field as possible to prevent alternate site burns.

PATIENT POSITIONING: LAPAROSCOPIC PELVIC SURGERY (SEE VIDEO 1-1)

Patient positioning for laparoscopic pelvic surgery has traditionally been the lithotomy position in ST. Although this allows the small bowel to fall away from the surgical site, affording increased working space and improving visualization, the position has numerous disadvantages. Chief among these are the risks to the patient as a result of the steep, inverted position, resulting in decreased perfusion pressure of the lower extremities and increased intracranial and intraocular pressures.

Keeping the patient safely secured to the operating table and preventing an intraoperative fall is also a major consideration. A number of devices and materials have been developed specifically for this application. Examples include vacuum bean bag immobilizers, high-friction gel or foam pads, and restraint systems such as the TrenGuard cervical bump (D.A. Surgical, Chagrin Falls, Ohio) (Fig. 1-2). In addition to these restraint methods, taping is often needed for extra support. Before skin preparation and draping, a full tilt test should be performed with the table in maximum Trendelenburg position to ensure the patient does not shift or slide. Familiarity with the patient securement system of choice is absolutely necessary to prevent slipping or falling.

In the lithotomy position, the legs should be well supported with heels firmly planted in surgical stirrups. Flexion at the hip and knees should be less than 90 degrees, and the lower leg should be pointed in line with the contralateral shoulder in the sagittal plane. The stirrups should not exert excessive pressure at the popliteal fossa, which could lead to compromise of popliteal vasculature. The stirrups should also be well padded at the fibular head to avoid peroneal nerve compression injury. "Candy cane" stirrups and knee crutches should not be used because these cannot safely position the legs for long robotic procedures. In ST position, the stirrups should be positioned as low as possible to prevent lower leg ischemia.

The challenges of ST positioning can be mitigated with some minor modifications and experience. At our institution, we use a split leg table during robotic-assisted laparoscopic prostatectomy. This avoids the risks of lithotomy positioning by keeping the legs straight on rotating bed attachments (Fig. 1-3). Moreover, we use a minimal Trendelenburg (MT) position—that is, just enough Trendelenburg inversion for the small bowel to fall out of the pelvis. Usually only 10 to 20 degrees of inversion is necessary (Fig. 1-4). In our experience, MT positioning is still a sufficient amount of inversion to clear the operative field while minimizing the deleterious physiologic effects of the ST position. Our method also requires less elaborate means of patient securement, decreasing time for operating room positioning and saving total operating room time.

PATIENT POSITIONING: LAPAROSCOPIC UPPER TRACT SURGERY (SEE VIDEO 1-2)

Minimally invasive kidney and adrenal surgery can be performed via a laparoscopic (transperitoneal) or retroperitoneoscopic approach. Either is acceptable, and the decision regarding approach should be based on surgeon training and

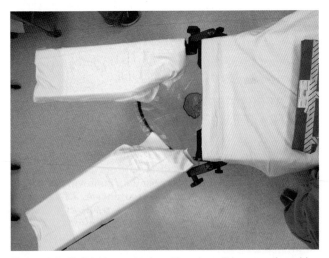

Figure 1-3. Split table mechanism. Use of a split leg operating table instead of lithotomy fins simplifies patient positioning for laparoscopic pelvic surgery while mitigating the risk of injuries from prolonged positioning in the lithotomy position.

experience. There are no prospective perioperative or postoperative outcome data supporting one approach or the other. Of course, many other factors are important in determining surgical approach and should be carefully considered, including tumor size and location, potential for intra-abdominal adhesions, and patient body habitus.

We use a modified lateral approach for all kidney and adrenal laparoscopic and robotic-assisted surgery (Fig. 1-5). This consists of the patient in a semisupine position, rotated laterally approximately 30 degrees. Rolled blankets or large gel rolls are used to support the patient's back in this position by placing them behind the patient from the shoulder to buttocks. In contrast to lateral positioning for open retroperitoneal surgery, jackknife (flexed) positioning and the kidney rest are not necessary and can potentially reduce the actual laparoscopic working space.

Towels, pillows, or foam donuts are used to support the head and cervical spine in neutral position. The patient's lower arm should be extended and supported on an arm board where it can be accessed as needed by the anesthesia team. The upper arm is slightly flexed and is supported with one folded pillow over the chest. Arm extension should be limited to 90 degrees or less to prevent a brachial plexus stretch injury. Foam-padded tape is used to secure the patient to the table, encircling the arms and securing the upper body and arms to the table. Pillows should be placed between the legs to keep the spine aligned. The dependent leg should be flexed at the hip and knee. The contralateral leg should remain extended with slight flexion at the knee and supported along its length with pillows. All bony protuberances such as the greater trochanter, head of the fibula, and lateral malleolus should be adequately padded with foam pads, gel pads, or egg crate foam.

Once appropriately positioned, the patient should be secured to the operating table and the table rotated a moderate amount to either side to ensure the body will not shift intraoperatively. If necessary during the case, the patient can still be rotated into a full flank position with movement of the operating table without undue stress on pressure points.

For retroperitoneoscopic surgery, the patient is typically placed in the full lateral flank position with the surgical site further rotated upward. Most surgeons choose to flex the table after positioning for retroperitoneoscopic surgery. With full flank position, an axillary roll should be positioned three fingerbreadths inferior to the axilla to reduce pressure on the axillary neurovasculature. The arms and legs can be secured in

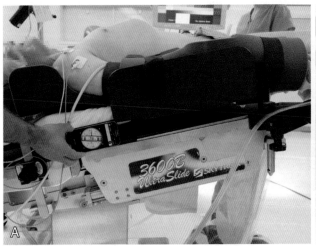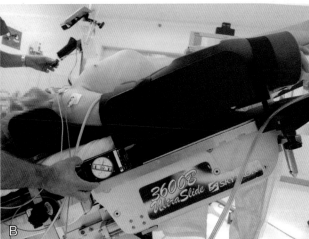

Figure 1-4. Minimal Trendelenburg positioning for laparoscopic pelvic surgery. **A,** Only 10 to 20 degrees of Trendelenburg are necessary to allow the small bowel to fall away from the pelvis. **B,** Steep Trendelenburg positioning confers additional risks while not significantly improving visualization.

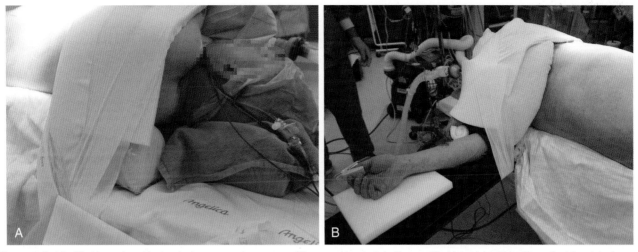

Figure 1-5. Modified lateral positioning for laparoscopic surgery of the upper tract. **A,** In the modified lateral position, the patient is rotated approximately 30 degrees with the surgical target elevated. The body is supported with gel rolls or rolled towels. **B,** The dependent arm is extended and supported on an arm board; the contralateral arm is extended and supported with a folded pillow. The dependent leg is flexed at the hip and knee, and the contralateral leg is supported along its length with a slight bend at the knee. A generous amount of foam-padded tape is then used to secure the patient to the table.

the same manner as described earlier for the modified flank position.

CONCLUSION

Preoperative preparation for laparoscopic and robotic surgery remains of vital importance because it will set the stage for a safe and effective surgery. Careful consultation with the anesthesia team and specialists in pulmonology and cardiology when appropriate remains crucial. The operating surgeon should understand physiologic changes associated with insufflation under these conditions. The surgeon should be present and guide preoperative positioning before laparoscopic and robotic cases. Early in one's learning curve, positional injuries can be more common as a result of long operative times. With experience, pelvic surgery can be performed without ST positioning, and upper tract surgery can be performed using a modified lateral position.

2 Laparoscopic/Robotic Camera and Lens Systems

Yasser A. Noureldin, Sero Andonian

It has been said that exposure is key for open surgery. Similarly, the imaging platform used in endoscopic surgery, whether it is laparoscopic or robotic-assisted laparoscopic surgery, is a key for success. In this chapter, the history of laparoscope and imaging systems is reviewed. In addition, the difference between analog and digital image processing is explained. Three-dimensional imaging systems in addition to the da Vinci robotic system (Intuitive Surgical, Sunnyvale, Calif.) are described. Furthermore, advances in different scopes and cameras including high-definition (HD) and augmented reality (AR) imaging systems will be explained.

HISTORY OF THE LAPAROSCOPE

Surgical scopes are among the oldest surgical instruments. The first illuminated scope, dubbed the *Lichtleiter* or "Light Conductor," consisted of a viewing tube, candle, and series of mirrors and was developed by Philipp Bozzini in 1804.[1] Because of its impracticality, the device did not find favor among the surgeons of the day. However, it served as a source of inspiration to other inventors. Antonin Jean Desormeaux was the first urologist to view inside the bladder, in 1855.[2] Using the principles of incandescent lighting, in 1867 Julius Bruck designed the first scope illuminated with an electrical light source. He used a platinum wire loop heated with electricity until it glowed. The main drawback to this design was the amount of heat generated by the light source, which could be conducted along the metal tubing of the scope to the tip. This heat represented a significant risk of burns to both the patient and the surgeon.[3] In 1877, Maximilian Nitze used a lens system to widen the field of view (FOV) and succeeded in creating the first cystoscope as an instrument to visualize the urinary bladder through the urethra.[4] The modern fiberoptic endoscope was invented by the British physicist Harold Hopkins in 1954.[5] Hopkins used the term *fiberscope* to describe the bundle of glass or other transparent fibers used to transmit an image. The main advantage of the fiberscope was that the illumination source could be kept away from the scope with significant reduction in the amount of heat transmitted to the scope tip. However, the resolution of the fiberscope was limited by the number of fibers used. Therefore in the 1960s Hopkins invented the rod-lens system, which he patented in 1977.[6] The rod-lens system used glass rods in place of air gaps, removing the need for lenses altogether, with resultant clarity and brightness that was up to 80 times greater than what was offered at the time (Fig. 2-1, *top*).[6] The rod-lens system remains the standard for currently used rigid endoscopes when high image resolution is required.[7] Over time, with advances in fiberoptics and magnifying lenses, sophisticated surgical scopes evolved. In the next two sections, developments in scopes and cameras are detailed.

SCOPES AND TECHNOLOGY

Since the 1960s, the classic laparoscope has been composed of an outer ring of fiberoptics used to transmit light into the body, and an inner core of rod lenses through which the illuminated visual scene is relayed back to the eye piece (Fig. 2-1, *top*).[5] The different types of laparoscopes are defined in terms of the number of rods, size of laparoscope, and angle of view. With regard to size, laparoscopes are available in the range of 1.9 mm to 12 mm, but 5 mm is the most common size for

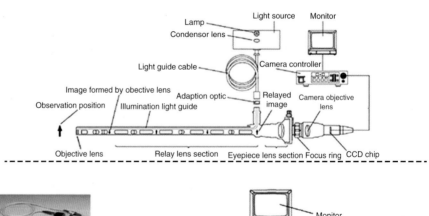

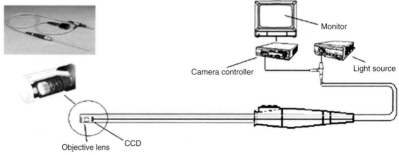

Figure 2-1. *Top,* Traditional rod-lens technology of Hopkins. *Bottom,* Videoscope technology. *CCD,* charge-coupled device. *(Courtesy Olympus America, Melville, NY.*

pediatric patients, and 10 mm is the most common size for adults. Furthermore, viewing angles between 0 and 70 degrees are possible, with 0 and 30 degrees being the most commonly used (Fig. 2-2). The 0-degree laparoscope offers a straight-on panoramic view. The 30-degree scope uses an angled lens, which can be used to view around corners, and can allow space for manipulation of laparoscopic instruments during surgery.

For a replication of the panoramic view of the human eye, which has a FOV of close to 180 degrees, the panomorph lens was recently developed. Whereas traditional laparoscopes

offer less than a 70-degree FOV, the panomorph lens uses multivisualization software to widen the FOV to 180 degrees (Fig. 2-3).[8] However, the panomorph lens is not commercially available yet.

Further miniaturization of the charge-coupled device (CCD) chip technology and digital imaging allowed the CCD chip camera to be placed at the distal end of the endoscope; therefore the image is immediately captured by the CCD chip, digitized, and converted into an electrical signal for transmission. These systems, called *digital video endoscopes*, allow the

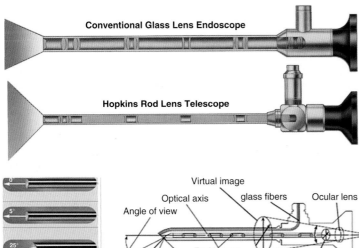

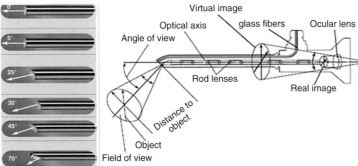

Figure 2-2. Anatomy of rigid telescopes with demonstration of the different angles of view. *(Top, Courtesy Karl Storrs GmbH & Co., KG, Tuttlingen, Germany; Bottom, from www.laparoscopy.am/index.php?mod=pages&act=show&menu_id=192#lap_1. Accessed March 22, 2015.)*

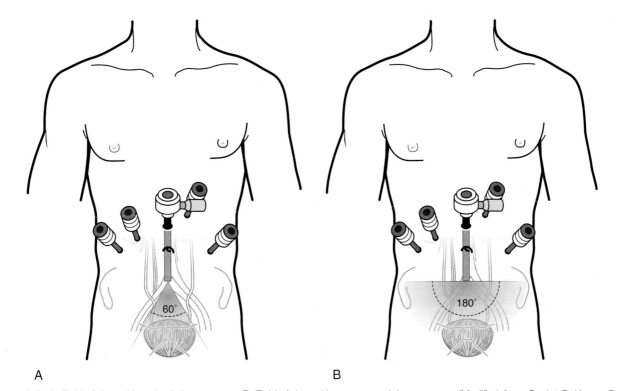

Figure 2-3. A, Field of view with a classic laparoscope. **B,** Field of view with a panomorph laparoscope. *(Modified from Roulet P, Konen P, Villegas M: 360° endoscopy using panomorph lens technology. Proc SPIE Int Soc Opt Eng. 2010 Feb 24;7558.)*

signal to be transmitted directly to an image display unit with minimal loss of image quality and distortion, and without the need to attach the camera head to the eye piece of the scope or the fiberoptic cable for light source[9-14] (Fig. 2-1, *bottom*). Therefore, digital flexible cystoscopes, ureteroscopes, and laparoscopes with durable deflection mechanisms have been developed (e.g., EndoEYE, Olympus America, Melville, N.Y.)[15-17] (Fig. 2-4).

CAMERAS AND TECHNOLOGY

Recent technologic advances—specifically improvements in how optical information is captured, transmitted, and produced as an image—have greatly enhanced laparoscopic surgery.[18-20] Initially, an optical image is converted to an electronic signal that has information regarding both color and luminescence. This signal is then transmitted to a video monitor, where it is scanned to produce an image on the screen.[20] The standard analog signal, in the form of the standard National Television Systems Committee (NTSC) video, uses a limited bandwidth

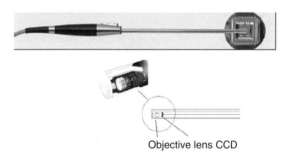

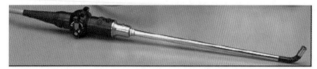

Objective lens CCD

Figure 2-4. EndoEYE technology. This technologic advance allowed for the development of the flexible laparoscope. *CCD,* charge-coupled device. *(Courtesy Olympus America, Melville, NY.*

that includes both color and luminescence information in a single or composite signal. There are many disadvantages to this system. First, processing of color and luminescence information separately and then combining both segments of information to create a video signal resulted in what is called *signal noise* or *cross talk.* This was accompanied by a decrease in resolution, grainy images, and loss of information around the edges of the video image. In addition, images and signals in the NTSC system are processed as voltage (Fig. 2-5, *A*). Therefore it is inevitable that small errors in recording and reproducing these voltages accumulate with each generation of video image. As a result, multiple copies of an analog image will reveal a decrease in quality of the video pictures.

Recently, digital imaging has revolutionized the process of image processing and display. A digital converter changes all video signals into precise numbers (i.e., 0 or 1) (Fig. 2-5, *B*). Once the video information has been digitized, it can be merged with other formats, such as audio or text data, and manipulated without any loss of information. This conversion to a digital signal prevents cross talk and image quality degradation. There are two formats of digital imaging.[9] The first is called *Y/C* or *super-video (S-video),* which allows the color and luminescence information to be carried as two separate signals with less cross talk, with cleaner and sharper images than those generated by composite signals. The second is known as the *RGB* (red-green-blue) format, which is also a component signal. The main difference from the Y/C format is that the video information (color and luminescence) is separated into four signals: red, green, blue, and a timing signal. In addition, each signal carries its own luminescence information, requiring four separate cables (red, green, blue, and sync). The separation of each video signal is performed electronically in the camera head. In contrast to the NTSC or Y/C format, the RGB format requires less electronic processing because the color and luminescence information are separate from the beginning. Therefore, RGB image quality is greatly enhanced when compared with the other two formats (NTSC and Y/C).

Analog medical cameras have been available since the mid-1970s; however, their use in operative applications was limited owing to their high weight and inability to be disinfected. Although the idea of coupling an endoscope with a camera was first described in 1957, it was impractical because cameras of the time were too large and cumbersome.[21] The situation

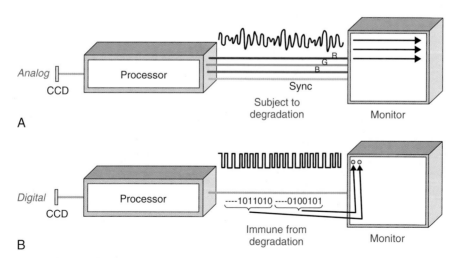

Figure 2-5. A, Representation of analog video imaging in which video signals remain as voltage waveforms. **B,** In contrast, digital video systems convert the analog video information to a digital format, which must be converted back to analog information before it is viewed on the video monitor. Conversion to a digital signal gives the digital video image immunity to noise buildup or image quality degradation. *CCD,* charge-coupled device. *(From Marguet CG, Springhart WP, Preminger GM: New technology for imaging and documenting urologic procedures.* Urol Clin North Am. *2006;33:397-408.)*

changed with the development of compact CCD cameras in the 1980s, when the endoscope could be coupled with CCD cameras and television (TV) monitors and the entire operating room team could watch the surgery. This allowed development of more complex laparoscopic instruments and procedures in which more than one hand is required to operate.[7]

Based on a silicon chip called a *charge-coupled device*, the first solid-state digital camera was invented. It consisted of a silicon chip covered in image sensors, known as *pixels*. It converts the incoming light from a visual scene into a digital signal that can be stored, processed, or transmitted with greater efficiency and reliability than with an analog camera. In addition, digital cameras are lightweight, fully immersible, sterilizable, and shielded from electrical interference that may be created by cutting or coagulating currents during laparoscopic procedures.[22]

A significant improvement in CCD camera technology has been the development of the three-chip camera, which contains three individual CCD chips for the primary colors (red, green, and blue) (Fig. 2-6). Color separation is achieved with a prism system overlying the chips.[23] This three-chip camera design produces less cross talk, with enhanced image resolution and improved color fidelity when compared with analog cameras.[24,25] Further development in digital camera technology was the invention of a single monochrome CCD chip with alternating red, green, and blue illumination to form a color image, rather than with three chips that had three separate color filters. This design reduces the space requirements[13] (Fig. 2-6). Recently, complementary metal-oxide semiconductor (CMOS) technology has replaced CCD sensor technology in the industry of digital endoscopes, with superior image resolution, better contrast discrimination, lower power usage, cheaper cost, and 50% weight reduction.[26-28]

The classic laparoscope does not have the ability to obtain high magnification and wide-angle images simultaneously. This represents a challenge when both close views and wide-angle images are required during sophisticated laparoscopic procedures.[29,30] The reason is that when high magnification is required, a laparoscope is advanced closer to the organ. However, this results in loss of angle of view. Therefore a multiresolution foveated laparoscope (MRFL) was recently introduced. With two probes (a high-magnification probe and a wide-angle probe), an MRFL system can capture images with both high-magnification close-up and wide-angle views (Figs. 2-7 and 2-8). At a working distance of 120 mm, the wide-angle probe provides surgical area coverage of

160×120 mm^2 with a resolution of 2.83l p/mm. Moreover, the high-magnification probe has a resolution of 6.35l pixel per millimeter (p/mm) and images a surgical area of 53×40 mm^2. The advantage of the MRFL camera system is that both high-magnification images and a wide FOV can be simultaneously obtained without the need for moving the laparoscope in and out of the abdominal cavity, thus improving efficiency and maximizing safety by providing superior situational awareness. In addition, the MRFL system provides a large working space with fewer laparoscopic instrument collisions because the laparoscope is held farther away because of the magnification.[31] In vivo evaluation verified the great potential of MRFL for incorporation into laparoscopic surgery with improved efficiency and safety.[31] However, this system is still not commercially available.

During traditional laparoscopic surgery, an assistant is needed to control the laparoscope. Directing an assistant to control the camera can be challenging and may prolong the operative time. Therefore the earliest master-slave robotic surgical platforms controlled the laparoscope, freeing the surgeon to operate both hands and eliminating the need to rely on expert surgical assistants. Autonomous camera navigation systems have been invented to automatically keep surgical tools such as forceps and graspers in view.[32-37] These systems use different methods for detecting operator intent and tracking the tool tips relative to the camera. These methods include "eye-gaze tracking," "instrument tracking," "kinematic tracking," "image-based tracking," "magnetic tracking system," and "inertial measurement unit."[38,39] Recently, Weede and colleagues developed a test system that applies a Markov model to predict the motions of the tools so that the camera follows them.[40,41] The system is trained with data from previous surgical interventions so that it can operate more like an expert laparoscope operator. Furthermore, Yu and colleagues proposed algorithms for determining how to move the laparoscope from one viewing location to another, using kinematic models of a robotic surgery system.[42]

Another device that has been recently developed to overcome the camera handling difficulties during laparoscopic or robotic-assisted surgery is the RoboLens (Sina Robotics and Medical Innovators Co. Ltd., Tehran, Iran). It is a robotic system that uses an effective low-cost mechanism, with a minimum number of actuated degrees of freedom (DOFs), enabling spheric movement around a remote center of motion located at the insertion point of the laparoscopic stem. Hands-free operator interfaces were designed for user control, including a voice command recognition system and a smart six-button

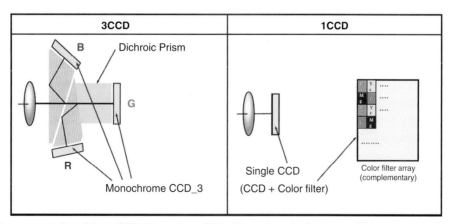

Figure 2-6. Schematic representation of three-CCD chip and one-CCD chip designs. Red, green, and blue are sent to three separate CCDs by a prism. *CCD*, charge-coupled device. *(Courtesy Olympus America, Melville, NY. From Lipkin ME, Scales CD, Preminger GM. Video imaging and documentation. In Smith AD, Preminger G, Badlan G, Kavoussi LR, eds.* Smith's Textbook of Endourology. *3rd ed. Oxford, UK: Wiley-Blackwell; 2012:19-37.)*

foot pedal (Fig. 2-9). The operational and technical features of the RoboLens were evaluated during a laparoscopic chole-cystectomy operation on human patients. RoboLens followed accurately the trajectory of instruments with a short response time.[43]

Currently, laparoscopic endoscopic single-site (LESS) surgery is a further refinement of minimally invasive laparoscopic procedures. The main difficulty is the limited space for the laparoscope and other instruments.[44] The miniature anchored robotic videoscope for expedited laparoscopy (MARVEL) is a wireless camera module (CM) that can be fixed under the abdominal wall to overcome crowding of instruments during LESS. The MARVEL system includes multiple CMs, a master control module (MCM), and a wireless human-machine interface (HMI). The multiple CMs feature a wirelessly controlled pan/tilt camera platform that enables a full hemispheric FOV

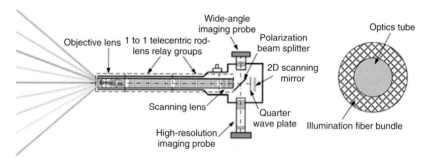

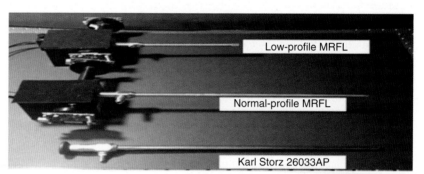

Figure 2-7. *Top,* Schematic layout of a dual-resolution, foveated laparoscope for minimally invasive surgery. The scope consists of a wide-angle imaging probe and a high-magnification probe. The two probes share the same objective lens, relay lens groups, and scanning lens groups. *Bottom,* Multiresolution foveated laparoscope (*MRFL*) prototypes in comparison with a commercially available standard laparoscope. *(From Qin Y, Hua H, Nguyen M. Characterization and in-vivo evaluation of a multi-resolution foveated laparoscope for minimally invasive surgery. Biomed Opt Express. 2014;5:2548-2562.)*

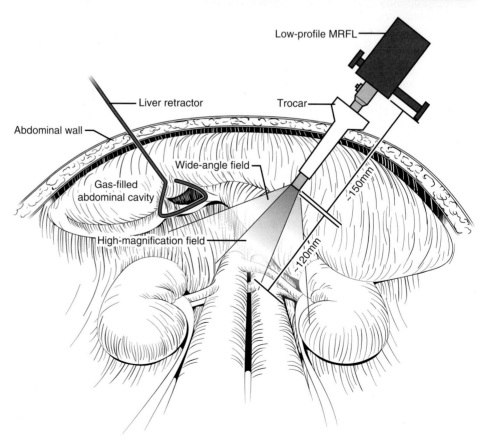

Figure 2-8. Conceptual idea for operation of MRFL in laparoscopic surgery. MRFL, multiresolution foveated laparoscope. *(From Qin Y, Hua H, Nguyen M. Characterization and in-vivo evaluation of a multi-resolution foveated laparoscope for minimally invasive surgery. Biomed Opt Express. 2014;5:2548-2562.)*

inside the abdominal cavity, wirelessly adjustable focus, and a multiwavelength illumination control system. The MCM provides a near-zero latency video wireless communication, digital zoom, and independent wireless control for multiple MARVEL CMs. The HMI gives the surgeon full control over

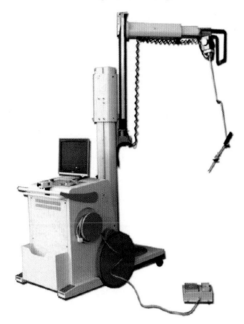

Figure 2-9. First prototype of designed robotic cameraman, RoboLens v1.1, in operational configuration. *(From Mirbagheri A, Farahmanda F, Meghdaria A, et al. Design and development of an effective low-cost robotic cameraman for laparoscopic surgery: RoboLens.* Scientia Iranica. *2011;18:105-114.)*

functionality of the CM. To insert and fix the MARVEL inside the abdominal cavity, the surgeon first inserts each CM into the end of a custom-designed insertion/removal tool (Fig. 2-10). A coaxial needle is used to secure the CM during insertion and removal. The CM is secured to the abdominal wall without use of a separate videoscope for assistance.[44] The surgeon can control the CM by a wireless joystick that controls the pan/tilt movement, illumination, adjustable focus, and digital zoom of all of the in vivo CMs. Each CM wirelessly sends its video stream to the MCM, which displays the images on high-resolution monitors.

Most recently, Tamadazte and associates introduced their Multi-View Vision System.[45] They tried to gather the advantages of stereovision, wide FOV, increased depth of vision, and low cost, without the need for either in situ registration between images or additional incisions. The system is based on two miniature high-resolution cameras positioned like a pair of glasses around the classic laparoscope (Fig. 2-11). The cameras are based on two 5-mm × 5-mm × 3.8-mm CMOS sensors with a resolution of 1600 × 1200 pixels, a frame rate of 30 frames/sec, a low noise-to-signal ratio, an exposure control of +81 dB, an FOV of 51 degrees with a low TV distortion (≤1%). This device is not more invasive than standard endoscopy, because it is inserted through the laparoscope's trocar.[45]

THREE-DIMENSIONAL VIDEO SYSTEMS

Two-dimensional video systems providing flat images are currently present in most operating rooms. The main disadvantage is the lack of depth perception. With advances in imaging technology, three-dimensional video techniques are now incorporated into laparoscopic or robotic-assisted surgery (Fig. 2-12). These systems simulate the human eye by using two cameras (right and left). Images of the right and left

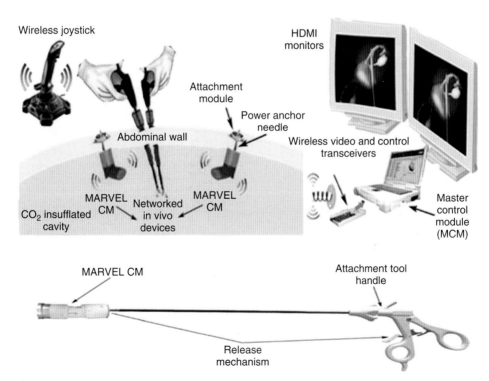

Figure 2-10. *Top,* Functional diagram of the MARVEL system, including the MCM and the MARVEL robotic CM. *Bottom,* Customized insertion removal tool used for attaching the MARVEL platform within the peritoneal cavity. MARVEL provides its own imaging during attachment, eliminating the need for a cabled laparoscope during any portion of the procedure. *CM,* camera module; *MARVEL,* miniature anchored robotic videoscope for expedited laparoscopy; *MCM,* master control module. *(From Castro CA, Alqassis A, Smith S, et al. A wireless robot for networked laparoscopy.* IEEE Trans Biomed Eng. *2013;60:930-936.)*

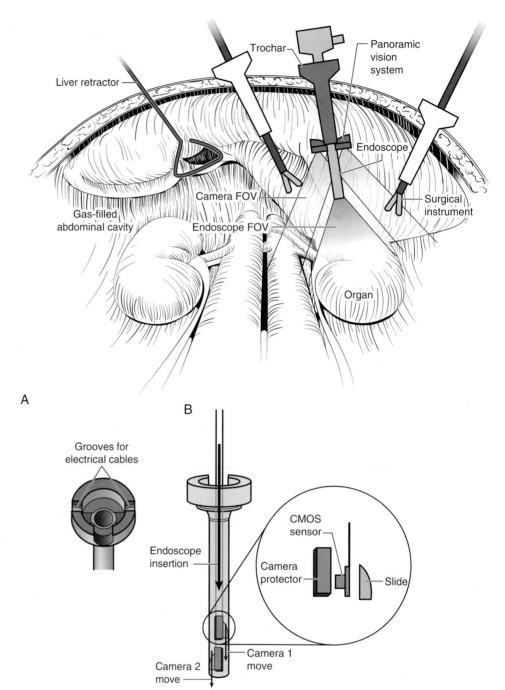

Figure 2-11. A, Schematization of the proposed concept of global vision system. **B,** Computer-aided design model of the proposed multiple-view device illustrating the different elements that compose the system. *CMOS,* complementary metal-oxide semiconductor; *FOV,* field of view. *(From Tamadazte B, Agustinos A, Cinquin B, et al. Multi-View Vision System for laparoscopy surgery.* Int J Comput Assist Radiol Surg. *2014;9:1-17.)*

cameras are alternated rapidly at a frequency of 100 to 120 Hz to display the three-dimensional image on the monitor. This method also is known as *sequential display procedure.* Most three-dimensional video systems function using four basic principles: (1) separation of the left and right eyes images, (2) image capture, (3) conversion of 60- to 120-Hz images, and (4) presentation of right and left images on a single monitor.[46,47] The three-dimensional image display may be accomplished with either polarizing glasses or active liquid crystal display glasses. In both cases, the brain fuses the right-sided and left-sided images on the appropriate imaging site, and in effect simulates depth. In fact, this technology is quite different from normal stereoscopic imaging, wherein the two independent images are shown to both eyes simultaneously.[23] The da Vinci robotic system uses another method of image display through mimicking the human eye's acquisition of images by presenting the two independent images to each eye using a fixed, head-mounted display.

True stereoscopic imaging favors the incorporation of three-dimensional imaging systems during laparoscopic or robotic-assisted surgical procedures.[48-50] The depth perception offered by three-dimensional endoscopic video systems facilitates complex minimally invasive laparoscopic procedures with better identification of tissue layers and easier suturing and knot tying.[51-53] Assessments of laparoscopic suturing and knot tying with three-dimensional endoscopic video systems have demonstrated a 25% increase in speed and accuracy compared with the standard two-dimensional endoscopic video systems.[54] Therefore incorporation of three-dimensional imaging into training for minimally invasive surgery may

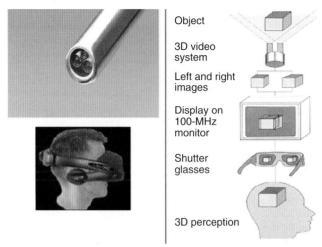

Figure 2-12. Three-dimensional (*3D*) stereoendoscope; schematic diagram of a three-dimensional video imaging system. The two images are projected on a screen, and the glasses bring the two together, giving the impression of a three-dimensional image. Alternatively, the separate images can be presented separately to the left and right eyes through a headset. This is currently available as part of the da Vinci robotic system and theoretically can be developed by means of a head-mounted display. *From Marguet CG, Springhart WP, Preminger GM. New technology for imaging and documenting urologic procedures. Urol Clin North Am. 2006;33:397-408.)*

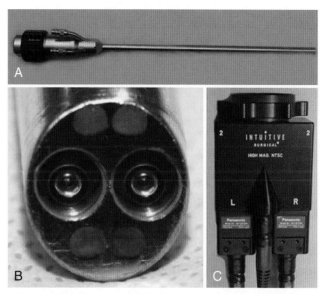

Figure 2-13. Photograph of da Vinci stereo endoscope **(A)** showing the two individual 5-mm endoscopes **(B)** and camera **(C)** with right and left optical channels. *(From Higuchi TT, Gettman MT. Robotic instrumentation, personnel and operating room setup. In Su LM, ed. Atlas of Robotic Urologic Surgery, Current Clinical Urology. New York: Humana Press; 2011.)*

shorten the learning curve and improve the performance of these procedures.[47,55]

However, it seems that this improvement in speed and accuracy is significant only when these tasks are performed by inexperienced surgeons rather than when performed by experienced laparoscopists who started training and gained their experience using the standard two-dimensional video systems. Furthermore, some studies suggest that the higher resolution and better luminescence offered by the two-dimensional video systems might be more advantageous than the depth perception offered by the three-dimensional endoscopic video systems.[56,57] In addition to the high cost of the three-dimensional video systems, they are associated with decreased image brightness and resolution, possibly because these video systems use two optical channels that are significantly smaller than a single-lens system in a standard two-dimensional 10-mm laparoscope. Moreover, because most three-dimensional video systems incorporate two separate camera systems, the camera head is significantly larger than with a single-camera system, which makes it awkward to work during minimally invasive procedures. Additional prospective studies are needed to compare surgical efficiency and surgeon fatigability with both systems.[48-50,56-58]

THE DA VINCI SURGICAL SYSTEM

The da Vinci is a "master-slave system" with three components: surgeon console, vision cart, and patient cart. It is available in four different models: standard, streamlined (S), S-HD, and S integrated (Si)-HD.[59,60] Images generated by the da Vinci models use stereoendoscopes to capture images from the surgical field. These images are generated by capturing two independent views from two 5-mm endoscopes fixed into the stereo endoscope and transmitting them into right and left optical channels to give a real-time high-resolution three-dimensional display (Fig. 2-13).[59] The endoscope is available in 0-degree, 30-degree upward, and 30-degree downward

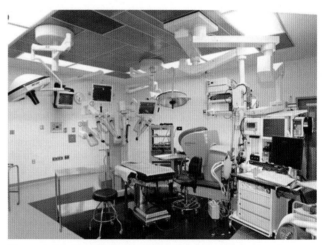

Figure 2-14. Photograph of operating room for the da Vinci S system. Several telemonitors are mounted from the ceiling, and a laparoscopic tower is mounted on a ceiling boom with the electrosurgical unit, insufflator, and light source. The room is also equipped with an integration system for DVD recording and telemedicine. *(From Higuchi TT, Gettman MT. Robotic instrumentation, personnel and operating room setup. In Su LM, ed. Atlas of Robotic Urologic Surgery, Current Clinical Urology. New York: Humana Press; 2011.)*

angles. Depending on the nature of intervention, the 30-degree downward endoscopes are typically used for most robotic pelvic procedures, whereas a variety of endoscopes are used for upper urinary tract interventions.

In the standard and S da Vinci models, the endoscope is connected to either a wide-angle (10× magnification with 60-degree view) or high-magnification (15× magnification with 45-degree view) camera head with right and left optical channels (Fig. 2-14). The HD da Vinci systems come with only one camera. The right and left optical channels are connected to two three-chip camera-control units (CCUs), with the camera head connected to an automatic focus control. Both the CCUs and the automatic focus control are integrated in the surgeon console. An additional advantage that has been introduced in the S-HD system is the addition of an HD camera and CCUs to increase resolution and aspect ratio. The first-generation HD system had a resolution of 720p (1280 × 720) with an aspect ratio of 16:9, which improved the viewing area by 20%. Another advantage is that the HD system also has a digital zoom that allows the surgeon to magnify the tissue without moving the endoscope. This could be performed by pressing the right and the left arrow keys on the left-side pod controls or depressing the camera pedal and moving the masters together or apart. The patient cart within the Si-HD da Vinci system was modified to integrate both the light source and CCU into a single connection, with the camera adjustments performed using the central touch pad or telemonitor and increased resolution up to 1080i (1920 × 1080).[61]

HIGH-DEFINITION LAPAROSCOPY

The high-quality image display systems are essential during endoscopic and laparoscopic surgery. However, the current analog NTSC, sequential color and memory (SECAM) and phase alternation line (PAL) monitors have limited resolution. Furthermore, previous studies demonstrated that the inherent optical quality of most endoscopes and CCD cameras exceeds the display resolution of standard TV.[62] High-definition television (HDTV) is one of the digital display systems with high image resolution and wide aspect ratio. HDTV pixel numbers range from 1 to 2 million, compared with the ranges of NTSC, PAL, or SECAM of 300,000 to 1 million. Therefore HDTV offers high image resolution with greatly enhanced image quality. For example, the European standard HD imaging chip resolution is 2,340,250 pixels, resulting in 1250 horizontal lines, and the most common HDTV formats used in the United States are 720p and 1080i, which correspond to 60 frames per second—double the value of conventional TV monitors. In terms of the aspect ratio (the width-to-height ratio of the screen), the HDTV format offers an aspect ratio of 16:9, which is greatly wider than that of the NTSC, PAL, and SECAM screens, which have an aspect ratio of 4:3. Recent studies have reported that HD laparoscopy had superior objective performance characteristics, in terms of superior resolution, increased image brightness, increased depth of field, and decreased image distortion, when compared with standard laparoscopy.[63] Therefore it enhances both diagnostic and therapeutic interventions.[25,57]

COMPUTER VISION (IMAGE-GUIDED) LAPAROSCOPIC AND ROBOTIC-ASSISTED SURGERY

Image-guided surgery (IGS) depends on AR image reconstruction, which involves integration of preoperative radiologic images with real-time intraoperative views. Therefore it provides the surgeon with a tool to reference preoperative image data to maintain orientation and see subsurface in formations that are not accessible through the ordinary imaging during laparoscopic surgery. One of the major potential advantages of AR is that it compensates for the loss of haptic feedback in laparoscopic and robotic-assisted surgery.[64]

The workstation of any AR imaging system imports preoperative computed tomography (CT), magnetic resonance imaging (MRI), or other volumetric images related to the patient. Then an initial calibration allows the system to settle on the transformation between CT image coordinates and the patient reference coordinates. The system uses a variety of graphical

means to inform the surgeon of the relationship between his or her tools and the corresponding three-dimensional volumetric data or patient models. Typically, the system displays several orthogonal slices of the volume data and some graphical indication of tool location.

For the surgeon to know how well the AR imaging system is working, the reliability of the system must be assessed in terms of precision and accuracy. The system is precise when it has low variance (i.e., returns the same measurement each time), and the system is accurate when its measurements are very close to a reference true value. Numerous metrics have been introduced to measure the reliability of AR imaging systems.[65]

There were different techniques for implementation of IGS and AR. First, real-time virtual sonography, which is based on synchronization of the preoperative CT or MRI images with intraoperative real-time sonographic imaging, was used to display three-dimensional reconstructed CT or MRI images. This technique was especially helpful for percutaneous renal and prostatic ablative procedures.[66,67] AR has been also applied to robotic-assisted partial nephrectomy. This system allows overlay of three-dimensional models constructed from preoperative CT scans onto three-dimensional intraoperative video recordings.[68] The major limitation of these systems is the accounting for organ motion and deformation. Gill and Okimura described a surgical radar and surgical body gravitational positioning system.[67] The surgical radar involved displaying color-coded zones over the real-time image of an intended surgical target. The trajectory of an instrument can be used to predict whether the current path of that instrument will violate an undesirable structure, such as a tumor. The surgical body gravitational positioning system allows for monitoring of real-time organ position. The surgeon can be alerted on how real-time movement of instruments can alter the line of excision to maximize normal tissue preservation and oncologic efficacy.[67]

Perhaps the most challenging new application for image-guided intervention will be in the field of natural orifice transluminal endoscopic surgery (NOTES), in which video cameras and miniature instruments are introduced into the body cavity via the mouth, rectum, or vagina with the objective of reaching the internal organs without leaving any scar. However, in 2006, the Natural Orifice Surgery Consortium for Assessment and Research (NOSCAR) identified a number of potential barriers to safe clinical implementation of NOTES.[69] One of the most challenging issues encountered in NOTES procedures is determining the orientation of the endoscope image.[70,71] Fortunately, AR imaging can accurately track the endoscopic camera and miniature surgical manipulation devices in space using miniature electromagnetic trackers and by accurately registering and fusing preoperatively acquired images of organs with the laparoscopic images and with intraoperative images such as those obtained by ultrasound.[72]

TELEMENTORING AND TELESURGERY

Advances in digital imaging, high-speed computer connections, and the widespread availability of the Internet have allowed a steady growth of telesurgery within urology.[73] Kavoussi and colleagues proved the concept when they published the findings of their initial laboratory experience with telerobotic-assisted laparoscopic surgery that took place on the other side of the globe.[74-78] Five patients underwent laparoscopic surgery in Rome while surgeons in Baltimore proctored the procedures in real time.[79] The telesurgical approach may afford improved patient care by allowing highly experienced surgeons to either perform or proctor less experienced laparoscopic surgeons who are geographically displaced.[73,78,80,81] Furthermore, this creates what is called *telementoring*—active real-time teaching between local and remote surgeons through videoconferencing.[81]

Urologic telementoring began in 1994, pioneered by a group at Johns Hopkins Hospital in Baltimore.[77,82] The authors initially established a remote site within the same hospital as the operating room (approximately 1000 feet away).[77] All the remote components were directly wired to their sources in the operating room. This preliminary system provided real-time video display from either the laparoscope or an externally mounted camera located in the operating theater. The remote surgical consultant communicated with the operating surgeon by duplex audio and telestration. In addition, the remote surgeon had control of the robotic arm, which manipulated the laparoscope. The authors then extended this system by adding a remote switch that activated the electrocautery for tissue cutting and hemostasis. With this initial equipment, remote presence surgical system procedures were performed in a controlled environment.[83] This work demonstrated that telementoring and remote presence surgery were effective and safe. However, it did not address a critical problem in the development of true telesurgery, that is, the transmission of the necessary data over long distances between medical centers.

The first truly telesurgical urologic procedure, a percutaneous renal access, was carried out on July 17, 1998 over a communications link between Baltimore and Rome, Italy (4500 miles). Previously, the Johns Hopkins robotics group had developed a purpose-built surgical robot for this procedure known as PAKY (Percutaneous Access to the Kidney).[84,85] An early version of this system with an active radiolucent needle driver was able to access the renal collecting system in more than 90% of attempts with a mean access time of 16 minutes and a mean of three needle passes. The next-generation PAKY had an active robotic arm with three DOFs for control of the access needle and a biplanar fluoroscopic imaging system for guidance. This system was then modified to allow a surgeon in Baltimore to control the robot located in Rome. Successful percutaneous access to a human kidney was accomplished within 20 minutes without complications using this system.[86] Substantial progress has been made in developing first-generation telesurgical systems that allow telementoring and limited active surgical assistance over great distances. These technologies, at the most basic level, should provide adequate visualization and transmission of the surgical procedure to the expert, and must allow two-way voice communication between the mentor and the mentee. In addition, they must be Health Insurance Portability and Accountability Act (HIPAA) compliant. More advanced tools allow for interactivity such as telestration and/or laser pointing on the operative field and should ideally be cost-effective.[87]

Recently, the InTouch or Visitor1 system (Karl Storz, Tuttlingen, Germany) was introduced. Although more expensive, this system allows for high-fidelity transmission with HIPAA compliance as a U.S. Food and Drug Administration–approved device with the elements of high-quality interactivity including laser pointing and telestration. The expert had a laptop that connected to the telementoring "robot" in the operating room. The robot is a device that was hanging from a boom that consisted of HD cameras, laser-pointing capabilities, and telestration on the screen. The expert could control the robot with a mouse and could move the camera and zoom in on the external view. Laparoscopically, the expert has no control of the camera but does have the ability to telestrate. This system was very easy to use and worked well. Unlike all other telementoring options, the two HD cameras situated on top of the Visitor1 make telementoring with this technology suitable for both laparoscopic and open surgery. Furthermore, the Visitor1 is also capable of helping with nonsurgical telementoring such as in the emergency room or clinics (Figs. 2-15 and 2-16). However, several significant technical and legal barriers must be surmounted before telesurgery can be widely accepted and incorporated into general urologic practice.[87]

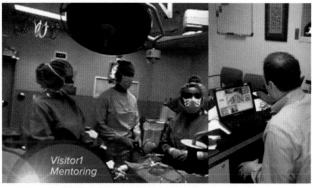

Figure 2-15. Dr. Ponsky acting as a mentor in Akron using the Karl Storz Visitor1 system to advise on a case in Denver. *(From Ponsky TA, Schwachter M, Parry J, et al. Telementoring: the surgical tool of the future. Eur J Pediatr Surg. 2014;24:287-294.)*

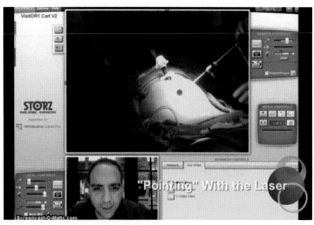

Figure 2-16. Dr. Ponsky in Colorado using the Visitor1 laser to point on a patient in Cleveland. *(From Ponsky TA, Schwachter M, Parry J, et al. Telementoring: the surgical tool of the future.* Eur J Pediatr Surg. *2014;24:287-294.)*

REFERENCES

1. Engel R. Philipp Bozzini—the father of endoscopy. *J Endourol.* 2003;17:859–862.
2. Desormeaux AJ. The endoscope and its application to the diagnosis and treatment of affections of the genitourinary passages. *Chic Med J.* 1867;24:177–194.
3. Shah J. Endoscopy through the ages. *BJU Int.* 2002;89:645–652.
4. Mouton WG, Bessell MD, Maddern MS. Looking back to the advent of modern endoscopy: 150th birthday of Maximilian Nitze. *World J Surg.* 1998;22:1256–1258.
5. Hopkins H, Kapany N. A flexible fibrescope, using static scanning. *Nature.* 1954;173:39–41.
6. Gow JG. Harold Hopkins and optical systems for urology—an appreciation. *Urology.* 1998;52:152–157.
7. Mirota DJ, Masaru Ishii M, Hager GD. Vision-based navigation in image-guided interventions. *Annu Rev Biomed Eng.* 2011;13: 297–319.
8. Roulet P, Konen P, Villegas M. 360° endoscopy using panomorph lens technology. *Proc SPIE Int Soc Opt Eng.* 2010 Feb 24:7558.
9. Knyrim K, Seidlitz H, Vakil N, et al. Perspectives in electronic endoscopy. Past, present, and future of fibers and CCDs in medical endoscopes. *Endoscopy.* 1990;22(Suppl 1):2–8.
10. Niwa H, Kawaguchi A, Miyahara T, et al. Clinical use of new video endoscopes (EVIS 100 and 200). *Endoscopy.* 1992;24:222–224.
11. Pelosi MA, Kadar N, Pelosi MA. The electronic video operative laparoscope. *J Am Assoc Gynecol Laparosc.* 1993;1:54–57.
12. Springhart WP, Maloney MM, Sur RL, et al. Digital video ureteroscope: a new paradigm in ureteroscopy. *J Urol.* 2005;173:428S.

13. Boppart SA, Deutsch TF, Rattner DW. Optical imaging technology in minimally invasive surgery. Current status and future directions. *Surg Endosc.* 1999;13:718–722.

14. Cuschieri A. Technology for minimal access surgery. Interview by Judy Jones. *BMJ.* 1999;319:1304.

15. Afane JS, Olweny EO, Bercowsky E, et al. Flexible ureteroscopes: a single center evaluation of the durability and function of the new endoscopes smaller than 9 Fr. *J Urol.* 2000;164:1164–1168.

16. Auge BK, Preminger GM. *Digital cameras and documentation in urologic practice. AUA Update Series XXI.* Linthicum, MD: American Urologic Association Press; 2002.

17. Levisohn PM. Safety and tolerability of topiramate in children. *J Child Neurol.* 2000;15(Suppl 1):S22.

18. Kennedy TJ, Preminger GM. Impact of video on endourology. *J Endourol.* 1987;1:75–79.

19. Litwiler SE, Preminger GM. Advances in electronic imaging for laparoscopy. *J Endourol.* 1993;7:S195.

20. Preminger GM. Video-assisted transurethral resection of the prostate. *J Endourol.* 1991;5:161–164.

21. Litynski GS. Endoscopic surgery: the history, the pioneers. *World J Surg.* 1999;23:745–753.

22. Flachenecker G, Fastenmeier K. High frequency interferences in video imaging systems during transurethral resection. *World J Urol.* 1988;6:8–13.

23. Hanna G, Cuschieri A. Image display technology and image processing. *World J Surg.* 2001;25:1419–1427.

24. Kuo RL, Preminger GM. Current urologic applications of digital imaging. *J Endourol.* 2001;15:53–57.

25. Kuo RL, Delvecchio FC, Babayan RK, et al. Telemedicine: recent developments and future applications. *J Endourol.* 2001;15:63–66.

26. Humphreys MR, Miller NL, Williams JC, et al. A new world revealed: early experience with digital ureteroscopy. *J Urol.* 2008;179:970–975.

27. Borin J, Abdelshahid C, Dean L, et al. The distal sensor digital flexible ureteroscope: an optical evaluation. *J Endourol.* 2006;20:199.

28. Andonian S, Okeke Z, Smith AD. Digital ureteroscopy: the next step. *J Endourol.* 2008;22:603–606.

29. Heemskerk J, Zandbergen R, Maessen JG, et al. Advantages of advanced laparoscopic systems. *Surg Endosc.* 2006;20:730–733.

30. Wu MP, Ou CS, Chen SL, et al. Complication and recommended practices for electrosurgery in laparoscopy. *Am J Surg.* 2000;179:67–73.

31. Qin Y, Hua H, Nguyen M. Characterization and in-vivo evaluation of a multi-resolution foveated laparoscope for minimally invasive surgery. *Biomed Opt Express.* 2014;5:2548–2562.

32. Ali SM, Reisner LA, King B, et al. Eye gaze tracking for endoscopic camera positioning: an application of a hardware/software interface developed to automate Aesop. *Stud Health Technol Inform.* 2007;132:4–7.

33. Lee C, Wang YF, Uecker DR, et al. Image analysis for automated tracking in robot-assisted endoscopic surgery. In: *Proceedings of the 12th IAPR International Conference on Pattern Recognition.* Jerusalem: Israel; October 9-13, 1994.

34. Wei GQ, Arbter K, Hirzinger G. Real-time visual servoing for laparoscopic surgery: controlling robot motion with color image segmentation. *IEEE Eng Med Biol Mag.* 1997;16:40–45.

35. Fortney DR. *Real-time color image guidance system.* Santa Barbara, CA: University of California at Santa Barbara; 2000.

36. Ko SY, Kim J, Lee WJ, et al. Compact laparoscopic assistant robot using a bending mechanism. *Adv Robot.* 2007;21:689–709.

37. Azizian M, Khoshnam M, Najmaei N, et al. Visual servoing in medical robotics: a survey. Part I: Endoscopic and direct vision imaging—techniques and applications. *Int J Med Robot.* 2014;10:263–274.

38. Mudunuri AV. *Autonomous Camera Control System for Surgical Robots.* Detroit, MI: Wayne State University; 2011. [master's thesis].

39. King BW, Reisner LA, Pandya AK, et al. Towards an autonomous robot for camera control during laparoscopic surgery. *J Laparoendosc Adv Surg Tech.* 2013;23:1027–1030.

40. Weede O, Bihlmaier A, Hutzl J, et al. Towards cognitive medical robotics in minimal invasive surgery. In: *Proceedings of the Conference on Advances in Robotics.* ; July 4-6, 2013. Pune, India.

41. Weede O, Monnich H, Muller B, et al. An intelligent and autonomous endoscopic guidance system for minimally invasive surgery. In: *Proceedings of the IEEE International Conference on Robotics and Automation.* Shanghai: China; May 9-13, 2011.

42. Yu L, Wang Z, Sun L, et al. Kinematics method of automatic visual window for laparoscopic minimally invasive surgical robotic system. In: *Proceedings of the IEEE International Conference Mechatronics and Automation.* August 4-7, 2013. Takamatsu, Japan.

43. Mirbagheri A, Farahmanda F, Meghdaria A, et al. Design and development of an effective low-cost robotic cameraman for laparoscopic surgery: RoboLens. *Scientia Iranica.* 2011;18:105–114.

44. Castro CA, Alqassis A, Smith S, et al. A wireless robot for networked laparoscopy. *IEEE Trans Biomed Eng.* 2013;60:930–936.

45. Tamadazte B, Agustinos A, Cinquin B, et al. Multi-View Vision System for Laparoscopy Surgery. *Int J Comput Assist Radiol Surg.* 2014;9:1–17.

46. Tan YH, Preminger GM. Advances in video and imaging in ureteroscopy. *Urol Clin North Am.* 2004;31:33–42.

47. Durrani AF, Preminger GM. Three-dimensional video imaging for endoscopic surgery. *Comput Biol Med.* 1995;25:237–247.

48. Chang L, Satava RM, Pellegrini CA, et al. Robotic surgery: identifying the learning curve through objective measurement of skill. *Surg Endosc.* 2003;17:1744–1748.

49. Dakin GF, Gagner M. Comparison of laparoscopic skills performance between standard instruments and two surgical robotic systems. *Surg Endosc.* 2003;17:574–579.

50. Renda A, Vallancien G. Principles and advantages of robotics in urologic surgery. *Curr Urol Rep.* 2003;4:114–118.

51. Garcia BJ, Greenstein RJ. True-stereoscopic video from monoscopic sources: the DeepVision system for minimally invasive surgery. *Virtual Real Syst Mag.* 1994;1:52.

52. Birkett DH. 3-D imaging in gastrointestinal laparoscopy. *Surg Endosc.* 1993;7:556–557.

53. Janetschek G, Reissigl A, Peschel R, et al. Chip on a stick technology: first clinical experience with this new videolaparoscope. *J Endourol.* 1993;7. S195.

54. Babayan RK, Chiu AW, Este-McDonald J, et al. The comparison between 2-dimensional and 3-dimensional laparoscopic video systems in a pelvic trainer. *J Endourol.* 1993;7. S195.

55. Chiu AW, Babayan RK. Retroperitoneal laparoscopic nephrectomy utilizing three-dimensional camera. Case report. *J Endourol.* 1994;8:139–141.

56. Hofmeister J, Frank TG, Cuschieri A, et al. Perceptual aspects of two-dimensional and stereoscopic display techniques in endoscopic surgery: review and current problems. *Semin Laparosc Surg.* 2001;8:12–24.

57. van Bergen P, Kunert W, Buess GF. The effect of high-definition imaging on surgical task efficiency in minimally invasive surgery: an experimental comparison between three-dimensional imaging and direct vision through a stereoscopic TEM rectoscope. *Surg Endosc.* 2000;14:71–74.

58. Herron DM, Lantis 2nd JC, Maykel J, et al. The 3-D monitor and head-mounted display. A quantitative evaluation of advanced laparoscopic viewing technologies. *Surg Endosc.* 1999;13:751–755.

59. Narula VK, Melvin SM. Robotic surgical systems. In: Patel VR, ed. *Robotic Urologic Surgery.* London: Springer-Verlag; 2007:5–14.

60. Bhandari A, Hemal A, Menon M. Instrumentation, sterilization, and preparation of robot. *Indian J Urol.* 2005;21:83–85.

61. Higuchi TT, Gettman MT. Robotic instrumentation, personnel and operating room setup. In: Su LM, ed. *Atlas of Robotic Urologic Surgery, Current Clinical Urology.* New York: Humana Press; 2011, 15-30 doi 10.1007/978-1-60761-026-7_2.

62. von Orelli A, Lehareinger Y, Rol P, et al. High-definition truecolour television for use in minimally invasive medical procedures. *Technol Health Care.* 1999;7:75–84.

63. Pierre SA, Ferrandino MN, Simmons N, et al. High definition laparoscopy: objective assessment of performance characteristics and comparison with standard laparoscopy. *J Endourol.* 2009;32:523–528.

64. Ukimora O. Image-guided surgery in minimally invasive urology. *Curr Opin Urol.* 2010;20:136–140.

65. Fitzpatrick JM, West JB, Maurer CR Jr: Predicting error in rigid-body point-based registration. *IEEE Trans Med Imaging.* 17:694–702.

66. Ukimora O, Gill IS. Image assisted endoscopic surgery. Cleveland Clinic experience. *J Endourol.* 2008;22:803–810.

67. Ukimora O, Gill IS. Image-fusion, augmented reality, and predictive surgical navigation. *Urol Clin North Am.* 2009;36:115–123.

68. Su LM, Vagvolgyi BP, Agarwal R, et al. Augmented reality during robot-assisted partial nephrectomy: toward real-time 3D-CT to stereoscopic video registration. *Urology.* 2009;73:896–900.

69. Rattner D, Kalloo A. ASGE/SAGESWorking Group on Natural Orifice Translumenal Endoscopic Surgery. *Surg Endosc.* 2006;20: 329–333.

70. Spaun GO, Zheng B, Martinec DV, et al. Bimanual coordination in natural orifice transluminal endoscopic surgery: comparing the conventional dual-channel endoscope, the R-Scope, and a novel direct-drive system. *Gastrointest. Endosc.* 69:e39–e45.

71. Swanstrom L, Swain P, Denk P. Development and validation of a new generation of flexible endoscope for NOTES. *Surg Innov.* 2009;16:104–110.

72. Cleary1 K, Peters TM. Image-guided interventions: technology review and clinical applications. *Annu Rev Biomed Eng.* 2010;12:119–142.

73. McFarlane N, Denstedt J. Imaging and the Internet. *J Endourol.* 2001;15:59–61.

74. Byrne JP, Mughal MM. Telementoring as an adjunct to training and competence-based assessment in laparoscopic cholecystectomy. *Surg Endosc.* 2000;14:1159–1161.

75. Janetschek G, Bartsch G, Kavoussi LR. Transcontinental interactive laparoscopic telesurgery between the United States and Europe. *J Urol.* 1998;160:1413.

76. Lee BR, Bishoff JT, Janetschek G, et al. A novel method of surgical instruction: international telementoring. *World J Urol.* 1998;16:367–370.

77. Moore RG, Adams JB, Partin AW, et al. Telementoring of laparoscopic procedures: initial clinical experience. *Surg Endosc.* 1996;10:107–110.

78. Rosser Jr JC, Herman B, Giammaria LE. Telementoring. *Semin Laparosc Surg.* 2003;10:209–217.

79. Micali S, Vespasiani G, Finazzi-Agro E, et al. Feasibility of telesurgery between Baltimore, USA and Rome, Italy: the first five cases. *J Endourol.* 2000;14:493–496.

80. Lee BR, Png DJ, Liew L, et al. Laparoscopic telesurgery between the United States and Singapore. *Ann Acad Med Singapore.* 2000;29:665–668.

81. Link RE, Schulam PG, Kavoussi LR. Telesurgery: Remote monitoring and assistance during laparoscopy. *Urol Clin North Am.* 2001;28:177–188.

82. Docimo SG, Moore RG, Adams J, et al. Early experience with telerobotic surgery in children. *J Telemed Telecare.* 1996;2:48–50.

83. Hodge Jr JG, Gostin LO, Jacobson PD. Legal issues concerning electronic health information: privacy, quality, and liability. *JAMA.* 1999;282:1466–1471.

84. Cadeddu JA, Stoianovici D, Chen RN, et al. Stereotactic mechanical percutaneous renal access. *J Endourol.* 1998;12:121–125.

85. Stoianovici D, Cadeddu JA, Demaree RD, et al. A novel mechanical transmission applied to percutaneous renal access. In: *Proceedings of the ASME Dynamic Systems and Control Division.* 1997. Available from http://citeseerx.ist.psu.edu/viewdoc/download? doi=10.1.1.17.2845&rep=rep1&type=pdf.

86. Lee B, Cadeddu JA, Stoianovici D, et al. Telemedicine and surgical robotics: urologic applications. *Rev Urol.* 1999;1:104–110.

87. Ponsky TA, Schwachter M, Parry J, et al. Telementoring: the surgical tool of the future. *Eur J Pediatr Surg.* 2014;24:287–294.

3 Basic Instrumentation

John Schomburg, Sean McAdams, Kyle Anderson

With ubiquitous adoption of laparoscopic surgery in many surgical disciplines, a wide variety of laparoscopic instruments are available in operating rooms. Herein we describe commonly useful laparoscopic instruments as well as instruments specialized for retroperitoneal laparoscopic urologic surgery. We focus our discussion on the following areas: graspers, scissors, needle drivers, retractors, energy instruments, suction and irrigation devices, and extractors. Access ports, closure devices, laparoscopes, and other instruments such as staplers and clip appliers are discussed elsewhere in this book.

DISSECTORS AND GRASPERS

A variety of laparoscopic grasping instruments are available. Instrument sizes vary in both diameter (3 to 10 mm) and length (20 to 45 cm). Although narrower instruments facilitate operations through smaller ports, they are less rigid and limited to single-action jaw movement compared with larger instruments, which can have dual-action jaw movement. Longer instruments, commonly referred to as bariatric instruments, are helpful in patients with a high body mass index or in cases with difficult access. Handle options include open ring, ratchet, pistol grip, coaxial, and bent wire handles (Fig. 3-1). Handles are available with or without locking mechanisms. Grasper tips are available in a variety of shapes and sizes (Fig. 3-2). Traumatic graspers use toothed forceps to attain a firm grasp on tissue but can damage it. Atraumatic graspers use serrated tips that cause less damage to vital structures. Graspers with disposable padded tips are also available; these are atraumatic in their grip and avoid the crushing forces often seen with metal-tipped graspers. Both single-use and reusable graspers are available. Reusable instruments feature interchangeable instrument tips and handle pieces. Some reusable instruments can also be disassembled to allow cleaning.

In addition to the rigid, straight graspers, more recent technical advances have led to the development of articulating laparoscopic instruments (Fig. 3-3). These are available from a variety of manufacturers and can facilitate single-site surgery and other complicated laparoscopic procedures.

SCISSORS

Both single-use and reusable scissors with a variety of tip shapes (straight, curved, and hook) are available. Most scissors can be connected to monopolar cautery devices to facilitate simultaneous ligation and coagulation. In addition, the scissor tips can be useful as a monopolar dissector without operating the scissor action. The instrument shaft is insulated to prevent damage to surrounding structures.

NEEDLE DRIVERS AND SUTURING INSTRUMENTS

Laparoscopic needle drivers are available in a variety of tip configurations (straight, curved, self-righting), insert types (carbide, serrated), and handles (finger, palm, pistol grip). Whereas needle driver configuration is driven by surgeon preference,

proper positioning of the needle in the jaws of the driver is critical to successful manipulation of the suture needle. Specific situations may vary, but in general the needle is ideally positioned in the tips of the jaws, pointed away from the body of the instrument, and gripped one quarter to one half of the way along the curve (Fig. 3-4).

Knots may be tied intracorporeally with a needle driver and grasper or extracorporeally with the assistance of a laparoscopic knot pusher (Fig. 3-5). For intracorporeal tying, suture tails should be trimmed to 7 to 12 cm; longer suture lengths can be more difficult to tie. For extracorporeal tying, a longer suture should be used.

Several devices are available to assist with intracorporeal suturing, including Endo Stitch (Covidien, Dublin, Ireland) and Sew-Right (LSI Solutions, Victor, N.Y.). These instruments feature a specialized needle and passing mechanism that is designed to facilitate both suturing and knot tying. Suture Assistant (Ethicon, Somerville, N.J.) is more similar to a traditional needle driver in passing the needle through tissue but features a specialized suture and tying mechanism to facilitate intracorporeal knot tying. Endoloop (Ethicon) is a preformed loop of Vicryl or polydioxanone (PDS) with a slip knot that can be used to efficiently ligate structures. Lapra-Ty (Ethicon) is an alternative to intracorporeal knot tying. Instead of tying a knot, an absorbable clip is applied to a tensioned 2-0, 3-0, or 4-0 Vicryl suture (Fig. 3-6). Lapra-Ty can prove particularly useful if a suture breaks and the end becomes too short to tie.

Although freehand suturing and knot tying are technically advanced skills, we generally prefer them over the suturing aids because they allow for more dexterity and finesse in movement as well as a much larger range of needle selection and suture material.

VASCULAR CLAMPS

Several instruments are available to assist with vascular control and clamping, including laparoscopic Satinsky clamps as well as bulldog clamps, which are inserted, applied, and removed with the aid of a specialized instrument (Fig. 3-7).

BIOPSY FORCEPS

Laparoscopic biopsy forceps are available in 5- and 10-mm sizes.

RETRACTORS

Although proper patient positioning and insufflation are critical first steps in exposing the operative field, intracorporeal retraction is often needed to displace organs for best visualization. Graspers can be used safely in most situations, but they are not appropriate in all cases and may damage organs or important structures.

A variety of laparoscopic retraction instruments are available, including the fan, PEER (Jarit Surgical Instruments, Hawthorne, N.Y.), and Diamond-Flex (Genzyme Surgical Products Corp., Tucker, Ga.), as well as disposable paddle retractors

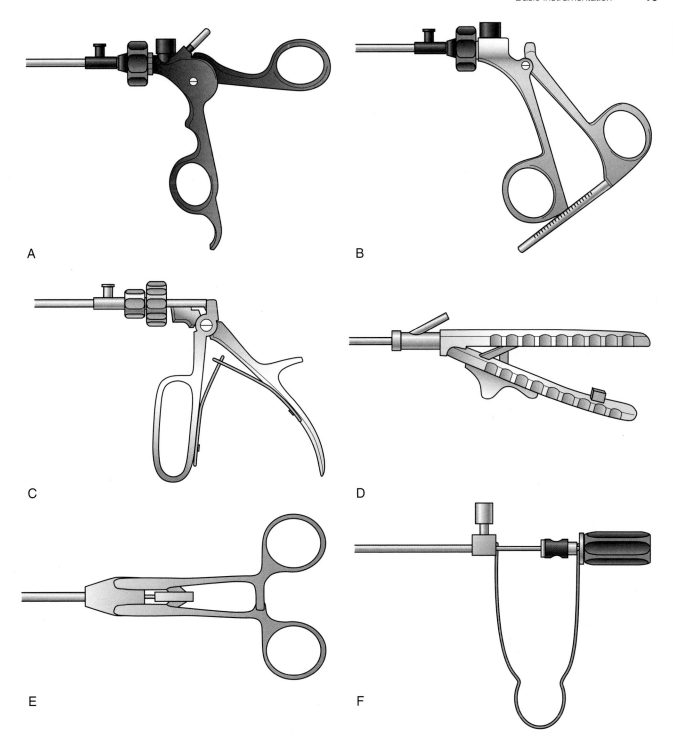

A

B

C

D

E

F

Figure 3-1. Common instrument handle configurations include **(A)** open ring, **(B)** ratchet, **(C)** pistol grip, **(D** and **E)** coaxial, and **(F)** bent wire handles.

(Fig. 3-8). Once the retractor is positioned, the assistant can either maintain the position or the instrument can be secured to an extracorporeal holding system (Fig. 3-9).

The fan retractor is a reusable instrument, available in 5- and 10-mm sizes. Once the instrument has been passed through a trocar, the blades of the fan are opened radially to provide a retraction surface. The PEER retractor is similarly reusable and available in 5- and 10-mm sizes. The PEER retractor opens into an H shape. The Diamond-Flex retractor

is a reusable 5-mm device. Once passed through a trocar, the tip flexes into a triangle shape, which provides a retraction surface. There are also multiple disposable paddle retractors, all of which provide a padded or soft surface for atraumatic retraction.

Alternatively, a locking grasper (such as an Allis clamp) passed through an appropriately positioned 5-mm port can be used to safely retract the liver or spleen by maintaining a locking grasp on the contralateral body wall or diaphragm (Fig. 3-10).

In certain situations, retraction can be achieved with a suture passed through the abdominal wall on a straight needle. To accomplish this, the surgeon passes a suture on a straight needle through the abdominal wall under direct vision. The suture is then passed around the structure to be retracted (such as the ureter) and then the needle is passed back through the abdominal wall. The needle is then cut off and the suture is tensioned by clamping the suture at the skin level (Fig. 3-11). Alternatively, a suture can be passed into the field through one of the trocars and grasped by a Carter-Thomason Needle Point Suture Passer (Cooper Surgical, Trumbull, Conn.) that is passed through the

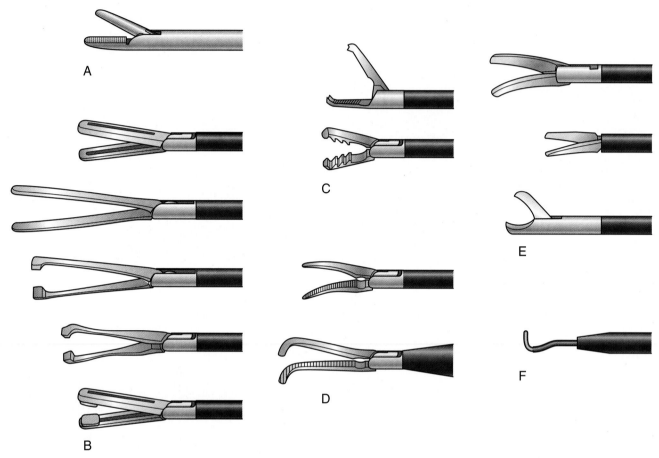

Figure 3-2. Common instrument tip configurations include **(A)** needle driver, **(B** and **C)** grasper (atraumatic and traumatic), **(D)** dissector, **(E)** scissor, and **(F)** cautery hook tips.

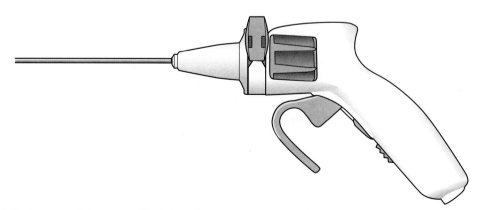

Figure 3-3. Articulating laparoscopic instrument (Cambridge Endo, Framingham, Mass.). Articulating laparoscopic instruments provide an additional axis of motion.

skin. Once the suture is outside the body, it can be secured with a clamp, taking care to protect the skin beneath the clamp.

ENERGY INSTRUMENTS

Many laparoscopic instruments allow delivery of energy for the purposes of tissue cutting and coagulation. Energy can be delivered to tissue by electrical current or ultrasonic vibrations. Before talking about specific instruments, it is helpful to understand each form of energy.

Monopolar Electrocurrent

Monopolar electrocurrent passes through tissue via the use of two electrodes at distant sites. Energy is dispersed from the active smaller electrode on the instrument to a larger return electrode, typically a grounding pad placed externally on the patient's skin. Given the much smaller size of the active electrode, current density is much higher versus the return

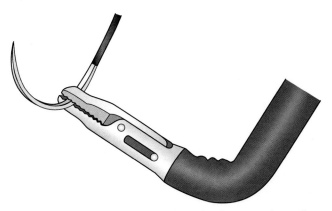

Figure 3-4. Ideal position of needle loaded on laparoscopic needle drive. The needle is positioned at the tip of the needle driver, grasped approximately one third of the distance from the swage with the tip of the needle canted away from the instrument.

electrode. This allows focal cutting and coagulation at the active electrode with no trauma at the return electrode. Common monopolar instruments include the shears and scissors and the hook.

There are several safety concerns with monopolar energy. Because the energy current passes through the shaft of the instrument, the shaft must be insulated. Any breaks or cracks in this insulation can result in conduction at the location of the defect, resulting in potential injury to bowel or blood vessels that may be in contact. Reusable instruments have an expected lifespan, and even new instruments should be thoroughly inspected for evidence of insulation defects. Direct coupling is another potential complication of monopolar energy. When the active electrode of a monopolar instrument comes in direct contact with a metal instrument or object, such as the laparoscope, a grasper, or a ligating clip, an electric arc allows for conduction of energy through this instrument or object. This can result in conduction to tissues that are outside the field of vision, and the possibility of unnoted injuries to critical structures. A less well-known but equally critical electrosurgical safety concern with monopolar cautery is capacitive coupling. Capacitive coupling is the induction of stray current to surrounding cannulas or instruments through the intact insulation of an active electrode. The concept of capacitive coupling is complex and beyond the scope of this text, but readers should know it is more likely to occur with monopolar cautery, with placement of a metal port inside of a plastic port (hybrid port), and with coagulation or high-voltage modes of energy delivery. All-metal or all-plastic ports will help avoid this phenomenon (Fig. 3-12). Finally, caution may be needed when monopolar cautery is used in patients with implantable electronic devices (e.g., a pacemaker or neurostimulator). Precautions to take in this setting include the preferential use of bipolar energy, or use of monopolar energy in short bursts at lower energy.

Bipolar Electrocurrent

Bipolar diathermy uses an active electrode and a return electrode in a single electrosurgical instrument with two small poles. Alternating current passes through target tissue that

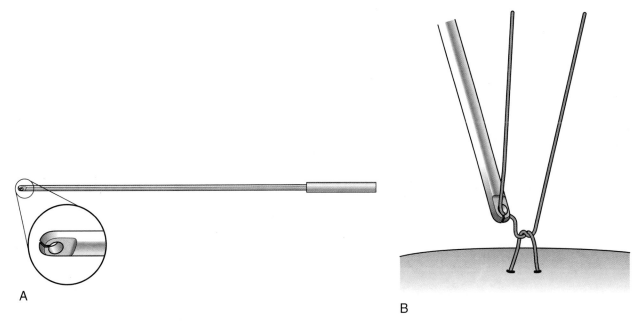

A

B

Figure 3-5. The laparoscopic knot pusher **(A)** facilitates laparoscopic knot tying **(B)** by allowing the throws to be made extracorporeally.

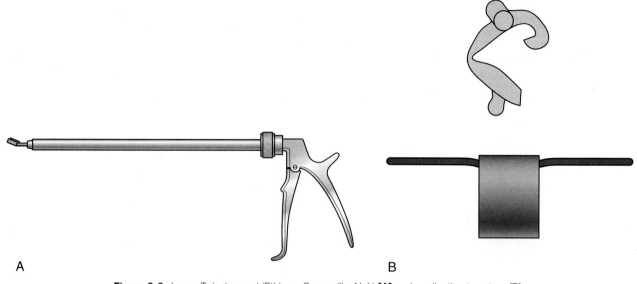

Figure 3-6. Lapra-Ty instrument (Ethicon, Somerville, N.J.) **[A]** and application to suture **(B)**.

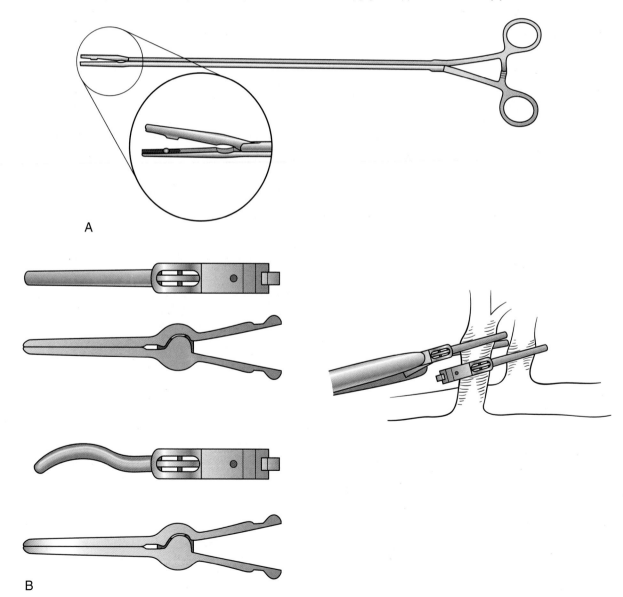

Figure 3-7. A, Bulldog clamp. **B,** Laparoscopic clamping performed with a bulldog clamp.

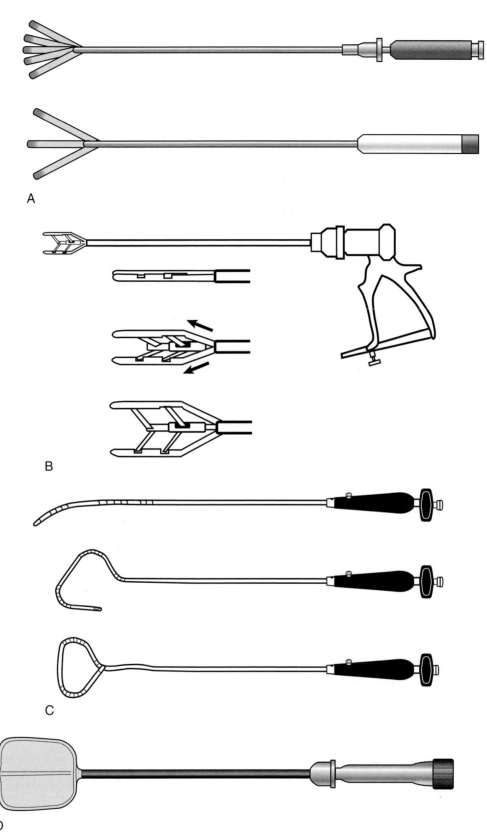

Figure 3-8. Retractor systems. **A,** The fan retractor houses several arrays that can be passed through a standard trocar and then opened to provide a wide surface for retraction. **B,** The PEER retractor (Jarit Surgical Instruments, Hawthorne, N.Y.) can be placed through a standard trocar and opened to provide retraction of organs, including the kidney, liver, spleen, and bowel, in a variety of situations. **C,** The Diamond-Flex Triangle retractor (Genzyme Surgical Products, Tucker, Ga.) is a 5-mm device that can be placed through a standard trocar. Once inside the abdomen, the handle can be tightened, pulling the tip into an angled, triangle shape with a large surface area for retraction. **D,** Endo Paddle retractor (Covidien, Dublin, Ireland).

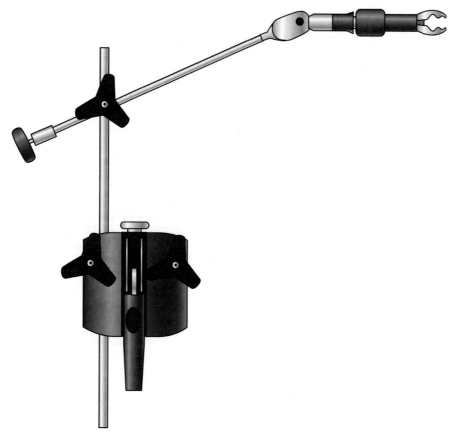

Figure 3-9. Extracorporeal retractor holding system attaches to the bedside to stabilize the Diamond-Flex retractor (Genzyme Surgical Products, Tucker, Ga.).

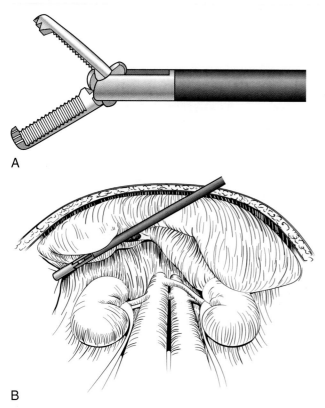

Figure 3-10. A locking Allis clamp **(A)** can be used to safely retract the liver or spleen by maintaining a locking grasp on the contralateral body wall or diaphragm **(B)**.

lies between these two poles. Because the two poles are close together, lower voltages are needed to achieve the same tissue effect compared with monopolar energy. The lower voltage results in less potential damage to surrounding structures and less chance of capacitive coupling. Several manufacturers produce bipolar forceps.

Ultrasonic Energy

Ultrasonic energy creates ultrasonic vibrations to generate heat that is then focally applied to cauterize or cut tissue. This energy is applied in combination with physical pressure from an instrument to seal vessels. The seal created allows a blood vessel stump to withstand supraphysiologic pressures without bursting. Ultrasonic energy instruments are typically disposable.

Vessel Sealing Devices

There currently exist several ultrasonic and bipolar electrosurgical instruments that seal blood vessels by using tissue-sensing technology (Fig. 3-13). There are several important factors when considering use of these devices. One should choose a device that permits sealing and ligation for the majority of the steps of a given case. Each of these instruments allows vessel ligation at slightly different speeds, although the slight differences are unlikely to affect operative case time. Also, these devices result in varying amounts of smoke production and thermal spread to adjacent tissues. Finally, the ergonomics and ease of operation for each instrument vary and may affect surgeon preference. With any such instrument, the operator should be aware that vessels are less likely to seal when under

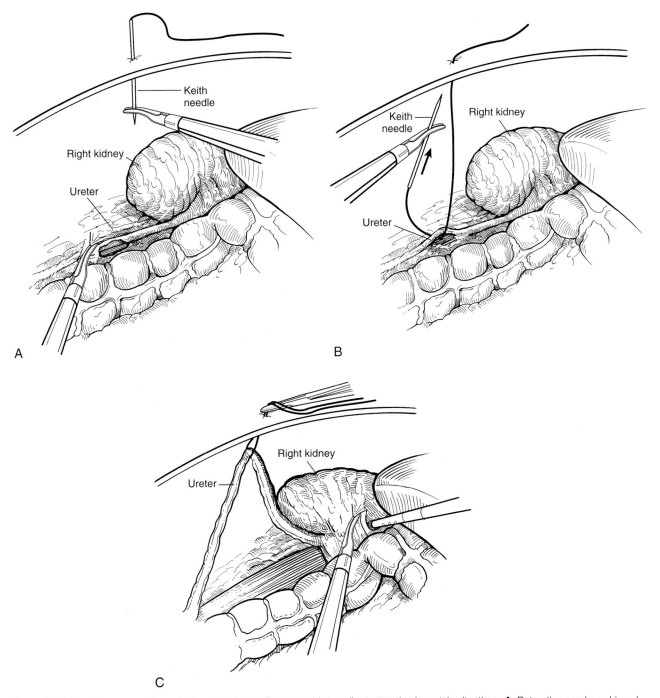

Figure 3-11. A suture passed through the abdominal wall can provide excellent retraction in certain situations. **A,** Retraction can be achieved without the insertion of an additional trocar site. When temporary retraction is needed, a straight needle with suture can be passed through the abdominal wall under direct vision. **B,** The needle is passed through or under the structure to be retracted. **C,** The needle is passed back through the abdominal wall, and the two strands are secured with a hemostat.

high tension, and that instruments may stick to sealed tissues after cutting. Accordingly, opening the jaws quickly or making other abrupt movements can lead to unnecessary tearing or bleeding. Select devices are discussed in the following sections.

Argon Beam Coagulator

Argon beam coagulators use the properties of electrosurgery and a stream of argon gas to improve the effectiveness of

the electrosurgical current. Argon gas is noncombustible and inert, making it a safe gas to use in the presence of electrosurgical current. The argon gas is ionized by the electrical current, making it more conductive than air. The highly conductive stream of argon gas provides an efficient pathway for delivering the current to tissue, resulting in hemostasis. Direct tissue contact is not required. Both ConMed (Utica, N.Y.) and Valleylab (Boulder, Colo.) make 28-cm long, monopolar instruments that fit 5-mm and 10-mm

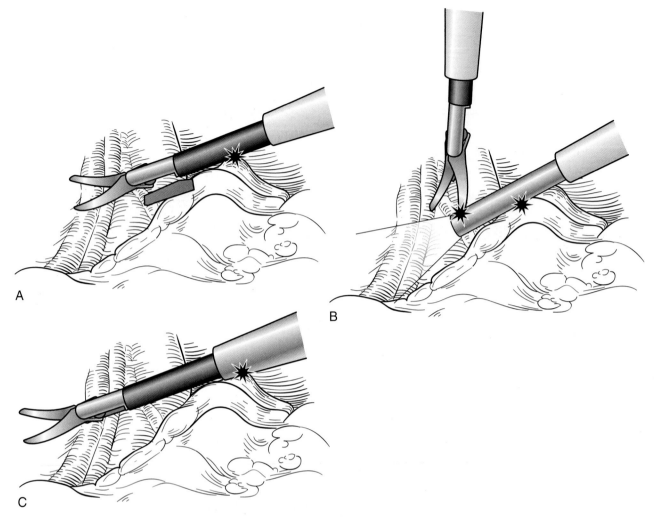

Figure 3-12. Risks with monopolar energy. **A,** Insulation defect. **B,** Direct coupling. The active electrode of a monopolar instrument comes in direct contact with a metal instrument or object, such as the laparoscope. **C,** Capacitive coupling. The induction of stray current to surrounding cannulas or instruments through the intact insulation of an active electrode. This effect results from current traveling through a cylinder and causing a charge to build until it discharges.

cannulas. Options for the tip include a needle electrode, a straight blade electrode, and a flat L electrode. An argon handset is required along with a supply of argon gas. Because the laparoscopic argon beam coagulator does not have an evacuation system, the pressure inside the abdomen can rise quickly above the desired level. Consequently, an insufflation port should be opened during coagulation (see Fig. 3-13, *A*).

Caiman (Aesculap, Tuttlingen, Germany)

Caiman electrosurgical instruments deliver radiofrequency (RF) energy to tissue within their jaws. Caiman claims its sealing instruments have the longest jaw of any RF device available. Also, the jaw is unique in that the tip of the instrument closes first to prevent tissue slippage. Five-millimeter and 12-mm sizes are available with several working lengths, and the 12-mm device also features an articulating jaw. The required Lektrafuse RF Generator provides power modulation in response to real-time tissue changes (see Fig. 3-13, *B*).

EnSeal (Ethicon, Somerville, NJ)

The EnSeal tissue sealing system uses bipolar energy delivered to tissue that is within the instrument's plastic jaws. The instrument can seal vessels of 1 to 7 mm. EnSeal claims to offer improved efficacy by using nanopolar thermostats embedded within the jaws of the device to monitor temperature and control the energy that is delivered to the tissue within its jaws. EnSeal now makes articulating tissue sealers that are compatible with 5-mm ports. The articulation facilitates a perpendicular approach to vessels in tight spaces, such as the retroperitoneum. The bottom jaw of the articulating instrument can also be used for spot coagulation (see Fig. 3-13, *C*).

Harmonic Scalpel (Ethicon, Somerville, N.J.)

The Harmonic Shears energy source is a high-frequency ultrasonic transducer that relies on a titanium blade vibrating at 55,000 cycles per second to break down protein in tissues and create a coagulum. The power setting is variable and

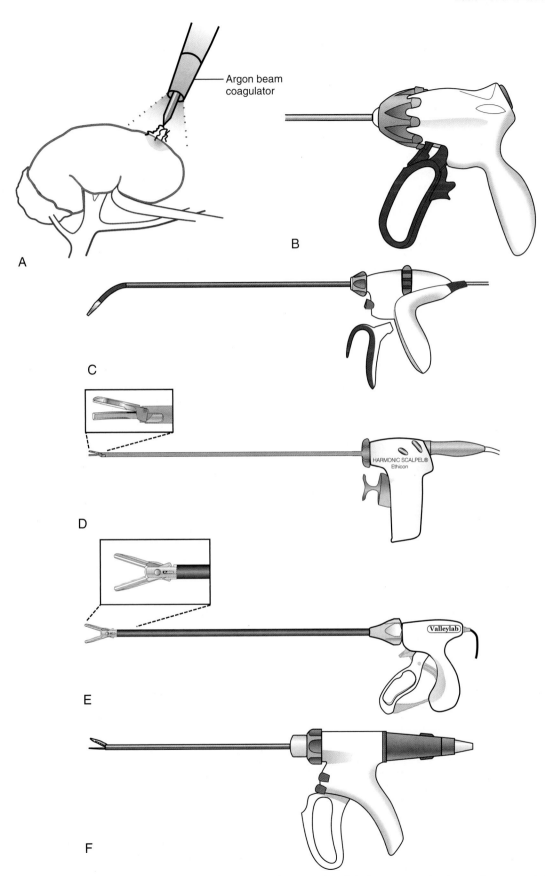

Figure 3-13. Vessel sealing devices. **A,** Argon beam coagulation uses the properties of electrosurgery and a stream of argon gas to improve the effectiveness of the current. The argon gas is ionized by the electrical current, making it more conductive than air. **B,** Caiman radiofrequency sealing device (Aesculap, Tuttlingen, Germany). **C,** EnSeal sealing device (Ethicon, Somerville, N.J.). **D,** Harmonic Scalpel (Ethicon, Somerville, N.J.). **E,** LigaSure device (Valleylab, Boulder, Colo.). **F,** Thunderbeat device (Olympus, Center Valley, Pa.). The tip delivers ultrasonic and bipolar energy and gives the options of seal and cut or seal only.

determines the vessel and tissue sealing time, along with the amount of tension the tissue is under and the pressure exerted on the tissue by the jaws. The newest version of this instrument is indicated for sealing vessels up to 7 mm. It performs at relatively lower temperatures compared with other electrosurgical instruments. The active blade is available in straight, curved, or hook shapes and can be used as a knife (see Figure 13, *D*).

LigaSure (Valleylab, Boulder, Colo.)

The LigaSure bipolar device delivers high current at a low voltage along with pressure from the jaws of the device to tissue. LigaSure is available in 5- and 10-mm sizes and is able to seal vessels up to 7 mm in diameter. Several configurations with different instrument tips are available in 37-cm and 44-cm shaft lengths. The system monitors the energy expended while denaturing the collagen and elastin within the vessel walls. A computer algorithm adjusts the current and voltage based on real-time measures of tissue impedance, resulting in delivery of a constant wattage over a broad range of tissue types. The average seal time is 2 to 4 seconds. The device enables cutting independent of sealing if desired. A monopolar version of this device is also available (see Fig. 3-13, *E*).

Thunderbeat (Olympus, Center Valley, Pa.)

A relatively new instrument, the Thunderbeat provides simultaneous delivery of bipolar and ultrasonic energies with the intent of increased efficiency. Bipolar electrodes are placed on both jaws, with one jaw being driven by ultrasonic energy in addition. The bipolar setting can be used independently for coagulation without cutting. Lengths of 35 and 45 cm are available, and all handpieces are 5-mm size (see Fig. 3-13, *F*).

SUCTION-IRRIGATION DEVICES

There are several suction-irrigation systems available, including the AHTO (Stryker, Kalamazoo, Mich.), StrykeFlow 2 (Stryker), Endopath PrOBE Plus II (Ethicon), and Epix suction-irrigation system (Applied Medical, Rancho Santa Margarita, Calif.). The Nezhat-Dorsey suction-irrigation tip is a reusable configuration.

All systems use a pump attached to a bag of irrigation fluid. There are two buttons on the handpiece: one activates the irrigation pump, and the other serves as a valve for suction. The suction can be connected to either wall suction or an independent suction unit.

In addition to clearing the operative field, the suction-irrigator can be effective for blunt dissection (Fig. 3-14). With the use of a second instrument to apply tension, the tip of the suction-irrigator can be applied with intermittent suction to help develop tissue planes bluntly.

The suction-irrigator tip can become clogged with coagulated blood, fat, or other tissues; however, irrigation will often clear the obstruction. One should ensure that the suction tip is clear before approaching critical portions of a case in which visualization by rapid fluid evacuation is necessary.

HYDRODISSECTOR

Waterjet hydrodissection is not commonly used but is described in some cases and continues to be actively

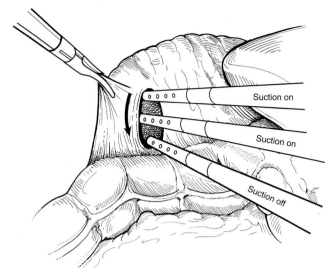

Figure 3-14. Use of a suction-irrigator as a dissecting instrument. The suction-irrigator can be effectively used for dissection when countertraction and intermittent suction are applied.

investigated. Commonly used in other disciplines, such as ophthalmology, the hydrodissector (Euromed, Schermwin, Germany) uses a thin stream of water under great pressure (30 atm) to act as a sharp instrument. In urology, the system has been described for use in partial nephrectomy as well as lymph node dissection.

EXTRACTORS

Endo Catch (Covidien, Dublin Ireland), Endo Pouch (Ethicon, Somerville, N.J.), Inzii (Applied Medical, Rancho Santa Margarita, Calif.), and LapSac (available with or without introducer) (Cook Medical, Bloomington, Ind.) are specimen retrieval devices designed for use in laparoscopy. The device serves to contain any specimen that is to be extirpated while minimizing the risk of spillage. The device is inserted through an appropriately sized trocar. The ring and bag are deployed by depressing the plunger. The specimen is placed into the bag with a grasper. Once the specimen is inside the bag, the bag is sealed and the deployment device is removed. The specimen bag is sealed by tightening a suture. The opposite end of the suture is clamped outside the body to facilitate easy retrieval once the abdomen is desufflated. At the end of the procedure, once the abdomen is desufflated, the specimen retrieval bag is removed from the body by extending one of the port incisions to accommodate the size of the specimen in the bag (Fig. 3-15). Of note, the specimen does not necessarily need to be retrieved through the same port through which it was deployed; the suture securing the bag can be delivered through an alternative port if that location is more desirable for the extraction incision. It is possible to place multiple retrieval devices through a single port if there are multiple specimens. Use of the port is permitted while a retrieval pouch is in situ, but caution should be used when inserting instruments and needles to ensure that damage to the pouch does not occur.

As noted in Table 3-1 the specimen retrieval devices are available in 5- to 15-mm port sizes, with larger devices able to accommodate larger volumes (180 to 1600 mL).

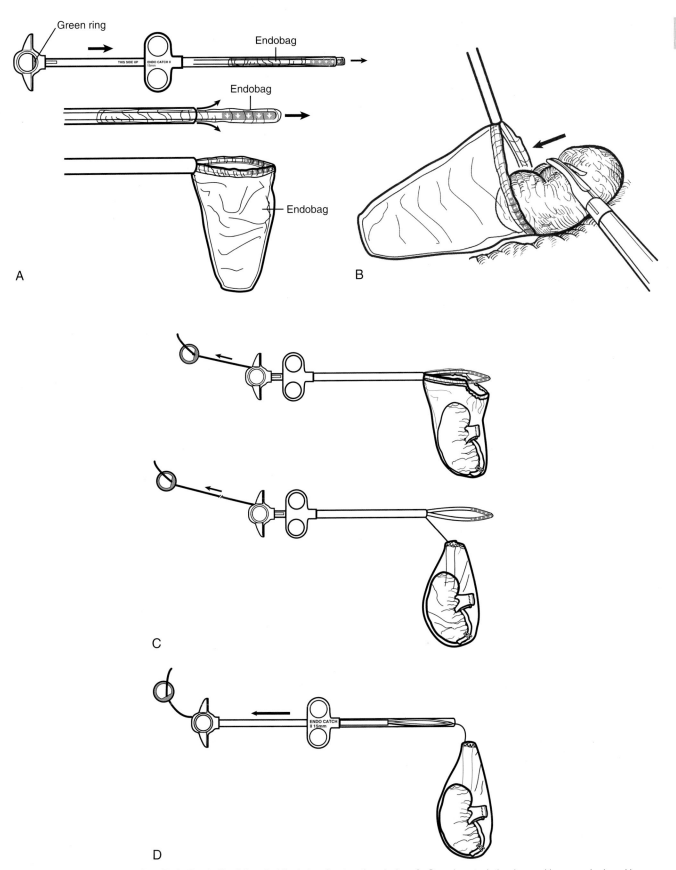

Figure 3-15. Deployment of an Endo Catch (Covidien, Dublin, Ireland) extraction device. **A,** Once inserted, the ring and bag are deployed by depressing the plunger. **B,** The specimen is placed into the bag with a grasper. **C,** Once the specimen is inside the bag, the bag is sealed and the deployment device is removed. **D,** The bag is later extracted through an extension of a port incision. Morcellation may be done within the bag to reduce the size of the skin incision.

TABLE 3-1 Extractor Specifications

Instrument	Manufacturer	Port Size	Bag Volume
Inzii Retrieval System	Applied Medical	5-12 mm	180-1600 mL
Endo Catch	Covidien	10-15 mm	220-1000 mL
Endo Pouch	Ethicon	10 mm	224 mL
LapSac	Cook	+/− 11-mm introducer	50-1500 mL

INTRACORPOREAL ULTRASOUND

Intraoperative intracorporeal ultrasound can be helpful during laparoscopic retroperitoneal procedures such as partial nephrectomy. Important features include color Doppler and an articulating head, as well as the ability to feed images into the operating room audiovisual system.

4 Stapling and Reconstruction

Stephen Y. Nakada, Necole M. Streeper

With the introduction of the laparoscopic nephrectomy in 1991 by Clayman and colleagues, advancements in minimally invasive surgical equipment have expanded the application of laparoscopic techniques to several urologic reconstructive-type procedures.[1] Laparoscopic stapling and clipping devices have been developed to provide more efficient alternatives to hand suturing to achieve hemostasis, tissue dissection, and tissue approximation. In spite of the availability of these devices and robotic platforms, it is also important for laparoscopic surgeons to develop intracorporeal suturing and knot tying skills in cases of device malfunction or unavailability. This chapter reviews the various clips, staplers, adjunct hemostatic agents, and suturing techniques required to perform non–robotic-assisted reconstructive laparoscopic urologic procedures.

CLIPS
Equipment

Occlusive clips are ideal for smaller vessels and provide a rapid, effective alternative for hemostasis. These clips are typically made of titanium and vary in size from 5 to 12 mm. Absorbable clips are available as well, and studies show no difference in adhesion formation between metallic and absorbable clips.[2]

An occlusive clip starts out in a V shape, and as it is applied, the tips close first from distal to proximal (Fig. 4-1). This ensures that the entire structure to be ligated is contained within the clip. Hem-o-lok, nonabsorbable polymer, ligating clips (Weck Closure Systems, Research Triangle Park, N.C.) are also available in four sizes (M, ML, L, XL), using 5- or 10-mm trocars (Fig. 4-2). These clips perform the same function as sutures by penetrating and locking through multiple layers of tissue. The engaging clip latching mechanism allows the surgeon to feel the clip lock close. Hem-o-lok clips are contraindicated in the control of the renal artery during donor nephrectomies owing to the risk of clip dislodgement.[3]

Occlusive clip appliers can be classified into the following categories: multiple or single load, and disposable or multiple use. Disposable clip appliers typically cost more than single-load reusable models, but the multiple-load feature makes their use much more efficient than withdrawing the instrument for each new clip to be placed. The majority of laparoscopic clip appliers used today are of the single-use and multiple-load variety, carrying 15 to 30 clips per unit (Table 4-1).

The diameter of the shaft generally depends on the size of the clips. In general, shafts of 5 mm are available for small clips, 10 mm for medium to large clips, and 12 mm for large clips. The Ligamax (Ethicon Endo-Surgery, Cincinnati, Ohio)

is a 5-mm shaft, single-use clip applier that is able to apply medium to large titanium clips. This is possible because its hinged jaws are retracted within the shaft until the handles are squeezed, and then the jaws advance and expand with a clip automatically loaded.

Present on all appliers are 360-degree rotating shafts that allow the tips to be placed around the target tissue at an ideal angle. Automatic loading clips are also available in many models, which immediately reload another clip into firing position. In addition, newer models may have a visual indicator showing the number of clips left.

Instrument Use

The vessel or other structure to be clipped should be dissected until the entire structure can be contained within the clip, without a significant amount of overlying tissue, to ensure maximum closure of the clip on the vessel. It is important to make sure the dissected window is large enough to accommodate the placement of several clips, with room to divide the structure with endoscopic scissors. Clips are typically used for small to medium-sized vessels, with one or two clips on either side before the vessel is divided.

Once the clip applier's jaws are completely around the structure, the handle is firmly squeezed until the clip is placed (Fig. 4-3). Then the clip applier is withdrawn at the same angle used for the approach to avoid accidentally displacing the clip. Additional clips are placed as necessary, and then the tissue is divided. A right-angle clip applier may be necessary to achieve the appropriate angle and may necessitate the use of a 10-mm trocar.

LINEAR STAPLERS
Equipment

Laparoscopic linear staplers are essential tools for the rapid division of tissue and vessels. The device deploys multiple,

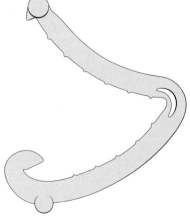

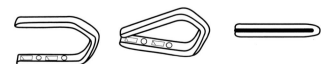

Figure 4-1. Standard laparoscopic clip closes from distal to proximal, with tips touching first.

Figure 4-2. Hem-o-lok (Weck Closure Systems, Research Triangle Park, N.C.) nonabsorbable polymer ligating clip.

TABLE 4-1 Disposable, Multiple-Load Single-Use Laparoscopic Clip Appliers

	Ligamax 5	10-mm Ligaclip	12-mm Ligaclip	Endo Clip	Endo Clip II	Endo Clip III	Acuclip Right-Angle
Manufacturer	Ethicon Endo-Surgery	Ethicon Endo-Surgery	Ethicon Endo-Surgery	Covidien	Covidien	Covidien	Covidien
Trocar size (mm)	5	10	12	5, 10	10	5	10
Number of clips	15	20	20	12-20	20	16	20
Sizes of clip	Medium/large	Medium/large	Large	Medium, Medium/large, Large	Medium/large	Medium/large	Medium/large
Clip loading	Automatic	Automatic	Automatic	Separate lever	Automatic	Automatic	Automatic

Ethicon Endo-Surgery, Cincinnati, Ohio; Covidien, Minneapolis, Minn.

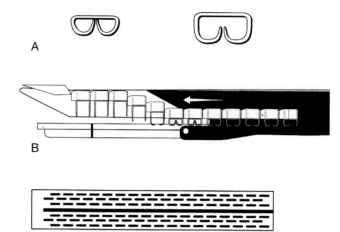

Figure 4-3. Clip ligation of a vessel. **A,** The jaws are closed until the tips meet, and then closed. **B,** Move proximally and repeat clip application to occlude the vessel.

Figure 4-4. Linear staplers. **A,** Vascular staple forms a tighter B shape than a regular or thick staple. **B,** Linear stapler jaws, side view. On firing of the stapler, staples are forced downward against the anvil and conform to their characteristic shape. The staples continue past the cut line to ensure hemostasis. **C,** Standard load: Three parallel rows of staples on either side of the cut line.

closely spaced, parallel rows of titanium staples. Most models require manually squeezing the handle three or four times to complete deployment of the staples and activating the knife to divide the tissue. There are newer models that have a battery-powered automatic device that allows for easier deployment and greater stapler stabilization with one hand.

Linear staplers can be broadly classified into cutting and noncutting staplers. Cutting staplers deploy loads with six intercalated rows of staples. With deployment of the stapler, staples are forced out of the load, through the tissue, and against an opposing anvil, closing back on itself (Fig. 4-4). After the staples are fired, a knife follows and divides the tissue, leaving three rows of staples on each side. The staple line extends past the range of the cutting knife to avoid incising nonstapled tissue (Fig. 4-4). Noncutting staplers, which fire three or four parallel rows of staples, are useful for closing enterotomies and repairing bladder injuries.

Laparoscopic linear cutting staplers are available in varying lengths (30/35, 45, and 60 mm), with most models offering an articulating head, which gives a greater range of angles for application from a fixed trocar. All models offer a 360-degree rotating shaft, which is essential for proper placement of the stapler. The size of the stapler requires the use of a 12-mm or larger trocar. Staplers today allow the same instrument to fire 8 to 25 separate staple-reloads before disposal (Table 4-2). The ETS-Flex stapler (Ethicon, Cincinnati, OH) is illustrated in Figure 4-5.

Staples come in different "loads"—mesentery/thin, vascular/thin, regular, regular/thick, thick, and very thick, with varying staple height from 2 to 4.4 mm—and are color-coded for easy recognition.

Instrument Use

It is important to dissect the structure to be stapled with a large enough window to accommodate the jaws of the stapler. Once this is done, introduce the stapler with its jaws closed through a 12-mm trocar under direct vision. Then rotate the shaft as needed, and use the articulating features to position the head of the stapler in correct alignment to the targeted structure.

Next, open the jaws of the stapler and pass the jaw holding the staple load through the window that has been developed. Advance the jaws of the stapler until the tips are beyond the far edge of the tissue, and close the jaws to the locked position. We use the 60-mm stapler and take the hilum en bloc during a nephrectomy rather than dissecting the vessels individually.[4] If no clips are used near the hilum, this is safe as long as the stapler closes. Make sure that you are able to visualize the tips of the stapler to ensure that only the targeted tissue is included within the locked jaws. If too much tissue is included, the jaws may not close properly, which will lead to incomplete deployment of the staples. There are safety switches built into each model that must be deployed before firing the staples.

After firing the staples, reopen the jaws before withdrawing the instrument from the staple site to immediately ensure that the staple line is intact. The stapler should be withdrawn under direct vision, and another load may be used if necessary. The proper use of the stapler is extremely important because malfunction can lead to devastating complications. Chan and colleagues reported a 1.8% stapler malfunction rate (10 of 565 cases) during laparoscopic nephrectomies performed over a 10-year period, with 7 of 10 malfunctions possibly attributed to misuse of the stapling device.[5]

TABLE 4-2 Linear Staplers

	Echelon Endopath	Endopath ETS-Flex Articulating	Echelon Flex Endopath	Echelon Flex Powered Endopath	Multifire Endo GIA 30	Multifire Endo TA 30	Endo GIA Universal	Endo GIA Ultra Universal
Manufacturer	Ethicon Endo-Surgery	Ethicon Endo-Surgery	Ethicon Endo-Surgery	Ethicon Endo-Surgery	Covidien	Covidien	Covidien	Covidien
Trocar size (mm)	12	12	12	12	12	12	12	12
Staple size(s)	Mesentery/thin, vascular/thin, regular, regular/thick, thick, very thick	Mesentery/thin, vascular/thin, regular, thick	Mesentery/thin, vascular/thin, regular, regular/thick, thick, very thick	Mesentery/thin, vascular/thin, regular, regular/thick, thick, very thick	2.0, 2.5, and 3.5 mm	2.5 and 3.5 mm	2.0, 2.5, 3.5, and 4.8 mm	2.0, 2.0-3.0, 3.0-4.0, and 4.0-5.0 mm
Staple length(s) (mm)	45 60	35 45	45 60	45 60	30	30	30, 45, and 60	30, 45, and 60
Articulating	No	Yes	Yes	Yes	No	No	Yes	Yes

Ethicon Endo-Surgery, Cincinnati, Ohio; Covidien, Minneapolis, Minnesota.

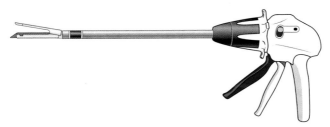

Figure 4-5. Endoscopic stapler (Ethicon, Cincinnati, Ohio).

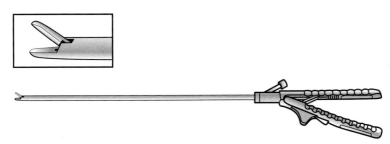

Figure 4-6. Standard laparoscopic needle holder (Ethicon, Cincinnati, Ohio).

LAPAROSCOPIC SUTURING

The introduction of occlusive clips and linear staples has greatly improved laparoscopic surgery. Despite these technologic advancements, it is important for the laparoscopic surgeon to learn simple interrupted and running suture closures.

Simple Stitch

To pass the needle, hold the suture with a needle driver near the swage of the needle. Larger curved needles may require passage through a 10-mm trocar instead of a 5-mm trocar. Sutures on 2-0 to 4-0 tapered needles are most commonly used with a cut length of approximately 8 cm for knot tying of an interrupted suture. Newer laparoscopic needle drivers mimic standard needle drivers (Fig. 4-6), and needles are similarly loaded.

On passing the needle, retract the tissue to provide countertension. The tip of the needle enters perpendicular to the tissue surface, and the needle should be passed through its arc to avoid damaging the targeted structure. When the needle tip emerges on the other side, it may be secured with graspers to prevent backslip of the tip into the tissue, or the needle may be advanced far enough that release of the needle driver allows for the tip to still be visualized. Once the needle driver has been released, the needle tip should be pulled through the rest of its arc.

Knot Tying

Laparoscopic knotting is broadly classified as extracorporeal or intracorporeal, with the latter being more commonly used. The square knot is commonly used and is demonstrated in Figure 4-7, A-D. Converting a square knot into a sliding knot is a useful skill for approximating tissues under tension (Fig. 4-7, E-H). After creating the slipknot, slide it into place on the tissue and convert it back to a square knot, throwing additional half-hitches to complete the knot.

Running Suture

The running suture line may be started with a simple stich or with a device such as the Lapra-Ty absorbable suture clip applier (Ethicon, Cincinnati, Ohio) (Fig. 4-8) or Hem-o-lok clip.[6,7] The Lapra-Ty device is nondisposable, uses a 10-mm port, and comes with clips for use with 2-0 to 4-0 coated Vicryl suture. Once the first anchoring stitch is placed, a running suture may be thrown to close the wound.

The Lapra-Ty absorbable or Hem-o-lok clip appliers may be used to place clips on the end of the suture in lieu of tying a finishing knot. To use this instrument at the end of a running stitch, pull the free end of the suture taut with a grasper and place a clip on the suture just where it exits the tissue

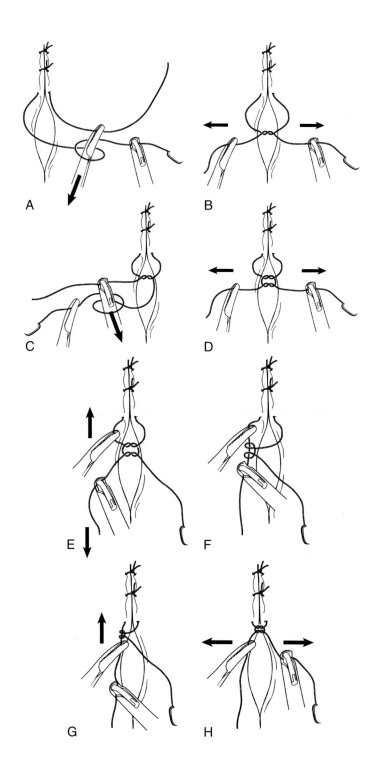

Figure 4-7. Intracorporeal square knot. **A** to **D,** Instrument tie formation of a square knot. **E** to **H,** Conversion of a square knot into a sliding knot.

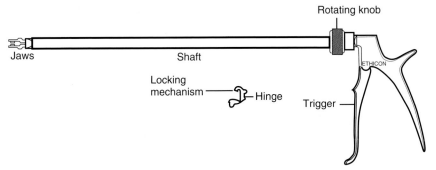

Figure 4-8. Lapra-Ty absorbable suture clip applier (Ethicon, Cincinnati, Ohio). The base unit is reusable and fits through a 10-mm port. The clip is hinged, as shown in the drawing, and locks when the handles are squeezed together.

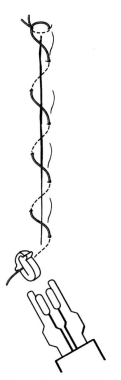

Figure 4-9. Lapra-Ty (Ethicon, Cincinnati, Ohio) used to finish a running suture, an alternative to tying a knot.

(Fig. 4-9). The alternative to clipping the suture is tying a knot at the end.

ADJUNCT HEMOSTATIC AGENTS
Fibrin Glue

Fibrin glue has been described as a hemostatic adjunct for laparoscopic reconstruction.[8-10] Brands include Tisseel (Baxter Healthcare, Deerfield, Ill.) and Evicel (Ethicon, Somerville, N.J.). Fibrin glue is made from the combination of fibrinogen and thrombin.

Thrombin Glue

The use of thrombin glue has been a useful adjunct agent to traditional reconstructive measures in maintaining hemostasis. FloSeal (Baxter Healthcare, Deerfield, Ill.), a hemostatic matrix, is a combination of collagen-derived particles and thrombin. It is applied to the bleeding tissue surface and the granules fill the wound, conforming to its shape. The high concentration of thrombin accelerates clot formation by converting fibrinogen into fibrin monomers, and the gelatin granules swell to produce a tamponade effect to provide hemostasis.[11] Surgiflo (Ethicon, Somerville, N.J.) is another commonly used gelatin matrix thrombin sealant that is mixed with sterile saline.[12]

Other Hemostatic Products

Surgicel (Ethicon, Somerville, N.J.) is a widely used absorbable hemostat derived from oxidized cellulose and comes in the form of a sheer weave material.[12] Surgifoam (Ethicon, Somerville, N.J.) is an absorbable gelatin sponge that is typically soaked in thrombin or saline before use as a hemostatic and conforms to irregular surfaces.

Figures 4-10 and 4-11 demonstrate how a combination of these products may be used for renal reconstruction during a laparoscopic partial nephrectomy. After simple running suture is placed to the base of the defect to control bleeding, FloSeal is applied to the defect through a 10-mm port (Fig. 4-10). Next, we introduce the suture to close the defect through a 10-mm port with a Hem-o-lok attached at one end. After throwing a stitch on one side of the renal capsule, we place a surgical bolster (typically made from Surgicel or Surgifoam) in the defect and secure it with a second throw of the suture. A second Hem-o-lok is applied after the suture is cinched up (Fig. 4-11). A Lapra-Ty clip may be placed on top of the Hem-o-lok to prevent slippage. This is repeated until the entire defect is closed.

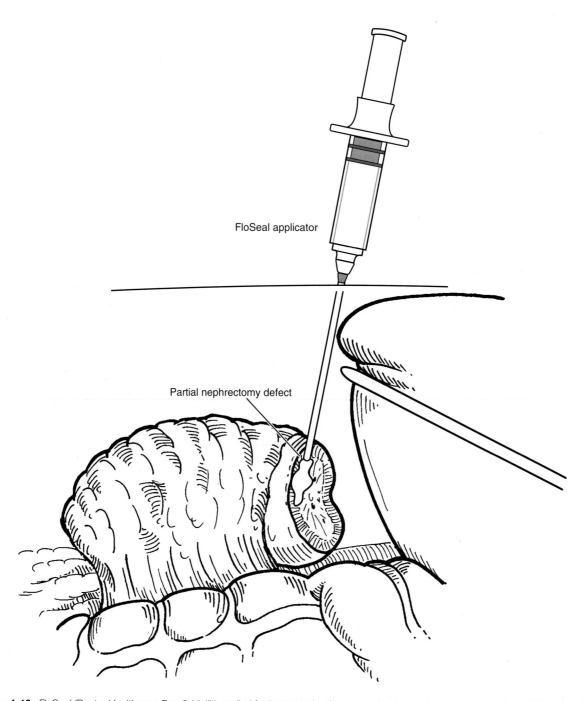

FloSeal applicator

Partial nephrectomy defect

Figure 4-10. FloSeal (Baxter Healthcare, Deerfield, Ill.) applied for hemostasis after removal of tumor during laparoscopic partial nephrectomy.

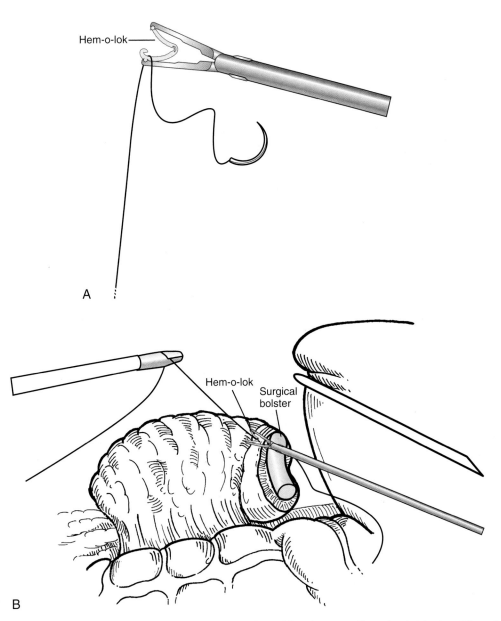

Figure 4-11. **A,** Laparoscopic suturing to close defect during laparoscopic partial nephrectomy. The suture is introduced through a 10-mm port with a Hem-o-lok clip on one end. After a stitch is thrown on one side of the renal capsule, a surgical bolster is placed in the defect and secured with a second throw of the suture. **B,** Hem-o-lok applier (Weck Closure Systems, Research Triangle Park, N.C.) places the second absorbable clip on the suture to tighten the suture and to secure the free end.

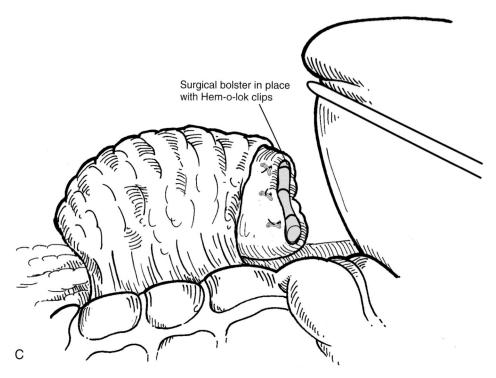

Surgical bolster in place
with Hem-o-lok clips

C

Figure 4-11, cont'd C, The tightened sutures secure the bolster in place, resulting in hemostasis at the cut surface of the kidney.

REFERENCES

1. Clayman RV, Kavoussi LR, Soper NJ, et al. Laparoscopic nephrectomy: initial case report. *J Urol.* 1991;146:278–282.
2. Ling FW, Stovall TG, Meyer NL, et al. Adhesion formation associated with the use of absorbable staples in comparison to other types of peritoneal injury. *Int J Gynecol Obstet.* 1989;20:362.
3. Friedman AL, Peters TG, Jones KW, et al. Fatal and nonfatal hemorrhagic complications of living kidney donation. *Ann Surg.* 2006;243:126–130.
4. Rapp DE, Orvieto MA, Gerber GS, et al. En bloc stapling of renal hilum during laparoscopic nephrectomy and nephroureterectomy. *Urology.* 2004;64(4):655–659.
5. Chan D, Bishoff JT, Ratner L, et al. Endovascular gastrointestinal stapler device malfunction during laparoscopic nephrectomy: early recognition and management. *J Urol.* 2000;164:319–321.
6. Orvieto MA, Lotan T, Lyon MB, et al. Assessment of the LapraTy clip for facilitating reconstructive laparoscopic surgery in a porcine model. *Urology.* 2007;69(3):582–585.
7. Shalhav AL, Orvieto MA, Chien GW, et al. Minimizing knot tying during reconstructive laparoscopic urology. *Urology.* 2006;68(3):508–513.
8. Eden CG, Coptcoat MJ. Assessment of alternative tissue approximation techniques for laparoscopy. *Br J Urol.* 1996;78:234–242.
9. Kram HB, Ocampo HP, Yamaguchi MP, et al. Fibrin glue in renal and ureteral trauma. *Urology.* 1989;33:215–218.
10. Jackson MR, Taher MM, Burge JR, et al. Hemostatic efficacy of a fibrin sealant dressing in an animal model of kidney injury. *J Trauma.* 1998;45:662–665.
11. Oz MC, Rondinone JF, Shargill NS. FloSeal Matrix: new generation topical hemostatic sealant. *J Card Surg.* 2003;18:486–493.
12. Galanakis I, Vasdev N, Soomro N. A review of current hemostatic agents and tissue sealants used in laparoscopic partial nephrectomy. *Rev Urol.* 2011;13:131–138.

5 | The da Vinci Surgical System

Michael H. Johnson, Mohamad E. Allaf

Integrating robotic technology into clinical medicine has been a sought-after goal for decades. This desire has manifested itself in a wide range of human-robot interfaces. On one end, fully automated surgical robots have been envisioned to perform techniques in the absence of human intervention. On the other, remote-controlled robotic technology offers a true master–slave relationship between human and robot. Although there have been many implementations of robotic-assisted surgical systems along this spectrum, the most successful and penetrant system has been the da Vinci Surgical System, which enables remotely controlled laparoscopic surgery.

PREDECESSORS OF THE DA VINCI SURGICAL SYSTEM

The first publicized use of robotics within surgery was ARTHROBOT in 1983. This instrument, used at the University of British Columbia in Vancouver, was developed by Dr. James McEwan and used by orthopedic surgeon Dr. Brian Day for arthroscopic procedures. In 1985, the PUMA 650, developed by Unimation, was used for computed tomography (CT)–guided stereotactic brain biopsies. PROBOT, developed in 1988 at Imperial College London, allowed for fully automated resection of prostatic tissue, after input from the urologic surgeon.

From these technologic developments arose the concept that remotely operated robots could be used to perform telesurgery. Backed by funding from the Defense Advanced Research Projects Agency (DARPA) and National Aeronautics and Space Administration (NASA), SRI International (founded as Stanford Research Institute) championed the initial efforts to develop surgical technologies that could be used in hazardous situations, such as the battlefield. Computer Motion, Inc. joined these research efforts and introduced the ZEUS system, a three-armed robot with AESOP (Automated Endoscopic System for Optimal Positioning), a voice-activated endoscopic arm (Figs. 5-1 and 5-2). The powerful capabilities

of this technology were demonstrated on September 7, 2001, when a 68-year-old woman in Strasbourg, France, underwent a successful cholecystectomy performed remotely in New York by Dr. Jacques Marescaux, later coined the "Lindbergh operation." Concurrently, Intuitive Surgical developed the da Vinci Surgical System, based on SRI research efforts, and obtained U.S. Food and Drug Administration (FDA) approval in 2000. Intuitive Surgical merged with Computer Motion, Inc. in 2003 to develop the earliest versions of the current da Vinci system.

EVOLUTION OF THE DA VINCI SYSTEM

Since its introduction into the surgical realm, the da Vinci system has undergone multiple iterations of improvement and optimization (Box 5-1; Figs. 5-3 to 5-7). Each system continues to have three general components: a surgeon's console, an endoscopic equipment and image processing tower, and the patient-side cart. The laparoscopic camera projects a three-dimensional image with up to 10× magnification to the surgeon's console and requires a specialized arm to control it. The additional robotic arms are capable of using a spectrum of laparoscopic tools, providing seven degrees of freedom for surgical tasks.

DA VINCI SAFETY MECHANISMS

The distance that the da Vinci Surgical System places between the patient and surgeon has justifiably produced safety concerns. As a result, multiple redundant safety checkpoints have been implemented. It is important to note that the da Vinci is a remote-controlled instrument without the ability to perform independent actions. Thus the safety checkpoints are centered on the correct interpretation and performance of surgeon-directed movements. Before any movement is requested from the robotic arms, checks are performed to ensure that the surgeon is positioned at the console. On the surgeon's console

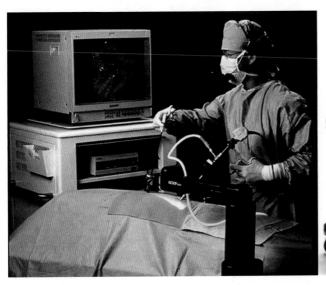
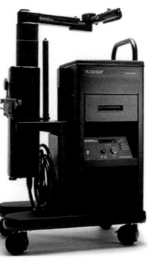

Figure 5-1. AESOP (Automated Endoscopic System for Optimal Positioning) system, a predecessor to the da Vinci Surgical System. *(From Regan JJ: Robotics and computers in minimally invasive spine surgery.* Spine Universe. *Montclair, NJ. http://bit.ly/1MFt8EX.)*

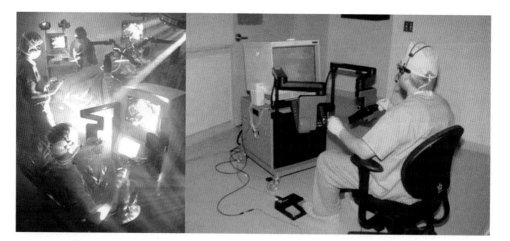

Figure 5-2. ZEUS robotic surgical system. (Right, *from Sung GT, Gill IS. Robotic laparoscopic surgery: a comparison of da Vinci and Zeus systems.* Urology. *2001; 58:893-898.* Left, *from https://spinoff.nasa.gov/spinoff2000/hm1.htm.*)

BOX 5-1   Iterations of the da Vinci System

da Vinci Standard Surgical System
- Introduced 1999
- FDA approval 2000
- Introduction of fourth arm 2003

da Vinci S system
- Introduced 2006
- Tile Pro multi-input display for integrated viewing of information
- Monitor built into patient-side cart
- Rapid instrument exchange

da Vinci Si system
- Introduced 2009
- Simplified user interface
- Dual console system
- Ergonomic upgrades
- High-definition camera
- Single-site instrumentation introduced 2011 (see Fig. 5-5)
- Firefly fluorescence imaging capabilities 2011 (see Fig. 5-6)
- EndoWrist One vessel sealer and stapler introduced 2012 (see Fig. 5-7)
- Surgical simulator

da Vinci Xi system (see Fig. 5-8)
- Introduced 2014
- Redesigned instrument architecture to allow for multiquadrant surgery and camera placement in any robotic arm
- Longer, thinner instrument arms to improve reach

FDA, U.S. Food and Drug Administration.

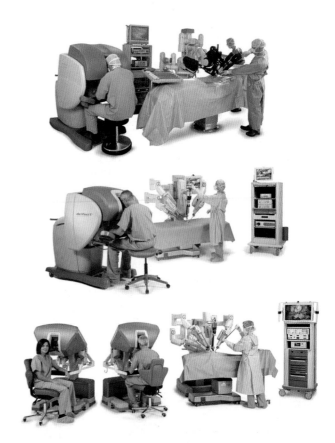

Figure 5-3. Evolution of da Vinci Surgical System: standard model (*top*, 1999), S (*middle*, 2006), and Si (*bottom*, 2009) systems. (*Copyright © Intuitive Surgical, Inc., Sunnyvale, CA.*)

screen, data are projected regarding the instruments being used, which arms are being controlled, and whether energy is being applied (Fig. 5-8).

The surgical arms of the patient-side cart have additional safety mechanisms. These include preventing manipulation of the robotic arms by the bedside operating room staff, unless an override button is pressed. On the other hand, when the arm is being controlled by the bedside operating room staff, the robotic arm is unable to be controlled by the surgeon at the console. For optimal functioning of EndoWrist instruments, each instrument has a predefined number of surgical cases for which it can be used, after which it requires replacement.

Should all else fail, there is a built-in feature to allow the machine to shut down to prevent undesired actions. Currently, the da Vinci system's software is not reprogrammable by users

and is not connected to the Internet in such a way that would allow for unwanted manipulation of the robotic technology.

ADOPTION OF DA VINCI SURGERY

Since its introduction, the da Vinci surgical system has expanded in both depth and breadth of use. Marketed for pelvic surgery, da Vinci was initially adopted by urologic and gynecologic surgeons. Since that time, the general surgery, colorectal, cardiac, thoracic, and otolaryngologic communities have also embraced the technology. This list is by no means

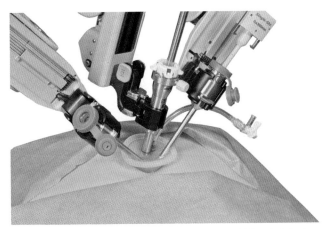

Figure 5-4. Single-site instrumentation for da Vinci Si Surgical System. *(Copyright © Intuitive Surgical, Inc., Sunnyvale, Calif.)*

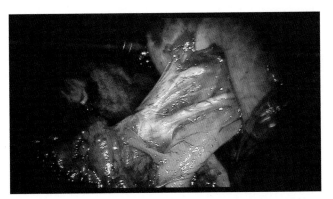

Figure 5-5. Firefly fluorescence for visualization of perfusion. In this case, the renal hilum is exposed with fluorescence detection within the renal arterial system. *(Copyright © Intuitive Surgical, Inc., Sunnyvale, Calif.)*

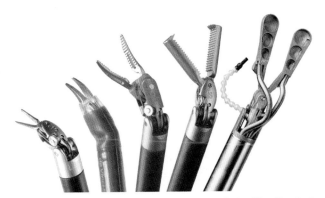

Figure 5-6. EndoWrist instruments. *(Copyright © Intuitive Surgical, Inc., Sunnyvale, Calif.)*

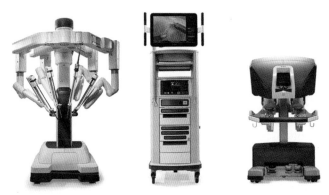

Figure 5-7. da Vinci Xi Surgical System (2014). *(Copyright © Intuitive Surgical, Inc., Sunnyvale, Calif.)*

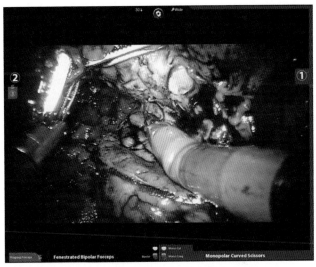

Figure 5-8. Robotic console view during partial nephrectomy. Instrument descriptions are displayed along the base of the screen, with blue highlighting when electrocautery is active. Camera information is displayed along the top of the screen. *(Courtesy Mohamad E. Allaf, Johns Hopkins Medical Institutions, Baltimore, Md.)*

exhaustive, with other surgical disciplines developing new uses for the surgical system.

Indeed, the adoption of robotic-assisted surgery by the urologic surgical community highlights the degree to which robotic surgery has been integrated into treatment strategies. Robotic-assisted laparoscopic radical prostatectomy (RP) was first introduced in 2001 for the treatment of prostate cancer. By 2003, 0.7% of radical prostatectomies were performed with da Vinci assistance. By 2010, this had increased to 42%.[1]

The da Vinci system's significant penetrance within pelvic surgery has extended into many other procedures, ranging from radical cystoprostatectomy with intracorporeal urinary diversions to inguinal lymphadenectomy for penile cancer to vasovasostomy for infertility.[2-4]

The reason for the rapid adoption and use of the da Vinci system has been multifactorial, with proponents emphasizing the system's improved dexterity and ease of use relative to traditional laparoscopic procedures. Some controversy does exist; critics have attributed adoption of this technology to aggressive marketing by the manufacturer as well as direct-to-consumer advertising.[5]

Within the realm of RP there remains some disagreement regarding the benefit of using the da Vinci system, but select studies have suggested clear advantages with respect to transfusion rates, length of hospital stay, overall complication rates, and even death. Two studies published in 2011 and 2013 compared results of minimally invasive robotic prostatectomy (MIRP) and open RP in large patient cohorts and confirmed these findings.[6,7] Studies are now emerging that reveal that the increased use of the da Vinci Surgical System in renal surgery has increased the rate of partial nephrectomy with a concomitant decrease in radical nephrectomy, suggesting that this technology has enabled surgeons to more successfully follow accepted guidelines by performing nephron-sparing surgery more often.[8]

DA VINCI SURGICAL SYSTEM IN RETROPERITONEAL SURGERY

Although the data regarding the comparative effectiveness of robotic-assisted prostatectomy remain mixed, the advantages of the da Vinci Surgical System are more clearly delineated within the realm of renal surgery. The first report of robotic-assisted laparoscopic nephrectomy was published in 2001.[9] Within 4 years, urologists had pushed the boundaries of this technology to perform nephron-sparing surgery.[10] Unlike robotic-assisted prostatectomy in which the reconstructive element of the case is distinct from the extirpative aspect, the robotic-assisted partial nephrectomy's critical steps—excision of the mass with subsequent renorrhaphy—are performed under the time-sensitive pressure of renal hilar clamping. Moreover, should the renorrhaphy be inadequate, severe bleeding may result and completion nephrectomy is more likely to be performed. Using multiple robotic arms, fluorescence imaging to delineate perfusion, and superior instrument articulation for performing the renorrhaphy, the da Vinci Surgical System has lowered the technical challenges associated with minimally invasive nephron-sparing surgery. As a result, more surgeons are able to perform these notoriously challenging procedures.

The familiarity with robotic-assisted renal surgery has also fostered more robotic retroperitoneal surgical techniques. Robotic-assisted laparoscopic adrenalectomy and pyeloplasty were initially reported in 2001.[11,12] The latter is now commonly used for ureteropelvic junction obstructions, with results comparable to those of open or laparoscopic surgery.[13] This surgical technique has also been adopted by the pediatric urology community, with robotic pyeloplasty being performed on 13.5% of pediatric patients as of 2010 and extending into the infant population (i.e., less than 10 kg).[14] For upper tract urothelial malignancy, robotic nephroureterectomy was first reported in 2006 and has emerged as a valuable tool, either for the nephrectomy, distal ureterectomy, lymphadenectomy, or for all aspects of the case. Finally, small case series data on robotic-assisted retroperitoneal lymphadenectomy for nonseminomatous germ cell cancer were reported in 2011; this use is gaining traction as surgeons become more comfortable with the technology and are able to provide comparable results to open or laparoscopic approaches.[15]

FUTURE OF THE DA VINCI SYSTEM

The proprietary nature of the da Vinci system may ultimately hinder research, development, and innovation. The developers of the system, however, are strongly positioned to develop exciting and helpful advances. Similar to the advent of laparoscopic surgery, the introduction of robotic-assisted technology represents a paradigm shift in the approach to surgery. The tight integration of robotic technology, computer technology, and surgeon expertise ensures that advancements in any of these fields will improve patient care. For example, improvements in optics, image processing software, and molecular imaging agents will help surgeons identify critical structures in real time. Increased emphasis on patient safety and surgical simulation will ensure that surgeons are maximally prepared for each case that they perform, and results will be objectively reviewed afterward. In addition, miniaturization of instruments and improvements in single-site techniques will allow for smaller or fewer incisions. Increasing research efforts into haptic feedback promise to augment all aspects of a surgeon's skill set.

CONCLUSION

In the 15 years since the da Vinci Surgical System received FDA approval, there have been remarkable advances and novel uses for robotic-assisted surgery. As a purely remotely controlled system, it has demonstrated the ability to improve surgical outcomes for the appropriately trained surgeon without the safety concerns inherent in automated devices. Its rapid adoption and penetration within retroperitoneal surgery are strong indicators that robotic-assisted surgical procedures will remain popular treatment choices for both patients and surgeons.

REFERENCES

1. Chang SL, Kibel AS, Brooks JD, Chung BI. The impact of robotic surgery on the surgical management of prostate cancer in the USA. *BJU Int.* 2015;115:929–936.
2. Pruthi RS, Nix J, McRackan D, et al. Robotic-assisted laparoscopic intracorporeal urinary diversion. *Eur Urol.* 2010;57:1013–1021.
3. De Naeyer G, Van Migem P, Schatteman P, Carpentier P, Fonteyne E, Mottrie A. Robotic assistance in urological microsurgery: initial report of a successful in-vivo robot-assisted vasovasostomy. *J Robot Surg.* 2007;1:161–162.
4. Dogra PN, Saini AK, Singh P. Robotic-assisted inguinal lymph node dissection: a preliminary report. *Indian J Urol.* 2011;27:424–427.
5. Alkhateeb S, Lawrentschuk N. Consumerism and its impact on robotic-assisted radical prostatectomy. *BJU Int.* 2011;108:1874–1878.
6. Liu JJ, Maxwell BG, Panousis P, Chung BI. Perioperative outcomes for laparoscopic and robotic compared with open prostatectomy using the national surgical quality improvement program (NSQIP) database. *Urology.* 2013;82:579–583.
7. Kowalczyk KJ, Levy JM, Caplan CF, et al. Temporal national trends of minimally invasive and retropubic radical prostatectomy outcomes from 2003 to 2007: results from the 100% Medicare sample. *Eur Urol.* 2012;61:803–809.
8. Patel HD, Mullins JK, Pierorazio PM, et al. Trends in renal surgery: robotic technology is associated with increased use of partial nephrectomy. *J Urol.* 2013;189:1229–1235.
9. Guillonneau B, Jayet C, Tewari A, Vallancien G. Robot assisted laparoscopic nephrectomy. *J Urol.* 2001;166:200–201.
10. Stifelman MD, Caruso RP, Nieder AM, Taneja SS. Robot-assisted laparoscopic partial nephrectomy. *JSLS.* 2005;9:83–86.
11. Horgan S, Vanuno D. Robots in laparoscopic surgery. *J Laparoendosc Adv Surg Tech A.* 2001;11:415–419.
12. Gettman MT, Peschel R, Neururer R, Bartsch G. A comparison of laparoscopic pyeloplasty performed with the da Vinci robotic system versus standard laparoscopic techniques: initial clinical results. *Eur Urol.* 2002;42:453–457. discussion 457–458.
13. Yanke BV, Lallas CD, Pagnani C, Bagley DH. Robot-assisted laparoscopic pyeloplasty: technical considerations and outcomes. *J Endourol.* 2008;22:1291–1296.
14. Monn MF, Bahler CD, Schneider EB, et al. Trends in robot-assisted laparoscopic pyeloplasty in pediatric patients. *Urology.* 2013;81:1336–1341.
15. Williams SB, Lau CS, Josephson DY. Initial series of robot-assisted laparoscopic retroperitoneal lymph node dissection for clinical stage I nonseminomatous germ cell testicular cancer. *Eur Urol.* 2011;60:1299–1302.

6 Considerations for the Assistant

Jeffery E. Piacitelli

Trends in health care predict increased use of assistants, or advanced practice providers (APPs), by physicians in the treatment and care of patients. For the urologist in the operating room, the use of these nonphysician providers to help with surgery can come with an increased unease because of liability from errors that cause harm to patients or staff. Although these concerns have not been supported by evidence at this time, suggestions are made about how to address this apprehension, and there are some recommendations on how to use the skills of the assistant while increasing safety in the operating room.

Indications for the present and near future of minimally invasive urologic surgery forecast that urologists will be increasingly likely to use assistants at the bedside in the operating room. The forces outside the operating room creating these conditions are the results of three trends for urologic health care in the United States. First, according to projections from the U.S. Census Bureau (www.census.gov/content/dam/Census/library/publications/2014/demo/p25-1140.pdf), over 55 million Americans will be older than age 65 years by 2020, and that number will increase annually to 80 million by 2050. Before 2030, those older than 65 years will constitute over 20% of the entire population and will continue to do so through at least 2050. As the population ages, urologic care will increasingly be required. Next, the Congressional Budget Office estimates that the expansion of health care under the Affordable Care Act (ACA) will increase the number of persons with insurance by an additional 32 million by 2017. Last, paralleling the aging population of the United States, data from the American Urological Association (AUA) predict that the number of urologists retiring from practice or decreasing the number of patients seen owing to semiretirement is projected to increase through 2025. Furthermore, owing to the 1997 Balanced Budget Act, the number of Accreditation Council for Graduate Medical Education (ACGME) urology residency slots remains fixed at 170; therefore the AUA reports that the number of graduates who achieve American Board of Medical Specialties (ABMS) certification will not be able to compensate for those retiring or for the increased demands for care placed on urologists. Measures to compensate for the coverage gap in urologic care will be manifold, including the decrease in prostate-specific antigen (PSA) screening, an increase in watchful waiting for prostate and kidney cancers, and increasing use of outside specialties such as primary care and interventional radiology for treatment of urologic conditions. Health professionals assisting the urologist in the operating room will vary in their roles and responsibilities and may include not only a urology resident or fellow but a physician assistant (PA) or advanced practice registered nurse (APRN). For the remainder of this chapter, both PAs and APRNs will be referred to as *advanced practice providers* (APPs).

In December 2014 the AUA released the Consensus Statement on Advanced Practice Providers (www.auanet.org/common/pdf/advocacy/advocacy-by-topic/AUA-Consensus-Statement-Advanced-Practice-Providers-Full.pdf), which outlines the professional organization's support for and guidelines for use of APPs. The remarks in the AUA statement are largely for the use of APPs by urologists in general; however, the application of practices and principles influencing their use should be extended into the operating room. The document states, "The official position of the AUA is that APPs work in a closely and formally defined alliance with a urologist that serves in a supervisory role. This physician-led, team-based approach provides the highest quality urologic care. As the physician-led, team-based approach evolves, so do the definitions of supervisory and collaborative models of care between physicians and APPs."

APPs are professionals with national certification and state licensing who usually fall into two groups. PAs are professionals who have become nationally certified and subsequently licensed by the state to practice under the supervision of a physician. An APRN is a nursing professional who, after completing a bachelor of science degree program, has some advanced training and becomes independently licensed by the state under the regulation of that state's board of nursing. Once national certification is obtained, an APP is allowed to assist the urologist in the operating room. The specific tasks that APPs are allowed to do are governed by state licensing and hospital operating room or surgical center bylaws. Surgeons and APPs are strongly encouraged to have a copy of applicable regulations and be familiar with them. The AUA Consensus Statement on APPs provides a well-written guide to the educational background, training, and certification required for each profession, in addition to links to related state-specific regulations.

The AUA Consensus Statement states, "The role of the APP in a urology practice is dependent on many factors, including academic versus private practice, large versus small group, APP experience, physician comfort level, and state laws. The supervisory/collaborative model in urology may be described as delegated autonomy. This autonomy process has a natural growth over time as the physician and the APP become accustomed to working together, which leads the team to provide the highest level of quality urological care." This is the case as well in the operating room with minimally invasive urologic surgery. Exercise of privileges will vary according to practice setting, regulation by agencies, and surgeon and APP dynamics. Although the questions of liability and coverage for urology residents and fellows are well defined, they are not as clearly defined for APPs.

The foremost concern when working with APPs is legal liability. The AUA frames the concern for urologists using an APP as follows: "The greatest risk for malpractice arises when practitioners engage in practice beyond their competency base either because of a lack of protocol, disregard for protocol, or inability to secure adequate collaboration or oversight. It is also important to remember that in any given environment, APPs are held to the same standards of practice as physicians; there are no separate guidelines for care outcomes that apply only for APPs." The Consensus Statement provides a discussion addressing whether use of an APP to give care resulted in any increase in legal liability and concluded that it did not, nor did it increase the costs of providing care or negatively affect the quality of care. However, as APPs are increasingly used, it can be expected that the rates of legal action will increase correspondingly. More important, the document makes general recommendations about how to reduce legal liability risks to the urologist, along with suggestions specific to the PA and APRN professions. Again, it is strongly recommended that this document be read and its suggestions followed. With regard to legal liability, APPs need to know explicitly what they are allowed to do and not allowed to do according to the surgeon and federal, state, local, and operating room requirements.

Understanding the federal, state, and hospital regulations that apply to assisting in the operating room is key to properly using the skills of an assistant. When operating room safety is truly the first priority, anxieties about legal liability, injury, and accidents and other concerns return to their proper proportions and places.

The safety of the patient and the team is the first priority. Culture drives behaviors, and behaviors determine outcomes. The operating room is a culture of safety, and as such it is locally owned and driven, with guidelines and recommendations in mind. I recognize that the goal of zero harm to patients or staff in the operating room is technically impossible while performing any surgery; however, it is the progress toward the perfection of zero harm that will help improve the culture, behavior, and outcomes. Safety for the patient often translates into safety for the rest of the surgical team in many areas, including improving communication among surgical team members, decreasing staff concerns over previously unidentified problems, and strengthening the operating room organizational culture. The surgeon should encourage the APP to spearhead the effort to maintain safety in the operating room. The desired outcome of delegating this to the APP is to allow the surgeon to concentrate his or her energies on taking care of the patient and functioning to the greatest degree as a team leader in the operating room. The assistant should become integrated into existing efforts of institutional "second-order" problem solving—identifying current problems and creating methods to avoid future harm. Some groups meet on a regular schedule to evaluate problems with the "Three Ws and How": (1) What happened? (2) Why did it happen? (3) What can be done to reduce the risk? and (4) How is it proved that the risk was reduced? Safety groups that examine questions such as these benefit from having a diversity of input from all groups of professionals and patients. An example of a scientific safety system that is becoming widely used and accepted is a Comprehensive Unit-based Safety Program (CUSP). It is likely that where you operate already has in place a safety program such as CUSP. A CUSP program in the operating room, as in other healthcare units, uses all stakeholders in safety, including patients, their families, and care administrators. The ideal behind use of a broad-based group is to include to the greatest degree possible those involved in care of the patient by drawing on the strengths of the varied perspectives. CUSP should do the following:

1. Educate on the scientific approach to safety.
2. Charge members with finding areas for improvement by asking questions that presume risk, such as "How will the next patient be harmed?"
3. Incorporate a senior administrative member who has the authority and ability to unite different units such as sterile processing, the preoperative unit, the postoperative unit, and the nursing floor.
4. Regularly review data to monitor safety problems, study and identify defects, and create safer systems for delivery of care. It is important that these recommendations come with a priority designation so that those with the greatest influence on safety and the most practicable can be implemented first.
5. Execute recommendations by using techniques and technologies for effective deployment of safety measures.

What a CUSP chooses to focus attention on depends on its members, and it may choose to incorporate outside safety guidelines—for example, those of The Joint Commission (TJC; formerly The Joint Commission on Accreditation of Healthcare Organizations [JCAHO]). Under its mission "to improve healthcare for the public," TJC established the National Patient Safety Goals (NPSGs) program in 2002 (https://www.jointcommission.org/the_joint_commission_mission_statement/). The NPSGs were established to help accredited organizations, such as hospitals and surgical centers, to address specific areas of concern with regard to patient safety. In the past, some goals have included areas of focus specifically affecting safety in the operating room. Examples of these include targeting the spread of infection secondary to multidrug-resistant organisms (MDROs), catheter-related bloodstream infections (CRBSIs), and surgical site infections (SSIs). TJC's new regulations for CRBSI and SSI prevention apply not only to hospitals, but also to ambulatory care and ambulatory surgery centers, and affect accreditation of those sites surveyed. The NPSGs now also include patient engagement efforts as well. Recommendations are based on feedback received by TJC and are updated on a routine basis in an effort to constantly improve safety. All current NPSG recommendations have direct bearing on minimally invasive urologic surgery. The NPSGs for 2015 are available at www.jointcommission.org/assets/1/6/2015_HAP_NPSG_ER.pdf.

One of the most important safety measures that can improve every laparoscopic and robotic-assisted surgical case is use of a checklist. This checklist is more than just a time-out to confirm the patient's name and date of birth. When done in a form like the United Nations World Health Organization (WHO) outline for a surgical safety checklist, it is a comprehensive three-phase safety check (see Fig. 6-1). The first phase, "Sign In," lists tasks that are to be completed before the induction of anesthesia. More important, the patient is actively involved in this phase to confirm his or her identity, if applicable; to undergo site marking with indelible ink; to confirm the surgical procedure; and to give surgical and anesthesia consent. Other risks are measured with the patient awake, such as allergies, airway, and blood loss. The second phase, "Time Out," is to be done before incision. This phase includes an introduction of staff and roles and an agreement by all present on the patient identification, procedure, and site. It should also cover the administration of appropriate antibiotics for prophylaxis and anticipated problems from the anesthesia, surgical, and nursing teams. The third and final phase is "Sign Out." This important phase records what procedure was done, the number and names of the specimens, and instrument and sponge counts. Also included are a report of postoperative concerns for the patient from surgical, nursing, and anesthesia teams. Notes should be made of any equipment problems and priority assigned for a safety concern to be addressed before the next case. This last item should also be reported to the CUSP team along with any other notes so that trends may be identified, tracked, and safety process solutions found. After the publication in 2008 of the WHO recommendations, the use of checklists in the operating room has been validated by many retrospective studies, notably reducing the frequency of wrong-site surgeries. There is also a subjective feeling that nursing staff are the most compliant of all the groups in using the checklist. Song and colleagues published their findings in a frequently cited article, "The second 'time-out': a surgical safety checklist for lengthy robotic surgeries" (www.ncbi.nlm.nih.gov/pmc/articles/PMC3689613). This was designed to function as "a checklist conducted three to four hours after the start of surgery" for the purpose of assessing safety and increasing communication among the operating room staff to address their specific concerns. It is a good example of what the WHO operating room checklist guidelines (Fig. 6-1) recommend for adapting a checklist to fit the purposes of a specific venue.

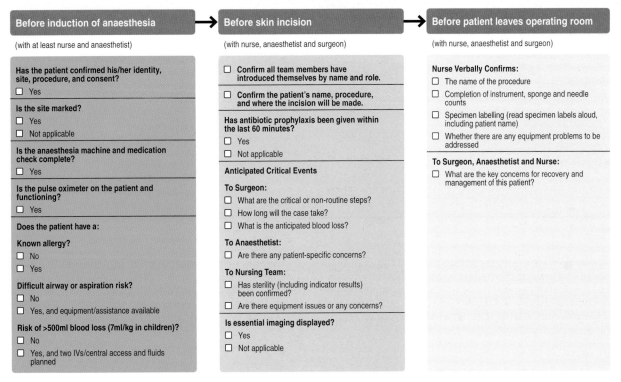

Figure 6-1. World Health Organization's Surgical Safety Checklist. *(Copyright © World Health Organization [WHO] 2009.)*

A portion of the AUA website is dedicated to safety as well. This section of the website highlights U.S. Food and Drug Administration (FDA) alerts and recalls pertinent to urologic devices, medicines, and herbal supplements. The AUA White Papers on safety give the organization's recommendations for anticoagulation and the prevention of catheter-related infections. The AUA Patient Safety page (www.auanet.org/resources/quality.cfm) gives notices regarding updates that affect patient care in the operating room, such as drug shortages and radiation exposure.

Surgical skills develop over time and with practice. Likewise, trust is built on the basis of honest and open communication among the APP, the surgeon, and the other members of the operative team, and develops over time and with practice. This book is full of detailed descriptions of minimally invasive urologic procedures, the indications and contraindications, patient positioning information, step-by-step descriptions of surgery, and information about postoperative recovery and potential complications, which are all interconnected. It is strongly suggested that APPs who are going to assist in any role avail themselves of the knowledge and experience available in this book and other resources. This chapter presents a list of safety resources for the APP (see Box 6-1). This book includes links to online videos in addition to standard reading resources. Surgeons will often take advantage of the many technologic devices in the operating room to make high-quality recordings of procedures as a way to improve their techniques. Regardless of how experienced or unexperienced an APP is with

assisting a particular surgeon with a certain case, recordings may be a very valuable learning resource for review. In addition to gross improvements in procedure and technique, these recordings may provide for small but important improvements that may be noticed or that otherwise may go unobserved during an operative case. The AUA provides a module on assisting with minimally invasive urologic surgery for continuing medical education (CME) credits; it is recommended that APPs avail themselves of this module on the AUA website at www.auanet.org/education/spotlight -on-surgical-assistance.cfm.

Because of national trends in health care, APPs are more likely to be used by urologists to assist in the operating room. One of the greatest concerns for doctors using APPs to care for patients is the increased liability for errors that they may make. Presently, this nervousness is not supported; it is suggested that to address apprehension and to make the best use of the assistant in the operating room, that the surgeon support the active involvement of APPs in safety efforts. All personnel would do well to note that the guidelines issued by bodies such as the AUA and WHO referred to in this chapter are changing to respond to contemporary concerns. As such, recommendations and references noted in this chapter may become obsolete—sometimes rapidly. As surgical techniques, staffing, and guidelines for safety inevitably change, the attitude of the entire surgical team with regard to safety must not. The first priority in the operating room is the safety of the patient and the team. APPs and others in the operating room should take ownership of safety on themselves to

---

BOX 6-1 Resources for the Advanced Practice Provider

- American Urological Association (AUA) Consensus Statement on Advanced Practice Providers (APPs)
  www.auanet.org/common/pdf/advocacy/advocacy-by-topic/AUA-Consensus-Statement-Advanced-Practice-Providers-Full.pdf
- United Nations World Health Organization (WHO) operating room checklist
  WHO Surgical Safety Checklist
  www.who.int/patientsafety/safesurgery/tools_resources/SSSL_Checklist_finalJun08.pdf?ua=1
- WHO operating room checklist manual
  World Alliance for Patient Safety Implementation Manual: Surgical Safety Checklist
  www.who.int/patientsafety/safesurgery/tools_resources/SSSL_Manual_finalJun08.pdf?ua=1
- The Joint Commission Goals, 2015
  The Joint Commission: Hospital National Patient Safety Goals 2015
  www.jointcommission.org/assets/1/6/2015_HAP_NPSG_ER.pdf
- Venous Thromboembolism (VTE) recommendations

Hospital Quality Alliance/Centers for Medicare and Medicaid Services (CMS) Surgical Care Improvement Quality Measures for Perioperative VTE prevention www.uptodate.com/contents/image?imageKey=HEME/50947&topicKey=ANEST%2F15077&source=outline_link&search=operating+room+safety&utdPopup=true
- AUA continuing medical education (CME) module for APPs on surgical assisting
  APN/PA Spotlight on Surgical Assistance
  www.auanet.org/education/spotlight-on-surgical-assistance.cfm
- AUA CME module for APPs on surgical assisting with robotics
  Urologic Robotic Surgery Course
  www.auanet.org/education/modules/robotic-surgery/module1.cfm
- AUA information on safety
  www.auanet.org/resources/quality.cfm
- Song JB, Vemana G, Mobley JM, Bhayani SB: The second "time-out": a surgical safety checklist for lengthy robotic surgeries
  www.ncbi.nlm.nih.gov/pmc/articles/PMC3689613

---

ensure that they are practicing within the legal limits of their profession and making every effort to ensure that the environment of the operating room is one of open communication of information to identify and resolve safety concerns. Assistants should be incorporated into efforts to track and address safety concerns to help prevent harm in the perioperative period. By doing so, it is believed that the urologist will make the best use of the skills of the APP, increase safety in the operating room, and decrease concerns for liability for harms done by the assistant.

7 Anesthetic Considerations for Laparoscopic and Robotic-Assisted Surgery

Judith Aronsohn, Jin Jung

Laparoscopic and robotic-assisted laparoscopic procedures are widely used in urologic surgery, conferring significant benefit to patients and improving outcomes. Benefits include less postoperative pain, faster recovery, shorter hospital stay, less blood loss, and lower incidence of postoperative wound infection.[1,2] Robotic-assisted surgery has increased dramatically worldwide and is now considered the standard of care in the United States for prostatectomies. Limited access to the patient, extreme Trendelenburg positioning, and an immoveable, docked robot present unique challenges for the anesthesia care team, particularly during crisis management.

The goal of anesthetic management is to provide optimal and safe surgical conditions while managing the pathophysiologic responses associated with laparoscopic surgery. This is a collaborative effort that requires effective and frequent communication with the surgical team and operating room staff. Protocols for rapid port removal and undocking the robot should be available and familiar to the team should a crisis situation arise.[3]

There are few absolute contraindications to laparoscopic surgery, and case reports and retrospective reviews document its safety in high-risk patients.[4-8] Laparoscopic surgery remains contraindicated in patients with increased intracranial pressure and nontreatable coagulopathy because of carbon dioxide (CO_2) insufflation and risk of uncontrolled bleeding. Ventriculoperitoneal shunt, congestive heart failure, and severe chronic obstructive pulmonary disease (COPD) are considered relative contraindications.

The ability of patients to tolerate prolonged, extreme positions, pneumoperitoneum, and CO_2 absorption must be weighed against the benefits of minimally invasive surgery for each patient.

PREANESTHESIA ASSESSMENT

Patients are ideally evaluated in a preoperative clinic to identify patient-specific and procedural risk factors, plan perioperative management, and optimize comorbid conditions. Routine, protocolized preoperative testing is expensive and has not resulted in improved patient outcomes.[9] The evaluation should include a focused physical examination, documentation of coexisting disease, and patient education on risks and potential strategies to minimize them. Additional testing and consultation should be tailored to the patient's comorbid conditions, functional capacity, and the surgical procedure. Further cardiac workup should follow current American College of Cardiology/American Heart Association (ACC/AHA) guidelines.[10] Patients considered at high risk should be counseled regarding the rare event in which a planned laparoscopic procedure must be converted to an open procedure.

PHYSIOLOGIC CHANGES

The physiologic changes that accompany laparoscopic surgery are caused by pneumoperitoneum, steep Trendelenburg position, CO_2 absorption, surgical procedure, and the patient's cardiovascular and pulmonary status.

Pneumoperitoneum

Pneumoperitoneum is established by insufflating the abdomen with CO_2, targeting intra-abdominal pressure (IAP) between 12 and 15 mm Hg. The increase in IAP displaces the diaphragm cephalad, decreasing pulmonary compliance and total lung volume. The head-down position does not appear to exacerbate these changes,[11,12] even in the morbidly obese.[13] Atelectasis and increased airway pressures result from reduced functional residual capacity and total lung compliance. These changes are well tolerated in healthy patients. Atelectasis may be more prominent in the elderly owing to increased closing capacity with age. Decreases in oxygen saturation can be treated with the judicious application of positive end-expiratory pressure (PEEP).[14] Recruitment maneuvers in addition to PEEP improve respiratory mechanics and oxygenation in healthy-weight and obese patients during pneumoperitoneum.[15]

Pressure-controlled ventilation is frequently used to lower peak airway pressure after insufflation of the abdomen, although it offers no hemodynamic benefit over volume-controlled ventilation during robotic-assisted radical prostatectomy.[16] Pulmonary barotrauma from increased plateau and airway pressures can lead to pneumothorax (PTX), pneumomediastinum (PMD), or pneumopericardium (PPM), particularly in patients with COPD.

Pneumoperitoneum increases systemic vascular resistance (SVR) and mean arterial pressure (MAP), with unpredictable effects on cardiac output (CO).[17,18] Increases in SVR are the result of mechanical as well as neuroendocrine responses to pneumoperitoneum.[19] IAPs above 12 mm Hg have been shown to decrease CO and increase SVR.[20] In hypovolemic patients, impairment of venous return by pneumoperitoneum may cause sudden or large decreases in blood pressure. Mechanical compression of the renal arteries and increased secretion of antidiuretic hormone and vasopressin decrease renal blood flow, glomerular filtration rate, and urine output.[21] Peritoneal stretching may cause severe bradycardia and even asystole owing to increased vagal tone (Table 7-1).

Carbon Dioxide Absorption

Carbon dioxide is commonly used for abdominal insufflation because it is highly soluble, chemically inert, colorless, inexpensive, and less combustible than air. Because of its high solubility, it is less likely than air (nitrogen) to cause clinically significant gas embolus. CO_2 is systemically absorbed during laparoscopy, causing hypercarbia. The degree of hypercarbia depends on CO_2 insufflation pressure and perfusion of the insufflation site and is higher in retroperitoneal surgery.[22] Hypercarbia can cause arrhythmias and contributes to increased SVR during laparoscopy. MAP, cerebral blood flow, and intracranial pressure are also increased. Mild hypercarbia can improve tissue perfusion through vasodilatation and by

TABLE 7-1 Cardiopulmonary Responses to Pneumoperitoneum Less Than 25 mm Hg

Measurement	Response
Heart rate	Increased or decreased
Stroke volume	Decreased
Mean arterial pressure	Increased
Systemic vascular resistance	Increased
Cardiac output	Decreased or unchanged
Central venous pressure	Increased
Functional residual capacity	Decreased
Respiratory compliance	Decreased
Peak airway pressures	Increased
PaO_2	Decreased or unchanged
$PaCO_2$	Increased
Cerebral blood flow	Increased
Intracranial pressure	Increased
pH	Decreased or unchanged

PaO_2, partial arterial oxygen tension; $PaCO_2$, partial pressure of carbon dioxide in arterial blood.

TABLE 7-2 Physiologic Changes in Steep Trendelenburg Position

Measurement	Response
Cardiac output	Increased or unchanged
Mean arterial pressure	Increased
Stroke volume	Increased
Mean pulmonary artery pressure	Increased
Pulmonary artery wedge pressure	Increased
Central venous pressure	Increased
Intraocular pressure	Increased

shifting the oxyhemoglobin dissociation curve to the right.[23] In healthy patients, excess CO_2 is easily eliminated by increasing minute ventilation 20% to 30%. However, hypercarbia-induced vasoconstriction in the pulmonary circulation may be poorly tolerated in patients with pulmonary hypertension.

Patient Position

Steep Trendelenburg position (25- to 45-degree head down) is necessary for proper surgical exposure during many urologic procedures. Instituting this position after abdominal insufflation significantly increases central venous pressure (CVP), MAP, CO,[24] and stroke volume,[25] as well as mean pulmonary artery pressure and pulmonary artery wedge pressure. These changes are well tolerated in healthy patients, and CO is preserved.[26]

Neurologic complications from cerebral edema after prolonged Trendelenburg position have been reported.[27] Although cerebral perfusion pressure in steep Trendelenburg is maintained in most cases,[24] Schramm and colleagues found impaired cerebral autoregulation in 23 patients undergoing robotic-assisted prostate surgery. Limiting the duration of steep Trendelenburg and keeping MAP within normal limits is a sensible strategy.[28]

Intraocular pressure increases with time in steep Trendelenburg.[29] However, no perioperative visual loss (POVL) has been attributed to steep Trendelenburg positioning alone in patients without preexisting ocular disease[30] (Table 7-2).

ANESTHETIC MANAGEMENT

General endotracheal anesthesia with neuromuscular blockade is the preferred technique for most major laparoscopic urologic procedures. Extreme patient positioning, prolonged abdominal insufflation, and patient discomfort make neuraxial techniques alone impractical. Although supraglottic devices

have been used successfully during laparoscopic cholecystectomies[31] and shorter gynecologic laparoscopic procedures,[32] their use in longer procedures requiring steep Trendelenburg positioning has not been sufficiently studied for them to be recommended.

Monitoring should include electrocardiography, noninvasive blood pressure, pulse oximetry, capnography, peripheral nerve stimulator, and temperature probe. Placing two blood pressure cuffs and two large-bore intravenous lines may be helpful when access to the patient is restricted. A central line is rarely indicated. Patients with significant cardiopulmonary disease may require invasive blood pressure monitoring for frequent arterial blood gas analysis.

Propofol is the most frequently used sedative-hypnotic for induction of general anesthesia, although other agents may be preferable in selected high-risk patients. Tracheal intubation and controlled mechanical ventilation are used to offset the effects of positioning, pneumoperitoneum, and CO_2 absorption. After the patient has been padded and positioned, all intravenous and monitoring lines should be tested and confirmed operational. Migration of the endotracheal tube (ETT) into the right mainstem bronchus has been reported in patients after abdominal insufflation in Trendelenburg position. The cause is cephalad displacement of the diaphragm and movement of the carina toward the relatively fixed ETT.[33,34] Securing the ETT immediately after the cuff passes the vocal cords may minimize this risk. Rechecking the position of the ETT after abdominal insufflation and placing the patient in Trendelenburg position are recommended. An orogastric tube is placed to deflate the stomach after the ETT is secured. Eyes should be protected with lubricating ointment, taped, and padded. Manipulation of the heavy, metal robotic camera occurs just above the patient's head, neck, and face. Protective preventative measures must be taken to pad or shield the patient's head in case of a dropped camera, lens, or other instrument.

Maintenance of anesthesia is accomplished through the use of an inhalational agent, opioid, and muscle relaxant. Alternatively, total intravenous anesthesia (TIVA) with propofol can be used in lieu of an inhaled anesthetic and is associated with less postoperative nausea and vomiting.[35] Although the choice of inhaled agent or TIVA is unimportant in most cases, the use of nitrous oxide is controversial. Concerns that it creates suboptimal operating conditions by causing bowel distention have led to infrequent use during laparoscopic procedures.

Insensible and third-space fluid losses are appreciably less for laparoscopic surgery compared with open procedures. Conservative intravenous fluid administration during robotic-assisted prostatectomy decreases the amount of urine obscuring the operative field and may also reduce the postoperative laryngeal edema resulting from prolonged steep Trendelenburg position.

POSTOPERATIVE MANAGEMENT
Pain Management

Although pain is often less after robotic-assisted laparoscopic surgery compared with conventional laparoscopy[36] and open procedures, opioids are often required in the postoperative period. Neuraxial opioids are frequently administered as part of an enhanced recovery protocol for major laparoscopic surgery.[37] Opioid analgesics are associated with a number of undesirable side effects, including nausea, vomiting, pruritus, urinary retention, respiratory depression, and delayed return of bowel function. Although there are no procedure-specific recommendations for pain management after major laparoscopic urologic surgery, opioid-sparing multimodal analgesia is gaining popularity to mitigate these side effects

TABLE 7-3 Commonly Used Analgesic Agents

Drug Name	Drug Class	Mechanism of Action	Side Effects
Morphine Fentanyl Hydromorphone Oxycodone Hydrocodone	Opioid	μ-Receptor agonist	Nausea, vomiting, pruritus, urinary retention, respiratory depression, constipation
Pregabalin Gabapentin	Anticonvulsant	$\alpha_2\delta$ Protein binding	Dizziness, somnolence, dry mouth, edema, blurred vision
Ketorolac Naproxen Ibuprofen Aspirin	Nonselective nonsteroidal anti-inflammatory	Cyclooxygenase antagonist	Bleeding, cardiovascular thrombotic events, gastrointestinal irritation, ulceration, renal impairment
Acetaminophen	Analgesic-antipyretic	Inhibition of prostaglandin synthesis in central nervous system	Hepatotoxicity, nausea, vomiting
Celecoxib	Cyclooxygenase-2–selective nonsteroidal anti-inflammatory	Cyclooxygenase-2 antagonist	Cardiovascular thrombosis, peripheral edema, dizziness, headache, abdominal pain, nausea, vomiting, renal impairment

TABLE 7-4 Commonly Used Antiemetic Agents for Postoperative Nausea and Vomiting

Drug Name	Drug Class	Mechanism of Action	Adverse Effects
Ondansetron Granisetron Dolasetron Palonosetron Tropisetron Ramosetron	5-Hydroxytryptamine ($5\text{-}HT_3$) antagonist	Central and peripheral selective $5\text{-}HT_3$ receptor antagonist	QT prolongation, serotonin syndrome, headache, malaise, fatigue, constipation
Aprepitant Fosaprepitant	Substance P/neurokinin-1 receptor antagonist	Substance P/neurokinin-1 receptor antagonist	Fatigue, constipation, weakness, hiccups, decreased serum oral contraceptives
Diphenhydramine Dimenhydrinate Cyclizine Meclizine Promethazine	H_1 antagonist	Competitive H_1 antagonist in gastrointestinal tract, anticholinergic	Central nervous system depression, tachycardia, palpitation, headache, restlessness, urinary retention, blurred vision
Dexamethasone	Glucocorticoid	Unknown	Hyperglycemia, increased risk of wound infections
Droperidol Haloperidol	Butyrophenone	Dopamine blockade at the chemoreceptor trigger zone	QT prolongation, anticholinergic effects, extrapyramidal symptoms, neuroleptic malignant syndrome, sedation, orthostatic hypotension
Metoclopramide	Benzamide	Dopamine antagonist in chemoreceptor trigger zone, increases acetylcholine receptor sensitivity in gastrointestinal tract, increasing motility	Extrapyramidal symptoms, neuroleptic malignant syndrome, depression, hypertension
Scopolamine	Anticholinergic	Histamine and serotonin antagonist, acetylcholine antagonist at parasympathetic locations in central nervous system	Delirium, tachycardia, constipation, dry throat, blurred vision, flushing

and promote early recovery.[38,39] Systemic steroids, pregabalin, nonsteroidal anti-inflammatory drugs, and cyclooxygenase-2–selective inhibitors have been used successfully before, during, and after surgery to decrease postoperative opioid requirements.[40] Local infiltration of port sites has been shown to be more effective at reducing postoperative pain when administered preemptively[41] (Table 7-3).

Transabdominal plane block has also been used as part of a multimodal strategy to improve postoperative pain outcomes in laparoscopic patients with varying degrees of success. Differences in surgical procedure, timing of block administration, and dose and volume of local anesthetic may contribute to these conflicting results.

Nausea and Vomiting

Refractory postoperative nausea and vomiting (PONV) is upsetting to patients and can result in delayed postanesthesia care unit (PACU) discharge, unplanned hospital admission, and increased healthcare costs.[42] Laparoscopic surgery is strongly believed to be a risk factor for PONV. Other patient-specific risk factors include young age, nonsmoking status, female sex, and history of PONV or motion sickness.[43] Anesthetic causes of PONV are the use of volatile anesthetics, nitrous oxide, and

postoperative opioids.[44] Modifying anesthetic technique, minimizing postoperative opioid consumption, and using effective antiemetic agents either alone or in combination can decrease risk. TIVA has been shown to decrease PONV risk by 25% in high-risk patients.[45] Recommended pharmacologic antiemetic agents for PONV prophylaxis include 5-hydroxytryptamine ($5\text{-}HT_3$) receptor antagonists, neurokinin-1 receptor antagonists, antihistamines, corticosteroids, butyrophenones, and anticholinergics.[42] The decision to use PONV prophylaxis should be based on patient risk factors, side effects of the antiemetics, and drug cost. Moderate- and high-risk patients may benefit from combination therapy using drugs that bind at different receptor sites. Drugs used for prophylaxis should not be repeated if rescue therapy becomes necessary[43] (Table 7-4).

COMPLICATIONS
Carbon Dioxide Embolism

Catastrophic CO_2 embolism leading to decreased CO and death is uncommon during minimally invasive surgery. Although the true incidence is unknown, it has been reported to occur in a variety of laparoscopic procedures. Various monitoring devices can help detect gas embolism; transesophageal echocardiography (TEE) is the most sensitive. Subclinical CO_2 embolism was discovered in 17% of patients undergoing laparoscopic radical prostatectomy when TEE was used for detection.[46] Kim and colleagues reported the presence of CO_2 embolism in 100% of patients undergoing total laparoscopic hysterectomy with TEE monitoring. None became hemodynamically unstable or sustained neurologic sequelae.[47] Clinically significant CO_2 embolism can cause cardiac arrhythmias, hypoxemia, hypotension, and cardiovascular collapse. End-tidal CO_2 may increase initially, then decrease with obstruction of the pulmonary vasculature by emboli. Treatment is aimed at preventing further gas entry, reducing the amount of gas entrained, and providing hemodynamic support. The abdomen should be deflated and the patient hyperventilated with 100% O_2 to correct hypoxemia and washout CO_2. Volume loading and the Valsalva maneuver may reduce further gas entry by elevating CVP. Vasopressors and inotropic agents are administered as needed. Placing the patient in the left lateral decubitus position and head down may prevent CO_2 from entering the pulmonary artery. A multiorifice central venous catheter can be used to aspirate gas from the right atrium or ventricle. Cardiopulmonary bypass and hyperbaric oxygen[48] have both been used successfully to treat critical cases involving gas embolism.

Well-Leg Compartment Syndrome

Well-leg compartment syndrome (WLCS) is a rare but devastating complication that can lead to myoglobinuria, renal failure, limb loss, and death. The reported incidence of lower limb compartment syndrome in patients undergoing pelvic surgery in the lithotomy position is 1 in 3500 cases.[49] Risk factors include prolonged surgery, pressure on the calves, elevation of the lower limbs with hyperflexion of the hips and knees, pneumoperitoneum, and Trendelenburg position.[50] Postoperative limb pain out of proportion to the clinical findings is a suggestive finding. Left untreated, WLCS leads to muscle ischemia, metabolic acidosis, rhabdomyolysis, and myoglobinuric renal failure. Chronic neuromuscular impairment, loss of limb, or death may result. Treatment consists of surgical opening of the affected compartments.

Patient Positioning

Trendelenburg position for prolonged periods of time has been associated with laryngeal edema requiring reintubation postoperatively.[51] Time-limited Trendelenburg position and conservative fluid management intraoperatively may help reduce this risk.

Shoulder braces, used to keep the patient from migrating cephalad while in steep Trendelenburg position, have resulted in brachial plexus injuries from compression and stretch.[51] Nonsliding (disposable egg crate) mattresses or chest straps are alternatives to shoulder braces, recognizing that chest straps may further decrease pulmonary compliance.

Ocular Injuries

The reported incidence of corneal abrasion in robotic-assisted laparoscopic prostatectomy is 3%.[52] Possible causes include chemosis and exposure keratopathy. Eye tape may separate when the conjunctiva becomes edematous during prolonged surgery in Trendelenburg position, drying the cornea. Chemical and mechanical injuries may also result in corneal abrasion.

POVL is rare after laparoscopic urologic surgery. It is more commonly reported after spinal fusion surgery and cardiopulmonary bypass but has been reported after robotic-assisted radical prostatectomy[53] and laparoscopic donor

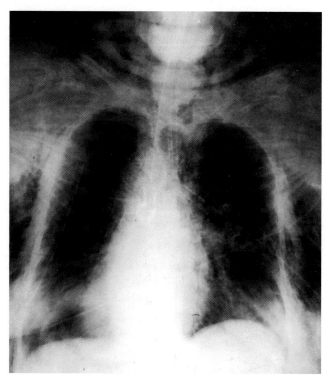

Figure 7-1. A patient with bilateral pneumothorax and subcutaneous emphysema who subsequently had hypotension and hypoxia and consequently required bilateral chest tubes.

nephrectomy.[54] Factors identified as increasing the risk for POVL include prolonged surgery, hemorrhage, hypotension, and hemodilution.[55]

Pneumothorax, Pneumomediastinum, and Pneumopericardium

PTX, PMD, and PPM are well-known complications of laparoscopic surgery and can result from a variety of causes (Fig. 7-1). Pleural or diaphragmatic injury during surgery, tracking of insufflated CO_2 along musculofascial planes, subcutaneous emphysema, and congenital defects in the diaphragm allow CO_2 to enter the mediastinal and pleural spaces (Fig. 7-2). Subcutaneous emphysema can occur in 20% to 60% of all laparoscopic cases[56] and is more likely to develop with the use of four or more trocars, prolonged increases in IAP, increased operating time, and increased volume of gas.[57] When severe, it can lead to significant hypercarbia during and after surgery. Intraoperative end-tidal CO_2 of 50 mm Hg or more has been found to be a risk factor for PTX and PPM. Other risk factors include operative times greater than 200 minutes and procedures near the diaphragm.[58-60] Most cases are subclinical and do not require aggressive treatment.[61] Rarely, patients with PPM exhibit signs and symptoms of acute myocardial ischemia or infarction after laparoscopy. Postoperative complaints of chest pain, diaphoresis, pallor, and shortness of breath accompanied by T-wave abnormalities on the electrocardiogram (ECG) are compatible with the diagnosis of PPM.[62] Treatment is supportive, with symptoms and ECG changes resolving within a few days.[63]

Increased airway pressure, hypercapnia, hypoxemia, absent breath sounds, and billowing of the diaphragm intraoperatively are suggestive of clinically significant PTX. Concomitant hemodynamic instability indicates the PTX is likely under tension. Some of these signs may be masked when surgery is performed using a valveless trocar system, delaying the diagnosis.[64]

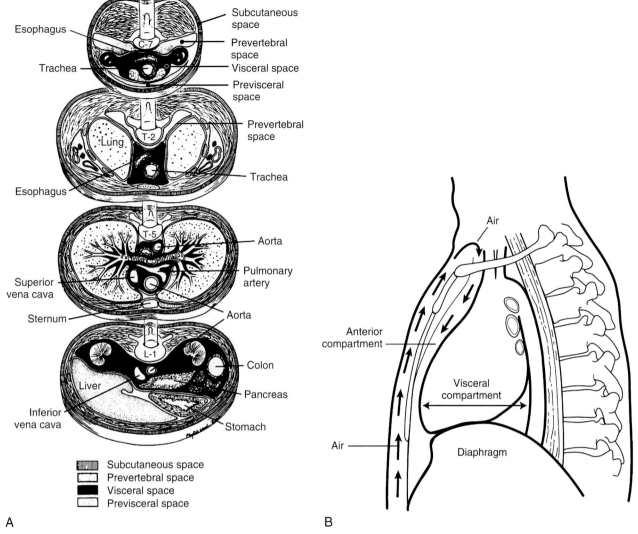

Figure 7-2. A, Cross-section cuts of different facial planes within the neck, chest, and upper abdomen. **B,** Gas extending from the retroperitoneum dissecting into the neck and visceral compartments. *(From Maunder RJ, Pierson DJ, Hudson LD. Subcutaneous and mediastinal emphysema: pathophysiology, diagnosis and management.* Arch Intern Med. *1984;144:1447-1453.)*

Treatment consists of immediate desufflation of the abdomen, hyperventilation with 100% oxygen, PEEP, and hemodynamic support. Severe compromise may require needle decompression or placement of a temporary drain. Owing to the high solubility of CO_2, hemodynamically stable, asymptomatic patients can be treated conservatively, regardless of the size of the PTX.[65,66]

TIPS AND TRICKS

The perioperative team should have a full understanding of the physiologic changes and adverse events that can occur during laparoscopic surgery.

Protocols for rapid port removal and undocking the robot during robotic-assisted laparoscopic surgery should be familiar to the team should a crisis situation arise.

The eyes and head must be protected against accidental trauma from the camera, lenses, cords, and instruments.

A multimodal approach to managing pain after laparoscopic procedures can reduce opioid requirements and minimize undesirable side effects associated with their use.

PONV prophylaxis should be based on patient risk, antiemetic side effects, and drug cost

---

REFERENCES

1. Veldkamp R, Kuhry E, Hop WC, et al. Laparoscopic surgery versus open surgery for colon cancer: short-term outcomes of a randomised trial. *Lancet Oncol.* 2005;6:477–484.
2. Varela J, Esteban V, Wilson S, Nguyen N. Laparoscopic surgery significantly reduces surgical-site infections compared with open surgery. *Surg Endosc.* 2010;24:270–276.
3. Cockcroft J. Anesthesia for major urologic surgery. *Anesthesiol Clin.* 2015;33:165–172.
4. Linden P, Gilbert R, Yeap B, Boyle K, Deykin A, Jaklitsch M, Sugarbaker D, Bueno R. Laparoscopic fundoplication in patients with end-stage lung disease awaiting transplantation. *J Thorac Cardiovasc Surg.* 2006;131:438–446.
5. Hsieh C. Laparoscopic cholecystectomy for patients with chronic obstructive pulmonary disease. *J Laparoendosc Adv Surg Tech A.* 2004; 13:5–9.
6. Gillory L, Meaison M, Harmon C, Chen M, Anderson S, Chong AJ, Chaignaud BE, Beierle EA. Laparoscopic surgery in children with congenital heart disease. *J Pediatr Surg.* 2012;47:1084–1088.
7. Cobianchi L, Dominioni T, Filisetti C, Zonta S, Maestri M, Dionigi P, Alessiani M. Ventriculoperitoneal shunt and the need to remove a gallbladder: time to definitely overcome the feeling that laparoscopic surgery is contraindicated. *Ann Med Surg (Lond).* 2014; 3:65–67.

8. Kang C, Halabi W, Chaudhry O, Nguyen V, Ketana N, Carmichael J, Pigazzi A, Stamos M, Mills S. A nationwide analysis of laparoscopy in high-risk colorectal surgery patients. *J Gastrointest Surg.* 2013;17:382–391.

9. Mantha S, Roizen M, Madduri J, Rajender Y, Naidu K, Gayatri K. Usefulness of routine preoperative testing: a prospective single-observer study. *J Clin Anesth.* 2005;17:51–57.

10. Fleisher LA, Fleischmann KE, Auerbach AD, et al. 2014 ACC/AHA guideline on perioperative cardiovascular evaluation and management of patients undergoing noncardiac surgery: a report of the American College of Cardiology/American Heart Association Task Force on practice guidelines. *J Am Coll Cardiol.* 2014;64:e77–e137.

11. Suh M, Seong K, Jung S, Kim S. The effect of pneumoperitoneum and Trendelenburg position on respiratory mechanics during pelviscopic surgery. *Korean J Anesthesiol.* 2010;59:329–334.

12. Rauh R, Hemmerling TM, Rist M, Jacobi KE. Influence of pneumoperitoneum and patient positioning on respiratory system compliance. *J Clin Anesth.* 2001;13:361–365.

13. Sprung J, Whalley D, Falcone T, Warner D, Hubmayr RD, Hammel J. The impact of morbid obesity, pneumoperitoneum, and posture on respiratory system mechanics and oxygenation during laparoscopy. *Anesth Analg.* 2002;94:1345–1350.

14. Meininger D, Byhahn C, Mierdl S. Positive end-expiratory pressure improves arterial oxygenation during prolonged pneumoperitoneum. *Acta Anaesthesiol Scand.* 2005;49:778–783.

15. Futier E, Constantin J, Pelosi P, Chanques G, Kwiatkoskwi F, Jaber S, Bazin J. Intraoperative recruitment maneuver reverses detrimental pneumoperitoneum-induced respiratory effects in healthy eight and obese patients undergoing laparoscopy. *Anesthesiology.* 2010;113:1310–1319.

16. Choi E, Na S, Choi S, An J, Rha K, Oh Y. Comparison of volume controlled and pressure controlled ventilation in steep Trendelenburg position for robot-assisted laparoscopic radical prostatectomy. *J Clin Anesth.* 2011;23:183–188.

17. O'Leary E, Hubbard K, Tormey W, Cunningham A. Laparoscopic cholecystectomy: haemodynamic and neuroendocrine responses after pneumoperitoneum and changes in position. *Br J Anaesth.* 1996;76:640–644.

18. Larsen J, Svendsen F, Pederson V. Randomized clinical trial of the effect of pneumoperitoneum on cardiac function and haemodynamics during laparoscopic cholecystectomy. *Br J Surg.* 2004;91:848–854.

19. O'Leary E, Hubbard K, Tormey W. Laparoscopic cholecystectomy: haemodynamic and neuroendocrine responses after pneumoperitoneum and changes in position. *Br J Anaesth.* 1996;76:640–644.

20. Ishizaki Y. Safe intraabdominal pressure of carbon dioxide pneumoperitoneum during laparoscopic surgery. *Surgery.* 1993;114:549–554.

21. O'Malley C, Cunningham AJ. Physiologic changes during laparoscopy. *Anesthesiol Clin North America.* 2001;1:1–19.

22. Streich B, Decailliot F, Perney C. Increased carbon dioxide absorption during retroperitoneal laparoscopy. *Br J Anaesth.* 2003;91:793–796.

23. Hager H, Reddy D, Mandadi G. Hypercapnia improves tissue oxygenation in morbidly obese surgical patients. *Anesth Analg.* 2006;103:677–681.

24. Kalmar A, Foubert L, Hendrickx J, Mottrie A, Absalon A, Mortier E, Struys M. Influence of steep Trendelenburg position and CO_2 pneumoperitoneum on cardiovascular, cerebrovascular, and respiratory homeostasis during robotic prostatectomy. *Br J Anaesth.* 2010;104:433–439.

25. Falabella A, Moore-Jeffries E, Sullivan M, Nelson R, Lew M. Cardiac function during steep Trendelenburg position and CO_2 pneumoperitoneum for robotic-assisted prostatectomy: a transoesophageal Doppler probe study. *Int J Med Robot.* 2007;3:312–315.

26. Lestar M, Gunnarsson L, Lagerstrand L, Wiklund P, Odeberg-Wernerman S. Hemodynamic perturbations during robot-assisted laparoscopic radical prostatectomy in 45 degree Trendelenburg position. *Anesth Analg.* 2011;113:1069–1075.

27. Pandey R. Unpredicted neurological complications after laparoscopic radical cystectomy and ileal conduit formation in steep Trendelenburg position: two case reports. *Acta Anaesthesiol Belg.* 2009;61:163–166.

28. Schramm P. Time course of cerebrovascular autoregulation during extreme Trendelenburg position for robotic-assisted prostatic surgery. *Anaesthesia.* 2014;69:58–63.

29. Awad H. The effects of steep Trendelenburg positioning on intraocular pressure during robotic radical prostatectomy. *Anesth Analg.* 2009;109:473–478.

30. Hoshikawa Y. The effect of steep Trendelenburg positioning on intraocular pressure and visual function during robotic-assisted radical prostatectomy. *Br J Ophthalmol.* 2014;98:305–308.

31. Maltby JR, Beriault MT, Watson NC, Liepert D, Fick GH. The LMA-ProSeal is an effective alternative to tracheal intubation for laparoscopic cholecystectomy. *Can J Anaesth.* 2002;49:857–862.

32. Teoh W, Lee K, Suhitharan T, Yahaya Z, Teo M, Sia A. Comparison of the LMA Supreme vs. the I-Gel in paralyzed patients undergoing gynaecological laparoscopic surgery with controlled ventilation. *Anaesthesia.* 2010;65:1173–1179.

33. Heinonen J, Takki S, Tammisto T. Effect of the Trendelenburg tilt and other procedures on the position of endotracheal tubes. *Lancet.* 1969;293:850–853.

34. Lobata E. Pneumoperitoneum as a risk factor for endobronchial intubation during laparoscopic gynecologic surgery. *Anesth Analg.* 1998;86:301–303.

35. Yoo Y, Sai S, Lee K, Shin S, Choi E, Lee J. Total intravenous anesthesia with propofol reduces postoperative nausea and vomiting in patients undergoing robot-assisted laparoscopic radical prostatectomy: a prospective randomized trial. *Yonsei Med J.* 2012;53:1197–1202.

36. Taylor E. Anesthesia for laparoscopic cholecystectomy. Is nitrous oxide contraindicated? *Anesthesiology.* 1992;76:541–543.

37. Tan M, Law LS, Gan TJ. Optimizing pain management to facilitate Enhanced Recovery After Surgery pathways. *Can J Anaesth.* 2015;62:203–218.

38. Saar M. Fast track rehabilitation after robot-assisted laparoscopic cystectomy accelerates postoperative recovery. *Br J Urol.* 2013;112:E99–E106.

39. Wong C, Gu X, Araki M, Shah C, Heider S, Raphaely S. Opioid-free analgesia following robot-assisted laparoscopic prostatectomy. *J Am Coll Surg.* 2013;217:152.

40. Trabulsi E, Patel J, Viscusi E, Gomella L, Lallas C. Preemptive multimodal pain regimen reduces opioid analgesia for patients undergoing robotic-assisted laparoscopic radical prostatectomy. *Urology.* 2010;76:1122–1124.

41. Joshi G, Bonnet F, Kehlet H. Evidence-based postoperative pain management after laparoscopic colorectal surgery. *Colorectal Dis.* 2013;15:146–155.

42. Ke R. A randomized, double-blinded trail of preemptive analgesia in laparoscopy. *Obstet Gynecol.* 1998;92:972–975.

43. Hill R, Lubarsky D, Phillips-Bute B, Fortney J, Creed M, Glass P, Gan T. Cost-effectiveness of prophylactic antiemetic therapy with ondansetron, droperidol, or placebo. *Anesthesiology.* 2000;92:958–967.

44. Gan T, Diemunsch P, Habib A, Kovac A, Kranke P, Meyer T, Watcha M. Consensus guidelines for the management of postoperative nausea and vomiting. *Anesth Analg.* 2014;118:85–113.

45. Apfel C, Kranke P, Katz M, Goepfert C, Papenfuss T, Rauch S, Heinek R, Greim C, Roewer N. Volatile anaesthetics may be the main cause of early but not delayed postoperative vomiting: a randomized controlled trail of factorial design. *Br J Anaesth.* 2002;88:659–668.

46. Apfel C, Korttila K, Abdalla M, Kerger K, Turan A, Vedder I, Zernak C. A factorial trial of six interventions for the prevention of postoperative nausea and vomiting. *N Engl J Med.* 2004;350:2441–2451.

47. Hong J, Kim W, Kil H. Detection of subclinical CO_2 embolism by transesophageal echocardiography during laparoscopic radical prostatectomy. *Urology.* 2010;75:581–584.

48. Kim C, Kim J, Kwon J, Choi S, Na S, An J. Venous air embolism during total laparoscopic hysterectomy: comparison to total abdominal hysterectomy. *Anesthesiology.* 2009;111:50–54.

49. McGrath B. Carbon dioxide embolism treated with hyperbaric oxygen. *Can J Anaesth.* 1989;36:586–589.

50. Mumtaz F. Lower limb compartment syndrome associated with the lithotomy position. *Br J Urol.* 2002;90:792–799.

51. Rao M, Jayne D. Lower limb compartment syndrome following laparoscopic colorectal surgery: a review. *Colorectal Dis.* 2011;13:494–499.

52. Phong S, Koh L. Anaesthesia for robotic-assisted radical prostatectomy: considerations for laparoscopy in the Trendelenburg position. *Anaesth Intensive Care.* 2007;35:281–285.

53. Danic M. Anesthesia considerations for robotic-assisted laparoscopic prostatectomy: a review of 1, 500 cases. *J Robot Surg.* 2007; 1:119–123.

54. Weber E, Colyer M, Lesser R, Subramanian P. Posterior ischemic optic neuropathy after minimally invasive prostatectomy. *J Neuroophthalmol.* 2007;27:285–287.

55. Metwalli A, Davis R, Donovan J. Visual impairment after laparoscopic donor nephrectomy. *J Endourol.* 2004;18:888–890.

56. Roth S. Perioperative visual loss: what do we know, what can we do? *Br J Anaesth.* 2009;103:i31–i40.

57. McAllister J, D'Altorio R, Snyder A. CT findings after uncomplicated percutaneous laparoscopic cholecystectomy. *J Comput Assist Tomogr.* 1991;15:770–772.

58. Ott D. Subcutaneous emphysema—beyond the pneumoperitoneum. *JSLS.* 2014;18:1.

59. Murdock C, Wolff A, Van Geem T. Risk factors for hypercarbia, subcutaneous emphysema, pneumothorax, and pneumomediastinum during laparoscopy. *Obstet Gynecol.* 2000;95:704–709.

60. Richard H, Stancato-Pasik A, Salky B, Mendelson D. Pneumothorax and pneumomediastinum after laparoscopic surgery. *Clin Imaging.* 1997;21:337–339.

61. Phillips S, Falk G. Surgical tension pneumothorax during laparoscopic repair of massive hiatus hernia: a different situation requiring different management. *Anaesth Intensive Care.* 2011;39: 1120–1123.

62. Abreu S, Sharp D, Ramani A, Steinberg A, Ng C, Desai M, Gill L. Thoracic complications during urological laparoscopy. *J Urol.* 2004; 171:1451–1455.

63. Ko M. Pneumopericardium and severe subcutaneous emphysema after laparoscopic surgery. *J Minim Invasive Gynecol.* 2010;17: 531–533.

64. Beaver J, Safran D. Pneumopericardium mimicking acute myocardial ischemia after laparoscopic cholecystectomy. *South Med J.* 1999;92(10):1002–1004.

65. Hillelsohn J, Friedlander J, Bagadiya N, Okhunov Z, Kashan M, Schwartzur M, Kavoussi L. Masked pneumothorax; a risk of valveless trocar systems. *J Urol.* 2013;189:955–959.

66. Msezane L, Zorn K, Gofrit O, Schade G, Shalhav A. Case report: conservative management of a large capnothorax following laparoscopic renal surgery. *J Endourol.* 2007;21:1445–1448.

8 Insufflators and the Pneumoperitoneum

Jaspreet Singh Parihar, Sammy E. Elsamra

Laparoscopy and the ever-expanding robotic-assisted techniques have revolutionized the field of minimally invasive surgeries. Pneumoperitoneum is the keystone that allows surgeon to create a visual field and working space necessary to conduct the operations. A basic understanding of the pneumoperitoneum process and its fundamental components is essential to create a safe and effective operating environment.

INDICATIONS AND CONTRAINDICATIONS

Pneumoperitoneum is an essential component in any transperitoneal laparoscopic surgery. Instillation of gas into the peritoneum allows distention of a potential space to safely visualize and manipulate tissues. It is a prerequisite for any contemporary transperitoneal laparoscopic or robotic surgery and hence indicated for any such procedure. Conversely, contraindications to laparoscopic surgery disqualify establishment of pneumoperitoneum. Uncorrectable coagulopathy, hypercapnia, intestinal obstructions, limiting working space, significant abdominal wall infections, hemoperitoneum or hemoretroperitoneum, generalized peritonitis, and suspected malignant ascites may preclude establishment of pneumoperitoneum.[1]

Fundamental to the development of adequate pneumoperitoneum is proper access to the peritoneal cavity. Clearly, without proper access, pneumoperitoneum may not be feasible. Ports and establishing access are discussed elsewhere in the text. Nonetheless, intra-abdominal adhesions from prior operations or inflammatory processes can increase the risk of inadvertent injury to the surrounding structures and make safe pneumoperitoneum difficult. Additional limiting factors include presence of abdominal mesh, cirrhosis, portal hypertension, morbid obesity, pelvic fibrosis, organomegaly, pregnancy, hernias, and vascular aneurysms, although recent evidence suggests improved safety.[2,3]

Of equal importance to the aforementioned patient-related factors are the surgical team elements. Clear understanding of the physiologic implications of pneumoperitoneum by the anesthesiologist and surgeon are critical. Furthermore, proper operative equipment should be readily available, along with trained ancillary staff members for troubleshooting common equipment malfunctions.

PATIENT PREOPERATIVE EVALUATION AND PREPARATION

Careful preoperative assessment of patient comorbidity is important when selecting candidates for a laparoscopic or robotic-assisted approach. For any complications related to access, pneumoperitoneum, or laparoscopic surgery to be minimized, a careful patient history and physical examination should be conducted. Inquiries should focus on the patient's medical conditions and prior surgical history including previous surgical approach, intraoperative or postoperative abdominal complications, and wound infections. The physical examination should also encompass an assessment of body habitus, presence of prior surgical scars, and abdominal hernias. Patients with chronic obstructive pulmonary disease (COPD) may benefit from baseline quantification of disease severity through arterial blood gas and pulmonary function testing.[4] Instead of carbon dioxide (CO_2), nitrous oxide or helium gas may be used for insufflation in patients who are intolerant to hypercapnia and subsequent acidosis.[5,6]

OPERATING ROOM CONFIGURATION

The operating room should be set up in a manner that maximizes surgical safety and efficiency of the task at hand. Specific floor diagrams for personnel and equipment will be procedure specific and are discussed elsewhere in this textbook. In general, all necessary equipment should be present in the operating room and tested to ensure proper functioning. The insufflator must be in clear view for the surgical team to monitor pressures at the beginning of the case and as needed during the case. It is important to check for readiness of the suction-irrigator unit and adequate insufflation gas supply. The insufflator unit should be checked for its preset settings, tubing equipment, and presence of gas flow. Furthermore, its alarms should be tested to confirm its safety mechanisms.

Specific techniques for establishing pneumoperitoneum are covered in greater detail elsewhere in this textbook. In brief, pneumoperitoneum can be initiated using open access techniques (Hasson technique, or through a hand port incision) as well as closed access techniques (Veress needle). Optimal access points for Veress needle access include the umbilicus, Palmer's point (midclavicular line subcostal, 3 cm inferior to the costal margin), and a site two fingerbreadths superior and medial to the anterior superior iliac spine. A Veress needle can also be used to confirm the absence of underlying adhesions by inserting it into an insufflated abdomen at an intended trocar site.

COMPONENTS OF THE INSUFFLATION SYSTEM
Insufflator Unit

An understanding of the insufflator system design and features is helpful for any laparoscopic surgeon. There are three components to the insufflation system: insufflator, tubing equipment, and insufflation gas. The role of an insufflator unit is to establish, monitor, and maintain a constant intra-abdominal pressure during laparoscopy. A variety of vendors offer insufflation systems (Table 8-1). Displayed on the face of the unit are modifiable settings for pressure and flow, alarm alerts, and real-time values for pressure, flow, and volume instilled (Fig. 8-1).

Initial insufflation of the abdomen should be started at a slow rate (1-2 L/min). Rapid rates risk rapid stretching of the peritoneum, which may precipitate cardiovascular dysfunction, such as hypotension, bradycardia, arrhythmia, and rarely cardiac arrest.[7-10] In such circumstances, the pneumoperitoneum should be immediately released, followed by cardiopulmonary resuscitative measures. After clinical stabilization and if appropriate, pneumoperitoneum may be reattempted with slow insufflation followed by maintenance of intra-abdominal pressures below 12 to 15 mm Hg.

During pneumoperitoneum, any leakage through the trocar or abdominal wall is sensed by the insufflator unit and compensated for by increased reinsufflation of the gas volume to maintain a preset intra-abdominal pressure. The patient should remain adequately anesthetized because abdominal wall contractions during pneumoperitoneum can unexpectedly increase intra-abdominal pressure up to 50 mm Hg.[11,12] Similarly, leaning on the patient's abdomen or placing heavy equipment can trigger automatic insufflator shutoff followed by pressure loss and time delay.[12]

In obese patients, maintaining a stable pneumoperitoneum becomes more critical because of greater resistance exerted by a thick abdominal wall as well as frequent instrument changes.[13] For such patients, high–flow rate insufflators may be better suited because they can deliver rapid insufflation of the lost gas volume. High flow rates can also help maintain pneumoperitoneum in emergent circumstances such as during bleeding requiring aggressive suctioning, during constant smoke evacuation, or during instances of a dislodged port cannula.

During high–flow rate settings, the intra-abdominal pressure will quickly rise to maintain a constant velocity. High-flow insufflators commonly use the overpressure insufflation principle, resulting in intermittent high peak intra-abdominal pressures during periods of insufflation despite a lower preset value. An advantage of this approach is rapid establishment of pneumoperitoneum; however, higher intermittent abdominal pressures and repeated peritoneal stretching may stimulate vagal responses, leading to various clinical sequelae. Low-pressure–principle insufflators do not exceed the preset value but require low resistance in the insufflation system.

Tubing Equipment

Insufflation gas is carried toward the trocar port via flexible tubing. Typically, it houses a disposable 0.3-micron gas filter to prevent any contaminants from entering the insufflator and gas storage cylinder.[14] Before pneumoperitoneum is initiated, the tubing toward the patient should be purged of room air to reduce the risk of mixed air-gas embolism.[15,16]

An important concept is that of resistance within the entire insufflation system. Minimizing the resistance of the system is perhaps of greater clinical significance than investing in costly high-flow insufflation units. Principles of gas flow have been described by the Hagen-Poiseuille law[17]:

$$\Phi = \frac{\pi \times r^4}{8 \times \eta \times l} \times \Delta P$$

where Φ = gas flow, r = radius, η = viscosity, l = length, and ΔP = pressure difference.

Accordingly, gas flow is dependent on changes in pressure and limited by the smallest diameter channel, such as Luer-Lok port connectors. Flow rate increase is exponentially dependent on the lumen, such that any increase in the radius of the lumen increases the gas flow rate to the fourth power. Consequently, the resistance of the system may be reduced through integration of large-diameter insufflation equipment such as gas filters, insufflation tubing, Luer-Lok connectors, and trocars.

There exists a risk of blood and/or irrigation contamination owing to transient negative pressure generated within the insufflator unit. Accordingly, the insufflator tubing should be disconnected before powering the unit on or off. The insufflator unit, typically housed in a device tower, should be positioned above the level of the patient because retrograde fluid flow into the tubing risks cross contamination between cases.[12] Furthermore, use of a large-capacity gas tank or a continuous central gas supply not only reduces case interruptions but also minimizes disruption of the pneumoperitoneum tent.

Insufflation Gas

Before recognition of potential compilations of air embolus and combustion, room air, oxygen, and nitrous oxide were used to establish pneumoperitoneum. Noble gases such as helium, xenon, or argon have been used in protocol studies; however, because of their poor solubility, these gases pose a serious risk of gas embolism.[5,18,19] At present, CO_2 is the most frequently used gas for insufflation, given its high solubility in blood and lack of combustion during electrosurgery. Its high diffusion coefficient allows rapid clearance from the body and decreases the consequences of gas embolism. Unlike CO_2, nitrous oxide (N_2O) has both anesthetic and analgesic properties without causing peritoneal irritation and cardiopulmonary side effects. Theoretical concerns regarding its failure to suppress combustion have limited its routine clinical use. However, contemporary evidence suggests its safety, especially in patients with compromised cardiopulmonary function or metabolic acidosis.[6,18,20]

TABLE 8-1 Examples of Laparoscopic Insufflators

Manufacturer	Product	Maximum Flow Rate
Karl Storz	Thermoflator, Endoflator	20-50 L/min
Olympus	UHI-4	45 L/min
SurgiQuest	AirSeal iFS System	40 L/min
Stryker	45L PneumoSure insufflator	45 L/min
Wolf	Laparoscopic CO2 Insufflator	40 L/min

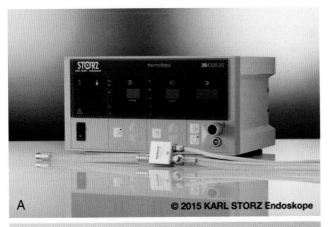

© 2015 KARL STORZ Endoskope

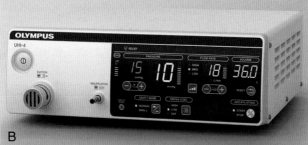

Figure 8-1. Examples of insufflator units and their control inputs. **A,** Karl Storz Thermoflator with display and heating element. **B,** Olympus UHI-4. (**A** © 2016. Photo courtesy KARL STORZ GmbH & Co. KG. **B** courtesy Olympus America, Center Valley, Penn.)

CO_2 is stored in high-pressure tanks in a liquid form. The temperature of the insufflated CO_2 is about 21° C, and it is low in humidity. This combination contributes to drying of the peritoneal surface and predisposes the patient to hypothermia.[17] Newer insufflation systems offer warmed (35° C) and humidified (95%) gas, which may prevent such complications. Furthermore, these features reduce lens condensation and perhaps decrease postoperative pain.[21,22]

Lens fogging during initial laparoscopy occurs because of a temperature and humidity difference between the abdominal cavity and the lens surface. A common remedy for lens fogging includes soaking the lens tip in a warm solution before introducing it into the abdominal cavity. Moreover, various antifogging kits are commercially available, such as Fog Reduction and Elimination Device (FRED; Covidien/Medtronic,

Minneapolis, Minn.), which uses isopropyl alcohol and surfactant mixture, or Clearify (Covidien/Medtronic, Minneapolis, Minn.), which offers a lens-warming hub containing defogging surfactant solution.

New Trocar Designs

Contemporary trocars use trap door valves that seal around laparoscopic instruments to prevent leakage of pneumoperitoneum. More recently, valveless trocars have been introduced, circumventing gas volume loss inherent in traditional trocars. AirSeal (SurgiQuest, Milford, Conn.) offers an insufflation system that allows a stable pneumoperitoneum to be maintained even in settings of aggressive suctioning and large open abdominal channels. Specialized access ports contain a series of high-pressure nozzles that direct CO_2 gas downward into the cannula, creating a horizontal air barrier (referred to as a vortex) and maintaining desired intra-abdominal pressure (Fig. 8-2). The continuous recirculation of CO_2 filters any surgical smoke through its external unit and allows for continuous smoke evacuation. Clinical observations suggest less fluctuation in intra-abdominal pressures in response to leakage or suction, less laparoscope lens smearing, and reduced overall CO_2 gas consumption. Furthermore, the valveless design aids in specimen and needle extraction[23-25] (Fig. 8-3).

A valveless trocar not only reduces the CO_2 lost during surgery, but it also allows a pop-off mechanism during increases in the intra-abdominal pressures such as during diaphragm movements of breathing or unexpected abdominal wall contractions. This recirculation of CO_2 results in a lower absorption intraoperatively. Consequently, this system may offer an advantage in patients with compromised cardiopulmonary functions.[25]

The vortex mechanism results in a better maintenance of pneumoperitoneum despite potential leakages. Whereas standard insufflators compensate for pressure loss by delivering boluses of gas, resulting in higher peak and lower trough pressures, the valveless trocar system recycles CO_2, resulting in less variation in the intra-abdominal pressure. Although this is beneficial in reducing variations in intra-abdominal pressure, it may mask intraoperative signs of an iatrogenic pneumothorax. The typical clinical features of such pneumothorax include increased end-tidal CO_2, diaphragm billowing, and a blunting of peak airway pressures. In a series of 850 transperitoneal laparoscopic cases using a valveless trocar system, 10 patients (1.2%) had pneumothorax, eight of which were delayed in diagnosis,[26] likely because of the lack of diaphragmatic billowing and peak airway pressure blunting associated with the valveless trocar system's vortex.

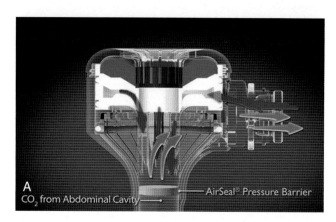

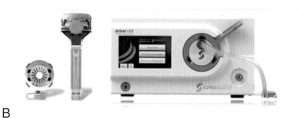

Figure 8-2. A, The AirSeal access port invisible air barrier system. **B,** A series of high-pressure nozzles directs CO_2 gas downward into the cannula, creating a horizontal air barrier (referred to as a vortex) that maintains desired intra-abdominal pressure. *(Copyright © 2015 SurgiQuest Inc., Milford, Conn.)*

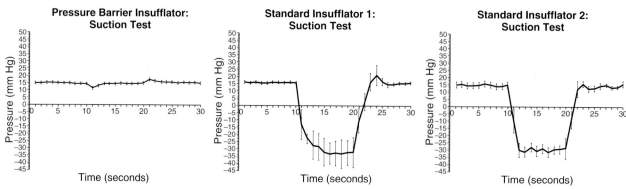

Figure 8-3. Variation of pressure based on aggressive suction test in vitro. Leftmost graph demonstrates minimal variation (AirSeal) compared with two standard insufflators. *(From Nepple KG, Kallogjeri D, Bhayani SB. Benchtop evaluation of pressure barrier insufflator and standard insufflator systems. Surg Endosc. 2013;27:333-338.)*

COMPLICATIONS

Pneumoperitoneum has been demonstrated to cause numerous alterations in normal physiology. Specific complications and the anesthetic considerations of laparoscopy are covered in further detail elsewhere in the text. General problems arising from insufflation and pneumoperitoneum are described here.

Increased intra-abdominal pressures have been associated with reduced venous flow in femoral vessels, liver, and kidney, as well as impaired cardiopulmonary function.[27] Hypercapnia or hypercarbia, defined as end tidal CO_2 levels above 45 mm Hg, may be observed and are caused by constant absorption of CO_2 during insufflation, leading to systemic acidosis. Accordingly, constant monitoring of cardiovascular parameters is crucial during any laparoscopic surgery. Most commonly, pneumoperitoneum is maintained at pressures of 12 to 15 mm Hg. Insufflation pressures of 10 to 12 mm Hg even for extended durations seem to have minimal clinical impact on intraoperative acid-base balance.[28] A 22% mean increase in the insufflated volume is noted when elevating the intra-abdominal pressure from 15 mm Hg to 20 mm Hg.[29] A recent study by Modi and colleagues reported on perioperative outcomes in 550 robotic prostatectomy patients in whom pneumoperitoneum pressures of 20 mm Hg were used. The results suggested no difference in outcomes when compared with matched cohorts using pressures of 15 mm Hg.[30]

Postoperative abdominal and referred shoulder pain caused by localized peritoneal irritation can be minimized by use of low insufflation rate, low-pressure pneumoperitoneum, and complete desufflation before port removal.[17,31] Subcutaneous and preperitoneal emphysema can be problematic with improper insufflation techniques. If significant, it can lead to hypercapnia necessitating increase in minute ventilation. Pneumomediastinum, pneumopericardium, and pneumothorax are all potential complications because the fascial planes allow for an extensive spread of insufflated gas. Gas embolism is a potential grave risk with improper intravascular insufflation. This can result in reduction of pulmonary blood flow and can progress to cardiovascular collapse. Incidence of gas embolism is lowest with use of CO_2 owing to its high solubility and can be minimized by routine aspiration of the Veress needle before insufflation is commenced. If recognized early, pneumoperitoneum should be immediately released, followed by left lateral decubitus (right side up) steep Trendelenburg position to prevent gas entry into the pulmonary artery. Aggressive cardiopulmonary resuscitation can be followed by aspiration of gas through central line access.

Transient pneumoperitoneum-related oliguria is commonly observed and may be more pronounced with higher intra-abdominal pressure and long case duration. It is often attributed to compression of renal vasculature and parenchyma as well as decreased venous return and cardiac output, with further contributions from antidiuretic hormones and plasma renin.

REFERENCES

1. Navez B, Navez J. Laparoscopy in the acute abdomen. *Best Pract Res Clin Gastroenterol.* 2014;28:3–17.
2. McGillicuddy JW, Villar JJ, Rohan VS, et al. Is cirrhosis a contraindication to laparoscopic cholecystectomy? *Am Surg.* 2015;81:52–55.
3. Neudecker J, Sauerland S, Neugebauer E, et al. The European Association for Endoscopic Surgery clinical practice guideline on the pneumoperitoneum for laparoscopic surgery. *Surg Endosc.* 2002;16:1121–1143.
4. Catheline JM, Bihan H, Le Quang T, et al. Preoperative cardiac and pulmonary assessment in bariatric surgery. *Obes Surg.* 2008; 18(3):271–277.
5. Makarov DV, Kainth D, Link RE, Kavoussi LR. Physiologic changes during helium insufflation in high-risk patients during laparoscopic renal procedures. *Urology.* 2007;70:35–37.
6. Tsereteli Z, Terry ML, Bowers SP, et al. Prospective randomized clinical trial comparing nitrous oxide and carbon dioxide pneumoperitoneum for laparoscopic surgery. *J Am Coll Surg.* 2002;195:173–179.
7. Jung KT, Kim SH, Kim JW, So KY. Bradycardia during laparoscopic surgery due to high flow rate of CO_2 insufflation. *Korean J Anesthesiol.* 2013;65:276–277.
8. Myles PS. Bradyarrhythmias and laparoscopy: a prospective study of heart rate changes with laparoscopy. *Aust N Z J Obstet Gynaecol.* 1991;31:171–173.
9. Cho EJ, Min TK. Cardiac arrest after gas insufflation for laparoscopic surgery: two case reports. *Korean J Anesthesiol.* 2005;49:712–715.
10. Dhoste K, Lacoste L, Karayan J, Lehuede MS, Thomas D, Fusciardi J. Haemodynamic and ventilatory changes during laparoscopic cholecystectomy in elderly ASA III patients. *Can J Anaesth.* 1996;43: 783–788.
11. Jacobs VR, Morrison Jr JE. The real intraabdominal pressure during laparoscopy: comparison of different insufflators. *J Minim Invasive Gynecol.* 2007;14:103–107.
12. Jacobs VR, Morrison Jr JE, Mundhenke C, Golombeck K, Jonat W. Intraoperative evaluation of laparoscopic insufflation technique for quality control in the OR. *JSLS: Journal of the Society of Laparoendoscopic Surgeons / Society of Laparoendoscopic Surgeons.* 2000;4(3):189–195.
13. Daskalakis M, Scheffel O, Weiner RA. High flow insufflation for the maintenance of the pneumoperitoneum during bariatric surgery. *Obesity facts.* 2009;2(Suppl 1):37–40.
14. Ott DE. Microbial colonization of laparoscopic gas delivery systems: a qualitative analysis. *JSLS.* 1997;1:325–329.
15. Air embolism and CO_2 insufflators: the need for pre-use purging of tubing. *Health Devices.* 1996;25:214–215.
16. High-flow laparoscopic insufflators. *Health Devices.* 1995;24: 252–285.
17. Jacobs VR, Morrison Jr JE, Kiechle M. Twenty-five simple ways to increase insufflation performance and patient safety in laparoscopy. *J Am Assoc Gynecol Laparosc.* 2004;11:410–423.
18. Menes T, Spivak H. Laparoscopy: searching for the proper insufflation gas. *Surg Endosc.* 2000;14:1050–1056.
19. Neuhaus SJ, Gupta A, Watson DI. Helium and other alternative insufflation gases for laparoscopy. *Surg Endosc.* 2001;15:553–560.
20. Rammohan A, Manimaran AB, Manohar RR, Naidu RM. Nitrous oxide for pneumoperitoneum: no laughing matter this! A prospective single blind case controlled study. *Int J Surg.* 2011;9:173–176.
21. Klugsberger B, Schreiner M, Rothe A, Haas D, Oppelt P, Shamiyeh A. Warmed, humidified carbon dioxide insufflation versus standard carbon dioxide in laparoscopic cholecystectomy: a double-blinded randomized controlled trial. *Surg Endosc.* 2014;28:2656–2660.
22. Herrmann A, De Wilde RL. Insufflation with humidified and heated carbon dioxide in short-term laparoscopy: a double-blinded randomized controlled trial. *Biomed Res Int.* 2015;2015:412618.
23. Nepple KG, Kallogjeri D, Bhayani SB. Benchtop evaluation of pressure barrier insufflator and standard insufflator systems. *Surg Endosc.* 2013;27:333–338.
24. Herati AS, Atalla MA, Rais-Bahrami S, Andonian S, Vira MA, Kavoussi LR. A new valve-less trocar for urologic laparoscopy: initial evaluation. *J Endourol.* 2009;23:1535–1539.
25. Herati AS, Andonian S, Rais-Bahrami S, et al. Use of the valve-less trocar system reduces carbon dioxide absorption during laparoscopy when compared with standard trocars. *Urology.* 2011; 77:1126–1132.
26. Hillelsohn JH, Friedlander JI, Bagadiya N, et al. Masked pneumothorax: risk of valveless trocar systems. *J Urol.* 2013;189:955–959.
27. Nguyen NT, Wolfe BM. The physiologic effects of pneumoperitoneum in the morbidly obese. *Ann Surg.* 2005;241:219–226.
28. Meininger D, Byhahn C, Bueck M, et al. Effects of prolonged pneumoperitoneum on hemodynamics and acid-base balance during totally endoscopic robot-assisted radical prostatectomies. *World J Surg.* 2002;26:1423–1427.
29. Adams JB, Moore RG, Micali S, Marco AP, Kavoussi LR. Laparoscopic genitourinary surgery utilizing 20 mm Hg intra-abdominal pressure. *J Laparoendosc Adv Surg Tech A.* 1999;9:131–134.
30. Modi PK, Kwon YS, Patel N, et al. Safety of robot-assisted radical prostatectomy with pneumoperitoneum of 20 mm Hg: a study of 751 patients. *J Endourol.* 2015;29:1148–1151.
31. Donatsky AM, Bjerrum F, Gogenur I. Surgical techniques to minimize shoulder pain after laparoscopic cholecystectomy. A systematic review. *Surg Endosc.* 2013;27:2275–2282.

9 Ports and Establishing Access into the Peritoneal Cavity

Daoud Dajani, Mohamed A. Atalla

For laparoscopic surgery, insufflation of the peritoneal cavity and establishment of entry ports must initially be completed. To achieve insufflation, the surgeon must first gain safe access to the peritoneal cavity. Several techniques of gaining access to the peritoneal cavity have been described involving various devices designed to minimize entry-related injury and complications. After pneumoperitoneum has been established, ports of entry and reentry are needed to allow retention of intraperitoneal gas and swift instrument exchange. To that end, different types of trocars have been introduced and continue to be modified to improve ease of placement and use. In this chapter, we review and describe the various available techniques and devices for accessing the peritoneum and maintaining access ports during laparoscopic surgery.

ESTABLISHING ACCESS TO THE PERITONEAL CAVITY

Veress Needle

In 1938, Hungarian surgeon Janos Veress invented a spring-loaded needle that consisted of a beveled-point cannula with incising capability (VER-FLOW; Sterylab, Milan, Italy) (Fig. 9-1). Inside the outer cannula, a blunt-tipped inner stylet would spring forward when encountered with a sudden decrease of tissue resistance. The decrease in tissue resistance correlates with entry into the peritoneal cavity. The deployment of the blunt inner stylet renders the needle into a blunt-tipped device that is safe to come into contact with intraperitoneal viscera. Although Veress did not use the device for that purpose, the needle quickly gained popularity as the preferred method for establishing pneumoperitoneum. The modern-day Veress needle has an external diameter of 2 mm and comes in varying lengths from 12 to 15 cm.

Points of Insertion

In the virgin abdomen, the umbilicus is an excellent site for needle insertion owing to the short distance between skin and peritoneum. Alternative points of insertion could be used after failure to establish safe access (after three attempts), in extremely thin or obese patients, in the presence of an umbilical hernia, or in the patient with prior midline or periumbilical incisions with expected midline adhesions. These alternative points of insertion can be used routinely based on surgeon comfort and preference.

Palmer's point (Fig. 9-2) is a point on the midclavicular line below the left subcostal margin that can be used as a point of Veress needle insertion. A mirror image point of Palmer's point on the right side also can be used. These points should be avoided with known hepatosplenomegaly, prior left or right upper quadrant surgery, or portal hypertension. Gastric decompression before peritoneal access is essential to help reduce the risk of gastric and duodenal injury.

An uncommonly used point of insertion is the ninth or tenth intercostal space along the anterior axillary line. This point has the advantage of the parietal peritoneum's natural attachment to the lower surface of the rib. Entry near the lower surface of the rib should be avoided, however, to avoid injury to the neurovascular structures. Pneumothorax, as well as injury to the stomach, liver, or spleen, has been reported with this approach. In the gynecologic literature, alternative access points include transuterine and trans–cul de sac paths, both with good results.

Insertion Techniques

Although some authors advocate lifting or stabilizing the anterior abdominal wall (such as with towel clips or with a manual rectus abdominis grasp) before Veress needle insertion, others downplay the necessity of the maneuver. Some surgeons prefer a skin incision before needle insertion. Angling of the needle at the time of insertion to 45 degrees in patients with a body mass index (BMI) of less than 30 kg/m^2 can help avoid major vascular injury.

Safe placement of a Veress needle into the peritoneal cavity can be confirmed by the following series of maneuvers:

- Measurement of the skin-to-peritoneum distance on preoperative imaging to help estimate the distance of needle advancement at the point of entry.
- Aspiration through the Veress needle after placement to confirm absence of vascular or visceral injury before insufflation.
- Performance of the saline drop test, which allows a drop of saline to passively pass through the lumen of the needle. A quickly disappearing saline drop confirms correct placement.
- Confirmation of a starting pressure of 9 mm Hg or lower at entry to confirm intraperitoneal placement.
- Other less commonly used maneuvers include reliance on the "hiss" sound test to confirm correct placement and the use of ultrasonography to identify possible adhesions before needle placement attempts.

Despite executing the safety maneuvers, complications of Veress needle placement may still occur. Known complications include abdominal wall bleeding; injury to major or minor vessels, the gastrointestinal tract, the liver, the spleen; and extraperitoneal insufflation. Those complications are rare and are reported to occur in about 1% of laparoscopic procedures.

Enhancements to a standard Veress needle have been described. These include a fitted sensor to detect the position of the tip of the needle as it enters the peritoneal cavity and a wider optical Veress needle that allows a semirigid minilaparoscope, allowing insertion of the needle under direct vision.

Open Access: Hasson Technique

Harrith M. Hasson first described this technique in 1971. The open technique (Fig. 9-3) is arguably the safest in the setting of prior abdominal surgery and adhesions. It can also be useful in pregnant patients or in those with a short distance between

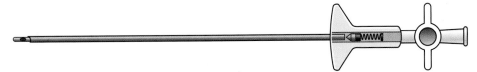

Figure 9-1. Veress laparoscopic insufflation needle.

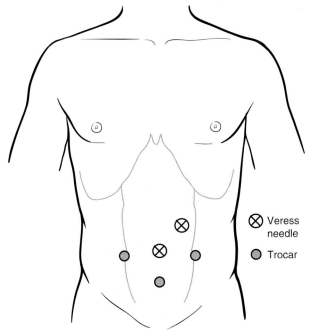

Figure 9-2. Veress needle insertion sites including the umbilicus and Palmer's point.

⊗ Veress needle

● Trocar

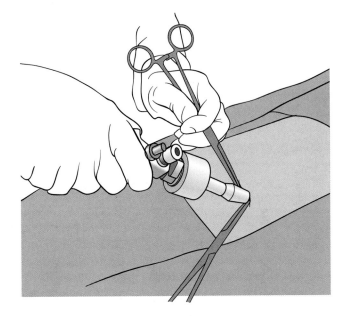

Figure 9-3. The Hasson technique. The Hasson trocar is placed through the incision after the fascia and peritoneum are incised in a controlled fashion.

the anterior abdominal wall and spine, such as children and extremely thin adults.

The steps of the Hasson technique are as follows:

- A skin incision is made in the desired location.
- The subcutaneous tissues are bluntly separated with adequate hemostasis.
- The fascia is incised, and stay sutures are placed on the divided fascial edges.
- The peritoneum is grasped and incised sharply.
- The surgeon's finger is used to confirm bowel safety.
- The Hasson trocar is placed through the incision, and the stay sutures are used to secure the port in place.
- The pneumoperitoneum is established through the port.
- The fascia is closed when the surgery is finished.

A balloon trocar can be used with the open technique as an alternative to the Hasson trocar. After trocar placement, the designated amount of air is injected into the internal retention balloon. An external sliding foam pad is positioned to maintain an airtight seal at the port site. The Hasson technique is generally considered a safe option with a complication incidence as low as 0.2%. However, its universal use is limited by the time required to accomplish access, particularly in obese patients.

Direct Trocar Entry

Direct trocar entry was first described in 1978 by Dingfelder. It consists of trocar entry before peritoneal insufflation. The technique relies on the translucency of the dilating tip, allowing trocar introduction under direct vision with a laparoscope in place. The safety of the technique requires sound familiarity

with abdominal wall anatomy and comfort with the appearance of each layer when viewed through an optical trocar and a gasless peritoneal cavity.

Some reported complications include bowel injury related to entry in 0.11% of patients and vascular injury in 0.01% of patients, with other series reporting higher complication rates. Other studies showed fewer complications with direct trocar entry than with Veress needle entry, indicating that direct trocar entry is a safe alternative to Veress needle insertion and perhaps is an underused technique. Its advantages also include the short time required for completion and the avoidance of complications related to blind insufflation. Yet, a survey of urologic surgeons revealed it is the least commonly used entry technique in urologic laparoscopic surgery.

The steps for direct trocar entry are as follows:

- The skin is incised below the umbilicus or in the subcostal region.
- The abdominal wall is lifted with clamps or with the surgeon's hand.
- The optical trocar is inserted under direct vision toward the pelvis with a laparoscope in place. Each layer is identified in sequence under vision.
- Insufflation is started through the trocar.
- The blade of the trocar is removed, and the laparoscope is reintroduced.

Indirect Laparoscopic Access

Indirect access into the peritoneal cavity is typically used for secondary trocar placement after peritoneal insufflation has

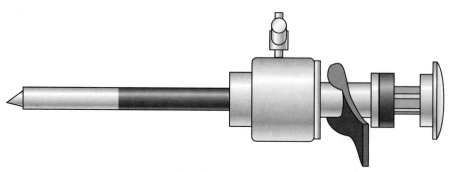

Figure 9-4. Reusable metal trocars.

been accomplished by one of the aforementioned techniques. A variety of disposable and reusable trocars can be used for that purpose.

LAPAROSCOPIC TROCARS

A laparoscopic trocar (also known as a port) is a hollow cylindric device that facilitates repeated access into the insufflated peritoneal cavity while maintaining a seal via an external valve mechanism. Most trocars also have a connector device for attachment to insufflation tubing. Each trocar is constructed of an outer cannula (or sheath) and an inner obturator for initial placement. Trocars typically fall into two categories: cutting (axial) and dilating (radial). Cutting trocars have a blade that is used to pass through the fascial layer. Cutting trocars have fallen out of favor because of increased risk of visceral or vascular injury. They also result in a larger fascial defect and thus are more likely to require fascial closure. Dilating trocars typically include a blunt-tipped obturator that allows insertion while resulting in a fascial defect that is smaller than half the diameter of the outer cannula. This allows avoidance of fascial closure in most situations. However, we recommend digitally examining the fascial defect of each trocar site (even those belonging to a dilating trocar) at the end of the procedure to assess the need for fascial closure.

Reusable Metal Trocars

Reusable metal trocars (Girish Surgical Works, Mumbai, India) (Fig. 9-4) have a stainless steel trumpet valve with an insufflation port. The valve ensures no gas loss after insufflation. The ports have easily detachable sleeves for expeditious replacement in case of damage or soiling. These ports are relatively inexpensive and are considered economical because they can be sterilized and reused.

Reusable Screw Trocars

Reusable screw trocars (Ackermann Instrumente Gmbh, Rietheim-Weilheim, Germany) (Fig. 9-5) are similar to the metal trocars but in addition are threaded on the surface of the outer cannula. Placement involves a twisting mechanism to penetrate tissue, eventually reaching the peritoneal cavity. The external threads also offer added stability, making the trocar more immobile during use.

Disposable Smooth and Ridged Trocars

Disposable smooth and ridged trocars (Thomson Surgicals, Bengaluru, India; Guangzhou T.K. Medical Instrument Co., Guangzhou, China) (Figs. 9-6 and 9-7) have similar insertion techniques and advantages to their reusable counterparts. As

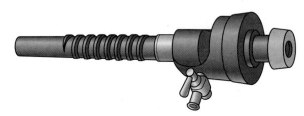

Figure 9-5. Reusable screw trocar with threading on the surface of the outer cannula.

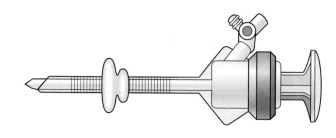

Figure 9-6. Disposable smooth trocars.

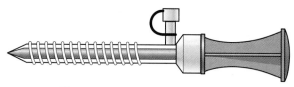

Figure 9-7. Disposable ridged trocars.

the name implies, they are single-use instruments and theoretically avoid the limitations of reprocessing and cross-infection.

Disposable Visual Trocars

Disposable visual trocars were introduced in the early 1990s and are very popular in urologic surgery. They are versatile for use as primary or secondary ports. The key feature of these trocars is the transparent distal tip found on the hollow obturator, which allows direct visualization of the entry process when used with a 0-degree laparoscope. Examples include the Visiport optical trocar (Tyco–United States Surgical, Norwalk, Conn.) and the Endopath Optiview optical trocar (Ethicon Endo-Surgery, Cincinnati, Ohio).

The Visiport (Fig. 9-8) is equipped with an internal blade that is advanced about 1 mm with every trigger squeeze, followed by retraction of the blade. The Visiport should be placed only into an insufflated abdomen (e.g., by Veress needle) to avoid the high risk of organ injury.

The Endopath Optiview trocar (Fig. 9-9) has a transparent outer cannula as well as a hollow obturator with a transparent tip. It can be placed either after preinsufflation with a Veress needle or with the gasless entry technique. When the trocar handle is twisted after the laparoscope has been introduced, the hydrophobic trocar tip dissects through the tissue layers under direct optical vision. Placing this trocar requires a certain amount of force and thus requires caution to avoid overshooting the entry motion into the peritoneal cavity.

Hasson Trocars

The Hasson trocar (Kii; Applied Medical, Rancho Santa Margarita, Calif.) (Fig. 9-10) consists of an outer cannula fitted with a cone-shaped sleeve, a blunt obturator, and occasionally a second sleeve to which stay sutures can be secured. This trocar is used during open laparoscopic entry as described earlier in this chapter.

Balloon Trocars

Balloon trocars (US Surgical, Norwalk, Conn.) are used mainly for retroperitoneoscopic surgery. A dilating balloon is first used to dilate the working space. A structural balloon trocar (Pajunk, EMT, Warriewood, Australia) (Fig. 9-11) is then placed to help maintain the seal. This balloon trocar is equipped with an inflatable balloon donut attached to the outer cannula that allows a sustainable seal when secured in place.

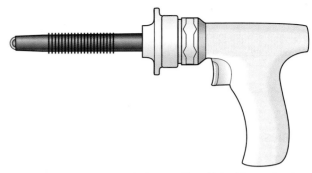

Figure 9-8. Visiport Plus optical trocar (Tyco–United States Surgical, Norwalk, Conn.).

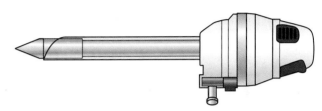

Figure 9-9. Endopath Xcel trocar with Optiview (Ethicon Endo-Surgery, Cincinnati, Ohio).

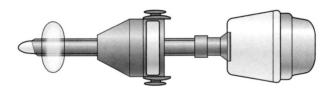

Figure 9-10. Kii balloon blunt-tip system (Applied Medical, Rancho Santa Margarita, Calif.) can be used for the Hasson technique.

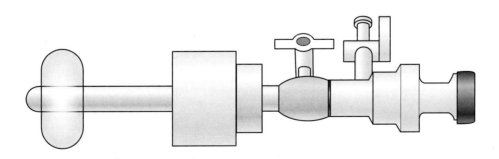

Figure 9-11. Blunt-tipped balloon trocar.

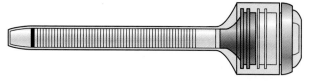

Figure 9-12. AirSeal trocar (SurgiQuest, Milford, Conn.).

Valveless Trocars

The AirSeal (SurgiQuest, Milford, Conn.) (Fig. 9-12) is a valveless trocar system that has the advantages of achieving a stable pneumoperitoneum (in spite of smoke evacuation) and smudge-free laparoscope introduction. A series of high-pressure nozzles direct the insufflation gas downward into the cannula until the desired pressure is achieved (Fig. 9-13). Once equilibrium is reached, a horizontal air barrier is created within the cannula with a continuous-flow circuit evacuating and filtering intraperitoneal gas, giving superior vision.

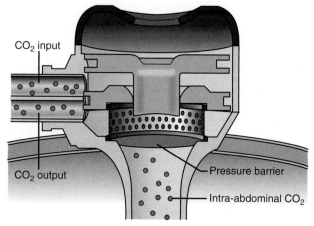

Figure 9-13. The AirSeal Dynamic Pressure system (SurgiQuest, Milford, Conn.) for smoke evacuation.

10 Retroperitoneal Access

Peter A. Caputo, Jihad H. Kaouk

The urologist's approach to retroperitoneal surgery has traditionally been through a flank or posterior incision to avoid violation of the peritoneal cavity. This approach also provides the most anatomically direct route to the organs of interest in the retroperitoneum. It was by adherence to this concept that urologists first founded retroperitoneoscopic surgery. Retroperitoneoscopic surgery was first described in 1979 and was then used only in the treatment of urolithiasis. In the early 1990s, transabdominal laparoscopy was first used for radical nephrectomy, which broadened the urologic scope of laparoscopic surgery and drew interest to the undertaking of more complex surgical procedures using laparoscopic technologies. Laparoscopic surgery was slowly adopted as a mainstay of treatment for both benign and malignant renal pathology. Now laparoscopy has become an essential technique in the modern urologist's armamentarium.

In a transabdominal approach, the anatomic planes of dissection are similar to open surgery, making this approach easier for the novice laparoscopic surgeon to overcome the learning curve of laparoscopy. The retroperitoneoscopic approach has a steeper learning curve and has been slow to be adopted by practitioners owing to the small working space it affords as well as the lack of easily recognized anatomic landmarks. However, retroperitoneoscopic surgery minimizes the occurrence of adjacent organ injury because there is little need for retraction or mobilization of adjacent organs. Furthermore, minimal or no manipulation of the peritoneal contents results in an earlier return of bowel function and shorter convalescence than with the transabdominal laparoscopic approach. The disadvantage of the technique is a higher incidence of injury to the great vessels or the renal hilum.

INDICATIONS AND CONTRAINDICATIONS

Retroperitoneoscopic surgery has been used for a vast spectrum of operative indications for both benign and malignant diseases of the adrenal gland, kidney, and urinary collecting system. Adrenalectomy, simple and radical nephrectomy, partial nephrectomy, nephroureterectomy, renal cyst decortication, renal ablative therapy, pyeloplasty, lymph node dissection, pyelolithotomy, and renal biopsy may be performed via a retroperitoneoscopic approach. In the setting of prior abdominal surgery, particularly ventral hernia repair involving mesh, the retroperitoneal approach offers a more facile and direct route to the operative area of interest. In the case of partial nephrectomy or cyst decortication, retroperitoneoscopic surgery also facilitates a more direct approach to very posterior tumors or cysts.

Contraindications specific to retroperitoneoscopic surgery are dense fibrosis of the retroperitoneal and perinephric fat as would be expected from recent infection, radiation, or recent surgery of the retroperitoneum or kidney.

PATIENT PREOPERATIVE EVALUATION AND PREPARATION

Thorough preoperative evaluation is paramount before retroperitoneoscopic surgery. History and physical examination should be directed toward evaluation of cardiopulmonary status and should elucidate the presence or history of coagulopathy, abdominal infection, or previous abdominal surgery. Review of radiographic images is also essential in surgical planning and will help distinguish the most ideal surgical approach.

Traditional bowel preparation is not necessary before retroperitoneoscopic surgery. A clear liquid diet the day before surgery will suffice.

PATIENT POSITIONING AND OPERATING ROOM CONFIGURATION

The patient is placed in the lateral decubitus position with attention to padding of all pressure points, in particular the feet, ankles, and knees. An axillary roll is used to prevent compression nerve injury and should be placed at the level of the areola in men or just inferior to the true axilla in women. The top arm should be gently supported at a 90-degree angle to the thorax and should not be moved too far laterally or abducted above the head. The operative table should be flexed to expose the ipsilateral abdomen. The kidney rest should be left in a neutral position to help avoid postoperative rhabdomyolysis. The kidney rest is to be raised only in select cases in which it is necessary to further expose the abdomen and retroperitoneum. The patient is secured to the table using silk tape and belt restraints.

Contrary to transabdominal laparoscopy, during retroperitoneoscopic surgery the surgeon stands facing the patient's back. If a robotic surgical system is being used, the robotic system is docked over the patient's forehead for the retroperitoneoscopic approach rather than from the patient's back or shoulder for the transabdominal approach.

CREATION OF RETROPERITONEAL WORKING SPACE AND TROCAR PLACEMENT (SEE VIDEO 10-1)

The foundation of retroperitoneoscopic surgery is based on the creation of an adequate working space within the retroperitoneum. The following section outlines trocar placement for both retroperitoneoscopic and robotic-assisted retroperitoneoscopic approaches.

Initially, a 1.5-cm horizontal incision is made for the first port. The incision is carried down to the level of the flank musculature. The flank musculature is split bluntly with the aid of S-shaped retractors until the lumbodorsal fascia is visualized. The lumbodorsal fascia is incised, allowing entry into the retroperitoneal space. Alternatively, visual laparoscopic entry to the retroperitoneum may be used. A 12-mm trocar with a visual obturator and laparoscope may be guided through the subcutaneous tissue, flank musculature, and lumbodorsal fascia into the retroperitoneum. Either method can safely establish a tract to the retroperitoneum and is used based on surgeon preference.

Next, blunt finger dissection is used between the kidney and along the posterior abdominal wall musculature (Fig. 10-1). The retroperitoneal working space is then created with balloon dilation by placing the balloon just ventral to the posterior abdominal musculature. Balloon dilation displaces the Gerota fascia and the kidney anteromedially

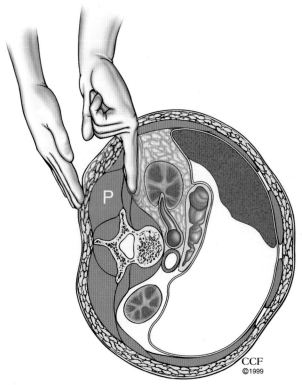

Figure 10-1. Blunt finger dissection between the kidney and along the posterior abdominal wall musculature (*P*). *(Reprinted with permission, Cleveland Clinic Center for Medical Art & Photography © 2015. All rights reserved.)*

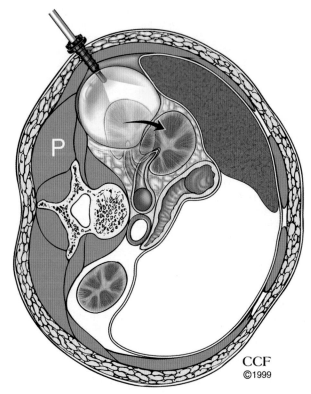

Figure 10-2. Balloon dilation displaces Gerota fascia and the kidney anteromedially. *P,* Posterior abdominal wall musculature. *(Reprinted with permission, Cleveland Clinic Center for Medical Art & Photography © 2015. All rights reserved.)*

(Fig. 10-2). The balloon dilator is removed and a 12-mm trocar is placed through the established tract. Pneumoretroperitoneum is achieved by insufflation with carbon dioxide to a pressure of 15 mm Hg. The remaining trocars should be placed under direct vision when possible; their position will vary slightly depending on the particular surgery being performed.

TROCAR PLACEMENT FOR THE RETROPERITONEOSCOPIC APPROACH

The aforementioned incision for the initial trocar is made just below the tip of the 12th rib. The second trocar is placed posteriorly below the 12th rib at the lateral border of the paraspinal muscle. Using the second placed trocar, further blunt dissection may be performed to clear space for the anterior third trocar. This is performed using a laparoscopic Kittner dissector to sweep the peritoneum medially, allowing the third trocar to enter the retroperitoneum unobstructed. The third trocar is placed just below the 11th rib between the midaxillary and anterior axillary lines (Fig. 10-3).

TROCAR PLACEMENT FOR THE ROBOTIC-ASSISTED RETROPERITONEOSCOPIC APPROACH

In the case of robotic-assisted surgery, the initial incision and trocar are placed 1 to 2 cm above the iliac crest in the midaxillary line. The second trocar (8-mm robotic trocar) is placed in the posterior-axillary line at a level 2 cm cephalad to the initial trocar site. The third trocar (8-mm robotic trocar) is placed in the anterior-axillary line at a level 1 cm cephalad to the initial trocar site. An additional 12-mm assistant trocar is placed 4 to 5 cm cephalad to the third trocar in the anterior-axillary line (Fig. 10-4).

If trocar placement under direct retroperitoneoscopic vision is not possible, the bimanual method can help guide the trocar. For the bimanual method, the finger of the surgeon's nondominant hand is inserted into the working space through the initial trocar site. Then with the dominant hand, the surgeon places the trocar through the abdominal wall into the retroperitoneum using the finger previously placed into the working space as a guide.

Having now developed a good retroperitoneal working space with careful placement of all trocars, we have set up our retroperitoneoscopic case for a successful surgery. From this point the primary procedure, whether adrenalectomy or partial nephrectomy, may be undertaken.

POSTOPERATIVE MANAGEMENT

Postoperative management for retroperitoneoscopic surgery focuses primarily on pain control and ensuring hemodynamic stability. Retroperitoneoscopic surgery avoids bowel manipulation and colon mobilization; this results in fewer gastrointestinal complications and allows for early feeding with lower rates of ileus. Patients may start a regular diet immediately after an uncomplicated retroperitoneoscopic surgery.

COMPLICATIONS

Unique intraoperative complications experienced during retroperitoneoscopic surgery exist. These intraoperative complications are associated with balloon dilator malfunction or failure to progress in surgery. Balloon dilator malfunction is quite rare since the introduction of balloon dilators manufactured specifically for retroperitoneoscopic surgery. Failure

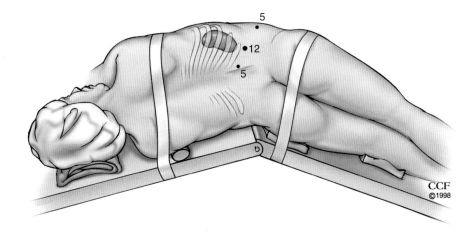

Figure 10-3. Trocar placement for the retroperitoneoscopic approach. *(Reprinted with permission, Cleveland Clinic Center for Medical Art & Photography © 2015. All rights reserved.)*

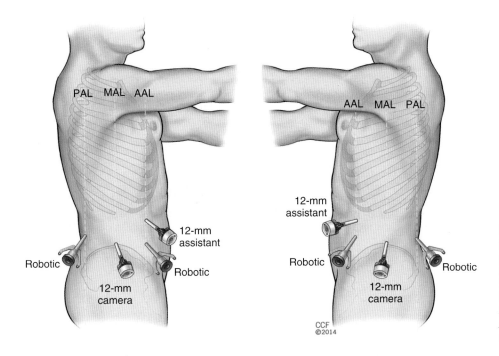

Figure 10-4. Trocar placement for the robotic-assisted retroperitoneoscopic approach. *AAL,* Anterior axillary line; *MAL,* midaxillary line; *PAL,* posterior axillary line. *(Reprinted with permission, Cleveland Clinic Center for Medical Art & Photography © 2015. All rights reserved.)*

to progress is usually a result of surgeon inexperience and secondary to inability to visualize landmarks or diminished working space from a violation in the peritoneum. A laceration of the peritoneum results in gas escape into the peritoneal cavity, effectively reducing the retroperitoneal working space. Inadvertent peritoneotomy does not necessitate conversion to open or transabdominal laparoscopic surgery. If working space is compromised, an additional port can be placed to aid with retraction of the peritoneum until the surgery is completed.

There is a slightly higher rate of subcutaneous emphysema experienced after the retroperitoneoscopic surgery. To prevent air leakage around the trocar and into the soft tissue structures, the surgeon must create an incision just wide enough to accommodate the trocar and ensure the trocar is not withdrawn during insufflation.

Postoperative hemorrhage after retroperitoneoscopic surgery can usually be managed conservatively because the hemorrhage is confined to the retroperitoneum and will create a tamponade.

TIPS AND TRICKS

- *Creation of retroperitoneal working space:* It is vital that the surgeon use the balloon in the correct space. To do this, blunt finger dissection is important. The dissection should be anterior to the psoas muscle and its enveloping fascia. The surgeon must be able to palpate the psoas. The balloon is then placed precisely into the location anterior to the psoas muscle fascia and posterior to the Gerota fascia.

- *Anatomic landmarks:* After creation of the retroperitoneal working space, the psoas muscle is the most important visual landmark. Once visualized, the psoas muscle should be positioned in horizontal orientation on the monitor throughout the remainder of the case.

- *Vascular identification:* To identify vascular structures, a search for pulsations along the medial aspect of the psoas muscle will be of great aid. Gentle undulating pulsations are characteristic of venous structures and likely represent the renal vein or inferior vena cava. Sharp bounding pulsations are characteristic of arterial structures and represent the renal artery or aorta.

11 Exiting the Abdomen and Closure Techniques

Bijan W. Salari, Debora Moore, Robert Moore

Laparoscopic surgery has reduced overall complication rates and minimized postsurgical recovery time; however, attention must be paid to the closure of laparoscopic ports on completion of the operative procedure. The rate of port site complications after conventional laparoscopic surgery is approximately 21 per 100,000 cases.[1] Complications include infection, dehiscence, trocar site hernia (TSH) of small bowel, entrapment of omentum, and incarcerated Richter hernia.[2] The incidence of TSH is 0.23% at 10-mm port sites and 1.9% at 12-mm port sites. This incidence increases to 6.3% for obese patients, defined as having a body mass index (BMI) greater than 30.[3] The current recommendation is that 10- and 12-mm port sites require fascial closure in all patients to prevent TSH. In children, port sites larger than 5 mm require fascial closure.[4] Several closure techniques have been described to reduce TSH complications, including hand closure and closure device techniques.

HAND CLOSURE

Hand closure of fascia offers advantages for the nonobese patient with minimal subcutaneous fat. This technique incorporates the fascia, but not the peritoneum, into the closure, and it may potentially result in increased procedure time, wound infection, wound dehiscence, and ascitic fluid leak when compared with other closure techniques.[4]

For prevention of injury to the underlying viscera, only the anterior fascia is reapproximated. To perform this closure, use two Army-Navy retractors to retract the skin and two Kocher clamps on either side of the fascia to facilitate exposure. Close the fascial layer with a 2-0 polyglycolic acid suture. A UR-6 tapered needle allows easy rotation to catch the fascia. Care should be taken to ensure no bowel is involved during passage of the suture. Passing the suture under direct laparoscopic visualization from an adjacent trocar is paramount.

To date, two needles have been designed specifically for closure of trocar ports: the TN needle (Ethicon Endo-Surgery, Cincinnati, Ohio) and the J needle (Ethicon Endo-Surgery). The TN needle is attached to a single-armed, 27-inch polydioxanone suture or coated polyglycolic suture in the 2-0 or 0 size. When using the TN needle, position it perpendicular to the fascial edge and roll up through the fascia. The J needles are double armed on an 18-cm strand of polydioxanone or coated polyglycolic suture in the 2-0 or 0 size. Insert the J needle parallel to the fascial edge and rotate 90 degrees through the edges of the fascia (Fig. 11-1).

CLOSURE DEVICE TECHNIQUES

Device closure systems include the Carter-Thomason device, the Endo Close device, and the Weck EFx device (Fig. 11-2).

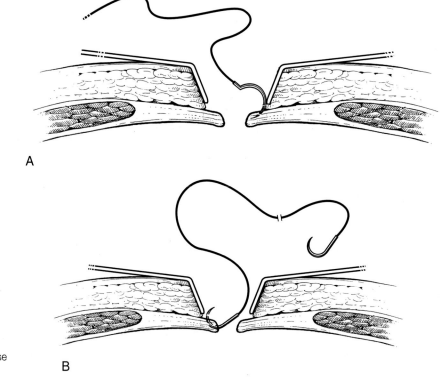

A

B

Figure 11-1. Hand closure. **A,** The single-armed TN needle (Ethicon Endo-Surgery, Cincinnati, Ohio) is inserted into the incision with the needle positioned perpendicular with the fascial edge. The needle is angled upward and rolled through the fascia. The opposite fascial edge is sutured in a similar manner. A figure-of-eight suture can be used as needed. **B,** The double-armed J needle (Ethicon Endo-Surgery is inserted into the trocar site parallel with the fascial edge and is then rotated 90 degrees through the fascia. A second J needle is passed through the opposite edge. Hand closure is recommended in the nonobese patient.

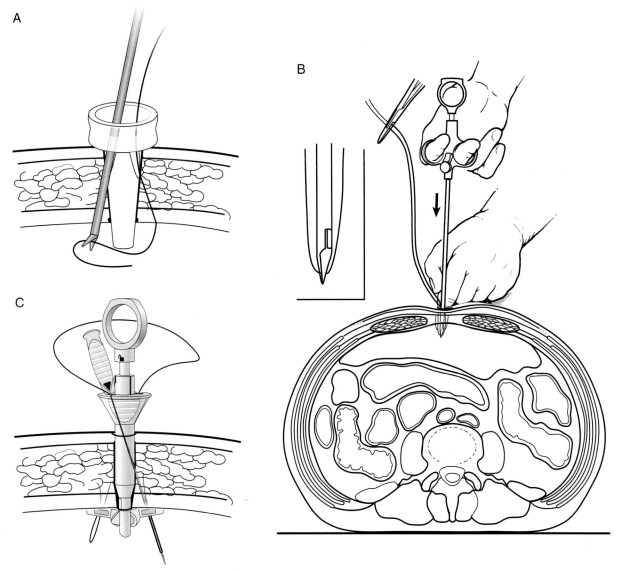

Figure 11-2. Fascial closure devices. **A,** The Carter-Thomason device technique begins by inserting the cone-shaped pilot guide into the port site defect. The hinged jaw is opened by retracting on the spring-loaded thumb handle, allowing placement of a suture. Under direct visualization, the needle passer is then placed through the guide channel, through the fascia and peritoneum. Once the suture passer enters the abdomen, retract the thumb handle to open the hinged jaw, and disengage the suture. Close the jaws, and withdraw the device through the guide channel. The suture passer is then placed on the opposite side of the Carter-Thomason pilot in the same fashion. Finally, release the thumb handle to secure the suture, and withdraw the suture passer. **B,** The Endo Close device works in a similar fashion to the Carter-Thomason device. It consists of a disposable, spring-loaded blunt stylet with a hook that retracts into a sheath as the 14-gauge needle is pushed through the abdominal wall. **C,** The Weck EFx device is a further modification of the Carter-Thomason device. It consists of the EFx device and a suture passer. The device uses approximation wings for improved stability and a silicone depth control pad that helps catch the suture inside the abdomen.

Carter-Thomason Device (See Videos 11-1 and 11-2)

The Carter-Thomason CloseSure System (Cooper Surgical, Trumbull, Conn.) consists of two components: a 5-mm or 10/12-mm, cone-shaped pilot guide and a single-action (only one arm moves; the other is fixed) hinged jaw at the end of a suture passer. This construction enables three degrees of freedom:

- Translational or in-and-out movement
- Rotational movement
- An end-effector jaw that allows it to grasp the suture

The closure technique begins with insertion of the cone-shaped pilot guide into the port site defect. Manipulate the pilot guide so that the plane of the guide channel holes are perpendicular to the fascial defect. Open the hinged jaw by retracting on the spring-loaded thumb handle. Place the end of a 2-0 polyglycolic acid suture within the hinged jaw and release the handle. The suture is now held within the jaw. Place the suture-loaded needle grasper, under direct visualization, through the guide channel. Pass through the fascia and peritoneum, entering the abdomen close to the camera. This optimizes visualization for finding and grasping the suture end during the second pass. Once the suture passer enters the abdomen, and one is comfortable with the suture position, retract the thumb handle to open the hinged jaw and disengage the suture. Close the jaws. Withdraw the device through the guide channel. Place the suture passer on the opposite side of the Carter-Thomason pilot guide, and enter the abdomen again. Open the hinged jaw by retracting the thumb ring and grasp the loop of suture previously left on the first pass. Use a grasper through another laparoscopic port to aid in passing the suture loop to the hinged jaw if having difficulty. Once the suture is secured within the jaws, withdraw the suture passer. Now both ends of the suture are outside the abdomen and can be secured with mosquito clamps to prevent inadvertent removal of the suture. Reinsert a trocar to maintain the pneumoperitoneum. Close the other ports in similar fashion. Once the surgeon is ready to exit the abdomen, the surgeon can remove the trocar and tie the ends of the suture together to complete the fascial closure.

Another technique that can be useful at times is the placement of the suture via digital guidance. The index finger of the nondominant hand occludes the abdominal wall defect to prevent loss of pneumoperitoneum and can be used to elevate the abdominal wall during closure. This finger also palpates the edge of the fascia to guide proper needle placement.

Endo Close Device

The Endo Close (Medtronic, Minneapolis, Minn.) works in a similar fashion to the Carter-Thomason device. It consists of a disposable, spring-loaded blunt stylet with a hook that retracts into a sheath as a 14-gauge needle is pushed through the abdominal wall.[3] This device has two degrees of freedom: translational (in and out) and rotational. Begin the technique by depressing the top button to open the hook, and place a 2-0 polyglycolic acid suture into the notched portion. Release the top button, which draws the hook inward and anchors the suture at the tip of the device. Insert the Endo Close through one side of the trocar site, incorporating both the fascia and peritoneum. Once the suture is within the abdomen, depress the button to drop the suture. Remove and reinsert the Endo Close device on the opposite side of the incision and depress the button to expose the notched end of the stylet. Keeping the hook exposed, snare or place with a grasper through another port the loop of suture into the device. Withdraw the device and suture together through the incision. This now leaves two free ends of suture outside of the abdominal cavity, and a knot can be tied to complete the fascial closure when suitable.

Weck EFx Device (see Video 11-2)

The Weck EFx Endo Fascial Closure System (Teleflex Medical, Research Triangle Park, North Carolina) is the newest system. It consists of two components: the EFx device and a suture passer. To use the device, load the suture passer with a size 0 suture. Pass the device into the defect. Twist the device handle to the unlock position, and pull the handle to open the approximation wings inside the abdomen. Manipulate the device so that the wings are perpendicular to the abdominal defect. Lock the device to stabilize it. Insert the previously loaded suture passer through the lateral guide channels down through the silicone depth control pads. The suture placement is now 1 cm lateral to the defect. Visually ensure the suture is captured by the pad. Remove the suture passer, load the other end of the recently placed suture, and repeat the aforementioned steps on the opposite guide. Unlock the device, press down on the ring handles to close the approximation wings, and remove the device from the port site. The surgeon is then able to tie the suture. The Weck EFx Closure System offers unassisted delivery and retrieval of sutures and uniform 1-cm closure in varying abdominal thickness and is reported

to be a more efficient method to capture all fascial layers to complete the fascial closure. Literature comparing use of the Weck EFx with the Carter-Thomason device on 72 trocar defects found mean fascial closure times of 1.6 minutes and 2.23 minutes, respectively.[5]

RADIALLY EXPANDING TROCARS

To avoid having to close trocar sites, one can choose to use radially expanding trocars (Step, InnerDyne, Sunnyvale, Calif.). These are nonbladed trocars that develop incisions parallel to muscle fibers and a narrower tract. The device consists of a 1.9-mm Veress needle surrounded by an expanding polymer sleeve. The blunt effect of the trocar placement results in not having to close the fascia, even for incisions up to 12 mm. The technique begins by first applying an expandable polymer sleeve over a Veress needle (Fig. 11-3). Pass a blunt-tipped fascial dilator through the polymer sleeve lumen. Use the nondominant hand to stabilize the trocar with upward traction on the polymer sleeve while inserting the fascial dilator and sheath. Radially expanding trocars are not superior to traditional trocars. Advantages of this system include elimination of sharp trocars, avoidance of blood vessel injury, less likelihood of causing visceral injury, and elimination of the need for fascial closure.[6] The downside is that significantly greater force is required for their insertion.[6]

FINAL SURVEY

When exiting the abdomen after a laparoscopic procedure, the surgeon must carefully perform a survey of the operative field, looking for signs of bleeding or visceral injury or entrapped bowel within the closure site. Large extraction sites must be evaluated at the end of the procedure after closure through inspection interiorly with the laparoscope. If no obvious injury is detected, insufflation pressures should be lowered to below 5 mm Hg to identify bleeding vessels that were occluded at higher pressures. Finally, irrigate the operative field, paying particular attention to the color of the returned fluid; if yellow-brown, consider a bowel injury as the source.

DESUFFLATION AND TROCAR REMOVAL

During desufflation of the abdomen, attention should be given to the sequence of removal of the trocars. This sequence ensures adequate closure of the trocar sites, facilitates evacuation of the pneumoperitoneum, and potentially minimizes procedure time.

The following sequence is recommended. After placing the fascial sutures at each of the 10/12-mm trocar sites, the surgeon should not tie the suture so that trocars can be reinserted to maintain the pneumoperitoneum. This optimizes visualization during the remainder of the closure process. Begin by removing 5-mm trocars under direct vision, enabling the use of 10/12-mm ports to visualize and control potential bleeding. Next, remove 10/12-mm trocars other than at the camera site, and tie the fascial sutures. Escaping gas from a 10/12-mm trocar site may indicate the need for additional sutures. One should plan to evacuate as much of the pneumoperitoneum as possible before removal of the last trocar.

Before removing the final 10/12-mm trocar with the camera, elevate it to the highest portion of the abdomen, which contains the greatest amount of gas (Fig. 11-4). Turn off the gas and disconnect it from the trocar. Move the trocar insufflation valve to the open position to allow the gas to escape. Apply external, manual pressure to the abdomen to facilitate evacuation. In addition, the anesthesia team can use manual ventilation to assist in removing any residual gas.

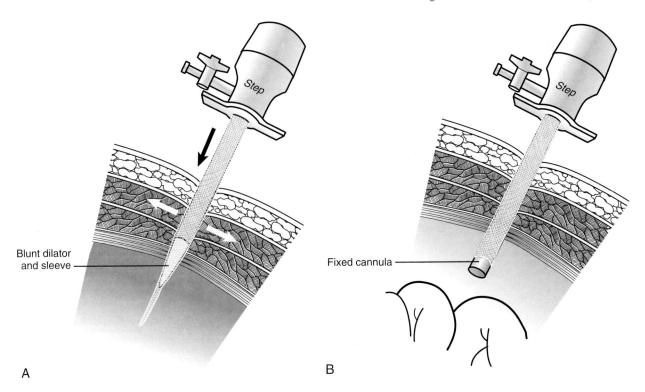

A

B

Figure 11-3. Radially expanding trocars. **A,** An expandable polymer sleeve is applied over a Veress needle. A blunt-tipped fascial dilator is subsequently passed through the polymer sleeve lumen. **B,** Use the nondominant hand to stabilize the trocar with upward traction on the polymer sleeve while the fascial dilator and sheath are inserted. This technique avoids having to close trocar sites.

When CO_2 is used as an insufflation agent, it is metabolized to carbonic acid and water on the peritoneal surface. Carbonic acid may cause diaphragmatic irritation, leading to postoperative shoulder, chest, or back pain. Residual pneumoscrotum or subcutaneous emphysema usually resolves within 24 to 48 hours.

Finally, pull up on the previously placed fascial sutures to place tension on the wound edges; this maneuver will prevent herniation as the trocar and laparoscope are removed. First, remove the trocar over the camera, leaving only the laparoscope in the abdomen so that a solid, not a hollow, instrument is the last piece of equipment to be withdrawn. A hollow trocar removed at the end of the procedure can allow a small piece of bowel or omentum to be pulled into the closure site. Slowly remove the laparoscope, inspecting the trocar tract for bleeding as the laparoscope is withdrawn. Tie the suture to complete the fascial closure.

SKIN CLOSURE

Irrigate the trocar sites and achieve adequate hemostasis of the skin edges before skin closure. After fascial closure, perform a subcuticular stitch with a 4-0 polyglycolic acid suture on a cutting needle, or staple depending on the desired cosmetic affect. Apply Steri-Strips or Dermabond (Ethicon LLC, San Lorenzo,

Puerto Rico) to the skin. Trocar sites can be closed using only Dermabond adhesives without subcuticular closure; this has been shown to be faster than subcuticular closure with suture. Steri-Strips should not be applied over Dermabond skin adhesives.

SUMMARY

- Inspection of the surgical field, evacuation of the pneumoperitoneum, and removal of the trocars are important steps in every laparoscopic procedure. Careful attention must be given to closing laparoscopic ports to prevent TSH.
- The steps in exiting the abdomen include the following:
  - Inspection of the operative site with the pneumoperitoneum below 5 mm Hg
  - Complete evacuation of the pneumoperitoneum to prevent postoperative discomfort from retained CO_2
  - Removal of all trocars under direct vision
- Salient points are as follows:
  - Trocar sites greater than or equal to 10 mm are closed on all patients.
  - Trocar sites greater than or equal to 5 mm are closed on pediatric patients.
  - Hand closure of trocar sites should be reserved for the normal BMI patient.
  - Use the closure technique that works best for you.

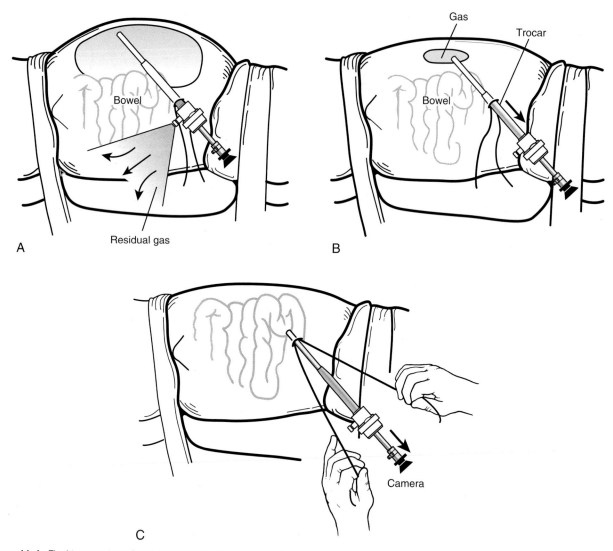

Figure 11-4. Final trocar removal and exiting the abdomen. **A,** All ports have been removed under direct vision, and all but the final 10/12-mm trocar sites have been closed with suture. The scope is directed to the area containing the residual pneumoperitoneum, and the insufflation port is disconnected, allowing escape of residual gas. Manual compression of the abdomen and deep inspirations administered by the anesthesia team can assist with expulsion of the vast majority of the residual gas. **B,** The trocar is retracted from the abdomen, leaving the scope in place. **C,** The scope is slowly retracted while the trocar site is inspected for bleeding. An assistant applies gentle traction to the previously placed fascial suture. After the scope exits the abdomen, the tension on the fascial suture immediately closes the defect, preventing herniation of bowel or omentum.

REFERENCES

1. Karthik S, Augustine AJ, Shibumon MM, Pai MV. Analysis of laparoscopic port site complications: a descriptive study. *J Minim Access Surg*. 2013;9:59–64.
2. Elashry OM, Nakada SY, Wolf Jr JS, Figenshau RS, McDougall EM, Clayman RV. Comparative clinical study of port-closure techniques following laparoscopic surgery. *J Am Coll Surg*. 1996;183:335–344.
3. Shaher Z. Port closure techniques. *Surg Endosc*. 2007;21:1264–1274.
4. Shetty A, Adiyat KT. Comparison between hand suture and Carter-Thomason needle closure of port sites in laparoscopy. *Urol J*. 2014;11:1768–1771.
5. del Junco M, Okhunov Z, Juncal S, Yoon R, Landman J. Evaluation of a novel trocar-site closure and comparison with a standard Carter-Thomason closure device. *J Endourol*. 2014;28:814–818.
6. Vilos GA, Ternamian A, Dempster J, Laberge PY. The Society of Obstetricians and Gynaecologists of Canada. Laparoscopic entry: a review of techniques, technologies, and complications. *J Obstet Gynaecol Can*. 2007;29:433–465.

12 Complications of Laparoscopic and Robotic-Assisted Surgery

Michael Siev, Louis R. Kavoussi

The benefit of any surgical intervention is weighed against the risk of complications. Although experience is of obvious importance, not even the most veteran surgeon is immune to complications that may occur during or after an operation. Many of the complications that may occur during laparoscopic or robotic-assisted retroperitoneal surgery are similar to those encountered with traditional open surgery. However, controlling these events requires a unique skill set. Moreover, some complications are unique to laparoscopy. Complications from laparoscopic or robotic-assisted procedures may arise from almost every aspect of the operation, and when complications do occur, early recognition and aggressive treatment are crucial to minimize subsequent morbidity to the patient. In this chapter, we review the potential complications that can occur in each of these areas. Strategies aimed at complication prevention, recognition, and treatment are discussed.

POSITIONING INJURY

Attention to patient positioning is of great import during laparoscopy in order to avoid postoperative orthopedic and neuromuscular injuries. Complications include sensory and motor deficits, neuralgias, back pain, and rhabdomyolysis. Such injuries are more common after retroperitoneal versus pelvic laparoscopic surgery, with an occurrence of 3.1% reported in the literature.[1] Careful attention to patient positioning is imperative to avoid compression or stretch injuries to the extremities, particularly the brachial plexus. Prevention includes using foam pads at pressure points, maintaining the head in the neutral position, and, when indicated, adding a properly placed axillary or chest roll. When the patient is in dorsal lithotomy position or split leg position, care must be exercised in maintaining a straight line from the patient's heel to knee to contralateral shoulder. Hip overextension must be prevented as well.

Rhabdomyolysis is a potentially serious complication of laparoscopic and robotic-assisted surgery. The incidence of clinical rhabdomyolysis after laparoscopic surgery in the flank position has been reported to be as high as 0.4% and is associated with several factors, including male gender, heavier weight, large muscle mass, longer operative times, and the use of a full flank or exaggerated lithotomy position.[1] Management includes intravenous hydration with or without alkalization.

Skin breakdown and pressure sores are also a potential complication secondary to patient positioning and are associated with the flank position and prolonged operative times.[2]

INSUFFLATION INJURY

Incorrect placement of a Veress needle can result in inadvertent insufflation of extraperitoneal spaces with subsequent extravasation of gas along tissue planes. The most common site of incorrect needle placement is the preperitoneal space (Fig. 12-1), resulting in an increased distance between the skin and peritoneal cavity, which may necessitate open trocar placement to gain access. Moreover, preperitoneal or retroperitoneal insufflant can pass between diaphragmatic fibers or alongside

the great vessels, causing pneumomediastinum, which, in turn, can lead to pneumopericardium or pneumothorax.[3]

Insufflation of the subcutaneous space can be a result of incorrect Veress needle placement or secondary to leakage of gas around trocars. The resultant subcutaneous emphysema is usually of no clinical consequence; once the procedure is complete, the gas is absorbed. However, extensive dissection of gas can lead to pneumothorax, pneumomediastinum, and hypercarbia. The risk of development of a pneumomediastinum increases when crepitus is noted extending up to the neck. Because of a continuum of fascial planes existing between the cervical soft tissue and mediastinum, the potential exists for gas to track upward into the neck and down into the mediastinum[4,5] (Fig. 12-2). Subclinical thoracic air collections have been reported in 5.5% of urologic laparoscopic procedures, which can often be managed conservatively because of the high solubility of CO_2.[6,7] However, if symptomatic pneumothorax or pneumomediastinum develops, the pneumoperitoneum should be discontinued and the ectopic gas evacuated.

A pneumothorax can also occur in the absence of subcutaneous emphysema. Insufflant can enter the pleural space through anatomic or congenital defects in the diaphragm. Complications of anesthesia and positive pressure ventilation,

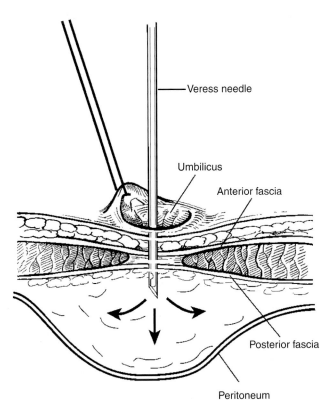

Figure 12-1. Insufflation of the preperitoneal space pushes the peritoneum away from the abdominal wall, making subsequent intraperitoneal access troublesome and impairing visualization.

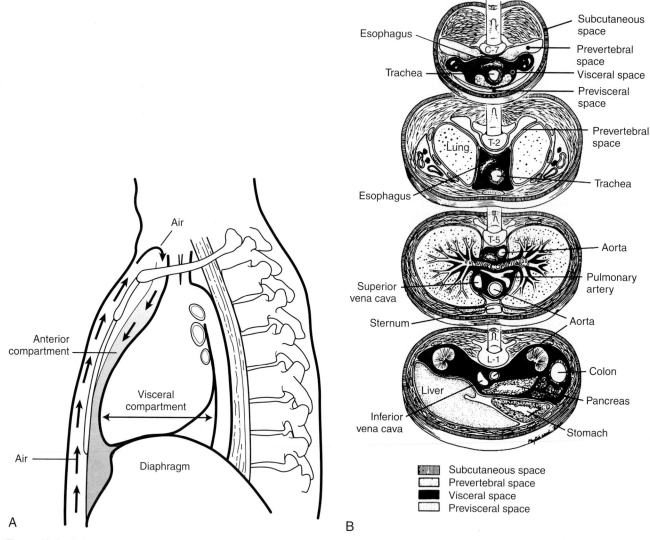

Figure 12-2. A, Anatomic fascial planes in the neck communicate with the subcutaneous tissue planes, allowing for egress of gas into the mediastinum. **B,** Compartments of the mediastinum. The viscera of middle compartment are in continuity with the neck and retroperitoneum.

as well as patient conditions such as emphysematous bullae, can also lead to the entry of air into the pleural cavity.[8]

After the pneumoperitoneum is successfully established, the presence of pressurized gas in the abdominal cavity has significant and variegated physiologic consequences that can result in complications. The cumulative response of the cardiovascular system during laparoscopy with CO_2 under moderate pressure (10 to 20 mm Hg) is usually sufficient for healthy individuals to tolerate pneumoperitoneum. However, patients with significant cardiovascular or pulmonary disease may not compensate sufficiently. In addition, careful attention to insufflation pressure is critical to avoid excessive tension and potential cardiovascular collapse.

Although appropriate ventilatory adjustments are usually sufficient to eliminate the increased CO_2 load that results from laparoscopy, in some patients CO_2 insufflation can produce profound hypercapnia. This can be exacerbated by subcutaneous emphysema and excessive intra-abdominal pressures. If severe, hypercapnia and acidosis can have significant depressive cardiac effects. Initial management consists of lowering the intra-abdominal pressure. If the anesthesiologist cannot adequately compensate, helium may be used or the procedure may need to be converted to open surgery.

Insufflation can also produce significant cardiac arrhythmias, including bradycardia, tachycardia, ventricular extrasystoles, atrioventricular dissociation, and nodal rhythms. Hypercapnia, as well as a vagal response to abdominal distention and peritoneal irritation, has been implicated. The use of atropine before insufflation may prevent these vagal reactions.[9]

A rare but potentially fatal complication related to the pneumoperitoneum is a gas embolism, which occurs most commonly during the induction of pneumoperitoneum. Although intravasation of gas as a result of the increased intra-abdominal pressure has been suggested as a cause, the most common cause is direct placement of a needle or trocar into a vessel or abdominal organ.[10,11] In a meta-analysis of nearly 500,000 laparoscopic procedures with closed access, the incidence of gas emboli was 0.0014%.[12]

Patient survival after gas embolism depends on rapid diagnosis and treatment. The diagnosis can be difficult, and there is often no warning before acute cardiovascular collapse, particularly during insufflation. When the size of the embolus increases, tachycardia, arrhythmias, hypotension, and increased central venous pressure may be noted. Hypoxia, hypercapnia, and cyanosis may also be evident. Electrocardiographic

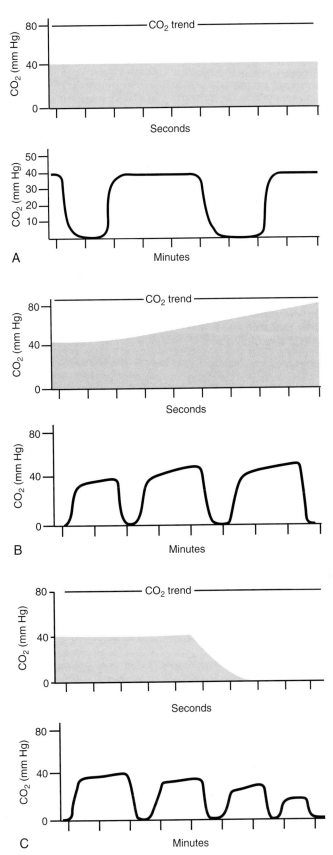

A

B

C

Figure 12-3. A, Graph showing a normal capnogram. **B,** Capnometry showing a gradual increase in end-tidal CO_2, which may be seen with chronic obstructive pulmonary disease, hypoventilation, and high insufflation pressures. **C,** Decrease in end-tidal CO_2 seen in pulmonary gas embolism and cardiac arrest.

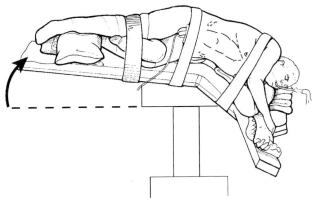

Figure 12-4. Position for suspected air embolism: left lateral decubitus and head down.

changes can include a right heart strain pattern, and auscultation may reveal the classic "mill wheel" murmur just before the acute event. Also, an acute decrease in measured end-tidal CO_2 measurements is noted as the embolism occludes the pulmonary trunk (Fig. 12-3). When an embolism is suspected, release the pneumoperitoneum and administer 100% oxygen. Place the patient in the left lateral decubitus position with the head down to move the gas away from the pulmonary artery (Fig. 12-4). Institute cardiopulmonary resuscitation, and place a central venous catheter in an attempt to aspirate the gas. Percutaneous or open evacuation of the gas may be indicated.[13-16]

CAUTERY INJURY

A thermal injury to tissue represents a serious complication because patients do not show symptoms of such injuries for several days postoperatively. Failure to recognize such an injury can result in significant morbidity. Prevention of burns depends on the careful use of electrocautery. Before using electrocautery, inspect all instruments, including robotic manipulators, to be certain that insulation is intact. Insulation defects can result in arcing of the electrocautery current between instruments. Moreover, when current is applied, the entire tip of the instrument must be kept within the visual field. Finally, be certain that the tissue to be cauterized is isolated from surrounding tissue to prevent inadvertent injury secondary to thermal conduction through tissue.

VASCULAR INJURY

Vascular injuries are among the most common and challenging complications of urologic laparoscopy, occurring in 2.8% of procedures.[17] Vascular injury can be a result of Veress needle and trocar placement or from trauma sustained during dissection. Many of these injuries are minor and are easily managed, whereas others have catastrophic potential. A thorough understanding of vascular anatomy and constant attention to maintaining orientation are critical to avoid vascular complications, and early recognition of such an event is key to minimizing the extent of injury.

Slight bleeding from the trocar or Veress needle access often resolves without intervention, though several maneuvers are available to control bleeding from abdominal wall vessels. If the bleeding is minor, apply electrocautery under direct vision. If the bleeding is brisk, pass a Foley catheter down the trocar, then inflate the balloon and put on traction to tamponade the bleeding vessel (Fig. 12-5). More significant

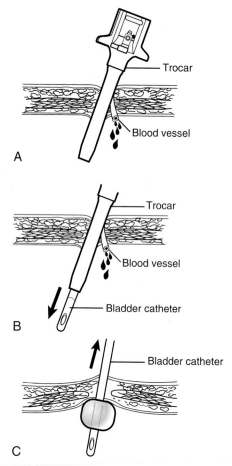

Figure 12-5. A, Placement of the trocar through an abdominal wall vessel can cause persistent bleeding that is not stopped with trocar placement. **B,** A bladder catheter is inserted through the trocar site. **C,** The catheter balloon is inflated and put on tension to tamponade the bleeding vessel.

bleeding may require sutures to achieve hemostasis. Pass a figure-of-eight suture using a Carter-Thomason needlepoint fascial closure device (Inlet Medical, Eden Prairie, Minn.) (Fig. 12-6). If this maneuver is unsuccessful, open exploration may be indicated.

Occasionally, abdominal wall or intra-abdominal vessel injury is not noted until the postoperative period. Hypotension or tachycardia associated with a decreasing hematocrit raises the suspicion of ongoing hemorrhage. Significant pain about a trocar site, ecchymosis, and a palpable paramedian mass are signs of a hematoma within the rectus sheath. Correction of any underlying coagulopathy is the initial step; continued hemodynamic instability, however, would warrant exploration for persistent bleeding.

Trocar placement can also result in major vessel injury and is related to the use of excessive force to advance the trocar. This is a particular risk with extremely thin patients; the great vessels can be deceptively close to the abdominal wall. Major bleeding may not be immediately recognized if the injury is confined to the retroperitoneum. When a major trocar injury is suspected, perform immediate laparotomy. Leave the trocar in place to help tamponade the vessel and aid in localizing the site of injury. Do not move the trocar, to prevent converting a puncture into a larger tear. Attempt to control bleeding proximally and distally. Moreover, it is important to mobilize the vessel and inspect the back wall for a possible through-and-through injury.

A mesenteric hematoma may occur as a consequence of trocar placement or dissection. If identified, closely monitor the hematoma. Evidence of expansion or compromise to bowel circulation warrants exploration.

Vascular injury can also occur during dissection. Each injury is individual and requires unique definitive treatment; however, general recommendations can be made. Most vascular injuries related to the upper urinary tract involve branches of the renal vein or vena cava, although arterial injuries are possible. Take care to avoid placing undue tension on veins during dissection of venous branches. It is important to realize that an instrument passed through a trocar site acts as a lever.

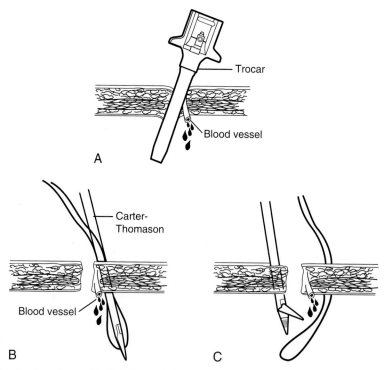

Figure 12-6. A, Persistent bleeding from trocar site. **B,** A figure-of-eight suture can be passed with the Carter-Thomason needlepoint fascial closure device (Inlet Medical, Eden Prairie, Minn.). **C,** The suture pass is effective in ligating a bleeding trocar site vessel.

Accordingly, significant torque can be generated at the tip of a given instrument (Fig. 12-7), whether laparoscopic or robotic. The lack of haptic feedback found on the robotic console can make it difficult to appreciate the torque being applied to the tissue. Be cautious, therefore, when positioning retractors on

viscera or the mesentery. Follow basic tenets of open surgery, such as the avoidance of past-pointing the tip of the scissors when cutting.

Endovascular gastrointestinal anastomosis (GIA) stapling devices are routinely used during laparoscopic nephrectomy for division of the renal vein or artery. Malfunction of such devices can cause significant vascular complications and has been reported to occur in 1.7% of cases.[18] Stapler malfunction is often secondary to preventable causes, not the primary device failure. Ensuring that no surgical clips or unintended tissue or vessels are within the stapler jaws is critical to help prevent stapler-related complications (Fig. 12-8).

The approach to management of a vascular injury depends on its location and severity. The surgeon must use personal judgment to rapidly determine whether the equipment or skills are available to repair a given injury laparoscopically. Random or blind placement of clips is often ineffective, clutters the operative field, and risks inadvertent narrowing or occlusion of a vital vessel. Dissection of surrounding structures often clarifies the site of bleeding.

Small venous bleeders can often be treated with electrocautery or clips. If a small tear or avulsion occurs in the renal vein or vena cava, make an attempt to grasp both ends of the tear with an atraumatic grasper. Alternatively, open a gauze pad, pass it through a trocar site, and use it to place pressure on the venotomy for 5 minutes.

Moderate bleeding may require suturing for repair. Place a freehand stitch with a pretied knot across the opening in a vessel (Fig. 12-9). Alternatively, use a Lapra-Ty absorbable clip (Ethicon, Somerville, N.J.) as a preformed knot

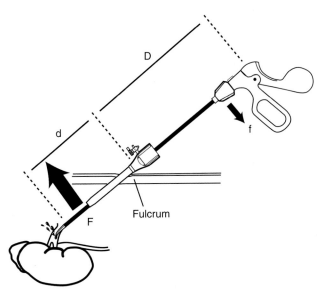

Figure 12-7. When an instrument enters the abdominal wall, the fixed skin site creates a lever through which force exerted on the skin can multiply. On the basis of the formula $F/f = D/d$, when $D > d$, the force at F can be much greater than the force at f and can result in injury.

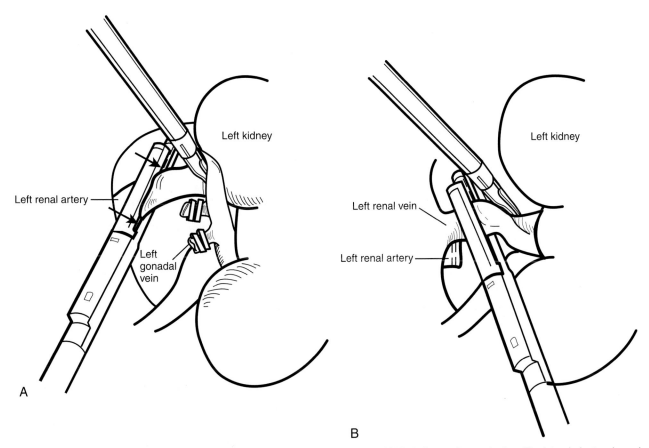

Figure 12-8. **A,** Correct placement of an endovascular gastrointestinal anastomosis (GIA) device on the renal artery. The intended artery is positioned inside the marks of the stapler jaws. Care must be taken to avoid clips if they have been placed on the renal vein branches. **B,** Placement of the endovascular GIA stapler on the renal vein ensures that it is not bunched in the jaws and that no clips are in the jaws.

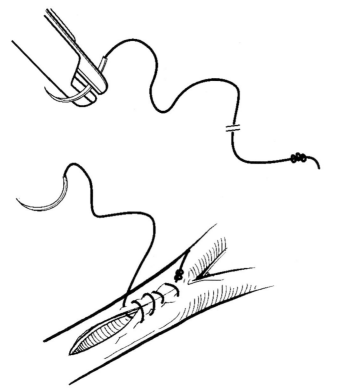

Figure 12-9. A knot is placed in the end of a suture cut to an appropriate working length, which is then passed through a trocar and used to rapidly close the defect.

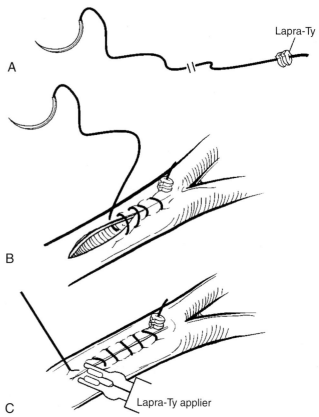

Figure 12-10. A, A length of suture approximately 8 to 10 cm is cut, and a Lapra-Ty absorbable clip (Ethicon, Somerville, N.J.) is placed on the end of the suture. **B,** The suture is passed to close the defect, and then upward tension helps control the bleeding. **C,** The suture is complete and a Lapra-Ty clip is placed on the opposite end to maintain tension and hemostasis.

(Fig. 12-10). Once the suture is passed, use another Lapra-Ty clip to secure the stitch, or use an automated suturing device to place a suture. With experience, arteriotomies can also be closed. However, when suturing, take care to avoid inadvertent narrowing or occlusion of the vessel. Compromise of major abdominal organs and the entire small bowel has occurred.

When brisk bleeding from a vascular injury is noted, use the irrigator-aspirator to help identify the source and aid compression. Increase intra-abdominal pressure to 20 to 25 mm Hg to help with tamponade as well as to compensate for aspiration of gas. Also, use a Foley catheter preloaded with a catheter guide to occlude the bleeding site (Fig. 12-11).

When significant bleeding that cannot be controlled laparoscopically is encountered, place the tip of an instrument on the area of bleeding as a marker and perform immediate laparotomy.

GASTROINTESTINAL INJURY

Injury to the stomach, intestine, gallbladder, liver, spleen, pancreas, and mesentery has been reported during laparoscopic procedures. Unfortunately, intestinal injury is often unrecognized intraoperatively, can have an atypical clinical presentation, and represents a potentially fatal complication. Bowel injury during laparoscopic procedures has an incidence ranging from 0.25% to 2.5% and is usually secondary to needle or trocar insertion or electrocautery.[17]

Gastric perforation is usually a result of trocar perforation of a distended stomach owing to esophageal intubation or mask ventilation. Thus, it is important to place an orogastric tube before access. Aspiration of succus or feces during access

may indicate penetrated bowel. A Veress needle injury may be managed conservatively as long as no leakage of enteric content is noted. When a trocar injury to bowel is noted, leave the trocar in place to help identify the site of injury. Small perforations may be approached laparoscopically, but extensive injuries in unprepared bowel may require open repair and diversion.

When detected intraoperatively, all bowel injuries should be repaired.[20] Intestinal burns may be more extensive than visually apparent. Therefore, perform a wide resection to ensure removal of all injured tissue.

Unfortunately, bowel injuries are often not recognized at the time of initial laparoscopic surgery.[21] The patient often is seen 2 to 7 days postoperatively with a persistent ileus and mild distention, vague abdominal discomfort, notable trocar site pain, nausea, or diarrhea. Peritoneal signs are commonly absent. Many patients have only a low-grade fever, and leukocytosis may not be present; in fact, many patients exhibit leukopenia. A complete blood count with manual differential usually demonstrates a left shift. A plain abdominal film may reveal an ileus pattern and free air; however, this finding is not helpful because the insufflant from the pneumoperitoneum may be visible for several days after laparoscopy. If the symptoms of bowel injury do not rapidly respond to conservative measures, undertake radiographic studies and surgical exploration as indicated.

Splenic and liver lacerations can be managed conservatively. Define the extent of the injury and pack the area with

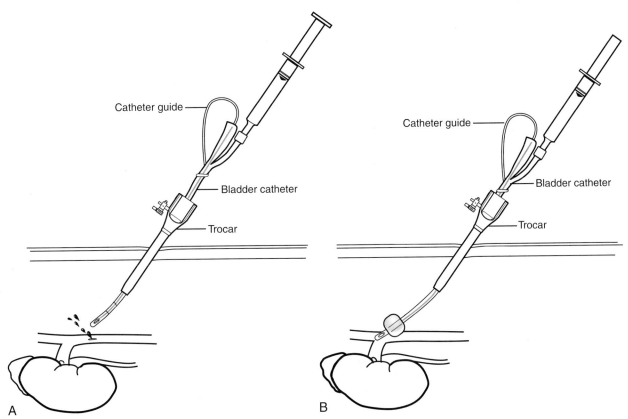

Figure 12-11. A bladder catheter with a catheter guide can be used to occlude major vascular bleeding. **A,** A catheter and guide are passed through the trocar to the site of bleeding. **B,** The balloon is inflated with 5 to 15 mL of water and pressure is placed on the bleeding site.

surgical cellulose (Surgicel [Ethicon]) or absorbable gelatin sponge (Gelfoam, Pfizer, Inc., New York, N.Y.). The argon beam coagulator is also invaluable in achieving hemostasis (Fig. 12-12).

The tail of the pancreas can be injured during left radical nephrectomy or adrenalectomy. If this injury is recognized intraoperatively, repair and drain it. Use the GIA stapler to excise the tail of the pancreas, if desired. If such an event is recognized in the postoperative period, place a drain and follow conservative management.

URINARY TRACT INJURY

Injuries to the bladder and urethra have been reported for laparoscopic surgery, primarily during gynecologic procedures. It is important to place a Foley catheter before gaining access in order to decompress the bladder. The bladder can be penetrated by the Veress needle or trocar. Such an event manifests as hematuria or gas inflating the Foley bag (Fig. 12-13).

Veress needle injuries to the urinary tract can be managed conservatively, but trocar or dissection injuries may require repair and catheter drainage. If a bladder injury is suspected, instill methylene blue or indigo carmine dye to help identify the site of injury, if desired.

Ureteral injuries usually manifest 1 to 5 days postoperatively. Leakage of urine can result in a urinoma, which causes localized pain, or can extravasate into the abdomen, resulting in peritoneal signs (Fig. 12-14). If such an injury is recognized intraoperatively, undertake endoscopic repair with stenting. Postoperative diagnosis may mandate stent placement, percutaneous drainage, and possible laparoscopic or open repair.

PLEURAL AND DIAPHRAGMATIC INJURY

Laparoscopic renal surgery carries a small but recognized risk of injury to the diaphragm and pleura during dissection or trocar placement, occurring in 0.6% of cases.[22] Diaphragmatic injury can occur during dissection of the upper pole of the kidney or adrenal gland or when mobilizing the liver or spleen (Fig. 12-15). Also, trocars placed above the ribs can violate the pleura and injure the lung. Special care must be exercised when placing trocars near the costal margin, such as in robotic-assisted partial nephrectomy, for fear of violating the diaphragm. Serious sequelae may result, becoming evident when the patient shows signs of a tension pneumothorax or pneumomediastinum.

Pay careful attention to the diaphragm at all times, especially with renal lesions close to the diaphragm, as well as when mobilizing the liver, spleen, or colon. Injury to the diaphragm or pleura may be recognized directly or suspected when the diaphragm is seen billowing into the surgical field, known classically as the "floppy diaphragm sign." Active communication with the anesthesiology team is critical because decreased oxygen saturation, increased airway pressures, diminished breath sounds, CO_2 retention, and hemodynamic instability are often key in making the diagnosis of pleural injury.

Once pleural injury is recognized, management depends on the stability of the patient. In the unstable patient, immediate release of the pneumoperitoneum and possible needle decompression of tension pneumothorax, or tube thoracostomy, is indicated. In the clinically stable patient, management may involve completion of the procedure with a reduced pneumoperitoneum (10 mg Hg) and close hemodynamic monitoring.

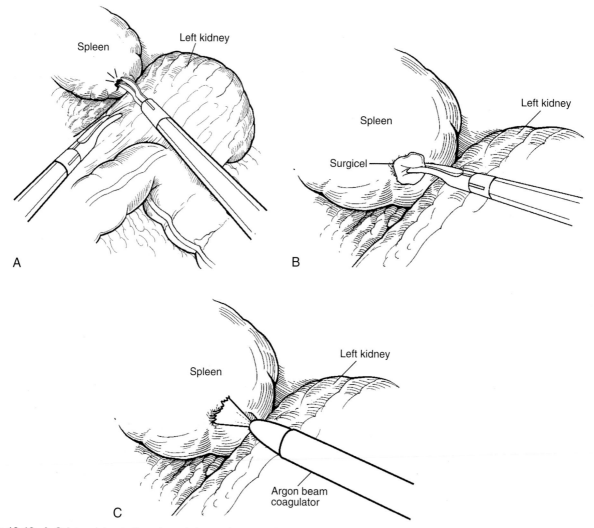

Figure 12-12. A, Scissors injury to the spleen during nephrectomy. **B,** Surgicel (Ethicon, Somerville, N.J.) is placed on the bleeding site and pressure is applied. **C,** An argon beam coagulator can also be used to achieve hemostasis.

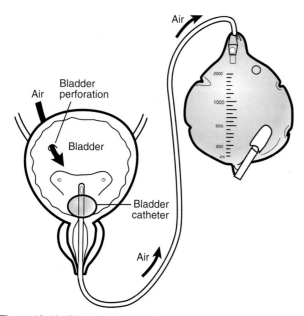

Figure 12-13. Bladder injury can allow intraperitoneal gas or blood to escape into the bladder catheter.

This will allow for better visualization of the injury with the specimen out of the field of view. After laparoscopic inspection of the pleural cavity to rule out direct pulmonary injury, perform closure of the diaphragmatic injury and pleurotomy with standard laparoscopic suturing or endoscopic suturing devices. Before securing the stitches, remove residual air from the pleural cavity using a suction device or by placing a 6-French central line into the sixth intercostal space.[22,23] Postoperative chest roentgenogram is necessary to rule out residual pneumothorax.

HERNIATION

In general, port site hernias are uncommon, with an incidence of less than 0.1%.[24] Because hernias are more likely to occur with larger trocars, attempt to close them when using ports greater than 10 mm placed anterior to the posterior axillary line. Herniation of bowel into the preperitoneal space (through a peritoneal defect with intact fascia) can occur. Therefore, attempt to close the peritoneum as well as the fascia. Incisional hernias at hand port sites after hand-assisted laparoscopy have also been reported with an incidence of 1.9%.[25] Take care when using a balloon device to create a working space in the retroperitoneum. If the balloon is inadvertently

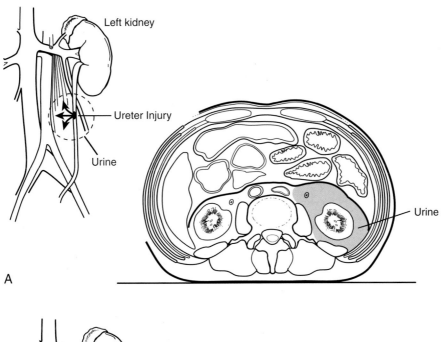

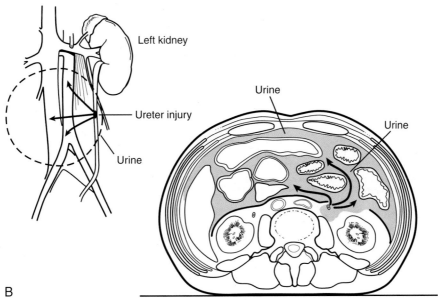

Figure 12-14. A, Ureteral injury can result in the development of a large retroperitoneal urinoma. **B,** If the peritoneum is not intact, peritonitis can result from seepage of urine and subsequent bowel irritation.

inflated within the fascia of the abdominal wall, a large defect may be created, resulting in hernia formation. Close all holes in mesentery to avoid a mesenteric hernia.

ROBOTIC-ASSOCIATED INJURY

Most injuries seen in robotic procedures are similar to those seen in their laparoscopic counterparts. However, certain adverse events are unique to robotic cases. Most can be prevented with vigilance. Extra care must be taken during trocar placement for robotic procedures to ensure that the robotic arms remain clear of the patient's head and limbs. Improper port placement may result in the extracorporeal section of manipulator striking the patient's head or limbs. Furthermore, once the robot is docked above the patient, the bed cannot be repositioned, because this could result in entrapment or

abdominal wall injury.[26] There have also been reports of excessive force resulting in instrument breakage.[27] Care must taken when using the manipulators.

SUMMARY

Complications are an inevitable part of surgical practice. With experience, the overall risks of laparoscopic surgery are equivalent to those seen with open surgical approaches. Laparoscopic renal surgery has well-defined potential risks that need to be discussed in detail with patients. To prevent, recognize, and treat complications, the laparoscopist must be thoroughly versed in the potential pitfalls that exist from preoperative planning to laparoscopic exit. Experience and attention to detail can help keep complication rates and patient morbidity to a minimum.

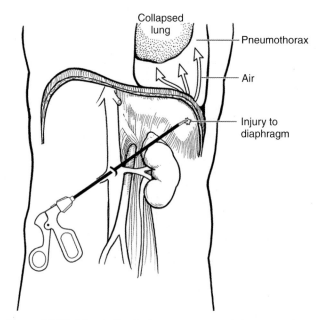

Figure 12-15. Injury to the diaphragm can occur during aggressive lateral dissection of the upper pole of the kidney, adrenal gland, or spleen. This injury is usually immediately apparent; the patient will rapidly show signs of increased peak airway pressures, difficulty with ventilation, and, if not corrected, tension pneumothorax.

REFERENCES

1. Wolf JS, Marcovich R, Gill IS, et al. Survey of neuromuscular injuries to the patient and surgeon during urologic laparoscopic surgery. *Urology.* 2000;55:831–836.
2. Stevens J, Nichelson E, Linehan WM, et al. Risk factors for skin breakdown after renal and adrenal surgery. *Urology.* 2004;64:246–249.
3. Wolf JS, Stoller ML. The physiology of laparoscopy: basic principles, complications and other considerations. *J Urol.* 1994;152:294–302.
4. Maunder RJ, Pierson DJ, Hudson LD. Subcutaneous and mediastinal emphysema: pathophysiology, diagnosis and management. *Arch Intern Med.* 1984;144:1447–1453.
5. Cooley JC, Gillespie JB. Mediastinal emphysema: pathogenesis and management. *Chest.* 1966;49:104–108.
6. Venkatesh R, Kibel AS, Lee D, et al. Rapid resolution of carbon dioxide pneumothorax (capno-thorax) resulting from diaphragmatic injury during laparoscopic nephrectomy. *J Urol.* 2002;167:1387–1388.
7. Abreu SC, Sharp DS, Ramani AP, et al. Thoracic complications during urological laparoscopy. *J Urol.* 2004;171:1451–1455.
8. Joris JL, Chiche JD, Lamy ML. Pneumothorax during laparoscopic fundoplication: diagnosis and treatment with positive end-expiratory pressure. *Anesth Analg.* 1995;81:993–1000.
9. Carmichael DE. Laparoscopy: cardiac considerations. *Fertil Steril.* 1971;22:69–70.
10. Morison DE, Riggs JR. Cardiovascular collapse in laparoscopy. *Can Med Assoc J.* 1974;111:433–437.
11. Ostman PL, Pantle-Fisher FH, Faure EA, Glosten B. Circulatory collapse during laparoscopy. *J Clin Anesth.* 1990;2:129–132.
12. Bonjer HJ, Hazebroek EJ, Kazemier G, et al. Open versus closed establishment of pneumoperitoneum in laparoscopic surgery. *Br J Surg.* 1997;84:599–602.
13. Wolf JS, Stoller ML. The physiology of laparoscopy: basic principles, complications, and other considerations. *J Urol.* 1994;152:294–302.
14. Gomar C, Fernandez C, Villalonga A, Nalda MA. Carbon dioxide embolism during laparoscopy and hysteroscopy. *Ann Fr Anesth Reanim.* 1985;4:380–382.
15. Shulum D, Aronson HB. Capnography in the early diagnosis of carbon dioxide embolism during laparoscopy. *Can J Anaesth.* 1984;31:455–459.
16. De Plater RM, Jones IS. Non-fatal carbon dioxide embolism during laparoscopy. *Anaesth Intensive Care.* 1989;17:359–361.
17. Parsons JK, Varkarakis I, Rha KH, et al. Complications of abdominal urologic laparoscopy: longitudinal five-year analysis. *Urology.* 2004;63:27–32.
18. Chan D, Bishoff JT, Ratner L, et al. Endovascular gastrointestinal stapler device malfunction during laparoscopic nephrectomy: early recognition and management. *J Urol.* 2000;164:319–321.
19. Deleted in review..
20. Reich H. Laparoscopic bowel injury. *Surg Laparosc Endosc.* 1992;2:74–78.
21. Bishoff JT, Allaf ME, Kirkels W, et al. Laparoscopic bowel injury: incidence and clinical presentation. *J Urol.* 1999;161:887–890.
22. Del Pizzo JJ, Jacobs SC, Bishoff JT, et al. Pleural injury during laparoscopic renal surgery: early recognition and management. *J Urol.* 2003;169:41–44.
23. Potter SR, Kavoussi LR, Jackman SV. Management of diaphragmatic injury during laparoscopic nephrectomy. *J Urol.* 2001;165:1203–1204.
24. Hashizume M, Sugimachi K. Needle and trocar injury during laparoscopic surgery in Japan. *Surg Endosc.* 1997;11:1198–2001.
25. Terranova SA, Siddiqui KM, Preminger GM, Albala DM. Hand-assisted laparoscopic renal surgery: hand-port incision complications. *J Endourol.* 2004;18:775–779.
26. Andonian S, Okeke Z, Okeke DA, Rastinehad A, Vanderbrink BA, Richstone L, et al. Device failures associated with patient injuries during robot-assisted laparoscopic surgeries: a comprehensive review of FDA MAUDE database. *Can J Urol.* 2008;15:3912–3916.
27. Park SY, Cho KS, Lee SW, Soh BH, Rha KH. Intraoperative breakage of needle driver jaw during robotic-assisted laparoscopic radical prostatectomy. *Urology.* 2008;71:168.e5–e6.

13 Laparoscopic and Robotic-Assisted Laparoscopic Pelvic Lymph Node Dissection

Ravi Munver, Leonard Glickman

Since its initial description in 1991, laparoscopic pelvic lymph node dissection (LPLND) has evolved from both a technical and a medical standpoint. The introduction of robotic-assisted technology has allowed the urologic surgeon to take advantage of the superior vision and control of the robotic system when performing robotic-assisted laparoscopic pelvic lymph node dissection (r-LPLND) for prostate cancer and bladder cancer staging. Pelvic lymph node dissection (PLND), in general, has been the subject of a great deal of debate regarding the extent of the dissection templates in high-risk prostate cancer, as well as the role for PLND in low-risk disease. Several predictive nomograms have noted that patients with prostate-specific antigen (PSA) levels below 10 ng/mL and Gleason scores below 7 are at a very low risk for lymph node involvement. Consequently, surgeons have questioned the need for PLND in this patient cohort. Other surgeons advocate for wider, more aggressive dissections than the standard dissection template in patients with higher risk disease. Conversely, there is greater consensus in the bladder cancer literature regarding the need for a wider dissection template to achieve an adequate therapeutic and diagnostic outcome after PLND.

INDICATIONS AND CONTRAINDICATIONS

LPLND is rarely indicated as an independent procedure separate from radical cystectomy or prostatectomy. The patients who may benefit from an independent LPLND include those who are at a high risk for having metastatic prostate cancer and are deciding among local therapies alone (radiation, perineal prostatectomy, or cryotherapy), systemic therapy (hormonal therapy), and multimodal therapy. Unfortunately, cross-sectional imaging studies such as computed tomography (CT) and magnetic resonance imaging (MRI) have very low sensitivities for detecting lymph node involvement, and therefore PLND remains the gold standard for lymph node staging. Therefore, patients with high-risk features, including a Gleason score of 8 or higher, suggestion of extracapsular extension on digital rectal examination or MRI, PSA level above 20 ng/mL, a positive seminal vesicle biopsy, or stage T2b or higher disease, may benefit from a staging PLND before committing to radical prostatectomy with its associated morbidity.

r-LPLND is primarily performed in conjunction with robotic-assisted laparoscopic prostatectomy based on the presence of preoperative risk factors of lymph node involvement. LPLND is also indicated in salvage procedures after failed radiation therapy, in patients undergoing robotic-assisted laparoscopic radical cystectomy, and rarely in patients with metastatic urethral and penile cancer.

Absolute contraindications to LPLND include bleeding diathesis, active infection, severe respiratory disease (chronic obstructive pulmonary disease [COPD]), and severe coronary artery disease. Relative contraindications to LPLND are often related to surgeon experience. These may include extensive prior surgery in the lower abdomen and pelvis (inguinal hernia repair with mesh), morbid obesity, iliac artery tortuosity or aneurysm, history of inflammatory bowel disorders (extensive diverticulitis, perforated appendicitis, and inflammatory bowel disease), and prior pelvic radiation.

PATIENT PREOPERATIVE EVALUATION AND PREPARATION

Before LPLND, routine laboratory tests should be performed, including a complete blood count, serum chemistry panel, coagulation studies, PSA testing, urinalysis, and urine culture. It is also critically important to determine whether the patient has any evidence of metastatic disease. Depending on the clinical indication, chest radiography, CT or MRI of the abdomen and pelvis, nuclear bone scan, and ProstaScint scan (Aytu BioScience, Inc., Englewood, Colo.) can be used to evaluate for the presence of metastatic disease. The patient is instructed to discontinue nonsteroidal anti-inflammatory medications, aspirin, and any other anticoagulants with sufficient time before surgery to allow for return to normal coagulation. All appropriate medical and cardiopulmonary clearances should be obtained. The patient is instructed not to eat or drink after midnight on the night before surgery. Preoperative bowel preparation is optional but may be more important in patients who have a history of prior abdominal surgery or inflammatory bowel disorders. The patient receives a perioperative dose of a first-generation cephalosporin antibiotic. Additional antibiotics with gram-negative and anaerobic coverage should be considered if prostatectomy or cystectomy is to be performed.

OPERATING ROOM CONFIGURATION AND PATIENT POSITIONING

Room configuration and patient positioning are, for the most part, similar for LPLND whether it is done as an independent procedure or as part of a radical prostatectomy or cystectomy. There are slight room configuration differences depending on whether a laparoscopic or a robotic approach is being used.

When an LPLND is performed, the patient is placed in either the supine position or in a low dorsal lithotomy position with a full-length gel pad mattress placed underneath. If the dorsal lithotomy position is chosen, careful attention is paid to minimize pressure along the lateral aspect of the knee where the common peroneal nerve lies. An r-LPLND is performed exclusively in the dorsal lithotomy position. Sequential compression devices are applied to the patient's legs to minimize the risk of deep venous thrombosis (DVT). The arms are carefully tucked and padded

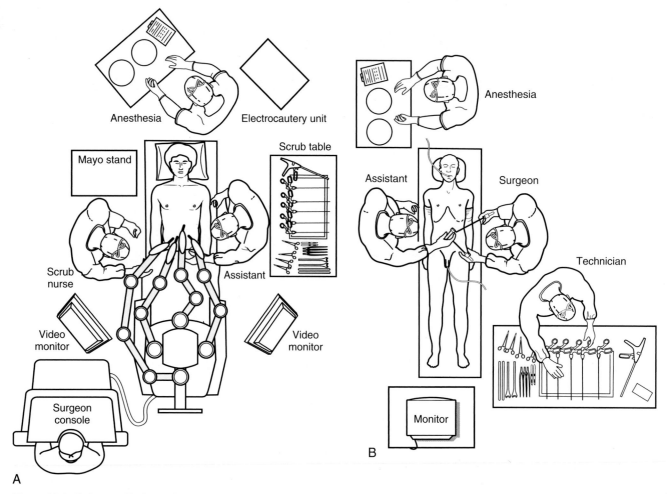

Figure 13-1. Patient positioning and room configuration. **A,** The operating room setup for a robotic-assisted dissection is shown. A gel pad mattress is placed on the operating room table. The patient is placed in a low dorsal lithotomy position with the legs secured in stirrups. The arms and hands are protected with egg crate pads and tucked at the patient's side. The surgeon sits at the robotic console, and the assistant surgeon stands on the patient's left if a right-sided four–robotic arm configuration is used. The patient is repositioned into steep Trendelenburg position after trocars have been placed. The robot is docked between the patient's legs. **B,** The setup for a laparoscopic dissection is shown. The patient is placed in the supine position. The surgeon stands on the side contralateral to the node dissection, and the assistant stands on the side of the node dissection. A monitor is placed at the foot of the bed. The table is placed in the Trendelenburg position.

along the patient's side in the neutral anatomic position with the thumbs pointing toward the ceiling. Attention is paid to ensure that the arms and hands are under no traction or pressure. A Foley catheter is placed once the patient has been prepared and draped when a PLND is performed in conjunction with radical prostatectomy or cystectomy. If only a PLND is being performed, then a urinary catheter is placed before preparation and draping.

For LPLND, the room is configured with the monitor at the foot of the bed, between the patient's legs (Fig. 13-1, *A*). The surgeon stands on the left side of the patient, and the surgical assistant stands on the patient's right side. For r-LPLND, the robotic patient-side cart is docked between the patient's legs, the operating surgeon sits at the robotic console, and the assistant surgeon stands on the side of the patient where there is only one robotic arm being used (Fig. 13-1, *B*).

TROCAR PLACEMENT

After the patient is prepared and draped in the standard sterile fashion, attention is turned toward peritoneal access.

A 12-mm skin incision is made superior to the umbilicus. Using either a Veress needle or the Hasson technique, access into the peritoneal cavity is obtained. Pneumoperitoneum is established with CO_2 gas to a pressure of 15 mm Hg. A 10/12-mm camera port is then placed through the supra-umbilical incision. If an r-LPLND is being performed, the 30-degree robotic laparoscope in the down position is inserted through the umbilical trocar. Alternatively, if an LPLND is being performed, the 10-mm, 30-degree laparoscope is used. A brief survey of the pelvis is then performed to evaluate for any trocar placement injuries and for the presence of any adhesions that may interfere with further port placement and to identify the location of the iliac vessels as surgical landmarks.

The remaining port locations are based on whether an r-LPLND or LPLND is being performed. When a robotic-assisted technique is used, our preference is to place an 8-mm robotic trocar approximately 7 to 8 cm (roughly one handbreadth) lateral to the level of the umbilicus on the right side. An additional 8-mm robotic trocar is placed one handbreadth further lateral on the right side, again at the level of the umbilicus. On the

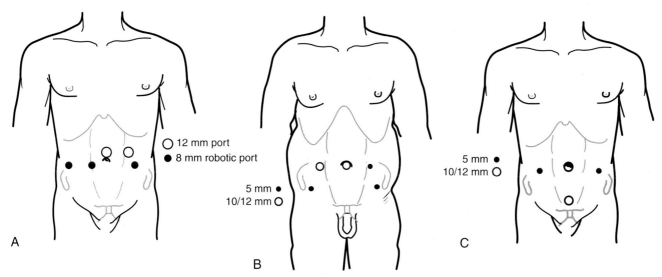

A

B

C

○ 12 mm port
● 8 mm robotic port

5 mm ●
10/12 mm ○

5 mm ●
10/12 mm ○

Figure 13-2. Port placement. **A,** An 8-mm robotic trocar is placed approximately 7 to 8 cm (roughly one handbreadth) lateral to the level of the umbilicus on the right side. An additional 8-mm robotic trocar is placed one handbreadth farther lateral on the right side at the level of the umbilicus. On the left side, a 10/12-mm assistant trocar is placed just superior to the level of the umbilicus approximately 6 to 7 cm from the midline. The third robotic, 8-mm trocar is placed on the left side approximately 10 to 11 cm (one and a half handbreadths) lateral to the umbilicus.
B, In the U configuration, five trocars are used. A 10/12-mm trocar is initially placed at the umbilicus and acts as the camera port. An additional 10/12-mm trocar is placed on the patient's right side 8 to 9 cm lateral and 2 to 3 cm caudal to the umbilical port. A 5-mm trocar is placed on the left side in a mirror image, and two additional 5-mm trocars are placed slightly lateral and caudal for retraction and suction. **C,** In the "diamond" configuration, two midline 10/12-mm trocars are used, one at the umbilicus and the other 4 to 6 cm superior to the pubic symphysis. Two 5-mm ports are placed on either side midway between the umbilicus and the anterior superior iliac spine.

left side, a 10/12-mm assistant trocar is placed just superior to the level of the umbilicus approximately 6 to 7 cm from the midline. Finally, the third robotic, 8-mm trocar is placed on the left side approximately 10 to 11 cm (one and a half handbreadths) lateral to the umbilicus. Alternatively, port placement for r-LPLND can be the mirror image of the aforementioned configuration if the surgeon's preference is to have two robotic arms on the patient's left side (Fig. 13-2, *A*).

Two port configurations can be used for LPLND. In the U configuration, a 10/12-mm port is placed on the patient's right side 8 to 9 cm lateral and 2 to 3 cm caudal to the umbilical port. Depending on the patient's anatomy, this port is brought into the abdomen just medial to the inferior epigastric vessels and just lateral to the medial umbilical ligament. A 5-mm port is placed on the left side in a mirror image, and two additional ports are placed slightly lateral and caudal for retraction and suction. Alternatively, a four-port diamond configuration can be used with two midline 10/12-mm ports, one at the umbilicus and the other 4 to 6 cm superior to the pubic symphysis, and two 5-mm ports midway between the umbilicus and the anterior superior iliac spine on either side (Fig. 13-2, *B* and *C*).

Once the ports have been placed, the operating room table is repositioned into steep Trendelenburg, allowing for gravity to move the bowel out of the pelvis and facilitating access to the pelvic lymph nodes. Occasionally there are sigmoid colon adhesions that need to be gently freed to gain better access to the left obturator fossa (Fig. 13-3).

PROCEDURE (SEE VIDEO 13-1)

PLND requires identification of crucial anatomic landmarks such as the medial umbilical ligament, the external iliac vessels, the vas deferens, and the internal inguinal ring

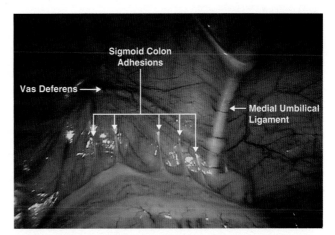

Sigmoid Colon
Adhesions

Vas Deferens →

← Medial Umbilical
Ligament

Figure 13-3. Access to the left obturator fossa is occasionally obscured by adhesions from the sigmoid colon to the pelvic side wall. The anatomic relationship among the sigmoid colon, medial umbilical ligament, and vas deferens is demonstrated. The sigmoid colon is carefully mobilized medially with athermal lysis of adhesions to expose the left obturator fossa in order to facilitate lymph node dissection.

to help facilitate dissection in the correct tissue plane to maximize lymph node yield and minimize complications (Fig. 13-4). The dissection begins with identification of the medial umbilical ligament. An incision with the robotic monopolar scissors is made in the posterior peritoneum lateral to the ligament and medial to the internal inguinal ring to uncover the underlying external iliac vein (Fig. 13-5). The incision is extended in a cephalad and medial direction

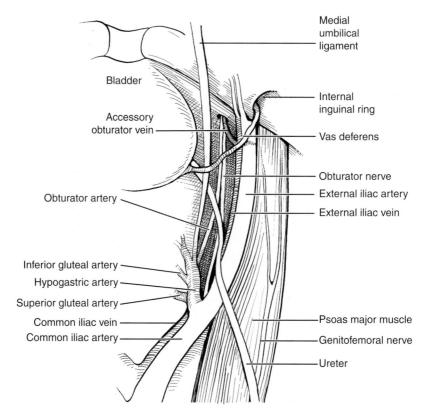

Figure 13-4. Illustration depicts important anatomic landmarks such as the medial umbilical ligament, vas deferens, internal inguinal ring, and external iliac artery and vein that should be identified before initiating the peritoneal dissection, to ensure entry into the correct surgical plane and avoid surgical complications.

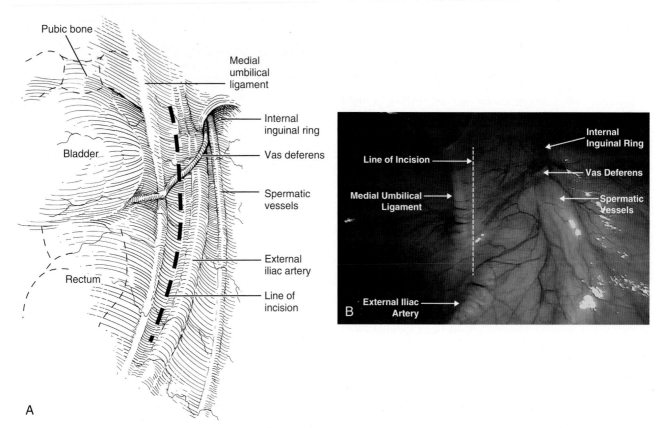

Figure 13-5. A, The dissection begins with an incision in the posterior peritoneum lateral to the medial umbilical ligament and medial to the internal inguinal ring. **B,** The dashed line in this intraoperative image of the right hemipelvis delineates the correct location of the incision in the peritoneum.

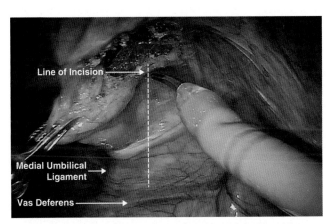

Figure 13-6. This image illustrates the initial dissection of the right side of the space of Retzius during a radical prostatectomy, which also serves to develop the medial border of the pelvic lymph node dissection.

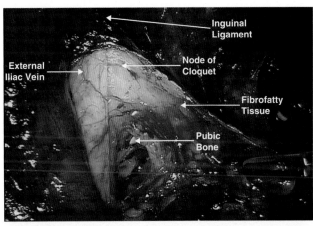

Figure 13-7. The left external iliac vein is dissected proximally to the level of the confluence with the internal iliac vein and distally to the inguinal ligament.

along the lateral aspect of the medial umbilical ligament as it becomes the obliterated umbilical artery and joins the hypogastric artery. Care should be taken to avoid injuring the ureter as it courses over the iliac vessels and into the pelvis. When the vas deferens is encountered during this dissection, it can be clipped, ligated, and divided, or it can be mobilized to allow for easier access to the lymph node packet in the obturator fossa. If the PLND is performed as part of a prostatectomy or cystectomy, the peritoneal dissection will have already been performed when the space of Retzius is developed (Fig. 13-6).

Once the peritoneum has been adequately mobilized, the next step is to identify the external iliac vein. In obese patients the iliac vein may be difficult to identify in the enveloping fibrofatty tissue. In these situations it may be beneficial to identify the external iliac artery by looking for its pulsation and dissecting medially until the vein is encountered. Occasionally the iliac vein may be collapsed owing to the pressure exerted by the pneumoperitoneum, making it difficult to define the borders of the vein. This problem can be resolved by temporarily decreasing the pneumoperitoneum to 5 mm Hg, allowing for the vein to fill with blood and thus making it easier to delineate the vein's borders.

In a standard template PLND, the vein is carefully dissected along its length toward its caudal limit defined by the node of Cloquet, or roughly where the vein dives under the inguinal ligament (Fig. 13-7). The cephalad extent of dissection is defined by the confluence of the hypogastric vessels with the external iliac vessels. Next, the medial border of the node packet will need to be defined and dissected when PLND is performed as an independent procedure. This is done by using the medial umbilical ligament to help define the medial node packet border. The decompressed bladder is retracted medially, which will allow for easier delineation of the node packet. Dissection is then carried out from the node of Cloquet distally, to the iliac bifurcation proximally. Simple blunt dissection is usually sufficient to develop the medial border. The medial dissection has usually already been performed during a radical prostatectomy or cystectomy when the space of Retzius is developed.

Attention is then turned toward dissection of the lateral border of the node packet. The fibrofatty and lymphatic

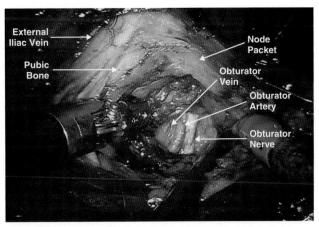

Figure 13-8. The left obturator node packet is gently retracted medially with the fourth arm of the robot, allowing for easier access to the pelvic side wall and the obturator fossa below. This exposure is crucial for the safe dissection of the obturator nerve and vessels.

tissue medial and inferior to the vein is grasped and pulled medially using the fourth arm of the robotic system. The assistant can aid in exposure by using the suction device to carefully retract the vein laterally. Blunt dissection is then performed inferior to the vein until the pelvic side wall is exposed. A good anatomic landmark for this is to expose the pubic bone and follow it to its inferior border where the side wall can be seen. The lateral border of the node packet is then developed caudally along the side wall until the pubic bone is encountered at the level of the node of Cloquet. The dissection is carried posteriorly until the obturator vessels and nerve are encountered (Fig. 13-8). Once the nerve has been identified, the distal extent of the node packet pedicle can be safely dissected with the angulation of the robotic instruments, or, alternatively, if an LPLND is being performed, a right-angle dissector can be used (Fig. 13-9). During this dissection, special attention should be paid to avoid the easily injured circumflex vessels (Fig. 13-10). The isolated distal pedicle of the node packet is then clipped using endoscopic locking clips and divided. It is essential to clip this tissue to

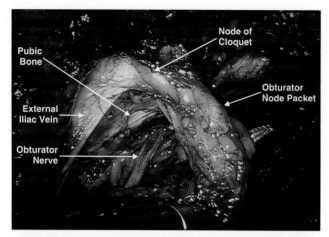

Figure 13-9. The distal aspect of the left node packet is dissected off of the obturator nerve. The articulating robotic instruments allow for easy delineation of the pedicle of the distal node packet.

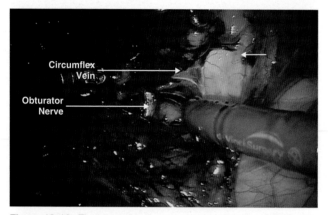

Figure 13-10. The circumflex iliac vein can be a source of troublesome bleeding during pelvic lymph node dissection if it is not identified and avoided. This image depicts the right circumflex vein.

minimize the risk of lymphatic leakage with possible lymphocele formation (Fig. 13-11, *A*).

The distal end of the node packet is then retracted anteriorly using the fourth arm of the robotic system, allowing for careful skeletonization of all lymphatic and fibrofatty tissue off of the obturator vessels and nerve. The node packet is then retracted superiorly and medially to facilitate dissection along the obturator vessels and nerve up to the level of the confluence of the hypogastric artery. During this dissection it is not uncommon to encounter an accessory obturator vein, which can arise anywhere between the bifurcation of the iliac vessels and the inguinal ligament. This accessory vein can be ligated and transected as necessary to facilitate lymph node dissection. Dissection of the proximal lymph node packet pedicle is performed with special care taken to avoid injury to the ureter or its blood supply. Once isolated, the proximal pedicle is ligated and transected (Fig. 13-11, *B*). The lymph node packet is then removed in its entirety either with a reusable 10-mm retrieval bag or by removal of the lymph nodes directly through the 10/12-mm trocar. Once the specimen has been removed, the obturator fossa is inspected for any bleeding. Electrocautery is used judiciously to achieve hemostasis (Fig. 13-12).

In the setting of a radical cystectomy, the boundaries of the PLND are expanded to include the genitofemoral nerve and pelvic side wall laterally, the bladder medially, the node of Cloquet inferiorly, and the aortic bifurcation superiorly. Posteriorly, the dissection includes complete skeletonization of the hypogastric artery, including its medial branches, as well as the area posterior to the obturator nerve and vessels. Ultimately, the node dissection should yield paravesical, pararectal, presacral, obturator, common iliac, external iliac, and internal iliac node packets. The dissection starts similar to the standard PLND; however the incision in the peritoneum lateral to the medial umbilical ligament is over the external iliac artery. The peritoneal incision is extended inferiorly to the pubic ramus and superiorly to the common iliac artery. During this dissection it is important to identify and preserve the ureter and the superior vesical artery. A split and roll technique is used to clear the fibrofatty tissue and lymphatics over the external iliac artery and vein. The aortic and vena cava

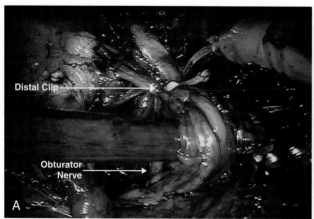

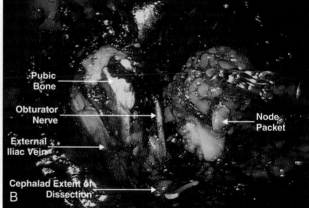

Figure 13-11. Endoscopic locking clips are best for ensuring proper ligation of lymphatic channels to avoid postoperative lymphocele formation. In this image (**A**), a clip is applied to the distal aspect of the left node packet (**B**).

bifurcations are then identified by moving cranially along the common iliac vessels. The presacral node packet is then meticulously dissected. Presacral venous branches should be avoided when performing this portion of the dissection because they are a frequent cause of troublesome bleeding. The bladder is then retracted medially to expose the internal iliac vessels. A similar split and roll technique is used to clear the lymphatic tissue over these vessels. Next, the obturator dissection is performed in the same fashion as described earlier (Fig. 13-13). It is critically important to maintain meticulous hemostasis throughout the node dissection. This is achieved with the use of bipolar, electrocautery, or clip ligation. In addition, close attention should be paid to ligate lymphatic channels to minimize the risk of lymphocele formation.

Attention is then turned toward the contralateral PLND, which is performed in a mirror-image fashion. The node packet is then removed, and the pneumoperitoneum is decreased to a pressure of 5 mm Hg. This will allow for

identification of any venous bleeding that can be promptly cauterized to achieve excellent hemostasis. After all obvious bleeding has been controlled, some surgeons prefer to place an absorbable hemostatic agent such as Surgicel (Ethicon, Somerville, N.J.) in the obturator fossa to aid in hemostasis; however, this is optional. A closed suction drain is then placed in the pelvis through one of the lateral 8-mm robotic trocar sites, or through one of the lateral 5-mm trocar sites if LPLND is being performed. The 10/12-mm trocar sites are then closed using a fascial closure device to minimize the risk of port-site hernia. The 8-mm trocars are then removed under laparoscopic vision to ensure there is no bleeding. An injectable anesthetic such as 0.25% bupivacaine is injected into the incision sites to aid in postoperative pain management. Finally, the skin is closed using either skin staples or absorbable 4-0 monofilament suture. The skin is dressed using Steri-Strips, gauze, and a waterproof, transparent adhesive film.

POSTOPERATIVE MANAGEMENT

Postoperative management depends on whether any concomitant procedures are being performed with the node dissection. Patients are typically discharged on the first postoperative day once they tolerate a diet if the node dissection is the only procedure performed. If the node dissection is performed concomitantly with radical prostatectomy or cystectomy, the postoperative management is dictated by the additional procedures. In all cases, the patient should be encouraged to ambulate early and to use the incentive spirometer to minimize the risk of a thromboembolic event or pulmonary complication, respectively.

COMPLICATIONS

Intraoperative complications for PLND are similar to those encountered in prostatectomy or cystectomy, including injury to vasculature, nerves, and adjacent organs. Vascular injuries include injury to the epigastric, external and internal iliac, and circumflex vessels. The genitofemoral and obturator nerves can be injured during the node dissection and therefore need to be identified and preserved. Finally,

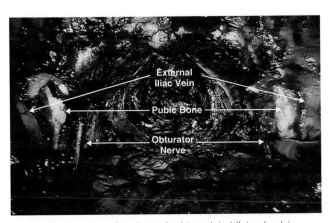

Figure 13-12. A completed standard template bilateral pelvic lymph node dissection should have the internal iliac vein, pelvic side wall, and obturator nerve and vessels cleared of all lymphatic tissue. This image is from a robotic-assisted radical prostatectomy procedure.

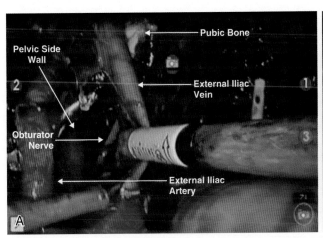 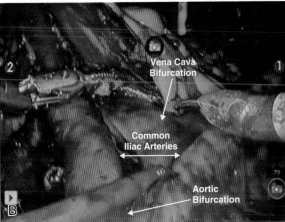

Figure 13-13. A, An extended pelvic lymph node dissection should include removal of all lymphatic tissue from the internal and external iliac vessels, and the obturator fossa. **B,** The extended dissection should also include lymphatic tissue enveloping the common iliac vessels as far proximal as the aortic bifurcation. *(Courtesy Dr. Lee Richstone, North Shore-Long Island Jewish Hospital, New Hyde Park, New York.)*

injuries to the ureter, bowel, and bladder are all possible during the dissection. Injuries should be identified and repaired appropriately intraoperatively to avoid significant morbidity associated with delayed recognition of these injuries. Consultation with appropriate surgical services may be needed to repair these injuries (e.g., general or vascular surgery).

Postoperative complications may include lymphocele, nerve palsies, hematomas, wound infection, ileus, small bowel obstruction, urinary retention, and DVT of the lower extremity. Neural injuries can include traction injury to the obturator nerve during dissection, or injury to peripheral nerves, such as the ulnar and peroneal nerves, as a consequence of suboptimal patient positioning. The risk of DVT can be reduced with the intraoperative and postoperative use of lower extremity sequential compression devices, as well as the postoperative use of prophylactic anticoagulation using subcutaneous heparin or enoxaparin in higher-risk patients. The risk of lymphocele formation is more commonly seen in extraperitoneal dissections. Most lymphoceles are asymptomatic; however, symptomatic lymphoceles can manifest with infection, leg edema or swelling, and DVT. Immediate management of infected lymphoceles typically consists of percutaneous drainage. Recurrent lymphoceles can be treated with aspiration sclerosis, or more invasive techniques such as open or laparoscopic marsupialization into the peritoneal cavity.

TIPS AND TRICKS

- Sometimes the external iliac vein cannot be identified. Because of the compressive effects of the pneumoperitoneum, the vein often appears flattened during laparoscopic surgery. The pneumoperitoneum can be temporarily decreased to 5 mm Hg to allow the vein to fill with blood to delineate the margins.
- If the internal inguinal ring cannot be identified, scrotal traction should move the spermatic cord and assist in identifying its entrance into the ring.
- On insertion of the laparoscopic port in the area of the inferior epigastric artery, significant bleeding may be encountered. Use a fascial closure device to place a suture medial and lateral to the bleeding inferior epigastric vessel above and below the area of bleeding. These can be pulled tightly with a clamp during the surgery and then tied down onto the epigastric vessels after the completion of the procedure.
- If the Foley bag becomes distended like a balloon, suspect bladder injury from dissection medial to the medial umbilical ligament. Identify bladder injury and repair with intracorporeal laparoscopic suturing techniques.
- There may be difficulty identifying the medial boundary of nodal dissection. In this situation, firmly grasp the medial umbilical ligament with a grasping device and move it back and forth to delineate the obliterated umbilical artery. Use this as a starting point to begin blunt dissection to identify the medial edge of the lymph node packet.

14 Laparoscopic and Robotic-Assisted Retroperitoneal Lymph Node Dissection

Ashraf S. Haddad, James Porter

Retroperitoneal lymph node dissection (RPLND) allows for the accurate diagnosis of retroperitoneal disease in patients with nonseminomatous germ cell tumor (NSGCT), thereby permitting stage-directed therapy. In patients with low-volume retroperitoneal disease, RPLND alone can be therapeutic and avoids the side effects and long-term toxicities of chemotherapy. The open approach for RPLND is well established but results in significant morbidity for these young, active patients and may deter them from surgery, resulting in two cycles of chemotherapy.

In an effort to reduce the side effects of RPLND, a minimally invasive approach through laparoscopic or robotic-assisted RPLND provides a less morbid alternative to the open operation, with the goal of re-creating the dissection of the open approach. Although technically challenging, minimally invasive RPLND has been shown to be safe and reproducible and results in substantially less pain and morbidity for patients with testicular cancer as compared with the open approach. Minimally invasive RPLND has also demonstrated the ability to cure patients with low-volume stage II NSGCT, thus avoiding chemotherapy and meeting the same criteria established for the open approach.

In this chapter, we describe the technical evolution of minimally invasive RPLND for the treatment of patients with NSGCT. Our goal is to provide the technical framework for performing minimally invasive RPLND and thereby allow more young men with testicular cancer to experience the benefits of this approach and avoid unnecessary chemotherapy.

INDICATIONS AND CONTRAINDICATIONS

The indications for minimally invasive RPLND are the same as those for open surgery. This includes patients with clinical stages I, IIA, or IIB NSGCT who demonstrate normalization of tumor marker status after orchiectomy. In general, patients with low-risk clinical stage I disease (no lymphovascular invasion and <50% embryonal carcinoma in the orchiectomy specimen) are best followed with surveillance because many of these patients will not require additional therapy. With significant experience, patients with residual postchemotherapy masses can be treated by minimally invasive RPLND. Minimally invasive RPLND would be contraindicated in patients who cannot tolerate pneumoperitoneum or those with pure seminoma and postchemotherapy residual masses. Prior abdominal surgery is a relative contraindication to minimally invasive RPLND, but the vast majority of such patients can be successfully treated after initial minimally invasive adhesiolysis.

A unilateral nerve-sparing approach can be performed laparoscopically for stage I disease (Fig. 14-1). Modified and full bilateral templates can be performed either laparoscopically or with the assistance of the robotic platform. With the expected desmoplastic reaction in postchemotherapy patients as well as for larger burdens of disease as in stage IIA and IIB,

some surgeons find the robotic systems to offer improved angles of dissection and help with vascular control in the event of bleeding from the area of dissection.

PATIENT PREOPERATIVE EVALUATION AND PREPARATION

The preoperative evaluation includes assessment of tumor markers α-fetoprotein (AFP), β subunit of human chorionic gonadotropin (β-HCG), and lactate dehydrogenase (LDH) and computed tomography (CT) imaging of the abdomen and chest. Patients with persistently elevated tumor markers are not candidates for RPLND and should receive chemotherapy. In addition to staging the extent of disease, imaging studies allow for identification of patient-specific anatomic variations that could influence the surgery, such as multiple renal arteries, a retroaortic renal vein that could be confused for a lumbar vessel, or even a reversed aorta and inferior vena cava (IVC) (Fig. 14-2).

Patient preparation includes bowel preparation with a clear liquid diet and ingestion of oral laxatives (magnesium citrate) the day before surgery. Patients are asked to avoid all anticoagulants and platelet inhibitors for 7 days before the procedure. Sperm bank storage is discussed with patients and encouraged in young men who have yet to father children. A type and screen is performed on all patients. For patients in whom a difficult dissection is anticipated, a type and crossmatch for 2 units of packed red blood cells may be indicated.

OPERATING ROOM CONFIGURATION AND PATIENT POSITIONING

After induction of general anesthesia and the administration of intravenous antibiotics, a Foley catheter and an orogastric tube are placed. Pneumatic compression devices are routinely used to prevent thromboembolic complications. Complete neuromuscular blockade is maintained throughout the procedure to allow for stable pneumoperitoneum.

Lateral Position

The lateral position can be used for both the laparoscopic and robotic approaches; however, our experience has evolved so that we use the lateral position for laparoscopic RPLND and perform robotic-assisted RPLND using the supine approach. The patient is placed in a 60-degree modified flank position and well padded with pillows and blankets (Fig. 14-3). The upper arm can be supported with an arm hammock or pillows or tucked close to the body in a praying position. Great care should be taken with positioning to ensure padding of all bony prominences because these procedures can take 5 to 6 hours. We have found patient fixation with a beanbag to be less than ideal because this creates a hard contact surface with the dependent side of the patient. Once the patient is positioned, the room is configured for the laparoscopic approach as in Figure 14-4. The surgeon and first assistant are anterior to the patient, and the second assistant is positioned at the patient's back, to allow tissue retraction through the laterally placed assistant trocar.

After the abdomen has been prepared and draped in a sterile manner, a Veress needle is placed at Palmer's point in the left upper quadrant for a left-sided case and approximately 5 cm below the right costal margin in the midclavicular line for a right-sided case. The right-sided modification of Palmer's point is used to avoid Veress needle passage into the right lobe of the liver. Initial CO_2 insufflation is then performed to a pressure of 20 mm Hg until all the ports are placed, after which insufflation is taken down to 12 to 15 mm Hg.

Supine Position

Robotic-assisted RPLND with the supine approach allows a full bilateral dissection for patients with stage I NSGCT found to have positive nodes on frozen section as well as for patients undergoing postchemotherapy RPLND. Patients are placed in the supine position with the arms padded and

tucked (Fig. 14-5). A full-size gel pad is placed in contact with the patient's back from shoulders to buttocks to prevent the patient from sliding once placed in Trendelenburg position. After insufflation is achieved via Palmer's point, the patient is placed in Trendelenburg position to allow the intestines to fall cephalad. If the da Vinci Si system (Intuitive Surgical, Sunnyvale, Calif.) is being used, the robot is brought in from the head of the bed over the patient's left shoulder and the assistant stands on the right side of the patient. If the procedure is performed with the da Vinci Xi system, the robot is side docked on the ipsilateral side of dissection and the assistant is positioned on the contralateral side.

TROCAR PLACEMENT
Laparoscopic Approach

The trocar configuration for laparoscopic RPLND is shown in Figure 14-6. A 12-mm camera port site is placed just cephalad to the umbilicus in the midline. A 5-mm left-hand port and 12-mm right-hand port are placed just lateral to the midline through the middle portion of the rectus muscle. A second 5-mm assistant trocar is placed just medial to the ipsilateral

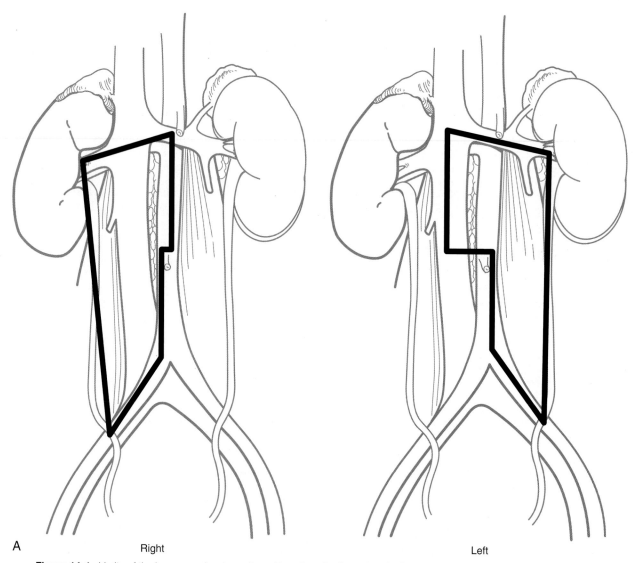

A   Right   Left

Figure 14-1. Limits of the laparoscopic retroperitoneal lymph node dissection. **A,** Clinical stage I: Unilateral modified templates.

anterior superior iliac spine (ASIS) and allows for tissue retraction by the second assistant. The 12-mm right-handed trocar is needed for clip appliers and placement of the extraction sac for lymph node removal. In general, the left-hand, right-hand, and camera trocars are placed more medially than for laparoscopic renal surgery because the dissection takes place around the great vessels in the midline. For right-sided dissections, an additional 5-mm port site can be used as for a liver retractor placed just inferior to the xiphoid process.

Robotic-Assisted Approach

da Vinci Si System

The trocar placement for the supine robotic approach is dependent on the type of robotic system that is available. The trocar configuration for the da Vinci Si system is shown in Figure 14-7. A 12-mm camera trocar is placed between the umbilicus and pubic synthesis in the midline position. An 8-mm trocar for the left robotic arm is placed medial to the right ASIS. The 12-mm assistant port is placed between these trocar sites. An 8-mm trocar for the fourth arm is placed medial to the left ASIS. Finally, an 8-mm trocar for the right

robotic arm is placed between the camera port and the fourth arm port site. There should be at least 7 to 8 cm between ports, if possible, to limit arm conflict.

The majority of the lymph node dissection takes place with this port configuration. However, to completely remove the spermatic cord from the inguinal canal, the robot is re-docked alongside the ipsilateral leg such that the camera is now facing toward the pelvis. The remaining robotic ports are also directed toward the pelvis and inguinal canal to allow complete removal of the cord to the previously placed suture from radical orchiectomy.

da Vinci Xi System

The da Vinci Xi robotic system is designed to allow multi-quadrant access without the need for re-docking or additional port placement. It also provides greater flexibility with regard to docking and allows side docking, which facilitates patient position and simplifies room configuration. This system is ideal for RPLND because it allows access from above the renal hilum to the inguinal canal without the need for re-docking or additional ports. Compared with the supine port placement with the da Vinci Si system, the da Vinci Xi system requires a

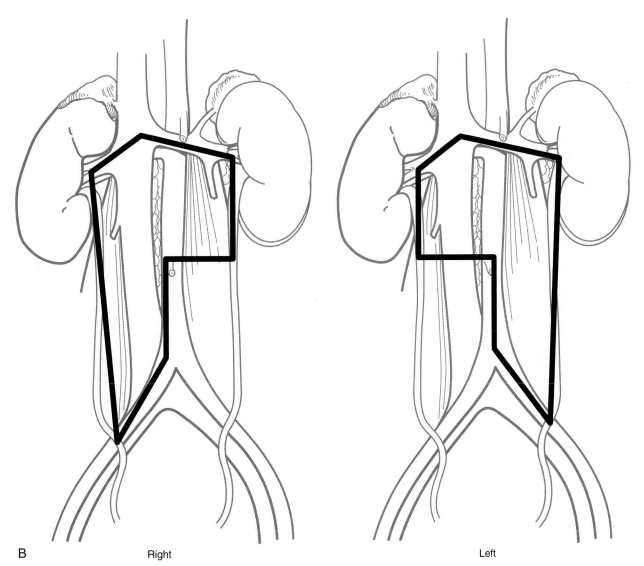

B   Right   Left

Figure 14-1 cont'd B, Clinical stage IIA and IIB: Bilateral modified templates.

Continued

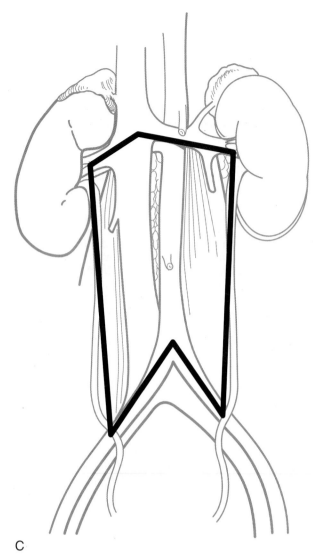

C

Figure 14-1 cont'd C, Postchemotherapy retroperitoneal lymph node dissection: Full bilateral template.

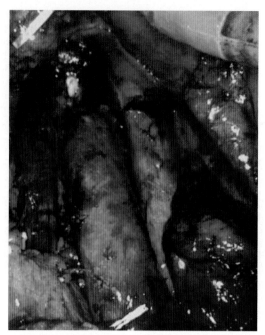

Figure 14-2. Imaging studies allow for identification of patient-specific anatomic variations that could influence the surgery, such as multiple renal arteries, a retroaortic renal vein that could be mistaken for a lumbar vessel, or even a reversed aorta and inferior vena cava.

linear port configuration (Fig. 14-8) to facilitate arm reach and to decrease external conflict. An angled, linear configuration (that depends on the side of the dissection) allows for easy access to the ipsilateral internal inguinal ring for removal of the spermatic cord.

For a right-sided procedure with the da Vinci Xi system, the 8-mm ports are aligned from the right lower quadrant toward the left costal margin, with the 12-mm assistant port placed in the left lower quadrant. For a left-sided dissection, the linear port arrangement is angled in the opposite direction and the assistant is placed in the right lower quadrant. The robot is docked from the ipsilateral side of dissection with the robot-guided docking system. The robotic arms are docked to the ports and the procedure is begun with a 0-degree lens and then converted to a 30-degree down lens once adequate exposure has been obtained.

PROCEDURE (SEE VIDEO 14-1)
Laparoscopic Technique

With the patient in the modified flank position as shown previously, a 30-degree laparoscope is placed through the camera port. The right-hand instrument is monopolar scissors or a monopolar hook cautery instrument; the left-hand instrument is an atraumatic grasper. Polymer locking clips are used to control large lymphatic channels, and titanium laparoscopic clips are used to control vascular structures. Care is taken to control all large lymphatic channels to prevent postoperative lymphatic leakage and potential chylous ascites.

On the right side, the dissection begins by incising the posterior peritoneum along the line of Toldt from the cecum to just beyond the hepatic flexure. This is followed by medial displacement of the ascending colon and duodenum, exposing the great vessels. The duodenum is kocherized until the head of the pancreas is mobile. The gonadal vessels are identified and clipped at the confluence with the great vessels and followed into the pelvis. The entire cord is removed with the cord stump, as indicated by retained suture, after dissection into the internal inguinal ring. The renal pedicle and the inferior mesenteric artery signify the upper and lower limits of resection, respectively. The modified template dissection of the right side includes the precaval, paracaval, retrocaval, and interaortocaval node packages. The split-and-roll technique is used to remove retrocaval nodal tissue. Nodal tissue posterior to the lumbar vessels is included in the resection; lumbar vessels are not transected unless it is necessary. Care is taken to clip all lymphatic channels to prevent lymph leakage, especially the large lymphatic channels crossing over the left renal vein. Fibrin glue is used as an extra safety measure to reduce lymphatic outflow. All excised tissues are removed in endoscopic extraction bags and sent for immediate frozen section analysis. If frozen section reveals tumor in the lymph nodes, then the procedure is converted to a full bilateral dissection. In our experience, this is best accomplished by repositioning and repreparing the patient for a left-sided dissection.

Left laparoscopic RPLND is performed with the patient in an approximately 60-degree flank right lateral decubitus position. The dissection begins with complete mobilization of the left colon and identification of the left gonadal vein entering into the left renal vein. The left gonadal artery is clipped at its

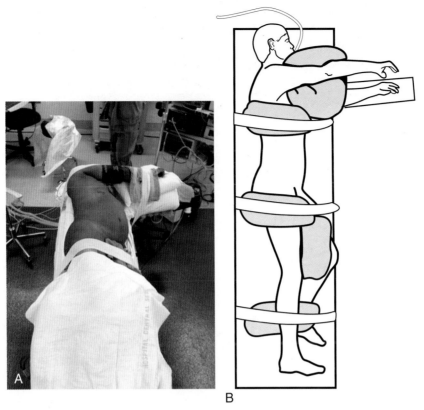

Figure 14-3. A, Lateral positioning for laparoscopic retroperitoneal lymph node dissection. **B,** The patient is placed in a 60-degree modified flank position and padded well with pillows and blankets.

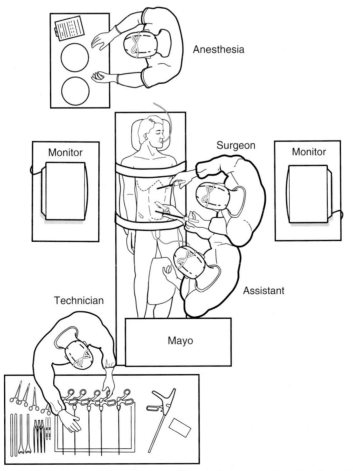

Figure 14-4. The surgeon stands on the side contralateral to the tumor. Two monitors are used so that all members of the team can observe the procedure. A laparotomy set is open and available for rapid access as needed to control severe bleeding.

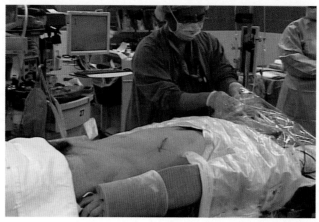

Figure 14-5. Supine positioning. The arms are padded and tucked at the sides.

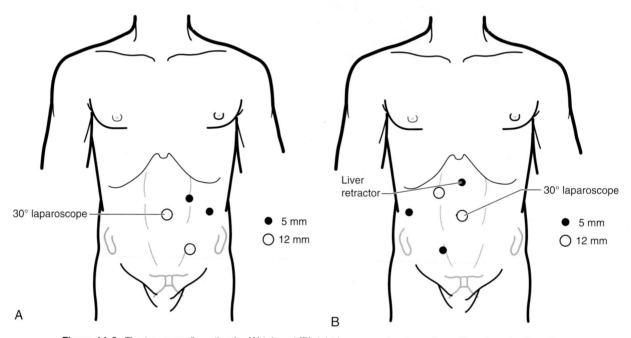

Figure 14-6. The trocar configuration for **(A)** left and **(B)** right laparoscopic retroperitoneal lymph node dissection.

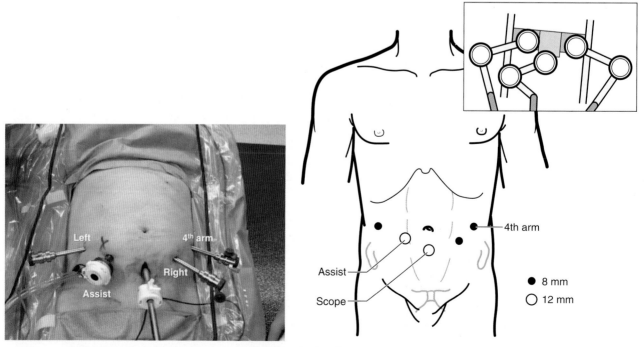

Figure 14-7. The trocar configuration for use of the da Vinci Si robotic system (Intuitive Surgical, Sunnyvale, Calif.).

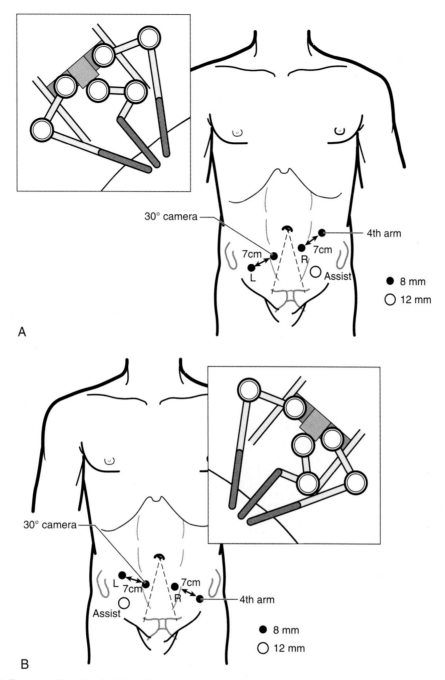

Figure 14-8. A, Trocar configuration for right-sided da Vinci Xi approach. **B,** Trocar configuration for left-sided da Vinci Xi approach.

origin on the aorta, and the artery and vein are dissected as the spermatic cord into the internal inguinal ring. The cord is completely excised as signified by the previously placed suture at radical orchiectomy. The lymphatic tissue lateral to the aorta is dissected first, beginning inferiorly where the left ureter crosses the iliac artery. The para-aortic tissue is dissected up to the left renal hilum, and the large lymphatic channels coursing over the left renal vein and under the left renal artery are controlled with clips. The preaortic tissue overlying the aorta is dissected from the inferior mesenteric artery up to the left renal vein. The retroaortic and interaortocaval nodes are removed using the same limits of dissection. All lymphatic tissue is removed using an endoscopic extraction sac and sent for frozen section analysis.

Robotic-Assisted Laparoscopic Retroperitoneal Lymph Node Dissection

Our initial experience with robotic-assisted RPLND was an extension of the laparoscopic approach; we used the lateral modified flank position with four robotic arms and the assistant placed medially. As with the laparoscopic approach, the lateral position limited access to the contralateral retroperitoneum, which became necessary in patients requiring bilateral dissection. We therefore transitioned to a supine approach for robotic-assisted RPLND, which provides exposure of the entire retroperitoneum and allows for a bilateral dissection.

Robotic-Assisted Retroperitoneal Lymph Node Dissection with da Vinci Si System

After the patient has been placed in moderate Trendelenburg position (15 to 20 degrees), the five-port configuration as shown in Figure 14-7, *B* is created and the robot is docked over the patient's left shoulder. This allows the robotic arms to be directed from the lower to the upper retroperitoneum. Initially, a 0-degree lens is used in the midline camera port, but after mobilization of the colon and exposure of the retroperitoneum, the lens is changed to 30-degree down.

The initial exposure of the retroperitoneum is the same whether it is a right, left, or bilateral dissection. The key to the supine approach is to use the posterior peritoneum and colon as a barrier to hold back the small bowel from falling into the retroperitoneum. The Trendelenburg position helps with this, but this is mainly accomplished by suspending the colon and posterior peritoneum from the anterior abdominal wall. This is performed by incising the posterior peritoneum medial to the cecum and carrying the incision cephalad toward the ligament of Treitz (Fig. 14-9). The cut edge of the posterior peritoneum is suspended with a 2-0 monofilament suture on a straight needle; this is brought up through the anterior abdominal wall. The same maneuver is performed on the left side as well, essentially creating a hammock that prevents the small bowel from entering the field (Fig. 14-10). For exposure of the renal vessels and upper retroperitoneum

to be provided, the fourth robotic arm can be used to retract the duodenum cephalad with the ProGrasp forceps (Intuitive Surgical, Sunnyvale, Calif.).

The aortic pulsation and IVC are identified, and for right-sided dissection the gonadal vein is identified at the IVC, where it is doubly clipped and divided (Fig. 14-11). The spermatic cord is then dissected caudally toward the inguinal canal, and the cord is removed at the end of the procedure when the da Vinci Si system is re-docked next to the ipsilateral leg. The vas is used as a handle to pull the spermatic cord out of the inguinal canal until the previously placed suture from the orchiectomy is identified (Fig. 14-12). The entire cord with the suture is then removed and sent as a specimen through the assistant port.

Attention is then turned to the caudal extent of the template. The lymphatic tissue is dissected where the ipsilateral ureter (Fig. 14-13) meets the iliac vessels, and clips are applied (Fig. 14-14). Lymphatic tissue is then dissected cephalad toward the ipsilateral renal hilum with the ureter marking the lateral extent of the template. Medially, the lymphatics overlying the IVC are split and the lymphatic tissue is dissected off the lateral border of the vena cava (Fig. 14-15). The cephalad extent of the lymph node packet is then dissected away from the renal hilum and clipped. The lymphatic tissue is then dissected off the posterior body wall and the undersurface of the IVC after careful identification of the sympathetic chain (which is preserved). The retrocaval lymph nodes are freed during this dissection. Care should be exercised while dissecting the lymph node tissue between the lumbar vessels and during anterior retraction of the IVC. Once freed, the paracaval and retrocaval lymph node packets are then placed in an endoscopic retrieval bag and removed through the assistant trocar. The tissue is sent for immediate frozen section analysis.

Attention is then turned to the interaortocaval lymph nodes, which are initially separated from the medial border of the vena cava and the medial border of the aorta. The cephalad extent of this lymph node packet is clipped as it travels underneath the left renal artery and the right renal artery. The cisterna chyli is usually encountered in this area, and care is taken to control this with clips. The remaining lymphatic tissues underneath the vena cava are then dissected with the interaortocaval packet as well (Fig. 14-16). The interaortocaval lymph nodes are dissected caudally to the level of the aortic bifurcation and then removed through the assistant port and sent for frozen section analysis.

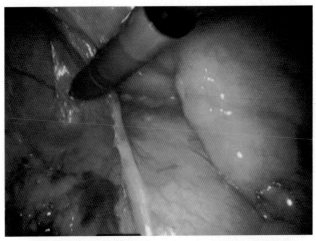

Figure 14-9. The initial exposure of the retroperitoneum.

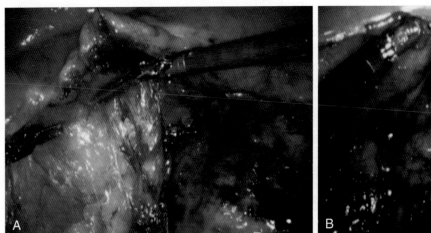
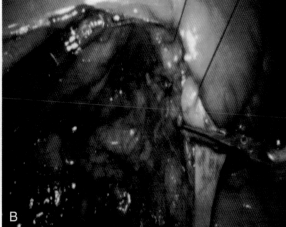

Figure 14-10. The cut edge of the posterior peritoneum is suspended with a 2-0 monofilament suture on a straight needle; this is brought up through the anterior abdominal wall. **A,** Right-sided suspension. **B,** Left-sided suspension.

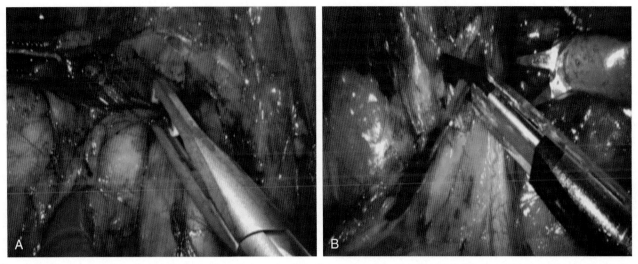

Figure 14-11. The gonadal vein and artery are dissected proximally to the great vessels and clipped. **A,** Clipping right gonadal vein. **B,** Clipping right gonadal artery.

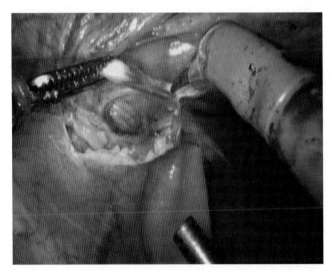

Figure 14-12. The vas is used as a handle to pull the spermatic cord out of the inguinal canal until the previously placed suture from the orchiectomy is identified.

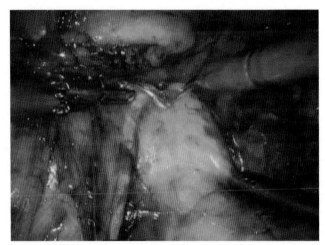

Figure 14-13. The ipsilateral ureter is the lateral border of the dissection.

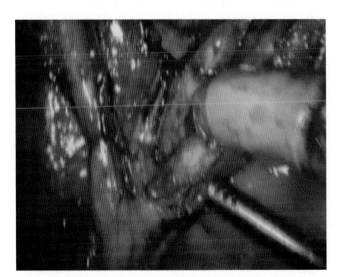

Figure 14-14. The inferior border of the template on the right side where the ureter crosses the iliac vessels.

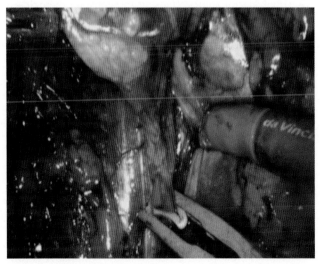

Figure 14-15. The lymphatics overlying the inferior vena cava are split and the lymphatic tissue is dissected off the lateral border of the vena cava.

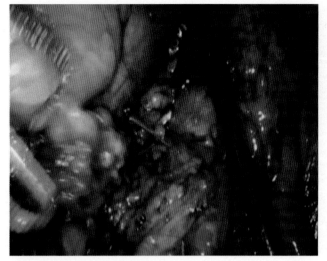

Figure 14-16. Interaortocaval lymph nodes are separated from the sympathetic nervous system fibers.

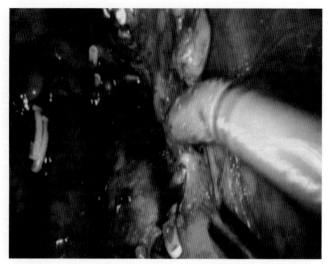

Figure 14-17. The dissection is carried caudally to the level of the inferior mesenteric artery.

The preaortic and para-aortic lymph node tissue is dissected beginning at the cephalad extent of the template, which is the renal hilum on the left side. Care should be taken to identify the large lymphatic channels crossing the left renal vein; they should be clipped to prevent lymphatic leak postoperatively. The lymphatic tissues anterior to the aorta are clipped as well and rolled off laterally, where they are dissected along with the para-aortic lymph nodes on the left side of the aorta. The left lateral limit of this dissection is the contralateral ureter. The dissection is carried caudally to the level of the inferior mesenteric artery (Fig. 14-17), where care is taken to dissect the para-aortic lymph nodes from the postganglionic fibers, as well as the preaortic nodes from the hypogastric plexus. This nodal packet is placed in an endoscopic retrieval bag and retrieved through the assistant port.

After hemostasis is confirmed, the previously placed sutures used to retract the bowel are removed, and the bowel is allowed to fall in its normal position. The robot is undocked at this time and re-docked alongside the ipsilateral leg; the spermatic cord is removed as described previously. All trocars are removed under direct vision and the carbon dioxide is evacuated. The 12-mm assistant trocar is closed with an interrupted No. 0 polyglactin suture. The skin incisions are then closed subcuticularly and dressed in a sterile manner. The orogastric tube is removed before recovery from anesthesia.

For a left-sided template dissection, the exposure is the same as for the right side. The dissection begins with identification and mobilization of the left gonadal vein and artery. The vessels are clipped proximally and dissected inferiorly as far as possible; they will be removed later in the procedure. Attention is then directed to where the left ureter crosses the iliac vessels. The para-aortic lymphatics are dissected cephalad up to the level of the inferior mesenteric artery, where the tissues are split and rolled, preserving the inferior mesenteric artery. The dissection is carried further to the renal hilum, and the sympathetic chain is identified laterally, preserving the postganglionic fibers. The proximal extent of the para-aortic tissues is controlled with clips at the level of the renal hilum. This packet is extracted and sent for frozen section analysis. The preaortic and interaortocaval tissues are then mobilized at the level of the inferior mesenteric artery and dissected cephalad to the left renal vein; the proximal extent of the lymphatics is controlled with clips. The lymph nodes are removed and sent for frozen section. As with the right-sided dissection, the robot is undocked and re-docked alongside the ipsilateral leg, and the remainder of the spermatic cord is removed from the inguinal canal down to the previous orchiectomy suture.

Robotic-Assisted Retroperitoneal Lymph Node Dissection with da Vinci Xi System

The major differences between RPLND with the da Vinci Si system and with the Xi system are the port configuration and the ability to remove the spermatic cord completely without having to re-dock the robot with the da Vinci Xi system. The da Vinci Xi port configuration is linear and angled depending on the side of dissection, as shown in Figure 14-8. This port configuration allows for a bilateral dissection when necessary and complete removal of the spermatic cord owing to the ability of the Xi system to work toward as well as away from the robot. The Xi system allows for easy access to all regions of the abdomen and is ideal for robotic-assisted RPLND. The dissection templates are the same for the da Vinci Xi and Si systems.

Nerve-Sparing Retroperitoneal Lymph Node Dissection

Nerve sparing should be considered in any patient requiring bilateral RPLND or in patients undergoing unilateral template RPLND who are at high risk for positive nodes and may require conversion to a bilateral dissection based on frozen section analysis. The key to successful nerve sparing, whether performed laparoscopically or robotically, is to identify the sympathetic chain laterally early in the dissection of the paracaval and para-aortic packets before injury to the postganglionic fibers can occur. The sympathetic chain is easily identified as being just lateral to where the lumbar vessels dive posteriorly. The large postganglionic fibers are then picked up coming off of the sympathetic chain, and the fibers are traced medially under the IVC on the right and on top of the aorta on the left. The fibers on the right side tend to be more numerous and more robust than on the left side, and care must be taken to avoid cautery during the dissection of the fibers. The postganglionic fibers are then traced to the hypogastric plexus, where the fibers form a network. Once the plexus is identified, the lymphatic tissue can be dissected from the nerve fibers.

POSTOPERATIVE MANAGEMENT

Pain management consists of around-the-clock acetaminophen with as-needed oral narcotics and intermittent breakthrough intravenous medications. The patient is encouraged to ambulate later that same day. The Foley catheter is removed the next morning. Patients are allowed to start a liquid diet the morning after surgery and then advanced to a low-fat diet, which is continued for 2 weeks after surgery to reduce the risk of chylous ascites. We routinely obtain a nutrition consultation to help with patient education on what is required for a low-fat diet. Most patients are stable for discharge on postoperative day 1. Patients are asked to avoid lifting anything heavier than 15 pounds and to avoid abdominal exercises for the first 4 weeks after surgery to prevent straining the incisions and potentially causing a hernia.

The pathologic results are discussed with patients in the clinic 1 week later. Patients found to have stage IIA or IIB disease are offered surveillance. Patients are followed with physical examination; serum AFP and β-HCG levels; and chest x-ray examination every 3 months for 2 years, every 6 months for years 2 to 5, and yearly thereafter. CT scan of the abdomen is performed yearly for the first 3 years.

COMPLICATIONS

The most common complication is chylous ascites. Depending on the degree of the ascites, conservative measures such as extending the duration of the low-fat diet and supplementing it with the use of diuretics can be curative. Otherwise, prolonged bowel rest and total parenteral nutrition might be in order. Rarely, patients may require re-exploration and ligation of a lymphatic channel to correct the ascites. Anejaculation is also a possible complication; however, it is quite uncommon with a nerve-sparing, modified template technique.

TIPS AND TRICKS

- For better exposure of the IVC and aorta during the robotic approach, the colon and small bowel can be retracted cephalad and out of the surgical field by tenting the posterior peritoneum with a 2-0 Keith needle with monofilament suture. Use two separate sutures for the best exposure.
- Identify the cisterna chyli between the IVC and aorta on the posterior body wall, and control this structure with clips to avoid postoperative lymphatic leakage.
- Identify the large lymphatic channels crossing anterior to the left renal vein, and be sure to clip them to prevent lymphatic leakage.
- Be mindful of the lumbar veins, which could be avulsed with placement of anterior retraction on the IVC during the retrocaval dissection.
- For sympathetic nerve preservation, identify the sympathetic chain laterally first and trace the postganglionic fibers medially to the hypogastric plexus. The postganglionic fibers on the right are more easily identified than on the left and course under the IVC on the way to the anterior surface of the aorta. Avoid electrocautery around the nerves.

15 Endoscopic Subcutaneous Modified Inguinal Lymph Node Dissection for Squamous Cell Carcinoma of the Penis

Jay T. Bishoff

The presence and extent of metastatic disease to the lymph nodes is the most important prognostic indicator of survival in patients with squamous cell carcinoma of the penis and has significant clinical application for cutaneous melanoma and vulvar cancer. Lymphadenectomy is often required in these disease processes for cancer staging and can also be curative when cancer is isolated to the penis and regional nodes. Serious, life-altering complications have been associated with inguinal lymph node dissection. Because of the substantial morbidity associated with inguinal lymphadenectomy, controversy surrounds the use of bilateral and prophylactic dissection.

In 2002, Dr. Ian M. Thompson conceived the idea of applying laparoscopic techniques in an endoscopic approach to the inguinal lymph nodes, with the hope of decreasing the morbidity associated with open surgery by preserving the continuity of the lymphatic and vascular supply to the overlying skin. Working together, we combined different techniques from subcutaneous endoscopic brow lift and saphenous vein harvest to formulate an approach using laparoscopic instruments for inguinal node dissection in staging penile cancer. The result of our work was the endoscopic subcutaneous modified inguinal lymphadenectomy (ESMIL) procedure, which mimics the same oncologic approach traditionally performed through an open incision.

We first explored the feasibility of this new procedure in several fresh cadaver studies; in 2003 a patient with T3, N1, M0 squamous cell carcinoma of the penis underwent the first ESMIL procedure.* Since our initial report, others have used the technique with great success and have applied the same technique to other cancers requiring inguinal node dissection. In all of the series, there has been less skin necrosis, less lymph edema, and fewer infections than with open surgery.

INDICATIONS AND CONTRAINDICATIONS

ESMIL is indicated when traditional inguinal lymphadenectomy would be required for staging squamous cell carcinoma of the penis. Patients with nonpalpable nodes or small (<1 cm) mobile nodes at high risk for inguinal node involvement are considered good candidates for endoscopic node dissection. Patients with pTa and pT1 G1 penile tumors will have positive nodes approximately 10% of the time, when inguinal nodes are not enlarged. Fifty percent of patients with pT2 tumors and G3 tumors will demonstrate positive inguinal lymph nodes.

Both stage and grade are predictive of nodal involvement. Verrucous carcinoma and carcinoma in situ are both associated with a low risk for nodal metastasis. However, 70% of

stage T2 cancers have positive nodes. G1 tumors have a 30% chance of spread to lymph nodes, whereas approximately 85% of patients with G3 tumors have inguinal node involvement. Because cross-drainage from the affected side to the contralateral side is a well-known occurrence, bilateral dissection is indicated in patients at high risk for metastatic disease (stage T2 or greater or G2 or G3 tumors).

Patients with large, fixed inguinal lymph nodes have a relative contraindication to ESMIL. In these patients it can be very difficult to dissect the superior aspect of fixed, matted lymph nodes with an endoscopic technique, and as a result they are better candidates for traditional open surgery.

PATIENT PREOPERATIVE EVALUATION AND PREPARATION

A complete metastatic evaluation should be performed before biopsy of the presenting penile lesion or partial penectomy when indicated. The presence of carcinoma of the penis is established with biopsy to determine the diagnosis, extent of invasion, presence of vascular invasion, and grade of the lesion before lymphadenectomy. Distant metastatic disease without lymph node involvement is rarely seen. However, distant metastatic spread to bone, brain, liver, and lung should be considered as part of the overall workup for penile cancer. Computed tomography of the pelvis and inguinal region can be helpful in determining the presence of large pelvic and inguinal nodes, especially in the obese patient.

Waist-high elastic stockings should be fitted and obtained before surgery. Preoperative intravenous antibiotics for skin flora coverage are given 60 minutes before the skin incision. A sterile preparation of the area is performed in the usual fashion.

OPERATING ROOM CONFIGURATION AND PATIENT POSITIONING

The operating room is configured so that all of the staff can view the procedure. The surgeon's monitor is placed on the contralateral side of the dissection, near the shoulder and arm of the patient. A second monitor is placed on the opposite side in the case of bilateral dissection or as needed for viewing by the entire team (Fig. 15-1).

The patient is placed in a supine position, with the ipsilateral knee flexed and hip abducted. The foot on the side of dissection is secured to the contralateral leg for a unilateral dissection, or both feet are secured together in the case of a bilateral procedure. A pad placed under the bent knee will help maintain the correct position during the case (Fig. 15-2).

TROCAR PLACEMENT

Before the first trocar is placed, the limits of the dissection are marked on the skin to preserve the orientation once the

---

* Bishoff JT, Basler JW, Teichman JM, Thompson IM. Endoscopic subcutaneous modified inguinal lymph node dissection (ESMIL) for squamous cell carcinoma of the penis. *J Urol.* 2003;169(Suppl 4): 78.

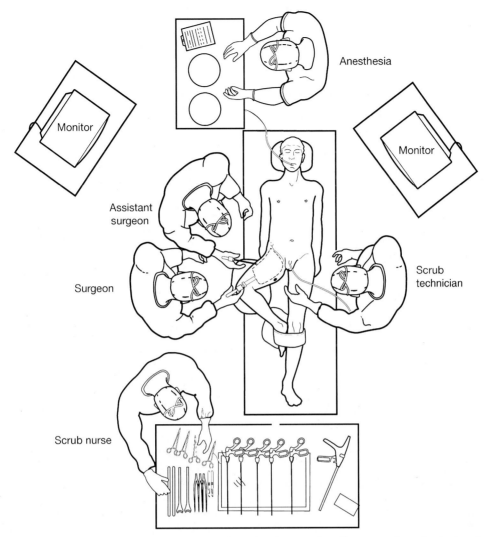

Figure 15-1. The operating room is configured so that all of the staff can view the procedure. The surgeon's monitor is placed on the contralateral side of the dissection, near the shoulder and arm of the patient. A second monitor is placed on the opposite side in the case of bilateral dissection or as needed for viewing by the entire team.

skin is distorted from the insufflation used to create the working space. A line is drawn from the pubic tubercle to the anterior superior iliac crest. The width of the area of dissection is approximately 11 to 12 cm, and the length is 15 cm down the medial thigh and 20 cm on the lateral thigh (Fig. 15-3).

Trocar placement is the same for the left and right sides. The trocars are placed just outside the delineated area of dissection. Initially, a 2.5-cm incision is placed over the saphenous vein 15 cm below the pubic tubercle. It is important to avoid making the incision any larger than 2.5 cm, to prevent CO_2 escape during the procedure once the trocar is inserted and the subcutaneous cavity insufflated. Sharp, fine scissors are used to develop the plane of dissection, elevating the skin from the deep membranous fascia and Scarpa fascia toward the area of dissection drawn on the skin for as far as the surgeon can see inside the lighted cavity. The laparoscope provides an excellent light source for the initial dissection. A blunt-tipped trocar is placed in the incision to create an airtight seal. The blunt-tipped trocar is ideal for this procedure because its unique internal balloon and foam collar create an excellent seal and leave a very small profile inside the area of dissection. This trocar will become the medial working trocar, and because

it is 10 mm, it can accommodate a retrieval sac to remove lymph node packets during the procedure. If a large nodal packet is placed in the sac and cannot be extracted through the trocar, the balloon on the trocar can be deflated and the packet (secured inside the retrieval bag) can be extracted directly through the incision. To prevent seeding of the trocar site, fatty and lymphatic tissue specimens should not be extracted directly through the skin incision without being placed inside an extraction sac.

A second 2.5-cm incision is placed outside the area of dissection approximately 16 cm inferior to the middle of the inguinal ligament. Scissors are used to establish the correct plane of dissection toward the first trocar until the two planes of dissection are joined and a second blunt tip trocar is placed. The laparoscope is usually placed through the second trocar during the procedure. The working space is insufflated to a pressure of 5 mm Hg.

A pair of endoscopic scissors or ultrasonic or bipolar cautery shears are used to dissect the inferior skin margin toward the edge of the surgical field so that the third trocar can be placed. A 5-mm threaded trocar is placed outside the area of dissection approximately 15 cm below the iliac crest (Fig. 15-4).

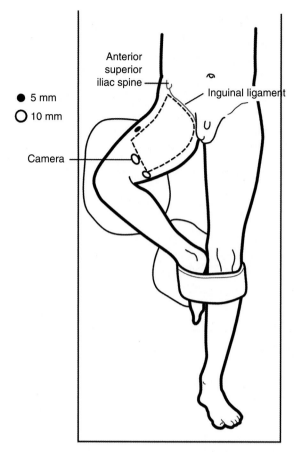

Figure 15-2. The patient is placed in a supine position, with the ipsilateral knee flexed and hip abducted. The foot on the side of dissection is secured to the contralateral leg for a unilateral dissection, or both feet are secured together in the case of a bilateral procedure. A pad placed under the bent knee will help maintain the correct position during the case.

PROCEDURE (SEE VIDEO 15-1)

Inguinal lymph nodes are divided into superficial and deep nodes. The superficial nodes are those located anterior to the fascia lata and the deep nodes posterior to the fascia lata. The inguinal lymph node dissection is carried 2 cm above the inguinal ligament superiorly, laterally to the sartorius muscle and medially to the adductor longus. The superficial nodes are located in four quadrants centered around the saphenofemoral junction: (1) nodes in the area of the superficial circumflex iliac vein; (2) nodes in the area of the superficial epigastric vein and the superficial external pudendal vein; (3) nodes located in the inferomedial quadrant around the saphenous vein; and (4) nodes around the insertion of the superficial circumflex iliac vein and the lateral accessory saphenous vein (Fig. 15-5).

The deep inguinal lymph nodes include the most cephalad node, known as the node of Cloquet, located in the area of the femoral vein and the lacunar ligament (Fig. 15-6).

The dissection begins above the Scarpa fascia anteriorly with removal of the tissue located between the skin and the fascia lata. Early in the dissection, the saphenous vein should be identified and preserved. If possible it is helpful to identify the borders of dissection medially at the adductor longus and laterally at the sartorius muscle edges. In some patients it can be difficult to identify these landmarks

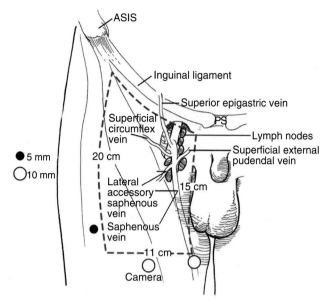

Figure 15-3. The limits of dissection are drawn on the skin. A line is drawn from the pubic tubercle to the anterior superior iliac crest. The width of the area of dissection is approximately 11 to 12 cm, and the length is 15 cm down the medial thigh and 20 cm on the lateral thigh. *ASIS,* anterior superior iliac spine; *PS,* pubic symphysis.

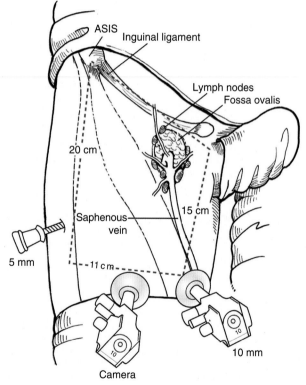

Figure 15-4. The trocars are placed just outside the delineated area of dissection. The first is placed approximately 15 cm below the pubic tubercle over the saphenous vein. A blunt-tipped trocar is placed in the incision to create an airtight seal. A second 2.5-cm incision is placed outside the area of dissection approximately 16 cm inferior to the middle of the inguinal ligament, and a second blunt-tipped trocar is placed. The laparoscope is usually placed through the second trocar during the procedure. A 5-mm threaded trocar is placed outside the area of dissection approximately 15 cm below the iliac crest. *ASIS,* anterior superior iliac spine.

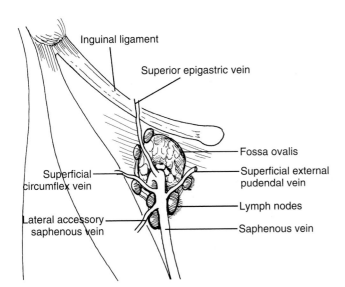

Figure 15-5. The superficial nodes are located in four quadrants centered around the saphenofemoral junction: (1) nodes in the area of the superficial circumflex iliac vein; (2) nodes in the area of the superficial epigastric vein and the superficial external pudendal vein; (3) nodes located in the inferomedial quadrant around the saphenous vein; and (4) nodes around the insertion of the superficial circumflex iliac vein and the lateral accessory saphenous vein.

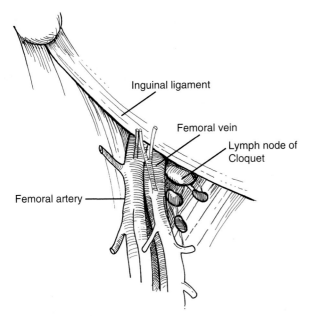

Figure 15-6. The deep inguinal lymph nodes are located under the fascia lata and include the most cephalad node, known as the node of Cloquet, located in the area of the femoral vein and the lacunar ligament.

without opening the fascia lata, but the margins marked on the skin will help in the dissection of the superficial nodal tissue. Subcutaneous vessels and saphenous branches can be divided with ultrasonic energy or electrocautery. Lymph node–bearing tissue is dissected from the fascia lata to the fossa ovalis.

As the dissection progresses toward the inguinal ligament, the external ring is identified and the fat and lymphatics in the area of the cord to the base of the penis medially are removed. The lymph node dissection is continued for 3 to 4 cm superior to the inguinal ligament. Once the nodal tissue and fat are removed from the external oblique and the inguinal ligament, the femoral vessels will be identified inside the femoral sheath.

To gain access to the deep nodes, the fascia lata is opened to the edge of the adductor longus medially and the sartorius muscle laterally. The triangular lymph packet within the femoral triangle is carefully removed. Opening the femoral sheath down toward the apex of the triangle will reveal the deep lymph nodes. Medial dissection will free the node of Cloquet. Any residual tissue between the femoral artery and vein is removed. Care is taken to prevent injury to the femoral nerve by limiting the lateral dissection to the femoral artery.

If the skin overlying the exposed vessels seems compromised in any way, the sartorius can be mobilized from the anterior superior iliac crest, with the use of ultrasonic or bipolar cautery, and transferred over the exposed vessels. Three or four size 2-0 polydioxanone (PDS) sutures are used to attach the sartorius muscle to the inguinal ligament.

At the end of the procedure a 7-mm Jackson-Pratt drain is placed inside the cavity to ensure drainage at the most dependent site of dissection. This can be placed through the 5-mm trocar site, or a new site can be chosen as needed. The two 10-mm trocar sites are closed with skin adhesive or subcuticular sutures. Once the skin adhesive is dry, a circular bandage is placed around the surgical area and held in place with an elastic bandage for 24 hours.

POSTOPERATIVE MANAGEMENT

Waist-high elastic stockings are placed and the patient is kept on bed rest for 5 to 7 days with the lower extremities elevated. Low-molecular-weight heparin or enoxaparin (Lovenox) is started after surgery and continued until the patient is fully ambulatory. The subcutaneous drain remains in place until daily output is less than 30 mL.

COMPLICATIONS

The diagnostic and therapeutic benefits of early inguinal lymphadenectomy should be measured against the potential morbidity associated with the procedure. Patients should be aware of the minor and major postoperative complications associated with this procedure (Box 15-1).

BOX 15-1 Postoperative Complications

MINOR COMPLICATIONS

1. Local wound debridement in clinics
2. Mild to moderate leg edema
3. Seroma formation not requiring aspiration
4. Minimal skin edge necrosis requiring no therapy
5. Scrotal edema

MAJOR COMPLICATIONS

1. Wound infection
2. Severe leg edema interfering with ambulation
3. Skin flap necrosis requiring skin graft
4. Deep venous thrombosis
5. Re-exploration or other invasive procedure performed in the operating room
6. Death

TIPS AND TRICKS

- Use of a lighted instrument or the light directed from the laparoscope will improve visualization of the initial dissection and establishment of the correct tissue planes during placement of the first two trocars.
- Entry into the correct plane of dissection with scissors facilitates dissection after trocars have been placed.
- Continuous flow of CO_2 allows rapid clearing of water vapor or smoke during dissection in the small working space.
- A working pressure of 5 mm Hg is sufficient to maintain visualization while avoiding spontaneous infiltration beyond the boundaries of dissection.
- Key landmarks should be readily identified, and transillumination of the skin facilitates orientation.
- Following the saphenous vein helps with identification of landmarks, but as many branches as possible should be preserved to decrease lymph edema in the lower extremity.
- Divide all tissue with ultrasonic energy or electrocautery to decrease the incidence of lymphatic leak.

16 Laparoscopic Simple Nephrectomy

Hassan G. Taan, Timothy D. Averch

In 1991, Clayman and associates reported the first simple laparoscopic nephrectomy on a 54-year-old woman with oncocytoma. Since the introduction of this revolutionary procedure, indications for laparoscopic renal surgery have expanded, and laparoscopic nephrectomy has gained worldwide acceptance as the preferred approach for most pathologic conditions of the kidney. Laparoscopic approaches to renal surgery allow for the safe removal of a nonfunctional, dysfunctional, or infected kidney while offering the benefits of decreased narcotic analgesia requirements, shorter hospital stay, improved cosmesis, and earlier return to complete activity compared with open approaches. The use of this minimally invasive technique for the removal of benign renal pathology has been verified at several institutions. Among minimally invasive tools, the robotic approach has not gained fame as laparoscopy has, because it failed to offer any obvious advantage over laparoscopy to justify the notoriously higher cost. This chapter focuses on simple laparoscopic nephrectomy via the intra-abdominal approach. The hand-assisted and retroperitoneoscopic approaches to nephrectomy can be applied to simple nephrectomy, but these methods are the subject of discussion in other chapters of this text.

INDICATIONS AND CONTRAINDICATIONS

Simple laparoscopic nephrectomy is the treatment of choice for many benign diseases of the kidney owing to the appeal of decreased perioperative pain and morbidity. Indications and absolute contraindications for laparoscopic simple nephrectomy are listed in Box 16-1.

To date, there is less clarity on the role of laparoscopy in the removal of kidneys affected by severe inflammatory conditions and adult polycystic kidney disease. Series have been reported of laparoscopic simple nephrectomy for xanthogranulomatous pyelonephritis, tuberculosis, and other inflammatory conditions. Advocates argue that laparoscopy, although more difficult in such cases, is possible and may result in improved outcomes in these patients. However, critics suggest that the increased level of difficulty, increased operative times, and increased risk of complications and rates of conversion to open surgery make laparoscopy in these patients unjustifiable. Inarguably, inflammatory conditions of the kidney make hilar dissection more difficult, and these patients are at higher likelihood for conversion to open procedure. These procedures should be attempted only by the urologist with vast experience in laparoscopy and on patients who understand the increased risks compared with open procedures.

In patients with an extensive history of prior abdominal surgery, the retroperitoneoscopic approach may be preferred. Abdominal cavities that have previously undergone surgery can present difficulties that increase operative time and complications. The retroperitoneal procedure gives the surgeon a more direct route to the diseased kidney while avoiding the potential adhesions and scar tissue.

Absolute contraindications to laparoscopic simple nephrectomy include uncorrected coagulopathy, untreated infection or sepsis, peritonitis, and hypovolemic shock. Although morbid obesity is not a contraindication to laparoscopic surgery, obese patients may be at increased risk for complications and open conversion. Anatomic and vascular anomalies of the kidney represent a challenge for the laparoscopic surgeon; however, surgery is feasible if the patient has undergone adequate preoperative imaging of the kidneys.

PATIENT PREOPERATIVE EVALUATION AND PREPARATION

Preoperative evaluation for simple laparoscopic nephrectomy consists of history and physical examination including inspection for prior surgeries, abdominal scars, and skeletal abnormalities. Laboratory tests include complete blood cell count, serum creatinine and electrolytes, clotting parameters, urinalysis and culture, and other tests as indicated depending on the patient's age and underlying comorbidities (e.g., electrocardiogram, chest radiograph). Typing and screening with preparation of two packed red blood cell units in anticipation of major bleeding is advisable. A clear liquid diet the night before surgery is recommended. If an extensive inflammatory reaction that will make the dissection more difficult is anticipated, a mechanical bowel preparation is also highly advisable. The informed consent should include the possibility of conversion to an open procedure.

A preoperative abdominal computed tomography (CT) scan is useful in evaluating the location, size, and disease of the kidney to be removed. Areas of perinephric stranding visualized on CT scan may indicate significant inflammation and dense adhesions, which render dissection more laborious and might increase the chance of conversion to open nephrectomy. In addition, cross-sectional imaging, particularly when coupled with intravenous contrast, will provide data on the vascular anatomy to the kidney, the presence of aberrant vessels or any mural calcifications, and the relationship of the kidneys to adjacent organs and will allow a rough estimate of the function of the contralateral kidney and adrenal gland.

OPERATING ROOM CONFIGURATION AND PATIENT POSITIONING

A beanbag can be placed on the operating table. After the induction of general anesthesia, place a Foley catheter and an orogastric tube to decompress the stomach. Secure eyes with patient safety goggles. Then roll the patient into the modified flank position with the side of interest up (i.e., for right-sided

BOX 16-1 Indications and Absolute Contraindications for Laparoscopic Simple Nephrectomy

INDICATIONS
- Multicystic dysplastic kidneys
- Nonfunction as a result of obstruction, infection, trauma, or stones
- Renovascular hypertension
- Xanthogranulomatous pyelonephritis (XGP)
- Renal tuberculosis
- Reflux nephropathy

ABSOLUTE CONTRAINDICATIONS
- Sepsis
- Untreated urinary tract infection
- Hypovolemic shock
- Peritonitis
- Uncorrected coagulopathy

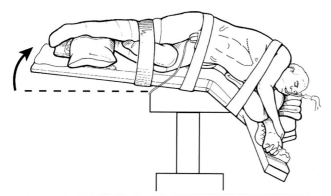

Figure 16-1. The patient is placed in a modified flank position. The umbilicus is placed over the break in the operating table and the patient is placed in a modified decubitus position with the hips and shoulders placed opposite the surgeon, as close to the far edge of the table as possible. This position allows the arms to be placed on the table in a "praying mantis" position or crossed over the chest with two pillows placed between them. Wide tape secures the chest and pelvis.

procedures, the patient lies on his or her left side). Place foam padding beneath all points of pressure created by contact with the operative table to avoid pressure injury. Place the umbilicus over the break in the table, and flex the table as shown in Figure 16-1. Use an axillary roll to prevent brachial plexus injury of the decubitus side arm. Position the arms on an arm board with a pillow or rolled blankets between them. Bend the bottom leg and place a pillow or blankets between the legs so that the top leg rests nearly parallel to the table. Generously use 3-inch cloth tape to tightly secure the patient at the hips and chest (Fig. 16-1). Roll the table in each direction with personnel at each side of the table to ensure adequate stabilization of the patient. Perform a sterile preparation over the entire abdomen in the event that conversion to an open procedure is required. A laparotomy instrument tray should be available in the operating room and ready at all times in case an emergent conversion to an open procedure becomes necessary.

TROCAR PLACEMENT

Trocar placement starts with insufflation of the peritoneal cavity. This can be achieved by inserting a Veress needle that helps inflate the abdomen, therefore rendering the insertion of the first trocar safe from injuring the bowel or other intraperitoneal

organs. Another method is the Hasson technique, which consists of a small incision and dissection to reach the peritoneum and open it to slide the first trocar under vision in an oblique direction.

The Veress needle is placed at the site of the initial trocar, which is usually lateral to the rectus muscle ipsilateral to the surgical site. With the patient situated in the lateral position, the bowel is displaced by gravity away from the site of the initial trocar. In patients with prior abdominal surgeries, place the Veress needle in a region away from prior surgical scars. To confirm intraperitoneal placement, connect a syringe to the Veress needle and aspirate. If there is no evidence of entry into the bowel or a major blood vessel, perform the drop test by placing saline into the Veress needle and watching it freely drop into the peritoneal cavity. To further confirm appropriate location, begin insufflation at low flow rates. Immediate rise of pressure indicates a wrong site of insufflation—most often still in the abdominal wall, which necessitates further advancement of the needle. Place the insufflator on the high flow setting after even distribution of air to an enlarging, tympanic abdomen and low intra-abdominal pressure are confirmed.

Once pneumoperitoneum is established, remove the Veress needle. Make a skin incision to accommodate a 12-mm trocar at the site of the needle puncture. Incisions that are too small can lead to use of excessive force to penetrate the abdominal fascia and, as a consequence, inadvertent trocar entry into underlying organs. Equally problematic are incisions made too large because they can lead to continuous air leakage and loss of pneumoperitoneum throughout the procedure. The visual obturator trocar is a safe option because it provides direct visualization of the fascial layers to gain initial trocar access. Place the laparoscope through the initial port and directly examine the abdominal cavity for injury from entry as well as adhesions to the abdominal wall.

In general, three-trocar configurations are used for laparoscopic simple nephrectomy. Figure 16-2 shows examples of trocar placement for right- and left-sided procedures as well as for trocar placement in obese patients. Shift the entire template laterally in obese patients to allow for optimal instrument movement.

Place the secondary trocars under direct visualization through the laparoscope so that the tip of the trocar is visualized in entirety as it penetrates the peritoneal lining. Place these ports in locations that are free of bowel adhesions. After placing the secondary trocars, take down adhesions with scissors or electrocautery. Various tools are available for dissection of tissues, including hook electrocautery, laparoscopic scissors, harmonic scalpel, curved Maryland dissector, suction-irrigator, right-angle dissector, and atraumatic bowel graspers.

PROCEDURE (SEE VIDEO 16-1)
Reflection of the Colon

Place the patient in the lateral position by rotating the operative table toward the surgeon. This position helps reflect the colon medially by use of gravity. Using an atraumatic bowel grasper in the left hand, pull the colon medially. If needed, make an incision at the white line of Toldt lateral to the colon using the laparoscopic scissors in the right hand (Fig. 16-3). Remain lateral enough to avoid damage to the colonic mesentery. Proper depth of the peritoneal incision is of utmost importance. Do not perform aggressive dissection posterior and lateral to the kidney at this part of the procedure. Concentrate on peeling the colon off the kidney at this time, rather than beginning to dissect the kidney away

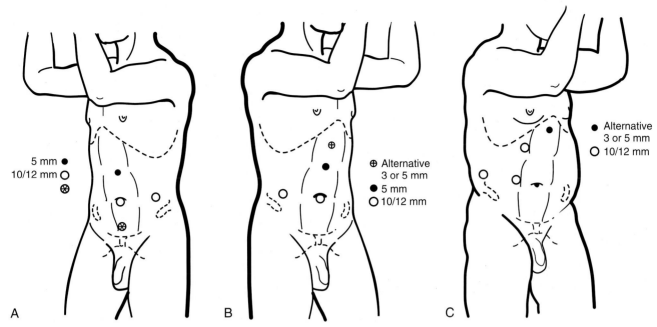

Figure 16-2. Trocar sites for left-sided **(A)** and right-sided **(B)** procedures. The first 10/12-mm trocar is placed lateral to the rectus at the level of the umbilicus and is used for dissection and placement of the endovascular gastrointestinal anastomosis. A second 10/12-mm trocar placed at the umbilicus is used for placement of the laparoscope. A 5-mm trocar inserted in the midline between the umbilicus and the xiphoid process is used for placement of various dissecting instruments. **C,** In obese patients, all trocars are moved laterally.

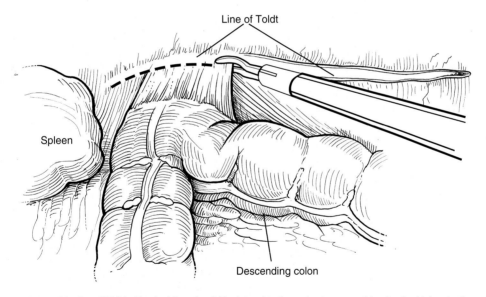

Figure 16-3. Incision of the white line of Toldt. The incision should be lateral to the colon to prevent inadvertent injury to the colon.

from the retroperitoneum. This is vital to further development of surgical planes because overdissection posteriorly will remove the attachments supporting the kidney, making dissection of the hilum extremely difficult.

Continue the line of the incision caudally to reach the bifurcation of the common iliac vessels and cranially to reach the lateral aspect of the spleen (left-sided procedure) or the liver (right-sided procedure) (Fig. 16-3). For left-sided procedures, the spleen can be troublesome owing to its attachments to the kidney and abdominal wall. Minimal tension secondary to aggressive retraction can lead to tearing of the splenic capsule. To avoid this, generously incise the lateral attachments that affix the spleen to the abdominal wall. After removing

these attachments, place gentle medial traction on the spleen and carry out the dissection in the superior direction. It is important to mobilize as much spleen as possible so that the spleen will fall medially along with the pancreas and colon. Be cautious not to incise too lateral to the spleen because the diaphragm can be injured.

For right-sided procedures, the white line of Toldt is incised to the bifurcation of common iliac vessels caudally as on the left side. The cranial extent of the incision follows a course lateral to the liver. Although caution should be exerted when retracting the liver to avoid tearing the capsule, the liver is anatomically more mobile than the spleen, making it less susceptible to traction injury.

On either side, make the lateral incision in a Y shape proceeding superior to the kidney. This allows the lienocolic or hepatocolic ligaments to be divided, further mobilizing the colon medially.

Dissection of the Ureter

The ipsilateral psoas muscle serves as a useful frame of reference in the localization of the ureter. The ureter is found at the medial aspect of the psoas, deep to the gonadal vein. Once the gonadal vein has been identified, sweep it medially with blunt dissection and identify the ureter. Use a blunt dissecting device such as the suction-irrigator to create a window posterior to the ureter, and anteriorly elevate the ureter (Fig. 16-4). Continue the anterior elevation of the ureter cranially until the renal hilum is identified (Fig. 16-5).

Dissection of the Hilum

Localize the renal hilum by placing anterior traction on the ureter and following the ureter in a cranial direction via blunt dissection. For left-sided procedures, the gonadal vein is also a useful anatomic landmark because it drains directly into the left renal vein. Identify the renal vein and make an incision in the Gerota fascia anterior to the vein. After accessing the vein, dissect it in its entirety, taking care to avoid inadvertent entry into the left adrenal vein (superomedial), the descending lumbar vein (posterior), or the gonadal vein (inferior). At this point, ligate the adrenal and gonadal veins using hemostatic clips (two clips on the proximal side and a single clip on the distal side of the incision).

For right-sided procedures, the gonadal vein is not as useful a landmark because it inserts directly into the inferior vena cava rather than the right renal vein. However, its anatomic position might require excessive manipulation, and exaggerated elevation can result at times in vein avulsion and significant blood loss. Follow the ureter cranially to the renal hilum. The duodenum and inferior vena cava are situated directly medial to the right renal vein. Identify these structures and dissect them medially to prevent inadvertent injury while isolating the renal vein. Also, avoid the adrenal gland, with its short adrenal vein entering the posterior surface of the vena cava, during dissection of the right renal hilum to prevent injury.

After isolation of the renal vein, the focus of the dissection changes to the renal artery, which is found posterior to the renal vein. Place indirect anterolateral traction on the kidney by lifting the suction-irrigator in the left hand after placing the device posterior to the ureter. Identify the renal artery posterior to the vein. Use a Maryland or right-angle dissector to separate the renal artery from the surrounding tissues. Some use blunt dissection, whereas others prefer hydrodissection using the irrigator-aspirator cannula. Once adequate length of the artery is established, apply metallic or Hem-o-lok clips (Weck Closure Systems, Research Triangle Park, N.C.) or an endovascular gastrointestinal anastomosis (GIA) tool (Endo-GIA, Covidien, Mansfield, Mass.) to occlude the flow through the artery. Ligate the artery, leaving at least two hemostatic clips on its proximal end if clips are used. Alternatively, the division of the artery can be performed with the endovascular GIA staple. On occlusion of the renal artery, the kidney becomes uniformly ischemic in appearance and soft. The ipsilateral renal vein becomes decompressed and flat. If these changes do not occur, the presence of an additional renal artery or arteries should be suspected.

Most surgeons prefer the endovascular GIA to control the renal vein; however, extra-large Hem-o-lok clips may also be used (Fig. 16-6). If the endovascular GIA is used, squeeze the grip confidently and deliberately in a single, smooth motion. Partial or staccato squeezing can lead to misfiring or locking of the device while on the vein and potentially dire consequences. Also, the application of clips on the renal vein closer to the hilum is discouraged because these can lead to

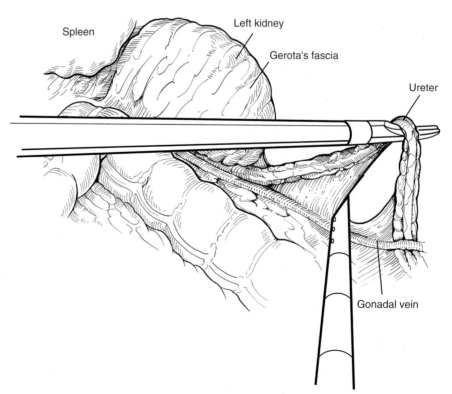

Figure 16-4. A curved dissector, in the left hand, is placed beneath the ureter and used to provide anterolateral elevation.

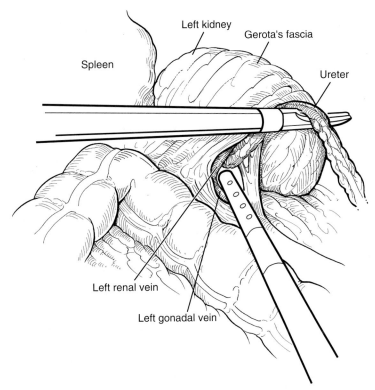

Figure 16-5. The ureter is followed to the lower pole of the kidney and then to the renal hilum. Thin medial attachments can be bluntly dissected with the tip of the irrigator-aspirator, revealing the edge of the renal vein.

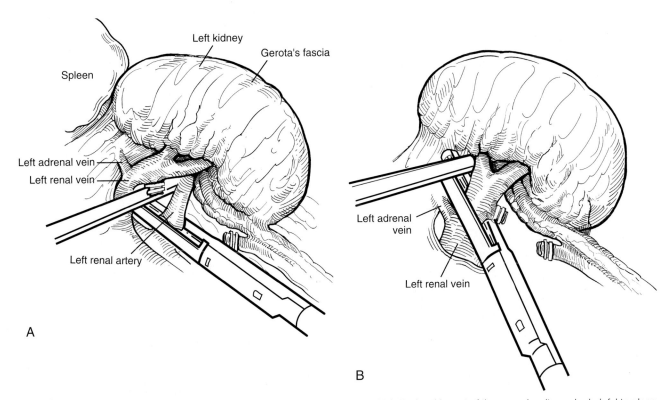

Figure 16-6. A, The artery is stapled first with the gastrointestinal anastomosis (GIA). During this part of the procedure it may be helpful to place the retracting instrument between the renal artery and vein. This will provide more arterial length and separate artery from vein. **B,** The renal vein is ligated lateral to the adrenal vein with the endovascular GIA. During a simple nephrectomy, it is often possible to divide the renal vein lateral to the gonadal vein, leaving both the gonadal and adrenal veins intact.

malfunctioning of the GIA. Furthermore, when applying the GIA onto the vein, visualize the tips of the instrument and ensure that there is no tissue within the tines other than the renal vein, including the renal artery or the staples applied on it. En bloc stapling of the renal hilum is widely used as well.

Dissection of the Superior Pole

The ipsilateral adrenal gland is spared with simple laparoscopic nephrectomy except in cases in which the gland is densely adherent to the upper pole of the kidney. Before removing the ipsilateral adrenal gland, confirm the presence of a normal-appearing contralateral adrenal gland on preoperative imaging.

Right-Sided Procedures

Free the upper pole of the right kidney from its peritoneal attachments by placing gentle superior traction on the liver. In cases in which the liver is extremely large or overlying the right kidney, place a fourth laparoscopic port to assist in retraction. Take care to avoid injury to the adrenal gland and its short vein to the posterior surface of the vena cava (Fig. 16-7). Connect the incision in the peritoneal attachments to that made lateral to the kidney during colon mobilization.

Left-Sided Procedures

Superior pole dissection on the left side often poses greater challenges to the surgeon than right-sided procedures. The spleen, pancreas, adrenal gland, colon, and diaphragm are in intimate relation to the left kidney. The plane of dissection must proceed immediately adjacent to the upper pole of the kidney. The harmonic scalpel, or bipolar cautery device, and a liberal amount of clips help in this dissection because problematic bleeding can be encountered in this region. Any retraction of the spleen must be gentle and in a superomedial direction. Retract the spleen only after adequate ligation of splenorenal attachments to prevent tearing of the delicate

splenic capsule. Furthermore, it is important to dissect lateral to the spleen in a superior direction so that the spleen can be safely retracted. Dissection should be in close proximity to the spleen and not too lateral to avoid injury to the diaphragm.

Incision of Gerota Fascia and Ureteral Ligation

After ligating the renal vessels and dissecting the superior pole, direct the dissection toward freeing the kidney from the Gerota fascia. Perform a superior incision through this fascia so that the renal capsule is visualized. Sweep the Gerota fascia off the kidney by placing posterior tension on the kidney with a blunt instrument while sweeping the fascia anteriorly with another. Continue the dissection by marching the instruments in a stepwise fashion through the developed tissue plane between the renal capsule and Gerota fascia inferiorly and posteriorly. Leave the ureter intact until after removal of the Gerota fascia from the kidney because the ureter prevents rotation of the kidney and facilitates retraction. When the dissection is complete, double clip the proximal ureter with clips and make an incision between the clips. The kidney is now entirely freed from any attachments and prepared for removal.

Entrapment and Specimen Removal

Remove the surgical specimen either intact or morcellated. Carry out morcellation by placing a sturdy impermeable bag through the umbilical port. The LapSac (Cook Medical, Bloomington, Ind.) is adequate for this purpose. Place the kidney inside the bag and morcellate with either the electronic morcellator or manual ringed forceps. Easily remove the bag containing the morcellated contents through the umbilical port incision.

Alternatively, place the specimen in a specimen retrieval bag such as the Endo Catch (Covidien, Mansfield, Mass.) via an extension of the umbilical port incision. Make an infraumbilical midline incision through the rectus fascia. Then close the laparoscopic ports with absorbable suture using a Weck EFx (Telefex Medical, Research Triangle Park, N.C.) device.

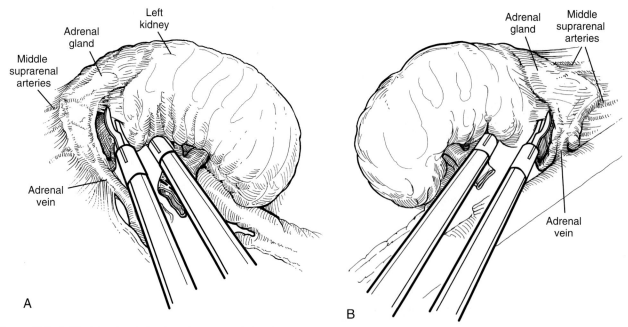

A

B

Figure 16-7. A, The left adrenal gland can be preserved during simple nephrectomy. Here, the left renal vein has been preserved and the dissection is continued directly on the capsule of the kidney. **B,** Preservation of the right adrenal gland. Caution must be exercised on the right so as not to avulse the short right adrenal vein from the vena cava.

Place a hand through the extraction incision if possible to prevent puncture injury to the underlying bowel by the closure tool.

POSTOPERATIVE MANAGEMENT

At the conclusion of the procedure, awaken the patient and remove the orogastric or nasogastric tube. Start clear liquids once the patient is fully awake, and gradually advance the diet to regular, as tolerated by the patient. Intravenous administration of ketorolac helps reduce the patient's discomfort and need for narcotic analgesia. The patient should begin early ambulation to prevent deep venous thrombosis as well as postoperative pulmonary complications. Obtain serum electrolytes the morning of postoperative day 1, as well as hemoglobin if excessive blood loss occurred during the procedure.

COMPLICATIONS

Be aware of the numerous complications of simple laparoscopic nephrectomy to promptly recognize and treat them should they arise.

Major vessel injury can occur with placement of the Veress needle or laparoscopic trocars. This injury is typically immediately noticed by seeing pulsatile blood return through the Veress needle or trocar. Open control and repair is an ideal approach to these injuries because blood loss can be severe and rapid.

Bowel injury is another potential complication and is, unfortunately, rarely recognized at the time of surgery. Bowel injury manifests as abdominal pain and peritonitis, port-site redness and tenderness, leukopenia, and diarrhea in the postoperative period. Perform abdominal CT scan if suspicion is raised for bowel injury based on these symptoms and signs.

Air embolism manifests as sudden hypoxia, hypercarbia, and a characteristic "mill-wheel" cardiac murmur. Once air embolism is recognized, place the patient in the head-down, right-side-up position and evacuate the embolism by central venous catheter.

Oliguria is common with pneumoperitoneum during surgery; discourage use of urine output as an indicator of intravascular volume status. Make the anesthesia team aware of this phenomenon so that the overadministration of intravenous fluids and the subsequent development of pulmonary edema do not occur.

Rhabdomyolysis can occur after prolonged procedures and has been associated with use of beanbag appliances used for patient stabilization. This can be minimized with liberal padding of all areas that come in contact with the operative table.

Additional complications include incisional hernia after intact specimen removal, prolonged ileus, cardiac events, pneumonia, pulmonary embolism, and brachial nerve injury.

NEWER APPROACHES IN LAPAROSCOPIC NEPHRECTOMY

The latest innovations applied in minimally invasive simple nephrectomies are natural orifice transluminal endoscopic surgery (NOTES) and laparoscopic endoscopic single-site surgery (LESS). LESS-nephrectomy (LESS-N) is a safe procedure in adequately selected patients. LESS-N has been considered a feasible alternative with the advantages of a single wound, less pain, a short recovery period, and better cosmetic results. Robotic-assisted surgery and LESS have been used as a combination in nephrectomy with results similar to those of laparoscopic single-site surgery. Studies and wider use are required to establish NOTES and LESS as potential alternatives to laparoscopic nephrectomy.

SUMMARY

Laparoscopic simple nephrectomy is a feasible and effective treatment option for benign renal pathologic conditions. This procedure offers a shorter hospital stay, decreased use of narcotic analgesia, better cosmesis, and an earlier return to full activity when compared with the open approach. The steps provided herein can be applied to most benign conditions of the kidney. Xanthogranulomatous pyelonephritis, tuberculosis, and other inflammatory conditions should be treated laparoscopically only by experienced surgeons.

TIPS AND TRICKS

- Careful positioning of the patient is essential to a successful procedure. Do not rush or neglect this aspect of the procedure.
- Ensure that the patient is adequately padded at all areas of contact with the operative table to prevent nerve injury, pressure sores, and rhabdomyolysis.
- If deciding to remove the ipsilateral adrenal gland, always stop to ensure that a contralateral adrenal gland exists.
- The ureter is a valuable retractor. If left intact, a blunt instrument can be used to elevate the ureter, and thus the lower pole of the kidney, allowing the surgeon to progress to the renal hilum.
- The harmonic scalpel is an indispensable instrument for dissection of the adrenal gland from the kidney as it controls bleeding from small vessels to the adrenal. It can, however, be replaced with the bipolar cautery device based on the availability and surgeon comfort.

SUGGESTED READINGS

Bercowsky E, Shalhav AL, Portis A, et al. Is the laparoscopic approach justified in patients with xanthogranulomatous pyelonephritis? *Urology.* 1999;54:437.

Capelouto CC, Kavoussi LR. Complications of laparoscopic surgery. *Urology.* 1993;42:2.

Clayman RV, Kavoussi LR, Soper NJ, et al. Laparoscopic nephrectomy: initial case report. *J Urol.* 1991;146:278.

Dunn MD, Portis AJ, Shelhav AL, et al. Laparoscopic versus open radical nephrectomy: a 9-year experience. *J Urol.* 2000;164:1153.

Fazeli-Martin S, Gill IS, Hsu TH, et al. Laparoscopic renal and adrenal surgery in obese patients: comparison to open surgery. *J Urol.* 1999;162:665.

Kim HH, Lee KS, Park K, et al. Laparoscopic nephrectomy for nonfunctioning tuberculous kidney. *J Endourol.* 2000;14:433.

Rassweiler J, Fornara P, Weber M, et al. Laparoscopic nephrectomy: the experience of the Laparoscopy Working Group of the German Urologic Association. *J Urol.* 1998;160:18.

Rassweiler J, Frede T, Henkel TO, et al. Nephrectomy: a comparative study between the transperitoneal and retroperitoneal laparoscopic versus open approach. *Eur Urol.* 1998;33:489.

17 Laparoscopic Radical Nephrectomy

Aaron H. Lay, Jeffrey A. Cadeddu

Radical nephrectomy has long been considered the gold standard surgical treatment for renal cell carcinoma. In the past two decades, nephron sparing surgery has become the standard for treatment of small localized renal masses 4 cm or smaller, with similar oncologic outcomes being achieved. Recently, focal ablative therapy is gaining acceptance as a viable alternative for poor surgical candidates. However, for larger tumors and in carefully selected cases with metastatic disease, radical nephrectomy is still the procedure of choice.

The first reported case of laparoscopic nephrectomy was in 1991. Since then, the technique has been refined to allow surgeons to remove kidneys with tumors larger than 10 cm and tumors with renal vein involvement. Laparoscopic radical nephrectomy can be performed by either a transperitoneal or a retroperitoneal approach. Hand-assisted technique is also an option. This chapter describes the more widely used transperitoneal approach.

INDICATIONS AND CONTRAINDICATIONS

Indications for laparoscopic radical nephrectomy include clinically staged T1 and T2 kidney tumors. Some patients with T3 disease including renal vein involvement may be candidates for the laparoscopic approach. Laparoscopic cytoreductive nephrectomy can also be performed in carefully selected patients with metastatic disease.

Absolute contraindications to the laparoscopic approach to radical nephrectomy are diminishing, though there are several important factors to consider before proceeding. Anatomically, extremely large tumors (>15 cm) may make the procedure difficult because of limited working space. Also, patients with tumor thrombus extending beyond the renal vein may be best served with an open approach for optimal control of the great vessels. Tumors that extend beyond the Gerota fascia, prior history of ipsilateral renal surgery, extensive intra-abdominal surgery, and perinephric inflammation may increase the chance for the need to convert to open surgery.

PATIENT PREOPERATIVE EVALUATION AND PREPARATION

The preoperative evaluation of a patient undergoing laparoscopic radical nephrectomy involves routine laboratory studies. Cross-sectional imaging with either computed tomography (CT) scan or magnetic resonance imaging (MRI) is required to delineate the anatomy. Renovascular anatomy can be better defined with three-dimensional reconstruction of the contrast-enhanced CT scan.

A chest radiograph is also necessary to assess for metastatic disease. In cases of cytoreductive nephrectomy, careful patient selection with Eastern Cooperative Oncology Group (ECOG) performance score of 0 or 1 and a brain MRI to rule out metastasis are essential to ensure optimal outcomes. If there is suspicion for a renal vein tumor thrombus, MRI is preferred to evaluate the extent of vein involvement preoperatively.

Contralateral renal function should be assessed before proceeding with a radical nephrectomy. Estimated glomerular filtration rate should be calculated, and appearance of the contralateral kidney on contrast-enhanced CT should be noted. In equivocal cases, a functional nuclear medicine scan can be considered.

The adrenal glands are also carefully evaluated. In general, attempts are made to spare the adrenal gland unless it is involved by local invasion of an upper pole tumor or by a metastatic deposit.

As with any surgical procedure, patient preparation begins with a thorough informed consent. In particular, patients undergoing laparoscopic radical nephrectomy should be informed of the risk for need to convert to an open procedure, although the risk is less than 5%.

Many surgeons prefer their patients to undergo a modest bowel preparation the day before the procedure. It helps by decompressing the colon during the transperitoneal approach. Type and screen is generally sufficient, although obtaining autologous or crossmatched blood before the procedure may be prudent in difficult cases.

OPERATING ROOM CONFIGURATION AND PATIENT POSITIONING

In the operating room, there should be at least two monitors available to allow visualization of the procedure by all members of the surgical team. The surgeon and the camera holder face the patient's abdomen; the scrub nurse and any other assistant face the patient's back. The primary monitor should be placed across the table from the surgeon at an appropriate height for optimal ergonomics (Fig. 17-1, *A*).

After the induction of general anesthesia and endotracheal intubation, an orogastric tube and a bladder catheter are placed. The patient is then positioned in a 30-degree modified decubitus position with the ipsilateral side up. The iliac crest overlies the break in the table. The ipsilateral arm is placed at the patient's side, secured, and padded. This arm can also be placed across the chest in a "praying" position. The bottom leg is bent slightly and pillows are placed between the legs. All potential pressure points are carefully padded, including the contralateral wrist, the elbow, and both legs and ankles. An axillary roll may be needed to prevent brachial plexus injury (Fig. 17-1, *B*).

The table is then flexed (optional) approximately 30 to 45 degrees to widen the space between the ipsilateral costal margin and the iliac crest. The patient is also placed in a slight reversed Trendelenburg position so the great vessels are in the horizontal plane. The patient is then secured to the table with wide tape over the chest, hips, and legs. Rotation of the bed is tested to ensure the patient is safely secured before surgical preparation and draping. The skin is prepared from the nipples to the pubis and from the paraspinal muscles to the contralateral rectus muscle.

TROCAR PLACEMENT

Intraperitoneal insufflation to 15 mm Hg is achieved with a Veress needle at the umbilicus with the table rotated slightly from the surgeon. In morbidly obese patients, the Veress needle can be inserted in the midclavicular line just off the costal margin.

In most cases three ports are sufficient to perform the procedure safely. On the right side, an additional port for the liver retractor is needed. For larger upper pole tumors, an additional port placed laterally may be helpful for upper pole and hilar dissection.

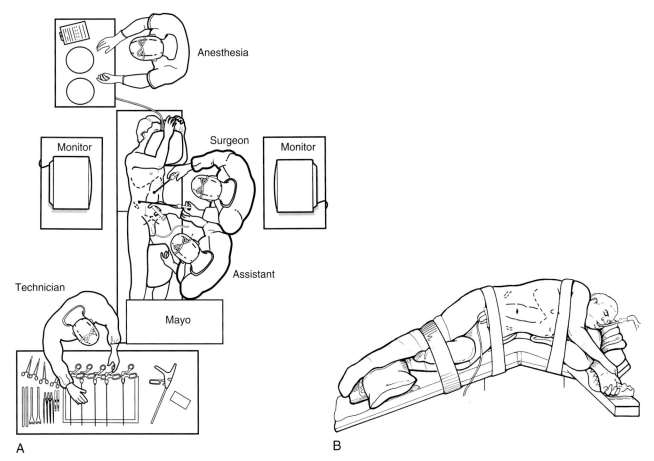

Figure 17-1. A, The operating room configuration includes two monitors, allowing visualization of the procedure by all members of the surgical team. The surgeon and camera holder stand on the contralateral side, facing the patient's abdomen; the scrub nurse and any other assistant stand facing the patient's back. *Mayo,* Mayo instrument table. **B,** The patient is positioned in a 30-degree modified decubitus position. The posterior iliac crest overlies the break in the surgical table, and the arms are flexed in a "praying" position. Pillows or an elevated arm board supports the ipsilateral arm. Care is taken to pad all potential pressure points, including the contralateral elbow and both legs and ankles. An axillary roll may be needed to protect the brachial plexus of the contralateral arm.

The first 10/12-mm port is placed through a periumbilical incision. An optical trocar is preferred to allow for endoscopic visualization while the trocar is introduced. The table is then rotated toward the surgeon such that the patient is at a flank position, 90 degrees to the floor. This will move the bowels medially and allow for better traction of the kidney later in the procedure. A second 10/12-mm port is then placed along the ipsilateral midclavicular line just caudal to the first port. A third port is then placed below the costal margin about one third of the way between the xiphoid and the umbilicus. For right-sided nephrectomies, a port is placed below the xiphoid for a liver tractor. The umbilical port is for the camera; the other two ports are for the surgeon. In obese patients, the ports need to be moved laterally to ensure that the instruments can complete the dissection (Fig. 17-2).

PROCEDURE (SEE VIDEOS 17-1 AND 17-2)

After successful port placement, the following steps are followed to complete the operation:

1. Incise the white line of Toldt to mobilize the colon medially.
2. Identify the gonadal vessels and the ureter.
3. Develop the posterior plane between the Gerota fascia and the psoas muscle.
4. Secure the hilum.
5. Dissect the upper pole, with or without the adrenal gland.
6. Divide the ureter.
7. Divide the lateral attachments.

8. Entrap the specimen.
9. Remove the specimen by extending the inferior trocar incision or the periumbilical trocar incision.
10. Fascial closure and skin closure.

Exposing the Retroperitoneum

A 5-mm atraumatic forceps and electrosurgical scissors are used to identify and incise the ipsilateral white line of Toldt. On the right side, this is carried from the hepatic flexure down to the right common iliac artery. The colon and mesentery need to be mobilized medially to expose the Gerota fascia and the retroperitoneum (Fig. 17-3). The right triangular and anterior coronary ligaments of the liver may need to be divided as well. The colonic mesenteric fat has a more pronounced yellow hue that is easily distinguishable from Gerota fascia and retroperitoneal fat. Be alert for the possibility of a retrocecal appendix that can be injured inadvertently during this portion of the procedure. The duodenum is then sharply mobilized until the vena cava is clearly visualized (Fig. 17-4).

For a left-sided radical nephrectomy, the white line of Toldt is incised similarly from the splenic flexure to the left common iliac artery. The splenorenal ligament and the splenophrenic attachments should be divided to properly mobilize the spleen medially (Fig. 17-5). The colon and mesentery should be rolled medially to the level of the anterior surface of the aorta.

When mobilizing the colon, grasp the peritoneum with atraumatic forceps to place the colon and mesentery under

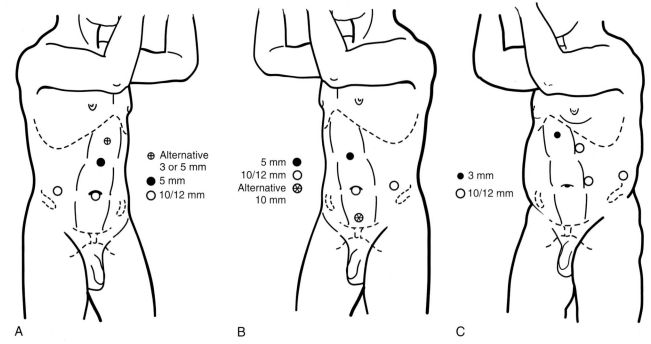

Figure 17-2. A, Port placement for a right nephrectomy. An optional fourth port (5 or 3 mm) to assist with liver retraction may be placed below the costal margin in the midclavicular line or in the midline below the xiphoid. **B,** Port placement for a left nephrectomy. An optional fourth port to assist with specimen elevation or medial retraction of the bowel is placed either in the midclavicular line below the costal margin (5 or 3 mm) or in the midline above the symphysis (10 or 5 mm). **C,** Port placement in the obese patient. The same configuration is used except that all primary trocars are positioned lateral to the rectus muscle.

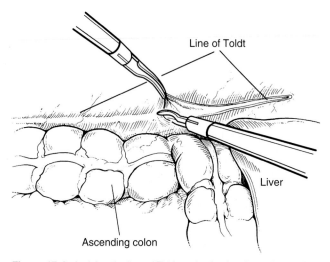

Figure 17-3. Incising the line of Toldt and reflecting the colon medially commences exposure of the specimen. In this illustration, the ascending colon is mobilized for a right-sided nephrectomy.

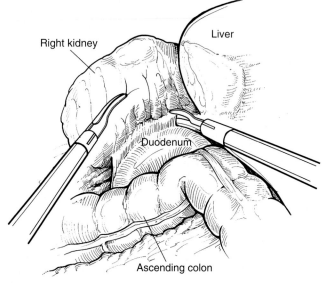

Figure 17-4. In a right-sided radical nephrectomy, the duodenum may be encountered after the colorenal attachments are divided. For the renal hilum, which invariably lies posterior to the second portion of the duodenum, to be exposed, a Kocher maneuver is used. Electrocautery must be used judiciously to avoid duodenal injury.

gentle tension. Use electrosurgical scissors to divide small vessels and achieve hemostasis. Blunt dissection can also be used with a blunt-tipped irrigator-aspiration device.

Be alert when using electrocautery near the bowel to avoid thermal injury. Also, be aware of the location of the colonic mesentery to avoid creating a mesenteric window during this portion of the procedure, which may result in troublesome bleeding from injured mesenteric vessels and could allow small bowel herniation in the future.

Identifying the Gonadal Vessels and the Ureter

After successful exposure of the retroperitoneum, the gonadal vessels are identified. The Gerota fascia is incised just lateral to the gonadal vein. The gonadal vein is then swept medially, and the ureter is identified within the retroperitoneal fat. The gonadal vessels are preserved whenever possible to prevent postoperative orchalgia or hydrocele, which can occasionally occur. Typically, the ureter is located lateral and deep to gonadal vein. The ureter along with retroperitoneal fat is then retracted laterally. The ureter is left intact at this time to aid in the exposure and dissection of the renal hilum (Fig. 17-6).

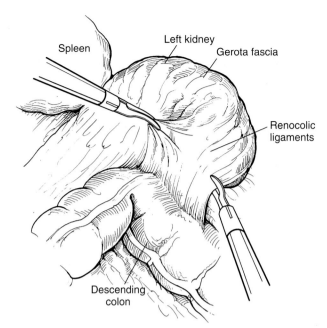

Figure 17-5. Division of the colorenal attachments during a left-sided nephrectomy allows full reflection of the splenic flexure and descending colon, as well as access to the retroperitoneum. Sharp and blunt dissection is used to release the colon medially.

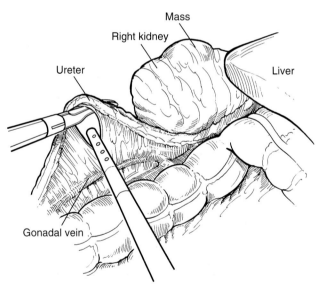

Figure 17-6. The ureter and gonadal vein are elevated with a grasper and mobilized cephalad. Blunt dissection with the irrigator-aspirator facilitates this maneuver.

The identification of the ureter can be difficult in certain cases. Occasionally, systematic inspection of the retroperitoneum is necessary, starting at the great vessels and working laterally. The ureter is located more medially than anticipated. Alternative techniques to identify the ureter in difficult cases include using atraumatic forceps to stroke and pinch the retroperitoneal fat to look for ureteral peristalsis. The ureter can also be found reliably caudally where it crosses the iliac vessels.

Developing the Posterior Plane

The ureter and retroperitoneal fat are retracted laterally and superiorly until psoas fascia is encountered. The posterior plane

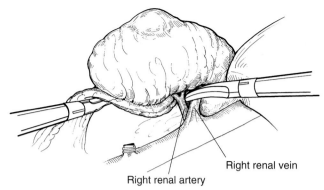

Figure 17-7. After mobilization of the lower pole and posterior attachments, the renal hilum is exposed.

between the Gerota fascia and the psoas fascia is generally avascular, and dissection to lift the specimen superiorly and laterally can be performed bluntly with an irrigator-aspiration device. While the specimen is lifted off the psoas fascia, the medial attachments are divided with electrocautery toward the renal hilum. We have found that commercial vessel-sealing products have been useful in this portion of the procedure. This dissection is carried out until the inferior edge of the renal vein is encountered (Fig. 17-7).

Securing the Hilum

The most hazardous step of this operation is securing the renal hilum. In our experience, dividing the hilum en bloc with a vascular stapler is safe and efficient and has not been shown to increase the risk of formation of arteriovenous fistulas. Accordingly, the individual renal arteries and veins are not dissected. The Gerota fascia superior to the renal hilum is incised with electrocautery so that the superior edge of the renal hilum is safely incorporated within the vascular stapler. If the adrenal gland is to be spared, then this dissection is performed just lateral to it, staying close to the adrenal gland to leave as much perinephric fat around the superior pole of the kidney as possible. It is important to note that for a left-sided nephrectomy, care is taken to preserve the adrenal vein and not incorporate it in the vascular stapler.

As mentioned previously, if there is a large upper pole tumor, an additional 5-mm port may be placed laterally at the level of the camera port. If the adrenal gland is to be removed with the specimen, the Gerota fascia is incised just lateral to the great vessels. For a left-sided procedure, make sure to secure the hilum proximal to the branching adrenal vein. For a right-sided procedure, secure the adrenal vein with clips as it branches off the vena cava.

Place the renal hilum on gentle tension by lifting the specimen laterally and superiorly. Pass a 10-mm endovascular gastrointestinal anastomosis (GIA) stapler through the 10/12-mm lower quadrant port. Close the jaws of the stapler to occlude the entire hilum and then divide. There should not be any resistance. It is critical to ensure that the jaws of the stapler are advanced entirely over the hilum (Fig. 17-8). If possible, avoid using and placing clips in the hilum because these can be hidden during subsequent stapling of the artery and vein, resulting in misfire of the stapler and severe venous or arterial bleeding.

Completing the Radical Nephrectomy

After the renal hilum is secured and divided, the upper pole dissection should be completed. If the adrenal gland is to be removed with the specimen, the superior, medial, and posterior attachments of the adrenal gland are divided along with

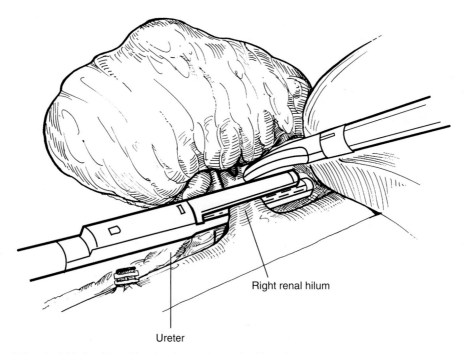

Right renal hilum

Ureter

Figure 17-8. The renal hilum is divided en bloc with an endovascular stapler. Note that the specimen is elevated with graspers to improve hilar exposure during placement of the stapler.

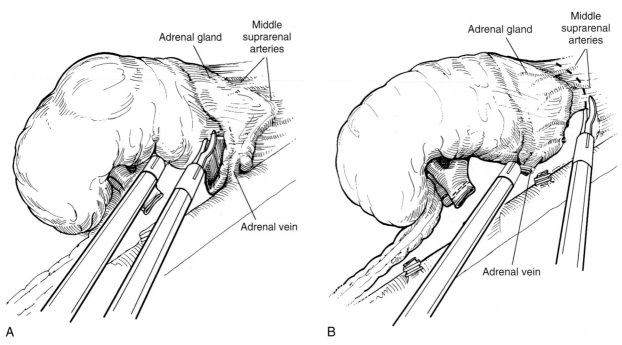

Adrenal gland

Middle suprarenal arteries

Adrenal vein

A

Adrenal gland

Middle suprarenal arteries

Adrenal vein

B

Figure 17-9. A, Adrenal-sparing right radical nephrectomy. Sharp cautery dissection is used to release all adrenocolic and adrenorenal attachments. Inferior retraction of the specimen facilitates exposure of this surgical plane. **B,** If the adrenal gland is to be included with right radical nephrectomy, the adrenal vein must be identified. This vein should then be divided either between clips or with an endovascular stapler to prevent avulsion injury at the vein's insertion on the vena cava. Superior attachments, including small adrenal arteries, are divided with electrocautery.

a cone of perinephric fat off the upper pole of the kidney. If the adrenal gland is spared, the kidney and perinephric fat are dissected off close to the adrenal gland to leave as much perinephric fat on the kidney as possible (Figs. 17-9 and 17-10).

After the upper pole attachments are divided, attention is turned to the caudal and lateral attachments. The ureter is divided between clips, and the perinephric fat off the lower pole of the kidney is divided to the body wall laterally. Finally,

pull the specimen medially and divide the remaining lateral attachments to complete the radical nephrectomy (Fig. 17-11).

To inspect the renal fossa for hemostasis, move the specimen to above the liver or spleen. Occasionally the specimen is too large and will need to be placed in the pelvis. Lower the pneumoperitoneum to 5 mm Hg and observe the operative field, paying close attention to the renal hilum, the adrenal bed, and any other potential sites for bleeding.

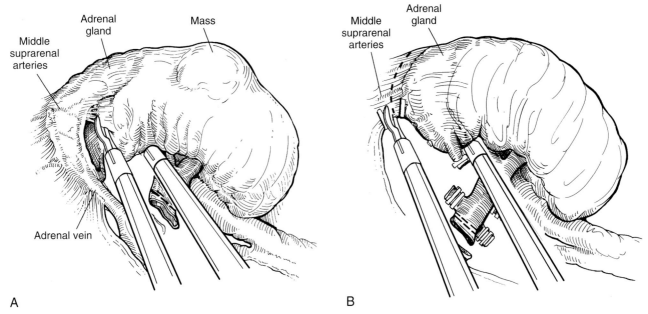

A B

Figure 17-10. **A,** Adrenal-sparing left radical nephrectomy. Sharp dissection and electrocautery are used to release all attachments between the adrenal gland and the kidney, colon, and spleen. Inferior retraction of the specimen facilitates exposure of this surgical plane. Note that the renal hilum was divided distal to the left adrenal vein. **B,** If the adrenal gland is to be included with left radical nephrectomy, the adrenal vein should be identified and divided between clips. Alternatively, the hilum can be divided with a stapler proximal to the left adrenal vein. Superior attachments, including small adrenal arteries, are divided with electrocautery.

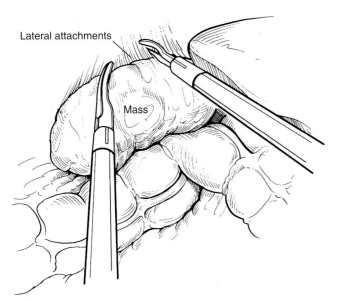

Figure 17-11. The lateral attachments to the side wall are divided. The kidney is pulled medially, and electrocautery along with blunt dissection with the tip of the irrigator-aspirator is used to free the kidney.

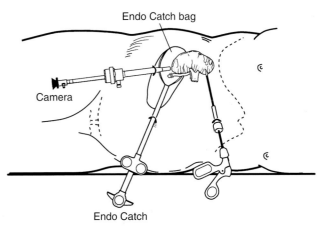

Figure 17-12. Placement of the specimen into an opened Endo Catch (Medtronic, Minneapolis, Minn.) device placed through the umbilical port site. Note that the camera is positioned in the lateral port and the specimen is maneuvered with a grasper through the upper midline port. The umbilical port is removed to accommodate the 15-mm Endo Catch device.

Entrapping the Specimen and Removal

A 15-mm endoscopic specimen sack is usually necessary to remove a radical nephrectomy specimen. The device is placed directly through the skin after the 10/12-mm port is removed and digitally dilated. The device is typically placed though the umbilical port site so the specimen can be extracted through a periumbilical incision for cosmetic reasons (Fig. 17-12). However, in obese patients, when the ports are moved laterally, the device is placed though the lower quadrant port and extracted through an extension of that incision.

Before placing the device into the abdomen, the specimen is grasped and placed above the spleen or liver. Once the bag

is introduced and deployed, use gravity to help drop the specimen into the bag. Pull the drawstring to close the bag after the specimen is in, and cut the string. Remember to close the ring under direct vision and withdraw the device from the abdomen, leaving the string outside the body.

At this time, the ports are removed under direct vision and the 10/12-mm ports are digitally inspected to ensure no fascial closure is required.

A 4- to 6-cm periumbilical incision is then made that incorporates the umbilical port incision. Alternatively, in obese patients, extend the lower quadrant port incision 4 to 6 cm. Open the fascia while carefully protecting the intra-abdominal structures (Fig. 17-13). Extract the specimen by pulling on the string, exerting gentle traction to get the bag through the incision. Avoid tearing or perforating the bag at this point by using

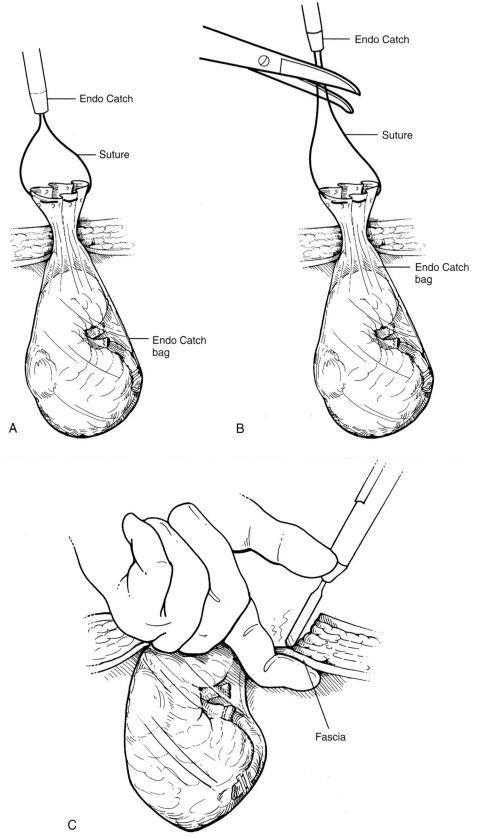

Figure 17-13. Removal of an intact specimen. **A,** Once the specimen is within the Endo Catch bag, the bag is cinched closed and the device and bag are withdrawn through the trocar site. **B,** The suture is cut to release the device from the bag. **C,** A 4- to 6-cm skin incision is made to extract the bag and specimen. The fascia is divided with electrocautery. The bag and specimen are protected during this maneuver by the surgeon's index finger positioned alongside them through the trocar site.

too much force; extend the incision as necessary. There is no role for morcellation in radical nephrectomy. Close the fascia and incision in a standard fashion.

POSTOPERATIVE MANAGEMENT

Pain is usually adequately controlled with minimal intravenous narcotics. The patient is started on a clear liquid diet after surgery, and then the diet is advanced to regular as tolerated the next day. The patient is encouraged to ambulate and the urethral catheter is removed the next day. In general, postoperative antibiotics are not necessary. Most patients are able to be discharged on the first or second postoperative day.

COMPLICATIONS

The potential complications of a laparoscopic radical nephrectomy have been well described. Large series have reported complication rates of around 10%. Access-related injuries include port-site hernias, abdominal wall hematomas, vascular injuries, and organ injuries. Intraoperatively, liver, spleen, bowel, and vascular injuries can occur. It is important to note that a general laparotomy set with vascular clamps and instruments must be readily available for each procedure. The surgical team should be prepared for emergent conversion to an open procedure secondary to vascular injuries or injuries to other organs.

Postoperative complications such as wound infections, incisional hernias, prolonged ileus, pneumonia, pulmonary embolus, and atrial fibrillation can also occur. Positioning injuries resulting in paresthesias and brachial nerve plexus palsy can occur and should be avoided by minimizing pressure points and properly securing and padding the patient.

TIPS AND TRICKS

- Set up the operation for success by positioning and securing the patient properly.
- Have imaging readily available and be familiar with the patient's vascular anatomy.
- Place additional 5-mm ports as necessary with little effect on cosmesis or pain.
- Do not mobilize the specimen laterally until the end because the lateral attachments stabilize the specimen and help with retraction and hilar dissection.
- Be cautious using cautery around bowel.
- Be sure that the jaws of the vascular stapler are completely across the hilum before firing; be prepared for equipment malfunction.
- Be meticulous with fascial closure and inspect all port sites before closure.

18 Nephroureterectomy

Armine K. Smith, Thomas W. Jarrett

Urothelial carcinoma can arise from any part of urothelium: bladder, renal collecting system, or ureter. The nomenclature of upper tract urothelial carcinoma (UTUC) is reserved for tumors that are localized to renal calyces or ureter. This is a relatively rare disease, representing only 5% to 10% of all urothelial cancers.

Reports from multiple comparative and one randomized study describe similar oncologic outcomes for laparoscopic and open extirpative surgery, with reduced perioperative morbidity favoring a laparoscopic approach. Because most upper tract urothelial tumors are not large or bulky, laparoscopic surgery is ideal for most patients, at least for the renal portion of a radical nephroureterectomy when the tumor warrants removal of the entire renal unit. There has been a recent shift in the paradigm for treatment of low-grade and low-stage tumors, for which consideration of endoscopic treatment may be given, but this discussion is beyond the scope of the chapter.

Once the extirpative management has been chosen, the surgical approach should be planned in a way that does not compromise oncologic control because UTUC is rarely able to be salvaged by adjuvant modalities. Accordingly, removal of an intact specimen is desirable to minimize the risk of tumor seeding from both the ureter and bladder. Laparoscopic nephroureterectomy can be performed by transperitoneal, retroperitoneal, hand-assisted, and robotic-assisted approaches, which are mostly dictated by surgeon's experience. In this chapter we describe the more widely used transperitoneal technique.

INDICATIONS AND CONTRAINDICATIONS

Radical nephroureterectomy with removal of bladder cuff is the gold standard for large, high-grade, and invasive urothelial tumors of the renal pelvis and proximal ureter. It is also a choice in the presence of large, multifocal, or rapidly recurring low-grade or noninvasive tumors.

Large bulky tumors with involvement of adjacent viscera or those cases requiring extended lymph node dissection in the hands of a less experienced laparoscopic surgeon may be better suited for the open approach. Other patient factors such as a prior history of ipsilateral or extensive abdominal surgery or the presence of a perinephric inflammatory process should prompt a consideration of a retroperitoneal or an open approach.

PATIENT PREOPERATIVE EVALUATION AND PREPARATION

The preoperative evaluation of a patient with a suspected upper tract tumor should include a complete history and physical examination and laboratory studies to include complete blood count, chemistry profile, and urine cytology. The upper tract collecting system should be evaluated by computed tomography (CT) urography, but if the patient is unable to undergo contrast administration owing to poor renal function or allergies, this may be replaced by a magnetic resonance imaging (MRI) urogram. If MRI is contraindicated or unavailable, CT without contrast or ultrasound of the kidneys supplemented with retrograde pyelography is an acceptable alternative. If a suspicious lesion is identified, a normal saline washing of the area is performed, followed by ureteroscopic biopsy of the tumor. Cystoscopy should always be performed to exclude bladder tumors.

In the setting of positive cytologic test results without an identifiable lesion, along with the upper tracts, one should consider the bladder and prostatic urethra as possible sites harboring cancer. If results of bladder evaluation were negative or if cytologic test results remain positive after successful treatment of the bladder, then one should proceed with evaluation of extravesical sites to include selective cytologic samples from each upper urinary tract as well as resection of a representative specimen of the prostatic urethra in men. Selective cytologic tests should preferably be done along with ureteroscopy to allow for direct visualization of the upper urinary tracts. However, because of the limitations of cytologic testing alone with false-positive results and the high risk for bilateral disease in the future, if selective cytologic test results are persistently positive in the absence of any ureteroscopic or radiographic findings or if the treatment is not well established, radical nephroureterectomy is not recommended.

Consideration of nuclear renal scan to evaluate the function of the contralateral kidney may help with the decision regarding an extirpative versus organ-sparing approach. Staging should include chest radiography or tomography and bone scan only in the presence of symptoms or elevated alkaline phosphatase or calcium. No bowel preparation is necessary, but the patient should be on a clear liquid diet the day before surgery.

OPERATING ROOM CONFIGURATION AND PATIENT POSITIONING

The operating room configuration for laparoscopic or robotic-assisted surgery is illustrated in Figure 18-1. The surgical team stands on the contralateral side of the patient, and the scrub technician stands at the foot of the patient's bed to facilitate access to the instrument table. Two towers with monitors are positioned, one on each side of the patient, to maximize visualization of the surgical progress by everyone involved in the operating room patient care.

If a transurethral approach is desired for bladder cuff removal, the patient is initially placed in the dorsal lithotomy position. If open distal ureterectomy or total laparoscopic or robotic-assisted technique is desired, or after the completion of the cystoscopic part, the patient is placed supine with the ipsilateral hip and shoulder rotated approximately 20 degrees (Fig. 18-2). The patient is secured to the table and can be easily moved from the flank position (nephrectomy portion) to the supine position (open portion) without repreparing the operative field. The table can be flexed to widen the distance between the costal margin and iliac crest, but we do not find this necessary in most cases. Once the patient is secured to the table, we test the stability of the position by rotating the table left and right. Finally, the ipsilateral flank and urethra are prepared and draped, and a Foley catheter is placed in the sterile field before insufflation of the abdomen.

TROCAR PLACEMENT

The abdomen is insufflated, and three or four trocars are placed as outlined in Figure 18-3, *A* and *B*, with the first usually being the lateral trocar. Subsequent trocars are placed under direct vision. With this configuration, the camera is kept at the umbilicus for the

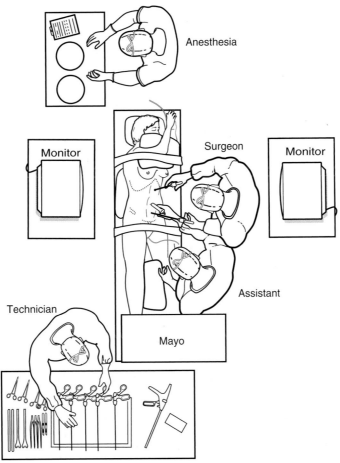

Figure 18-1. The surgeon and assistant stand on the contralateral side of the table with the scrub person at the foot of the table. *Mayo,* Mayo instrument table.

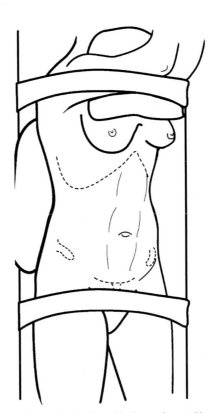

Figure 18-2. For laparoscopic nephroureterectomy, the patient is placed in the supine position with the ipsilateral arm across the chest. The patient is secured to the table and may be rotated during the procedure to the contralateral side.

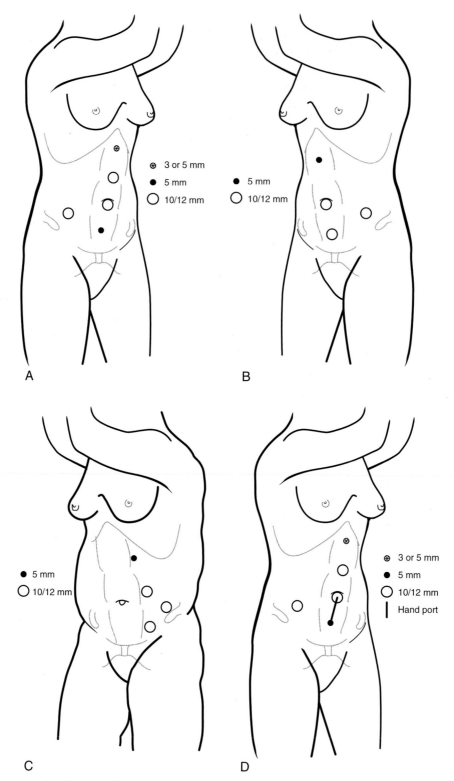

Figure 18-3. The trocars are placed in the midline for most patients. Port placement: **A,** left nephroureterectomy; **B,** right nephroureterectomy. **C,** In obese patients, ports should be shifted laterally. **D,** For hand-assisted nephrectomy, hand port should be placed caudally to help with distal ureterectomy and bladder cuff excision.

entire procedure. The upper midline and lateral trocars are used by the surgeon for the dissection of the kidney and the proximal half of the ureter. The lower midline and lateral trocars are used for the dissection of the distal ureter. On the left side, dissection of the distal ureter may require placement of the fourth trocar. A 3-mm trocar just below the xiphoid can be helpful in retracting the spleen and liver for left- and right-sided nephrectomy,

respectively. In obese patients, shifting of the trocars may be necessary to achieve optimal visualization (Fig. 18-3, *C*). If a hand-assisted approach is chosen, the hand port site should be placed so that it can be used for the dissection of the distal ureter and open bladder cuff as indicated (Fig. 18-3, *D*).

For robotic-assisted surgery, proper port positioning is paramount to success (Fig. 18-4). Docking the robot, the surgeon places the left arm in port 1 and the right arm in port 2; the fourth arm is placed in port 3 and used for retraction. Once the nephrectomy portion has been completed, the retraction instrument is moved to port 1 and left arm to port 3 for distal ureter and bladder cuff dissection.

PROCEDURE (SEE VIDEO 18-1)
Nephrectomy with Mobilization of the Ureter

The peritoneum is incised along the white line of Toldt from the level of the iliac vessels to the hepatic flexure on the right and to the splenic flexure on the left (Fig. 18-5). The colon is moved medially by releasing the renocolic ligaments while leaving the lateral attachments of the Gerota fascia in place to prevent the kidney from "flopping" medially. The colon mesentery should be mobilized medial to the great vessels to facilitate dissection of the ureter, renal hilum, and local lymph

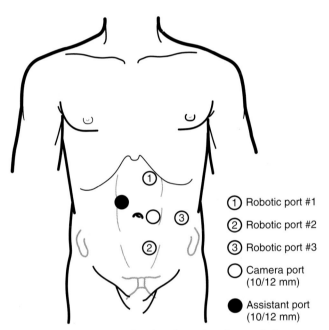

1 Robotic port #1
2 Robotic port #2
3 Robotic port #3
○ Camera port (10/12 mm)
● Assistant port (10/12 mm)

Figure 18-4. In robotic-assisted nephroureterectomy, robotic arms can be shifted among ports for nephrectomy and distal ureterectomy or bladder cuff excision portions.

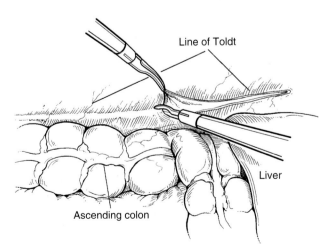

Line of Toldt

Liver

Ascending colon

Figure 18-5. The lateral attachments of the colon are divided along the white line of Toldt.

nodes as needed (Fig. 18-6). To expose the renal hilum, on the right side, it is necessary to perform a Kocher maneuver to deflect the duodenum medially (Fig. 18-7, *A*); on the left side, mobilize the pancreatic tail. Division of the splenorenal ligament is imperative to avoid the injury to the spleen and achieve mobility of the upper pole of the kidney (Fig. 18-7, *B*). The proximal ureter is identified, just medial to the lower pole of the kidney, and dissected toward the renal pelvis, avoiding skeletonization and maintaining copious periureteral fat if any tumor is located in this area (Fig. 18-8). If an invasive ureteral lesion is suspected, the dissection should include a wide margin of tissue. The renal hilum is identified, and its vessels are exposed with a combination of blunt and sharp dissection. The artery is ligated and divided by use of a stapling device with a vascular load or multiple clips. The renal vein is then divided in a similar fashion (Fig. 18-9). With vascular control ensured, most prefer to ligate the ureter with a clip, and the kidney is dissected free outside the Gerota fascia. As described for nephrectomy, the adrenal gland does not need to be removed routinely. Adrenal gland removal should be considered for high-grade and invasive lesions in the vicinity of the adrenal gland. The ureteral dissection is continued distally as far as is technically feasible, keeping in mind that the ureteral blood supply is generally anteromedially located in the proximal third, medially located in the middle third, and laterally located in the distal third. If distal limits of the dissection are below the level of the iliac vessels (Fig. 18-10), the remainder of the procedure can easily be completed through a lower abdominal incision. The specimen is placed in the pelvis, and the renal bed is inspected meticulously for bleeding.

Lymphadenectomy appears to have prognostic and therapeutic value in patients with invasive disease and should be performed in each patient. The extent of lymphadenectomy has been under debate, but at minimum it should include regional lymph nodes. For renal pelvis and proximal or middle ureteral tumors, this includes the ipsilateral renal hilar nodes and the adjacent para-aortic or paracaval nodes (Fig. 18-11, *A*). For distal ureteral tumors, this includes pelvic lymph nodes (Fig. 18-11, *B*).

Open Distal Ureterectomy with Excision of Bladder Cuff

The patient is moved to the supine position, which can usually be done without repreparation, and a low midline Pfannenstiel or Gibson incision is made (Fig. 18-12). The choice of incision largely depends on the tumor location, the body habitus of the patient, and the most caudal level of ureteral dissection attained during the laparoscopic portion. The Gibson incision is preferable when the distal ureter cannot be freed laparoscopically to the level of the iliac vessels.

The bladder cuff removal is performed by transvesical (Fig. 18-13, *A*), extravesical (Fig. 18-13, *B*), or combined approach. Any of these methods is acceptable, provided that the whole ureter, including the intramural portion and the mucosa of the ureteral orifice are removed with the surgeon's visual confirmation of complete resection. For the extravesical approach, the distal ureter is freed toward the bladder to the point of intramural ureter. Gentle traction on the ureter and full bladder may aid in this step; however, for adequate access to the entire intramural ureter, the lateral pedicle of the bladder (obliterated artery; superior, middle, and inferior vesical arteries) must be ligated and divided (Fig. 18-14). Care must be taken to avoid uncontrolled entry to the urinary tract. A cuff of bladder is removed en bloc with the ureter by applying a clamp to the bladder wall and excising the full intramural portion of the ureter, taking care to stay away from the contralateral ureteral orifice (Fig. 18-15). In the transvesical approach, after an anterior cystotomy is made, a feeding tube is inserted in the

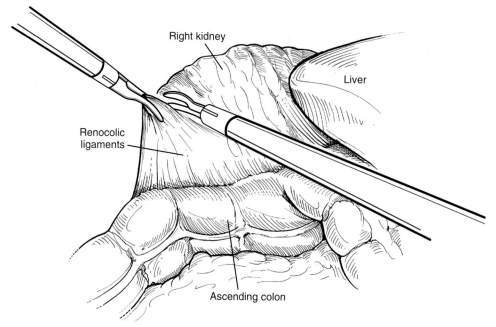

Figure 18-6. The renocolic attachments are freed from the kidney to expose the retroperitoneum.

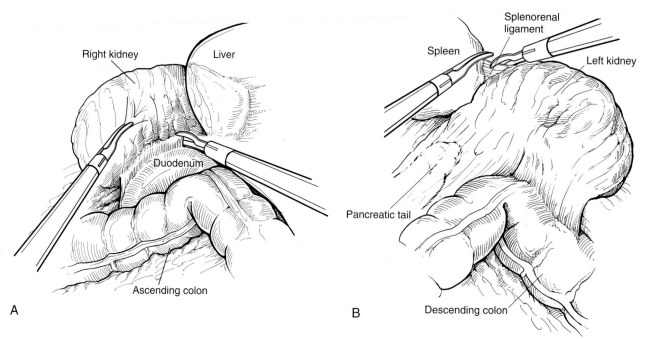

Figure 18-7. A, The Kocher maneuver mobilizes the duodenum away from the renal hilum. **B,** Division of the splenorenal ligaments allows mobilization of the upper pole of the left kidney.

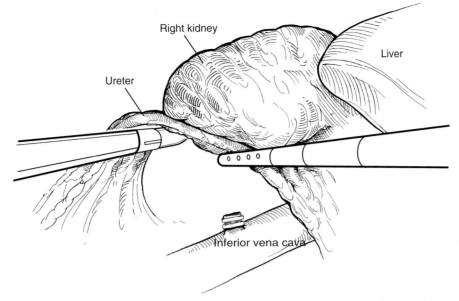

Figure 18-8. Ureter with ample periureteric tissue is mobilized distally toward iliac vessels.

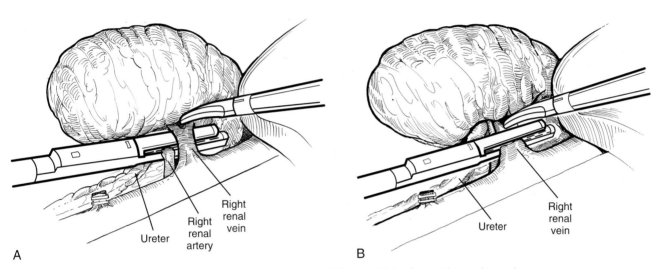

Figure 18-9. The renal artery **(A)** and vein **(B)** are divided with an endovascular stapler.

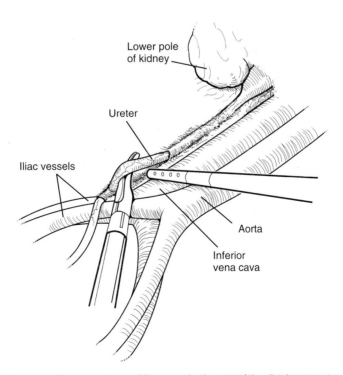

Figure 18-10. Once the ureter has been mobilized to the level of iliac vessels, the rest of the distal ureterectomy can be easily completed through a low abdominal incision.

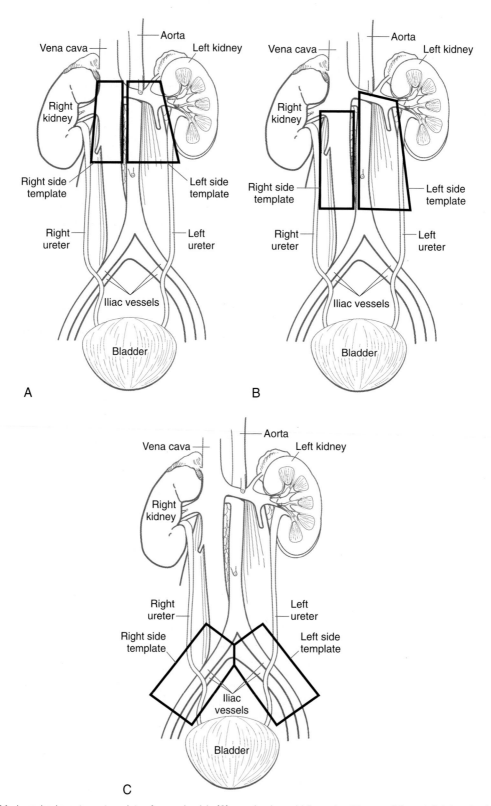

Figure 18-11. Lymphadenectomy templates for renal pelvis **(A)**, proximal or middle ureteral tumors **(B)**, and distal ureteral tumors **(C)**.

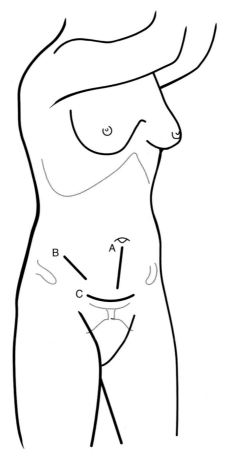

Figure 18-12. Low midline or Pfannenstiel incisions are adequate for dissecting the most distal ureter. A Gibson-type incision may provide better visualization of the midureter.

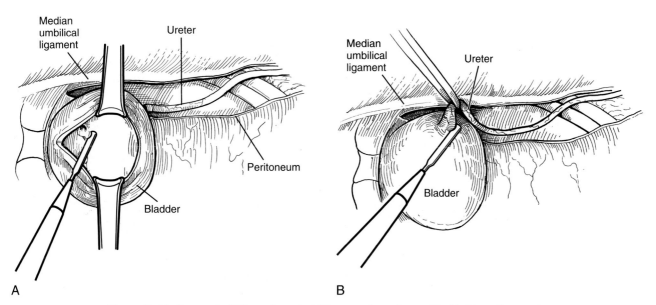

Figure 18-13. Transvesical **(A)** or extravesical **(B)** approach can be used for bladder cuff removal.

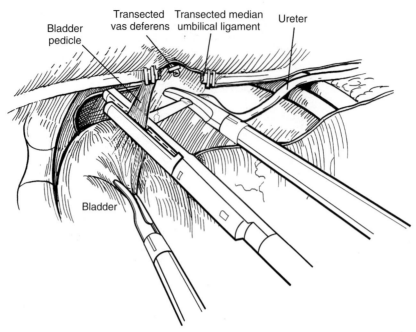

Figure 18-14. For extravesical approach, the ipsilateral pedicle of the bladder can be ligated to allow adequate access to the entire length of the distal ureter.

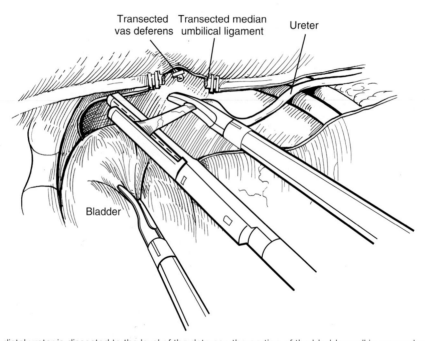

Figure 18-15. Once the distal ureter is dissected to the level of the detrusor, the portion of the bladder wall is grasped and excised with the distal ureter, taking care to stay away from the contralateral trigone.

ureteral orifice and sutured to bladder wall to both occlude the orifice and provide traction for excision of the intramural portion of the ureter. Intravesical dissection of the ureter is then performed, including a traditional 1-cm mucosal area around the orifice (Fig. 18-16). A wider margin can be taken if a gross tumor is seen protruding from the orifice; and if invasive intramural tumor is suspected, an en bloc partial cystectomy may be required to ensure negative margins. Frequently the ureter can be dissected completely intravesically to the level below the iliac vessels, avoiding the need to perform open dissection of the ipsilateral bladder and pedicle. Cystotomy defects are closed in two layers with interrupted or running absorbable sutures:

the first layer should incorporate mucosa, and the second layer should include detrusor muscle and adventitia. A Foley catheter is placed and maintained for 5 to 7 days, and a suction drain is left in the perivesical space.

Laparoscopic Distal Ureterectomy

If one is to consider a total laparoscopic procedure or to minimize the open distal portion, the ureteral dissection needs to continue to the level of the bladder. The patient is placed in the Trendelenburg position to move the bowel contents out of the pelvis. The peritoneal incision is extended from the level of the iliac vessels into the pelvis lateral to the bladder and medial to the medial umbilical ligament (Fig. 18-17). The vas deferens in male patients and the round ligament in female patients is clipped and divided if exposure is limited. The ureter can then be traced between the bladder and the medial umbilical ligament down to its origin at the bladder. Optimal exposure of the entire intramural ureter is gained by division of the lateral pedicle of the bladder, allowing medial rotation of the bladder and exposing the entire length of the ureter (Fig. 18-18). The bladder cuff may be dissected extravesically, freeing the ureter from the surrounding detrusor muscle; alternatively, opening the bladder immediately around the ureteral orifice allows direct visual confirmation for complete resection of the bladder cuff (Fig. 18-19). Yet another alternative during a complete extravesical approach is flexible cystoscopy in confirming complete ureterectomy and patency of the contralateral ureteral orifice.

Robotic-Assisted Laparoscopic Nephroureterectomy

With the increased use of robotic devices in urologic surgery, robotic-assisted nephroureterectomy has become a feasible alternative to more traditional open or laparoscopic techniques. The availability of the da Vinci S system (Intuitive Surgical, Sunnyvale, Calif.) with longer instruments and improved range of motion with less arm clashing has allowed performance of the surgery without the need to re-dock the robot or reposition the patient for the distal ureterectomy portion. For extravesical dissection of the ureter, a distended bladder is helpful in tracing the ureterovesical junction. Once the distal ureter is dissected out of the detrusor, the bladder can be emptied. Placement of stay sutures medial and lateral to the incision site of the ureterovesical junction aids in subsequent reconstruction of the bladder (Fig. 18-20).

Advances in laparoscopy have lessened the impact of the other described methods of bladder cuff removal, such as transvesical ligation and detachment, intussusception (stripping), and transurethral resection of the ureteral orifice or "pluck" technique. Because of concerns about tumor seeding of extravesical space and the potential of leaving behind a portion of the intramural ureter, these techniques are no longer widely used.

Our choice remains the transvesical approach because it does not add much time or morbidity to the procedure and allows easy identification and extraction of the whole length of the distal ureter with an oncologically reasonable margin of bladder cuff.

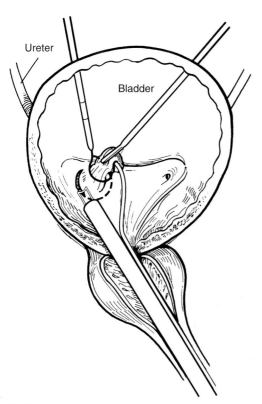

Figure 18-16. In the transvesical approach, a feeding tube inserted in the ipsilateral ureteral orifice is sutured to bladder mucosa and may be used as a guide and traction in dissecting the intramural ureter in its entirety.

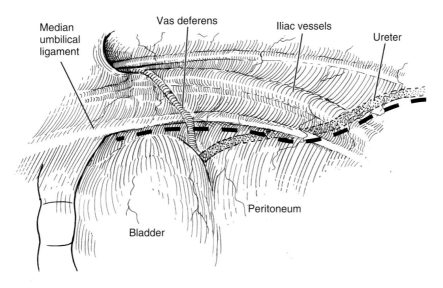

Figure 18-17. For laparoscopic distal ureterectomy, the peritoneal incision is extended deep into the pelvis over the iliac vessels and medial to the median umbilical ligament.

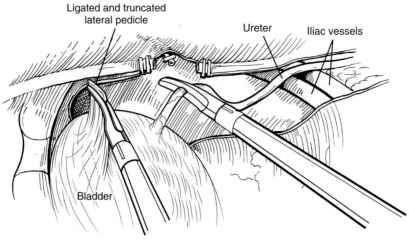

Figure 18-18. Ligation of the lateral pedicle rotates the bladder medially and exposes the whole distal ureter to the level of the detrusor.

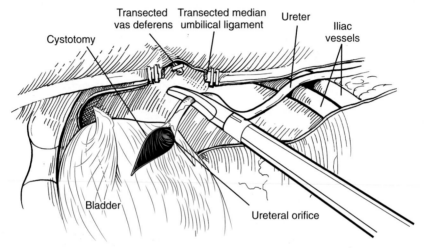

Figure 18-19. Laparoscopic extravesical excision of the bladder cuff may be aided by cystotomy extending to the ureteral orifice.

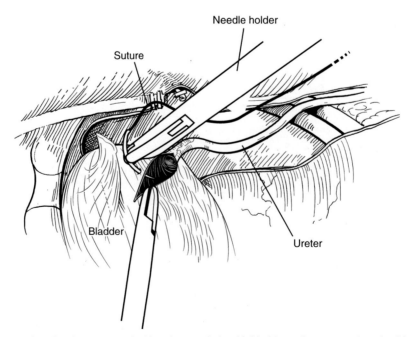

Figure 18-20. Sutures placed at the ureterovesical junction may help with bladder wall reconstruction after bladder cuff excision.

POSTOPERATIVE MANAGEMENT

We favor early ambulation and feeding in the immediate postoperative period. Patients are encouraged to ambulate starting in the evening of the day of surgery. A clear liquid diet is introduced on postoperative day 1, with advancement of the diet as appropriate, with evidence of bowel function return. Pain management includes intravenous opioids, with rapid transition to oral medicines once the patient is able to tolerate diet. Prophylactic antibiotic duration should be limited to less than 24 hours in the perioperative period. The drain is kept in place until outputs drop below 200 mL in 24 hours. Before removal of the drain, we routinely send drain fluid for a creatinine level, which should correspond with serum levels when no leak is present. Usually the drain is removed before the patient's discharge, but in the presence of urine leakage it can be kept in place until the leakage resolves. Patients are discharged home on postoperative day 2 or 3 when tolerating a regular diet with adequate pain control on oral medication.

Given the evidence for the role of perioperative intravesical instillation in reducing bladder tumor seeding, we perform cystography on postoperative day 1 and, if there is no evidence of extravasation, give a mitomycin instillation. A Foley catheter is left in place for approximately 5 days for women and 7 days for men. An office-based cystogram may be obtained on the day of planned removal to confirm lack of extravasation but is not necessary. Routine antibiotic administration postoperatively in the setting of an indwelling catheter is not recommended in a non-immunocompromised patient, but patients may be given a prescription for a 3-day regimen of antibiotic to be taken before the catheter removal.

The propensity of upper tract tumors for multifocal recurrence and metastatic spread with more dysplastic lesions makes follow-up complicated. Postoperative evaluation must routinely include evaluation of the bladder, the contralateral urinary tract, and extraurinary sites for local and metastatic spread. A follow-up regimen is thus dependent on the time from surgery and the potential for metastatic spread. For pathologic stage T2 tumors, this should include cystoscopy every 3 months for 1 year, then at increasing intervals. Imaging of the upper tract collecting system is performed at 3- to 12-month intervals, accompanied by cross-sectional abdominal imaging and chest radiographs.

COMPLICATIONS

Immediate postoperative complications, as in any major abdominal surgery, include ileus, wound infection, cardiac and respiratory events, and deep vein thrombosis. Postoperative stay and rates of the need for blood transfusion favor the laparoscopic approach. Urinary extravasation has been reported and usually can be managed with prolonged catheterization and percutaneous drainage.

Late complications include tumor seeding and intravesical recurrence and have been reported for both open and laparoscopic nephroureterectomy. These are associated with distal ureter management and are increased when the distal ureter is not removed in its entirety.

TIPS AND TRICKS

- In high-grade or invasive tumors, a more radical approach should be taken with excision of wide margins of tissue when possible in the area of the tumor. Lymphadenectomy should be anticipated at the time of hilar dissection.
- We prefer an open approach for the distal ureter and bladder cuff. Extravesical techniques have left concerns for retained ureter and possible distal recurrence. If the ureteral dissection can be reached below the iliac vessels, this can usually be done through a low midline incision and a transvesical approach. The patient can be repositioned to the supine position without repreparation to facilitate this portion of the procedure.
- Urothelial cancer will seed nonurothelial surfaces, so every effort should be made to maintain a closed system and prevent tumor spillage. This is of less concern with low-grade disease. However, many cases of low-grade disease are upgraded to high grade on final pathology reports.

SUGGESTED READINGS

Li WM, Shen JT, Li CC, et al. Oncologic outcomes following three different approaches to the distal ureter and bladder cuff in nephroureterectomy for primary upper urinary tract urothelial carcinoma. *Eur Urol.* 2010;57:963–969.

Ni S, Tao W, Chen Q, et al. Laparoscopic versus open nephroureterectomy for the treatment of upper urinary tract urothelial carcinoma: a systematic review and cumulative analysis of comparative studies. *Eur Urol.* 2012;61:1142–1153.

Parsons JK, Varkarakis I, Rha KH, et al. Complications of abdominal urologic laparoscopy: longitudinal five-year analysis. *Urology.* 2004;63:27–32.

Roupret M, Hupertan V, Seisen T, et al. Prediction of cancer specific survival after radical nephroureterectomy for upper tract urothelial carcinoma: development of an optimized postoperative nomogram using decision curve analysis. *J Urol.* 2013;189:1662–1669.

Siegel R, Naishadham D, Jemal A. Cancer statistics, 2013. *CA Cancer J Clin.* 2013;63:11–30.

Simone G, Papalia R, Guaglianone S, et al. Laparoscopic versus open nephroureterectomy: perioperative and oncologic outcomes from a randomized prospective study. *Eur Urol.* 2009;56:520–526.

Smith AK, Lane BR, Larson BT, et al. Does the choice of technique for management of the bladder cuff affect oncologic outcomes of nephroureterectomy for upper tract urothelial cancer? *J Urol.* 2009;181:133–134.

Stifleman MD, Hyman MJ, Shichman S, Sosa RE. Hand-assisted laparoscopic nephroureterectomy versus open nephroureterectomy for the treatment of transitional-cell carcinoma of the upper urinary tract. *J Endourol.* 2001;15:391–395.

Wolf Jr JS, Bennett CJ, Dmochowski RR, et al. Best practice policy statement on urologic surgery antimicrobial prophylaxis. *J Urol.* 2008;179:1379–1390.

19 Laparoscopic Partial Nephrectomy

Sam J. Brancato, Steven F. Abboud, Peter A. Pinto

HISTORY OF PROCEDURE

There will be an estimated 61,000 new cases of renal cell carcinoma (RCC) diagnosed in 2015. The incidence of RCC has continued to increase by 1.4% per year over the last decade. Surgical resection remains the gold standard treatment for RCC. Partial nephrectomy has been used to treat RCC with comparable oncologic outcomes to open radical nephrectomy in select groups of patients.

Laparoscopic partial nephrectomy has evolved significantly since Clayman and colleagues introduced the procedure in 1992 for benign disease. The benefits of such an approach include marked improvement in postoperative course and period of convalescence compared with open surgery. Currently, its indications have expanded to include malignancy. The key principles for successful application of this procedure are the same as in open surgery: secure vascular control, limited renal ischemia, and hemostasis.

INDICATIONS AND CONTRAINDICATIONS

Absolute indications for partial nephrectomy include surgical-sized lesions in patients with a solitary kidney or bilateral renal lesions. The increased risk of chronic kidney disease in patients undergoing radical rather than partial nephrectomy has influenced guidelines in favor of partial nephrectomy when feasible. Relative indications include renal lesions associated with hereditary syndromes, such as von Hippel-Lindau disease, hereditary papillary RCC, or Birt-Hogg-Dube syndrome, in which there is a risk of future development of ipsilateral or contralateral lesions. Relative indications also exist for solitary lesions in patients at risk for future renal deterioration (e.g., hypertension, diabetes). Partial nephrectomy for sporadic, unilateral, localized lesions in patients with a normal contralateral kidney was previously considered an elective indication; however, it has become the standard of care for small, exophytic lesions.

Contraindications to laparoscopic partial nephrectomy include renal vein or inferior vena cava thrombus, considerable tumor size, and direct tumor extension. Relative contraindications for laparoscopic partial nephrectomy include centrally located renal lesions, lymphadenopathy, history of prior ipsilateral renal surgery, and bleeding diathesis. Although there is no absolute size criterion, tumors smaller than 4 cm have a decreased recurrence risk and overall survival advantage when compared with tumors larger than 4 cm.

PATIENT PREOPERATIVE EVALUATION AND PREPARATION

Before laparoscopic partial nephrectomy, a detailed history and physical examination are undertaken. The anesthesiologist sees the patient for preoperative evaluation and clearance for surgery. The laboratory evaluation includes urinalysis and routine serum chemistries, including creatinine and liver function tests. Depending on the site and size of the tumor, type and screen or crossmatch should be obtained. Standard radiographic imaging includes abdominal computed tomography (CT) or magnetic resonance imaging (MRI).

We do not routinely require patients to undergo a mechanical bowel preparation before surgery. Preoperative prophylactic antibiotics should be administered within 60 minutes of surgical incision.

Sequential compression devices are placed and 5000 units of subcutaneous heparin is administered before induction. An orogastric or nasogastric tube is used for gastrointestinal decompression to maximize the operating space. A Foley catheter is placed after induction.

For lesions that extend into the renal collecting system, some recommend cystoscopic placement of an ipsilateral ureteral catheter through which dilute indigo carmine or methylene blue may be injected to facilitate intraoperative identification and repair of collecting system injuries. Others have not found that this improves their ability to detect or manage injuries to the collecting system.

OPERATING ROOM CONFIGURATION

The operating room configuration is dependent on the laparoscopic approach to be used. As is customary, the anesthesia machine should be at the head of the bed and the scrub nurse and sterile instruments opposite the surgeon to facilitate passage of instruments.

For the transperitoneal approach, the surgeon and camera-holding assistant stand on the side facing the patient's abdomen, and the viewing monitor is placed opposite them behind the patient. Some surgeons prefer to have an operating assistant stand opposite them. In such a case, the viewing monitor is placed so as to allow unobstructed viewing by the surgeon and camera-holding assistant. Similarly, a second viewing monitor may be placed opposite the operating assistant to the right or left of the surgeon to allow for unobstructed viewing, with care taken to not restrict the surgeon's ability to move. For the retroperitoneal approach, the setup is the same, except that the surgeon and camera holder stand at the patient's back (Fig. 19-1).

The choice of laparoscopic approach (transperitoneal versus retroperitoneal) is largely dependent on tumor position, patient's surgical history, and surgeon preference. Posterior or posterolateral tumors are easily approached retroperitoneally, but the transperitoneal approach is often used because it is most familiar to laparoscopists.

Placing the patient in the modified flank position greatly aids in the dissection by allowing the bowels to fall away from the kidney. Both approaches can be performed at 60 degrees of lateral tilt. However, for a laparoscopic retroperitoneal approach, a full 90-degree tilt allows for easier establishment of the pneumoretroperitoneum. Mild elevation of the kidney rest with either approach is used by some. Slight flexion of the bed allows adequate separation of the costal margin and iliac crest.

Emphasis is placed on use of foam padding at all patient pressure points, including the head and neck, axilla, arms, hip joint, knees, and ankles. It is also advisable to provide slight flexion at the joints to prevent inadvertent hyperextension during the procedure. We prefer securing the upper arm

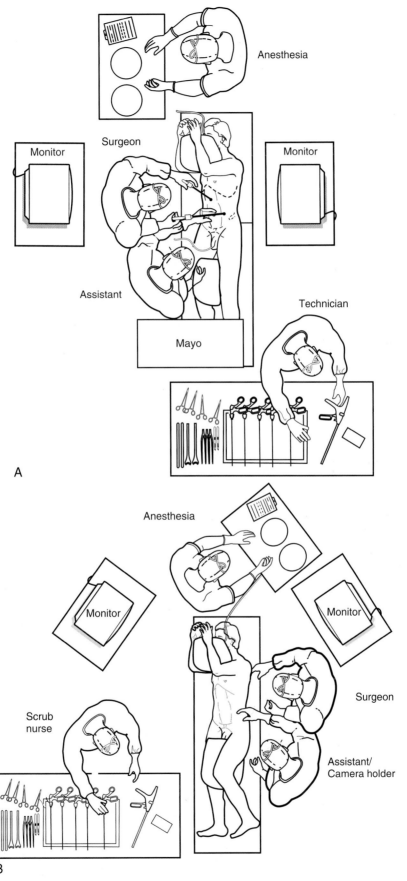

Figure 19-1. **A,** Operating room configuration for laparoscopic transperitoneal nephron-sparing surgery. The patient is in a modified lateral position. *Mayo,* Mayo instrument table. **B,** Operating room configuration for laparoscopic retroperitoneal nephron-sparing surgery. The patient is in a full lateral position.

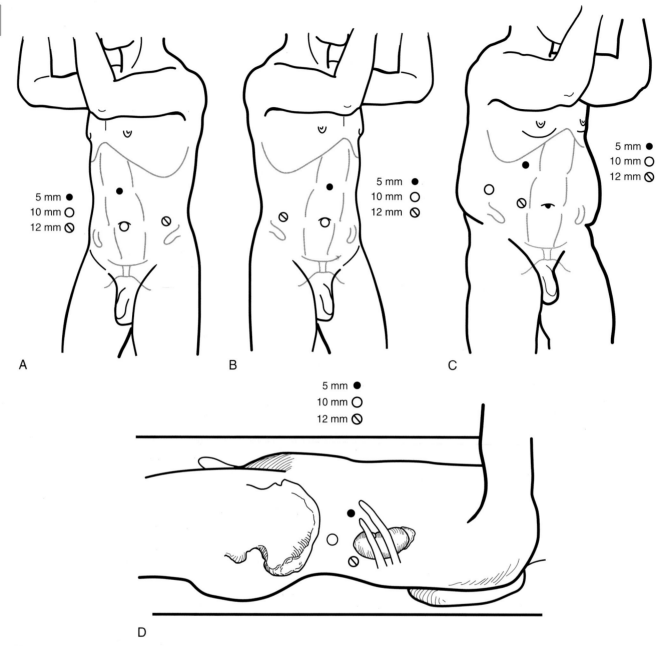

Figure 19-2. A, Trocar placement for left-sided transperitoneal laparoscopic nephron-sparing surgery. **B,** Trocar placement for right-sided transperitoneal laparoscopic nephron-sparing surgery. **C,** In the obese patient, the entire trocar configuration is shifted so that what would have been the umbilical trocar is in line with the umbilicus but placed lateral to the rectus muscle. **D,** Trocar placement for retroperitoneal laparoscopic nephron-sparing surgery.

between egg crate foam cushions and placing it across the patient's nipple line with a slight upward bend at the elbow. In all cases, secure the patient to the table using a safety belt or wide, strong adhesive tape, taking care to protect the skin from tape damage. Before preparation and draping, tile the table to ensure that the patient is fastened securely (see Fig. 19-1).

TROCAR PLACEMENT

We establish pneumoperitoneum with the Veress needle technique. Trocar placement is dependent on the intended laparoscopic approach. For simplicity, we use a three-trocar placement technique for intraperitoneal and retroperitoneal approaches that may be used interchangeably for right- or left-sided

approaches. For the transperitoneal approach, a 10-mm camera trocar is placed at the umbilicus. The remaining ports are placed: a 10/12-mm trocar lateral to the rectus abdominis muscle in the midclavicular line, and a 5-mm trocar approximately two fingerbreadths below the xiphoid process in the midline. An additional 5-mm trocar cephalad to the subxiphoid may be placed for liver retraction on the right or a 10/12-mm trocar in the midline below the umbilicus for Satinsky clamp placement if laparoscopic bulldog clamps are not being used. For obese patients, laterally shift the trocars toward the kidney (Fig. 19-2).

For the retroperitoneal approach, place the laparoscope through a 10-mm balloon-tipped trocar located just below the tip of the 12th rib. Then dilate the working space by inflating

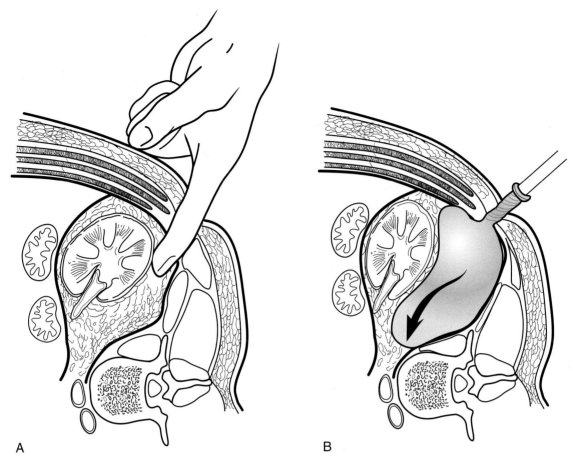

A   B

Figure 19-3. A, In the retroperitoneal approach, an incision is made off the tip of the 12th rib, large enough to allow placement of the index finger into the retroperitoneal space. The surgeon's finger is used to develop a space above the psoas muscle, posterior to the kidney.
B, A handmade or commercially available balloon is placed posterior to the kidney, and 300 to 500 mL of fluid or air is inserted to create the working space.

the balloon. After anterior deflection of the peritoneum, place a 5-mm trocar in the anterior axillary line two fingerbreadths above the iliac crest and below the tip of the 11th rib. Posteriorly place a 10/12-mm trocar in the angle between the 12th rib and the spinous musculature. A 5-mm assistant port may be placed in the upper anterior axillary line if needed (Fig. 19-3).

PROCEDURE (SEE VIDEO 19-1)
Transperitoneal Approach

The dissection is started by incising the white line of Toldt to deflect the colon medially. This often requires sharp release of the splenorenal or hepatorenal ligaments, depending on the operative side and location of the lesion. As the colon is deflected, the plane between the anterior Gerota fascia and the posterior mesocolon is developed. The psoas muscle is then identified, along with the overlying ureter and gonadal vein, which can be traced upward toward the renal hilum. On the right side, the duodenum is then kocherized. Dissect the renal hilum to the extent that a Satinsky or bulldog clamp can be easily placed when needed (Fig. 19-4).

The Gerota fascia is incised and the kidney is defatted at least 5 mm away from the lateral-most extent of the lesion to expose the renal capsule (Fig. 19-5). Intraoperative ultrasound is used to determine the depth and margins of the renal tumor, in additional to assessing for the presence of additional

lesions (Fig. 19-6). The capsule is scored with electrocautery circumscribing the mass (Fig. 19-7). The renal hilum is then clamped (if necessary) and the time is recorded (Fig. 19-8). Sharply incise the scored line of the renal capsule using cold scissors, and resect the tumor with the assistance of the suction cannula for countertraction and maintenance of a clear operative field (Fig. 19-9). This technique facilitates the proper plane of parenchymal dissection, preventing violation of the tumor capsule as well as recognition of the renal collecting system. Once freed from attachments, the mass is placed into a 10-mm Endo Catch (Medtronic Minimally Invasive Therapies, New Haven, Conn.) that is brought in through the 10/12-mm working port. The specimen is left in the abdomen for retrieval after completion of the renorrhaphy.

Assess for violation of the collecting system by injecting methylene blue via the ureteral catheter that was placed at the beginning of the procedure. If a defect is noted, it is oversewn with 3-0 Vicryl suture in a figure-of-eight fashion (Fig. 19-10). Transected vessels that are identified in the partial nephrectomy bed are closed in a similar manner.

A hemostatic agent, such as FloSeal or Tisseel (Baxter Healthcare Corporation, Westlake Village, Calif.), is injected into the parenchymal defect (Fig. 19-11). The parenchymal renorrhaphy is performed with 1-0 Vicryl suture. A Lapra-Ty clip (Ethicon, Cincinnati, Ohio) is preplaced on the tail end of the suture to serve as a pledget. Renal parenchymal stitches are placed over a Surgicel (Ethicon, Cincinnati, Ohio) bolster. The suture is

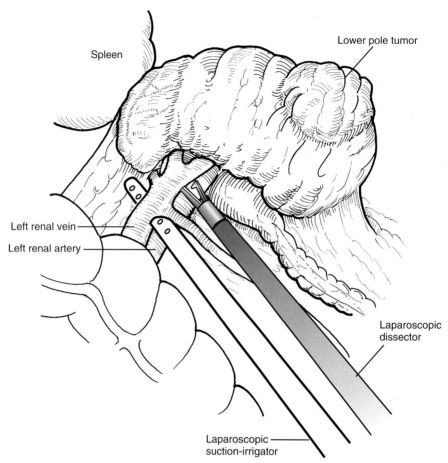

Figure 19-4. Careful dissection of the renal artery and renal vein allows complete occlusion and hilar control of the blood vessels to create a bloodless field for dissection of the renal mass.

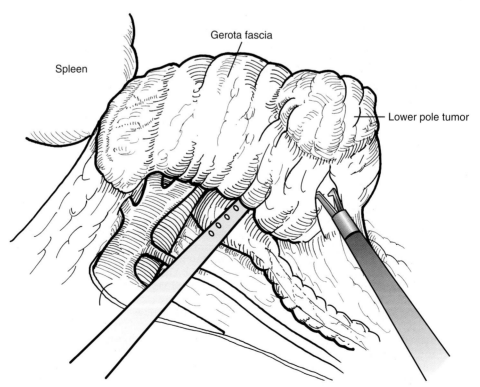

Figure 19-5. The Gerota fascia is opened near the renal mass, and the surface of the uninvolved kidney is identified.

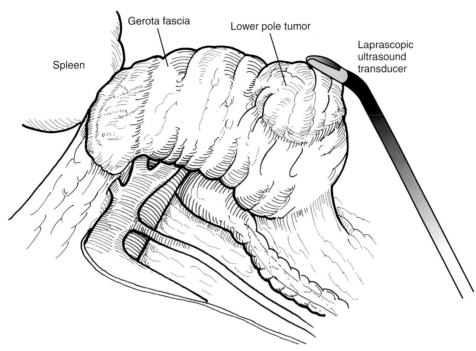

Figure 19-6. When the tumor is not readily identified on visual inspection or is endophytic, laparoscopic ultrasound is used to locate the mass.

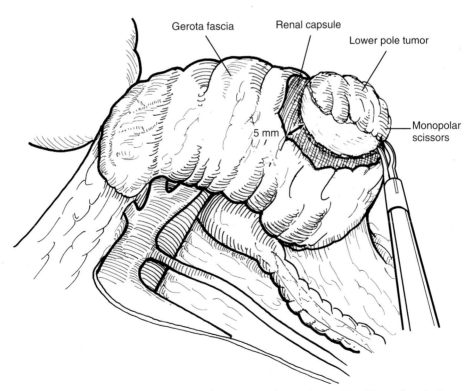

Figure 19-7. Electrocautery from closed monopolar scissors used to score renal parenchyma at least 5 mm from the tumor to delineate the intended line of dissection.

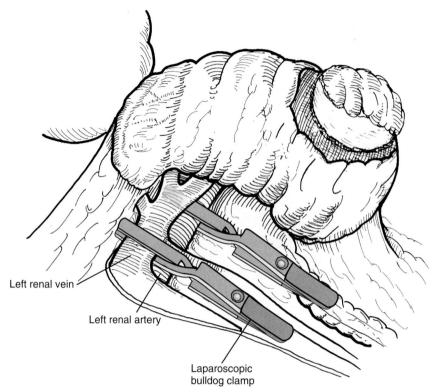

Figure 19-8. Vascular clamps are placed individually on both the renal artery and vein, or the renal hilum can be occluded with a vascular clamp inserted through a separate trocar site.

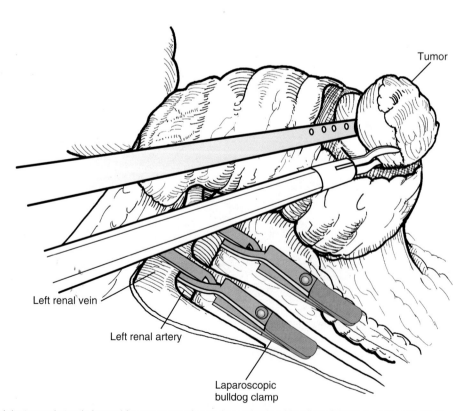

Figure 19-9. The irrigator aspirator tip is used for countertraction and to maintain a bloodless field while cold scissors are used to excise the lesion.

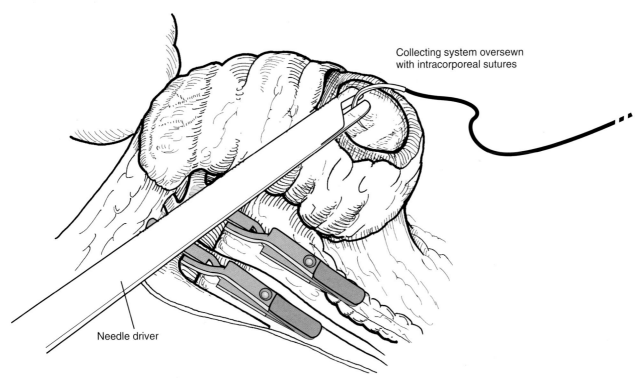

Collecting system oversewn
with intracorporeal sutures

Needle driver

Figure 19-10. Entry into the collecting system is common and can usually be seen without assistance. Some surgeons place an open-ended catheter at the beginning of the procedure and use retrograde injection of methylene blue to identify sites where the collecting system has been transacted. Collecting system injury is repaired with 4-0 absorbable suture. The Lapra-Ty clip (Ethicon, Cincinnati, Ohio) can be placed on the end of the suture as a knot, and a second clip is applied to secure the suture.

tightened, compressing the bolster firmly, and another Lapra-Ty clip is placed on the exiting suture flush with the parenchyma to compress the edges of the renal defect (Fig. 19-12).

The vascular clamp jaws are opened, but not removed, to assess the degree of hemostasis from the partial nephrectomy bed. Once the surgeon is satisfied, the clamp is carefully removed under direct vision. The Gerota fascia is closed with 3-0 Vicryl in a running fashion. A closed suction drain is placed in the paracolic gutter adjacent to the kidney, and the specimen is extracted through the 10/12-mm port.

A Carter-Thomason CloseSure System (Cooper Surgical, Trumbull, Conn.) is used to close the 10/12-mm trocar sites under direct vision to ensure no vital structures are entrapped. The pneumoperitoneum is released, and the skin incisions are closed with 4-0 Monocryl in a subcuticular fashion.

Retroperitoneal Approach

Make a 15-mm incision in the Petit triangle, just below the tip of the 12th rib, and extend the dissection downward through the lumbodorsal fascia and into the retroperitoneal space with the aid of a clamp. Bluntly dissect this space with the tip of a finger along the psoas muscle posterior to the kidney. Next, place a 12-mm balloon dilating trocar through this tract, and further expand the retroperitoneal space with balloon inflation. Introduce a 10-mm camera via this trocar, and establish a pneumoretroperitoneum of 15 mm Hg. Expand and cinch the trocar cuff to the skin to prevent CO_2 leakage. View pertinent structures for orientation and to exclude entry trauma: the psoas muscle with overlying intact fascia and ureter, inferiorly; intact Gerota fascia surrounding the kidney, cephalad; and intact peritoneal membrane, anterior. Place the other trocars as described previously, and further expand

the retroperitoneal space by bluntly sweeping the peritoneum anteriorly (see Fig. 19-3).

Retract the kidney upward and cephalad while bluntly dissecting it off the psoas fascia. The pulsation of the renal artery is then evident and guides the approach to its dissection. Dissect the renal artery and vein to the point of allowing easy placement of bulldog clamps when needed. Next, use intraoperative ultrasound to verify the location and extent of the renal lesion. Enter the Gerota fascia away from the area of the lesion, and remove the lesion as described for the intraperitoneal approach after clamping the vessels.

Regardless of laparoscopic approach, minimize warm ischemia time to less than 30 minutes (maximum 1 hour) because clamp times within this period do not appear to result in long-term renal dysfunction.

Postoperative Management

Important immediate postoperative considerations include, but are not limited to, monitoring of vital signs and quantity and content of drain output. Continued renal hemorrhage may manifest as persistent or sanguineous drain output, hematuria, or unstable vital signs. Delayed bleeding may occur up to 30 days postoperatively.

We recommend early ambulation to minimize the risk of deep venous thrombosis (DVT); however, 24 hours of postoperative bed rest is routinely prescribed by others. Furthermore, we restrict strenuous exercise for 4 to 6 weeks to allow adequate healing of the partial nephrectomy bed.

If a ureteral catheter has been placed, it should be removed immediately postoperatively. The Foley catheter stays in overnight. Note whether drain output increases after Foley catheter removal because this may indicate a urine

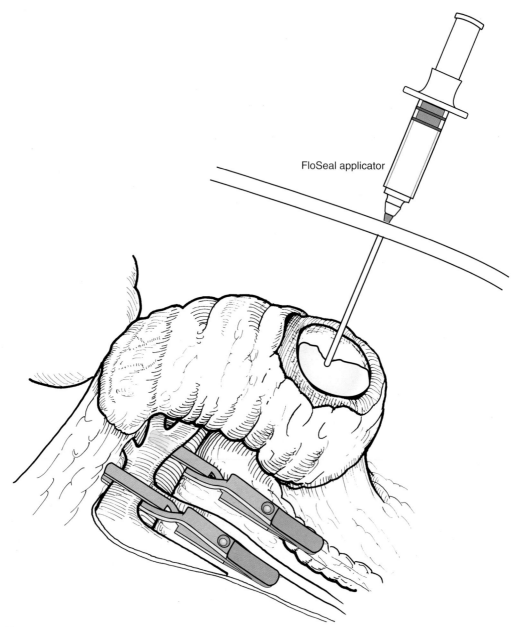

FloSeal applicator

Figure 19-11. Hemostatic and sealing fibrin product is applied to the surface of the kidney with a laparoscopic applicator through a trocar near the kidney.

leak from a persistent or unrecognized collecting system injury.

Monitoring of the drain fluid creatinine concentration may help differentiate peritoneal fluid from urine and assist in deciding on drain removal. Remove the drain only when the fluid content is consistent with peritoneal fluid in color and chemical composition.

COMPLICATIONS

In general, complications after laparoscopic partial nephrectomy can be divided into intraoperative and postoperative categories. Overall complication rates were well documented in a prospective randomized trial (European Organisation for Research and Treatment of Cancer [EORTC] 30904), with the most common being hemorrhage and urinary leakage. Intraoperative hemorrhage is invariably a result of inadequate vascular control

technique. Some have found that laparoscopic bulldog clamps, which are often used for the retroperitoneoscopic approach, provide suboptimal vascular occlusion when compared with Satinsky clamps. We have not found this to be true. However, Satinsky clamps are not infallible. In addition to clamp failure, failure to identify and control multiple renal arteries also may result in intraoperative hemorrhage. Furthermore, anatomic factors including proximity to the collecting system and tumor size influence the risk for perioperative hemorrhage. In a multicenter study of 730 elective partial nephrectomies, the rates of blood transfusions for tumors smaller than 4 cm and larger than 4 cm were 6.3% and 14.8%, respectively. Smoking (odds ratio [OR] 3.5) and American Society of Anesthesiologists (ASA) score below 3 (OR 2.9) are also patient-related risk factors for blood transfusion. If the hemorrhage cannot quickly be controlled, conversion to open surgery is indicated. Postoperative complications directly attributable to the laparoscopic technique are

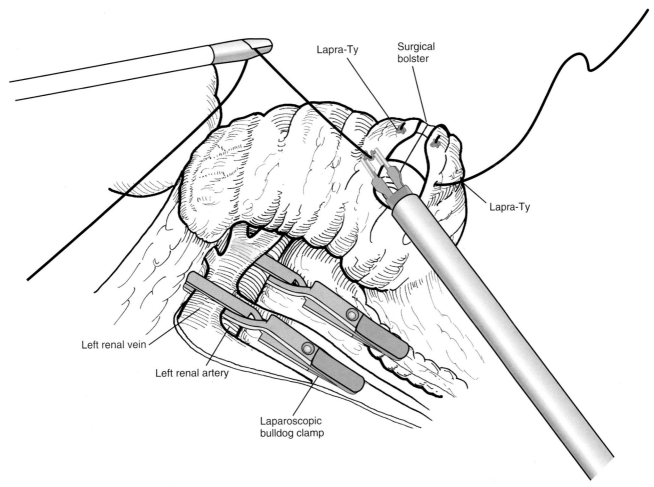

Figure 19-12. A hemostatic bolster can be formed by rolling Surgicel (Ethicon, Cincinnati, Ohio), tying each end with an absorbable suture, and placing it in the kidney defect. For large resections, two or more of these bolsters may be necessary. The kidney defect is then approximated with absorbable suture passed approximately 1 cm from the edge of the renal capsule. Lapra-Ty clips (Ethicon, Cincinnati, Ohio) can be used to secure both ends of the suture. However, the surgeon must guard against excessive tension on the suture, which can cause the Lapra-Ty to pull through the renal capsule into the kidney.

also typically related to hemorrhage or renal collecting system injury. Delayed spontaneous hemorrhage after partial nephrectomy occurs in approximately 6% of patients and has been described as occurring up to 14 days postoperatively. Bed rest with spontaneous resolution, segmental arterial embolization, and completion nephrectomy are typical treatment measures, depending on the severity of hemorrhage.

Renal collecting system injury also occurs intraoperatively with urinary leakage in approximately 4% to 5% of cases. Proximity to the collecting system and tumor size greater than 2.5 cm are associated with postoperative urinary leakage. Furthermore, the importance of renal pelvic anatomy has been recognized, leading to the development of a renal pelvic anatomy score (RPS). The RPS is defined as the percentage of renal pelvis inside the renal parenchyma volume, categorized as intraparenchymal (>50%) or extraparenchymal (<50%) renal pelvis. Intraparenchymal renal pelvic anatomy is associated with higher risk of urinary leakage and can be used to guide planning.

Such injuries may not be immediately recognized. The aforementioned techniques to identify such injuries are available. Most surgeons recommend immediate closure of large defects, but opinions differ on the need to close smaller ones.

Significant renal collecting system leaks usually manifest in the perioperative period as persistent drain output consistent with urine. Delayed presentation of unrecognized leaks manifests as urinomas, symptomatic or asymptomatic. Management in the perioperative period may consist of collecting system decompression via ipsilateral ureteral stenting or Foley catheter replacement, or simple prolongation of the drainage period. Urinomas may be managed by percutaneous drainage, by observation with ureteral stenting, or by observation alone, depending on size and symptoms.

Other less commonly occurring serious complications include ureteral injury, renal dysfunction, and vascular injuries.

TIPS AND TRICKS

- For obese patients, it is often helpful to shift all trocar positions laterally to place them closer to the kidney. This often obviates the need for extra-long instruments and for placing undue torque on the trocars with upward retraction. Care should be taken to avoid injuring the epigastric vessels.
- Grasping Gerota fascia with Debakey forceps and providing careful upward retraction of the kidney often facilitates hilar identification and dissection.
- Use of Lapra-Ty clips on each end of the sutures decreases warm ischemia time by obviating the need for tying.

SUGGESTED READINGS

Allaf ME, et al. Laparoscopic partial nephrectomy: evaluation of long-term oncological outcome. *J Urol.* 2004;172:871–873.

Bhayani SB, et al. Laparoscopic partial nephrectomy: effect of warm ischemia on serum creatinine. *J Urol.* 2004;172:1264–1266.

Campbell SC, et al. Guideline for management of the clinical T1 renal mass. *J Urol.* 2009;182:1271–1279.

Finelli A, Gill IS. Laparoscopic partial nephrectomy: contemporary technique and results. *Urol Oncol.* 2004;22:139–144.

Hafez KS, Fergany AF, Novick AC. Nephron sparing surgery for localized renal cell carcinoma: impact of tumor size on patient survival, tumor recurrence and TNM staging. *J Urol.* 1999;162:1930–1933.

Jeldres C, et al. Baseline renal function, ischaemia time and blood loss predict the rate of renal failure after partial nephrectomy. *BJU Int.* 2009;103:1632–1635.

Johnston 3rd WK, Wolf Jr JS. Laparoscopic partial nephrectomy: technique, oncologic efficacy, and safety. *Curr Urol Rep.* 2005;6:19–28.

Liu ZW, et al. Prediction of perioperative outcomes following minimally invasive partial nephrectomy: role of the RENAL nephrometry score. *World J Urol.* 2013;31:1183–1189.

Ljungberg B, et al. EAU guidelines on renal cell carcinoma: 2014 update. *Eur Urol.* 2015;67:913–924.

Patard JJ, et al. Morbidity and clinical outcome of nephron-sparing surgery in relation to tumour size and indication. *Eur Urol.* 2007;52:148–154.

Ramani AP, et al. Complications of laparoscopic partial nephrectomy in 200 cases. *J Urol.* 2005;173:42–47.

Richstone L, et al. Predictors of hemorrhage after laparoscopic partial nephrectomy. *Urology.* 2011;77:88–91.

Scosyrev E, et al. Renal function after nephron-sparing surgery versus radical nephrectomy: results from EORTC randomized trial 30904. *Eur Urol.* 2014;65:372–377.

Stroup SP, et al. RENAL nephrometry score is associated with operative approach for partial nephrectomy and urine leak. *Urology.* 2012;80:151–156.

Surveillance, Epidemiology, and End Results Program (SEER). *SEER stat fact sheets: kidney and renal pelvis cancer;* 2015. [cited 2015; National Cancer Institute. Available from: http://seer.cancer.gov/statfacts/html/kidrp.html.

Tomaszewski JJ, et al. Renal pelvic anatomy is associated with incidence, grade, and need for intervention for urine leak following partial nephrectomy. *Eur Urol.* 2014;66:949–955.

Van Poppel H, et al. A prospective randomized EORTC intergroup phase 3 study comparing the complications of elective nephron-sparing surgery and radical nephrectomy for low-stage renal cell carcinoma. *Eur Urol.* 2007;51:1606–1615.

20 Laparoscopic Live Donor Nephrectomy

Paras H. Shah, Michael J. Schwartz

INDICATIONS AND CONTRAINDICATIONS

Donor nephrectomy is unique among surgeries performed in urology. Unlike most procedures offered to our patients, there are no discrete medical indications—it is elective in the truest sense of the word. In addition, there are no direct health benefits for the donor patient other than the reward of knowing that they have provided a life-changing gift to the transplant recipient, whether it be a family member, friend, or individual previously unknown to them. The patient must be willing to be a kidney donor, competent to consent, and completely confident in the decision.

Contraindications to laparoscopic donor nephrectomy include uncorrected coagulopathy, the presence of medical renal disease, and active infection. There are also relative contraindications including history of renal stone disease, and other considerations include the presence of any significant medical comorbidities that could affect long-term renal function, presence of communicable disease (e.g., human immunodeficiency virus [HIV], hepatitis), and good mental health. Prior abdominal surgery is not a contraindication to donor nephrectomy, but the extent and nature of the prior surgery must be carefully considered when discussing risks of the procedure and may influence the surgical approach. The presence of microscopic hematuria is not a contraindication to renal donation, provided appropriate urologic evaluation to rule out malignancy or significant stone disease is performed preoperatively. Upper urinary tract imaging (ultrasound, computed tomography [CT], or magnetic resonance imaging [MRI]), urine cytology, and cystoscopy are the critical elements of the microscopic hematuria workup. Nephrology evaluation and possible renal biopsy can also be considered if there is a suspicion of early medical renal disease as the cause of the microscopic hematuria.

The evolution of protocols for recipient immunosuppression has also allowed for the expansion of the donor pool such that ABO incompatibility and positive crossmatch are not necessarily prohibitive. Donor swap and donor chain programs are also making transplants possible when they may not have been feasible otherwise.

PATIENT PREOPERATIVE EVALUATION AND PREPARATION

Evaluation of prospective kidney donors involves a multidisciplinary approach to ensure both physical and mental health and is typically coordinated through the transplant team. The goal of donor screening is primarily to determine whether renal function would be significantly compromised by donor nephrectomy. Internists, nephrologists, radiologists, and donor surgeons are most commonly involved. Additional medical subspecialists may also be required if there are specific elements in the patient's medical history that may play a role in the perioperative course or in determining suitability for kidney donation. As the pool of potential donors expands to include patients with advanced age or prior history of malignancy, subspecialists are playing an increasing role in the donor evaluation process.

If a volunteer for renal donation is found to be a suitable candidate for donor nephrectomy, CT angiography is performed to assess renal size and vascular and ureteral anatomy. The imaging plays the most critical role in determining which kidney will be selected for donation. Institutions and surgeons may have their own criteria for selecting the donor kidney. At some centers the left side is almost always preferred owing to the longer renal vein, even in the presence of multiple renal arteries. Others prefer to select the kidney with simpler arterial anatomy to minimize the need for vascular reconstruction. At our center, nuclear renal scans to assess differential function are not typically performed, and assuming a symmetric nephrogram phase on CT angiogram, renal size is used as a surrogate to estimate differential renal function. Ureteral duplication is occasionally encountered but does not strongly influence the choice of kidney for donation.

Mechanical bowel preparation is not used in our center before donor nephrectomy. Patients are currently being asked to drink clear liquids in the afternoon and evening on the day before surgery. The patient is given a single dose of prophylactic antibiotic in the operating room within 1 hour before incision.

OPERATING ROOM CONFIGURATION AND PATIENT POSITIONING

Laparoscopic donor nephrectomy can be performed with either a transperitoneal or a retroperitoneal approach, a choice that is the main determining factor influencing operating room configuration. A transperitoneal approach means positioning the patient in either a modified or full flank position. At our center, we use a modified flank position with the side of donation elevated 20 to 30 degrees with gel bumps placed to support the scapula and hip (Fig. 20-1). It is not necessary to flex the operative table or use a kidney rest or axillary roll in this position. The patient's legs are slightly flexed at the knee with a pillow under the knees for support. Foam padding is placed around the ankles to eliminate pressure on the heels. The arm contralateral to the donor side is left out, perpendicular to the operative table on an arm board, which allows easy access for the anesthesiologist. The ipsilateral arm is gently folded across the patient's chest, above the costal margin to allow exposure to the full abdominal wall. Sequential compression devices are placed for deep venous thrombosis prophylaxis before the induction of anesthesia. The patient is secured to the table with wide silk tape with towels or foam pads to protect the patient's skin. A Foley catheter is placed. The kidney extraction site is also marked before putting the patient in modified flank position to avoid anatomic distortion when the patient is rotated. Usually a mini–Pfannenstiel incision 4 to 5 cm in length is adequate. Upper and lower body warming devices are used to maintain the patient's temperature.

The laparoscopic tower accommodating the monitor and light source are placed on the side of kidney donation; the primary surgeon and assistant stand on the contralateral side facing the abdomen. The equipment required for insufflations, suction, and cautery are placed at the discretion of the surgeon, and typically at our center are placed behind the surgeon

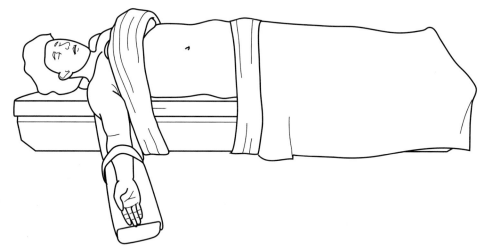

Figure 20-1. Patient positioned for transperitoneal left laparoscopic donor nephrectomy.

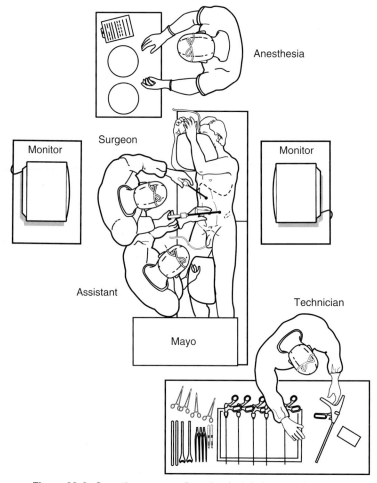

Figure 20-2. Operating room configuration for left donor nephrectomy.

and assistant. The surgical technician stands at the elevated hip, and the instrumentation table is at the foot of the operative table. A standard laparoscopic drape with side pockets is used (Fig. 20-2).

For a retroperitoneal approach, the patient is positioned in a full flank position with the donor side facing up. An axillary roll is used, and the table is flexed to expand the space between the anterior superior iliac spine and the costal margin. For this approach, both arms are out in front of the patient, with the lower arm resting on an arm board perpendicular to the table, and the other resting either on stacked blankets or on a purpose-built arm rest. Wide silk tape is used to secure the patient in position with towels or foam strips to protect the patient's skin. Upper and lower body warming devices are used to maintain the patient's temperature.

The laparoscopic tower is positioned in front of the patient in this configuration, opposite the surgeon and assistant, who stand at the patient's back. The insufflation device, cautery, and suction equipment remain at surgeon discretion. The surgical technician stands opposite the surgeon at the hip, with the instrumentation table at the foot of the operative table. The extraction site for a retroperitoneal approach may be in the flank, or a mini–Gibson incision may be used, but the site does not necessarily have to be marked before positioning.

TROCAR PLACEMENT
Transperitoneal Approach

A Veress needle is placed through the umbilicus to achieve insufflation to 15 mm Hg. Three trocars are initially placed, including an 11-mm umbilical port to accommodate the camera, a 6-mm subcostal working port, and a 12-mm working port 2 cm medial and superior to the anterior superior iliac spine on the side ipsilateral to the donor kidney (Fig. 20-3). Additional trocars may be necessary in some cases for the purpose of retraction, depending on internal anatomy and the patient's body habitus. Shifting the trocars laterally may be necessary if the patient is overweight or obese. A suprapubic trocar may also be used to insert a specimen bag at the time of extraction, as a working port for retraction, or to aid in the ureteral dissection.

Retroperitoneal Approach

A working space posterior to the kidney must be developed before trocar placement for a retroperitoneal approach. There are several well-established techniques for creating this space. First, a 12- to 15-mm incision is made off the tip of the 12th rib. A fingertip may then be used to push into the retroperitoneum, posterior to the kidney, and a sweeping motion of the finger allows for a small

space to be created. The surface of the psoas muscle, the kidney, or both can often be palpated with the fingertip and can aid in initial dissection. Then, with either the tip of a surgical glove attached to a catheter or a purpose-built trocar with a balloon at the tip, the space is further expanded by insufflating the tip of the glove or balloon. A camera port is then inserted and the space is inspected. Further blunt dissection with the tip of the laparoscope may also be performed to additionally expand the space as needed. Once adequate space is developed, two additional working trocars are placed under laparoscopic vision. A 5-mm or 12-mm trocar is placed in the midaxillary line, two to three fingerbreadths above the anterior superior iliac spine. The second trocar, also either 5 or 12 mm in size, is placed at the junction of the 12th rib and erector spinae muscle.

TRANSPERITONEAL LEFT LAPAROSCOPIC DONOR NEPHRECTOMY (SEE VIDEOS 20-1 AND 20-2)
Colon Mobilization and Deflection

After initial port placement, the surgery is begun by incising the white line of Toldt (Fig. 20-4). For this step, our instruments of choice are laparoscopic DeBakey forceps for retraction and monopolar cautery shears. This allows medial mobilization of the colon by developing the avascular plane between the mesentery and Gerota fascia with a combination of blunt and sharp dissection (Fig. 20-5). The kidney

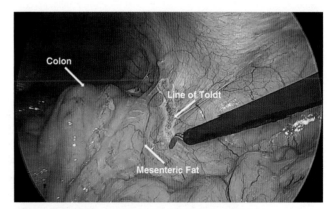

Figure 20-4. An incision is made along the line of Toldt to permit medial deflection of the colon.

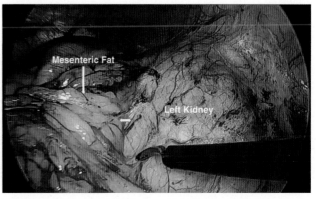

Figure 20-5. Mesenteric fat is dissected off Gerota fascia to facilitate medial mobilization of the colon. A plane between the mesenteric fat and Gerota fascia is developed (*double arrow*).

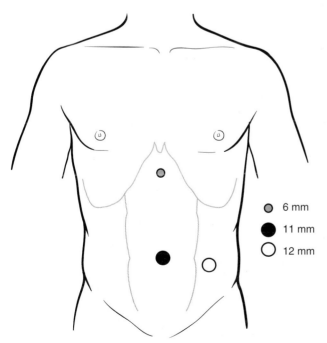

6 mm
11 mm
12 mm

Figure 20-3. Trocar placement for transperitoneal left laparoscopic donor nephrectomy: 11-mm umbilical trocar (camera), 6-mm subxiphoid trocar, and 12-mm left lateral trocar.

capsule may or may not already be visible at this point, depending on the volume of perinephric fat. Care is taken at this point to avoid entry into Gerota fascia, preservation of which facilitates dissection. Is it also recommended to avoid dissecting posterolateral to the kidney at this point to prevent the kidney from falling medially and obscuring the hilar vessels. The colon is reflected to allow adequate exposure of the kidney and ureter down to the level of the common iliac vessels.

Mobilization of the Spleen and Pancreas

The splenorenal and splenocolic attachments are divided with LigaSure (Medtronic, Minneapolis, Minn.), facilitating exposure of the upper pole (Fig. 20-6). Once divided, the plane medial to the upper pole and adrenal gland is further developed and the spleen and pancreas fall together toward

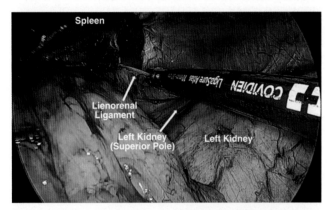

Figure 20-6. The lienorenal ligament is divided and the spleen is medialized to allow mobilization of the superior pole of the kidney.

the midline. Partially rolling the surgical table toward the surgeon can facilitate both the dissection and exposure along the medial aspect of the kidney and will maximize visualization of the renal hilum. A paddle retractor may also be used through a suprapubic trocar if visualization of the hilum is not sufficient.

Location of the Gonadal and Main Renal Veins

The left gonadal vein and ureter should be visible at this stage. If not, they are most easily located just below the lower pole of the kidney (Fig. 20-7, *A*). Developing the plane between the posterior portion of the kidney and underlying psoas muscle is undertaken at this time (Fig. 20-7, *B*), which allows for gentle traction on the hilar vessels and significantly accelerates their safe dissection. The gonadal vein is traced superiorly to the left renal vein (Fig. 20-8, *A*) and ligated with 10-mm titanium clips before division (Fig. 20-8, *B*). Care must be taken to allow for adequate space along the renal vein to accommodate the endovascular stapling device such that the clips are well away from the jaws of the stapler. It is recommended to dissect the renal vein as completely as possible at this point to ensure ample length and space for the stapler before placing gonadal vein clips.

Upper Pole Dissection

This step may be undertaken either before or after renal hilar dissection. Moving between hilar dissection and the upper pole may also be useful, depending on the anatomy specific to the case. Best exposure of the renal artery is usually gained after the upper pole is free. The Gerota fascia may be entered just above the renal vein, and the surface of the renal capsule is exposed. A plane may then be developed between the upper pole and the adrenal gland to preserve the adrenal (Fig. 20-9). We prefer to perform this phase of the operation with a

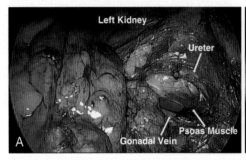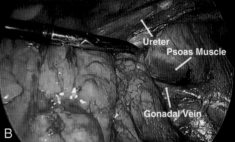

Figure 20-7. The ureter is identified below the lower pole of the kidney **(A)** and placed on anterior traction **(B)**, allowing a plane to be developed between the ureter and the psoas muscle fascia in an inferior-to-superior direction toward the renal hilum.

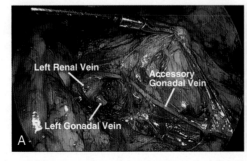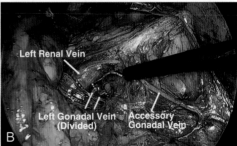

Figure 20-8. During a left laparoscopic partial nephrectomy, the left gonadal vein can be identified originating off of the left renal vein **(A)**. The vein may be clipped at its origin to facilitate hilar dissection **(B)**.

suction-irrigator device in the left hand and the LigaSure in the right. A combination of blunt dissection and LigaSure cautery aids in moving through this portion of the operation very efficiently. It is critical to be cognizant of arterial branches that may be encountered during this dissection, which are often present just above the renal vein medial to the lower tip of the adrenal gland.

Renal Arterial Dissection

Careful inspection of the preoperative CT angiogram is critical to minimize risk of unintentionally ligating any secondary

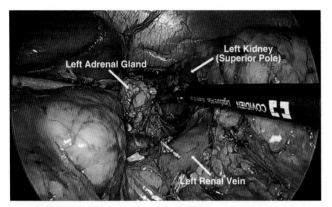

Figure 20-9. The adrenal gland is dissected off the superior pole of the kidney.

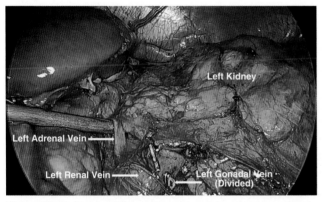

Figure 20-10. During a left laparoscopic partial nephrectomy, the adrenal vein can be identified originating off of the left renal vein. The vein is clipped and divided to facilitate mobilization of the adrenal gland off the superior pole of the kidney.

arterial branches during the dissection. All renal arteries are end arteries, and a portion of the donor kidney function may be lost if this were to occur. Before full dissection of the artery or arteries can occur, care must also be taken to ligate any remaining venous branches (Fig. 20-10). These include the adrenal and lumbar veins. Blunt dissection with the suction-irrigation device is often helpful in identifying these vessels, followed by the right angle dissector to prepare them for ligation. Depending on their size, titanium clips or the LigaSure device may be used for ligation of these vessels. The artery may then be skeletonized with the use of the laparoscopic DeBakey forceps or 10-mm right angle dissector (Fig. 20-11). Efforts should be made to expose the artery as close to its origin at the aorta as possible.

Ureteral Dissection

The ureter is again located just below the lower pole and is freed from surrounding connective tissue down to the level of the common iliac vessels. This length is quite adequate for the transplant recipient because the ureter is often trimmed by the transplant surgeon to minimize the risk of ureteral ischemia at the anastomosis. To that end, it is very important not to skeletonize the ureter too aggressively during dissection in order to preserve blood supply.

Lateral Dissection and Removal of Perinephric Fat

At this stage the only remaining attachments of the kidney are the renal hilar vessels, ureter, and posterolateral connective tissue. The Gerota fascia is entered to free the kidney from the perinephric fat intracorporeally (Fig. 20-12). Bipolar cautery (LigaSure) is typically used to complete this task. This is also the phase of the operation at which we prefer to administer intravenous mannitol. Although evidence for the use of mannitol is limited in the human population, it has the theoretical benefit of minimizing ischemic damage by acting as both a free radical scavenger and an osmotic diuretic.

Preparation of Extraction Site

The kidney is now ready for extraction, and the extraction site is prepared before ligation of the ureter and hilar vessels. The previously marked mini–Pfannenstiel incision is made and the rectus fascia is cleared of the overlying subcutaneous fat. The fascia is opened in the midline, but the peritoneum is left intact. A 15-mm port is then placed through the peritoneum to accommodate the specimen bag. Readiness of the transplant surgeon and back table to receive the kidney is confirmed.

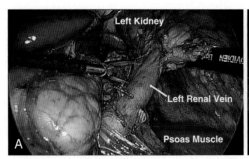
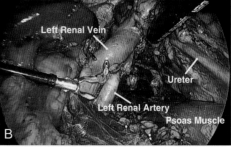

Figure 20-11. The hilar vessels are placed on slight anterior traction to facilitate skeletonization of the renal vein **(A)** and artery **(B)**.

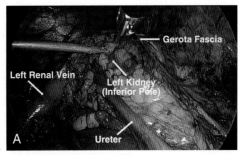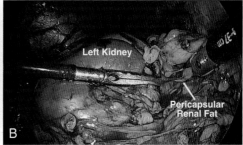

Figure 20-12. Perinephric fat is dissected off the kidney capsule by entering Gerota's fascia (**A**) and clearing the kidney of the surrounding perinephric fat (**B**).

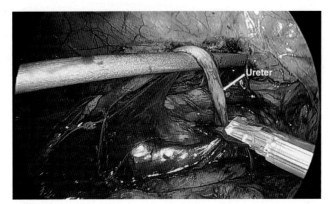

Figure 20-13. The ureter is dissected down to the level of the common iliac vessel bifurcation, at which point the ureter is clipped and divided.

Ureteral Ligation

If the ureteral length is not considered adequate, the suprapubic 15-mm port can facilitate further distal dissection of the ureter. It is then clipped and divided (Fig. 20-13).

Hilar Ligation

The renal artery is ligated first, with either an endovascular stapling device or three or four 10-mm titanium clips (Fig. 20-14, *A*). Hem-o-lok clips (Weck Closure Systems, Research Triangle Park, N.C.) are specifically recommended against and are contraindicated because they have been associated with bleeding complications and death. Maintaining anterior traction on the kidney helps to ensure maximum arterial length. The vein is then ligated, also with the endovascular stapler (Fig. 20-14, *B*).

Kidney Extraction

The kidney is placed into an Endo Catch bag (Medtronic, Minneapolis, Minn.) (Fig. 20-15) and immediately removed through the prepared mini–Pfannenstiel incision extraction site. It is placed in ice slush, and the cold preservation process is initiated by the transplant surgical team.

Closure

Closure of the incision involves suturing the rectus fascial defect. Reapproximating the peritoneum or rectus muscle bellies is at the discretion of the surgeon. The abdomen is then reinsufflated and inspected. The whole surgical bed should be inspected, with careful attention paid to the ligated renal vessels, adrenal gland, spleen, pancreas, and ureteral stump.

Any residual bleeding should be controlled, and the colon can be returned to its normal position. Any cutting trocar sites 10 mm or larger are closed at the level of the fascia with either a suture passing device under laparoscopic vision or externally placed sutures. Surgical drains are not necessary unless there is suspicion or confirmation and repair of pancreatic injury.

TRANSPERITONEAL RIGHT LAPAROSCOPIC DONOR NEPHRECTOMY

Trocar placement and most of the surgical steps are identical and mirror images of those for left laparoscopic donor nephrectomy. One difference is the more common need for an additional trocar for liver retraction. If needed, liver retraction may be performed with a 5-mm trocar placed in the anterior axillary line, through which the assistant may pass a retracting device. Alternatively, a 3-mm trocar placed in the subxiphoid region can be used to pass a locking grasper. By passing this under the inferior liver edge and grasping the peritoneum laterally, liver retraction is accomplished. It is critical to fully inspect the liver for injury throughout the procedure. Argon beam coagulation may be used in most cases of liver injury to ensure hemostasis.

Medial Exposure

During right laparoscopic donor nephrectomy, exposure of the renal hilum typically requires mobilization of the duodenum. After incising the white line of Toldt and deflecting the colon medially, the duodenum becomes visible. Sharp dissection should be used to divide the lateral attachments of the duodenum, which allows for exposure of the right renal hilar vessels and vena cava (Fig. 20-16). It is important to avoid cautery when mobilizing the duodenum to minimize the risk of thermal injury, which can be a cause of devastating surgical morbidity.

Interaortocaval Dissection of the Right Renal Artery

If there is an early branch point of the right renal artery, it may be necessary to perform an interaortocaval dissection to minimize the need for vascular reconstruction on the part of the transplant surgeon. Further medial mobilization of the duodenum and paddle retraction through a suprapubic trocar facilitate this exposure (Fig. 20-17). Before ligating the artery, it is important to ensure that the entire length of the renal artery is freed of surrounding connective tissue and vascular structures, especially posterior to the vena cava. Leaving attachments in this area may significantly prolong warm ischemia time if additional postligation dissection is required. If the right renal artery has no early branches, the artery may be dissected lateral and posterior to the vena cava, also with the use of an accessory trocar to allow for traction on the vena cava. This will

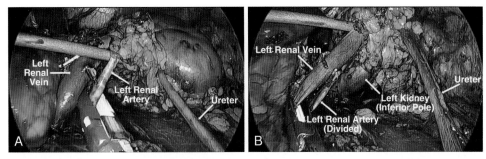

Figure 20-14. Control of the renal hilum is obtained with the vessels placed on anterior traction. For a left laparoscopic donor nephrectomy, the renal artery **(A)** and renal vein **(B)** are divided with an endovascular stapling device.

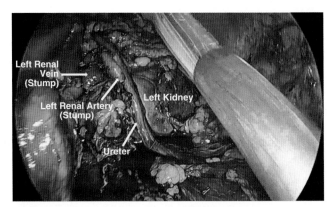

Figure 20-15. The kidney and ureter, free from all attachments, are placed in a specimen bag.

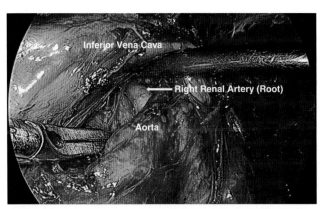

Figure 20-17. Interaortocaval dissection of the right renal artery is performed in a patient with early arterial branches. The vena cava is placed on anterior traction with the suction-irrigator device.

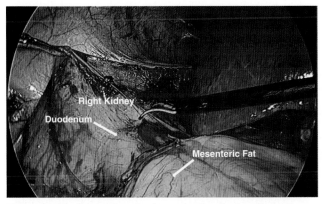

Figure 20-16. Sharp dissection is used to free the lateral attachments of the duodenum in a right laparoscopic donor nephrectomy.

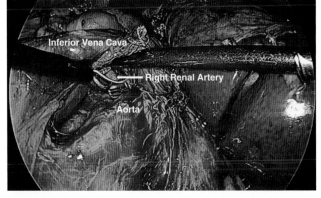

Figure 20-18. The right renal artery is ligated at its origin with multiple 10-mm titanium clips and divided.

aid in rolling the vena cava slightly medially and maximizing arterial length.

Right Renal Hilar Ligation

When ligating the right renal artery in the interaortocaval space, it is best to avoid endovascular stapling devices. Deploying a stapler in this region may cause the tips to be immediately against a vertebral body, and firing the stapler in this state may cause significant shear force on the artery. This may result in stapler misfire and hemorrhage. Using three or four 10-mm titanium clips at the most proximal section of the right renal artery allows for precise ligation with no shear forces on the

vessel (Fig. 20-18). The renal vein is ligated with an endovascular stapling device with the kidney on traction to maximize venous length.

RETROPERITONEAL LAPAROSCOPIC DONOR NEPHRECTOMY

There are fewer landmarks in the retroperitoneum and the working space is smaller, potentially making the dissection more challenging. However, there may be advantages to this approach in certain cases where it may be of benefit to avoid the peritoneum. Some surgeons also prefer this approach to transperitoneal donor nephrectomy.

Identification and Dissection of the Renal Hilar Vessels

Because of the paucity of landmarks, it is critical to maintain the camera with the horizon parallel to the psoas muscle, often the only initial visible landmark. To begin the dissection, the kidney is placed on anterior traction, and the pulsation of the renal artery is identified. The vessel is skeletonized, and the vein is then identified behind the artery and similarly freed of its surrounding connective tissue and vascular structures. It is imperative to circumferentially free the vein to avoid inadvertent ligation of adjacent structures when it comes time to ligate the renal hilar vessels. During a left-sided retroperitoneoscopic donor nephrectomy, this requires ligation and division of the gonadal, adrenal, and lumbar branches associated with the main left renal vein. Typically, this is best accomplished with 10-mm titanium clips.

Ureteral Dissection

The ureter is most easily identified with the kidney on anterior traction, just below the hilar vessels at the level of the lower pole. Dissection can then be carried out distally, preserving as much of the connective tissue and associated vascular supply as possible down to the level of the common iliac artery.

Removal of Perinephric Fat

The Gerota fascia may now be entered to separate the kidney from its surrounding fat. Depending on the body habitus and age of the patient, this step may require minimal dissection or may be quite tedious. Usually this step is accomplished with the use of the LigaSure device and grasping forceps to provide countertraction. The monopolar shears may also be intermittently valuable if the fat is particularly adherent. It is ideal to separate the fat from the kidney as completely as possible to minimize the size of the extraction site required. In addition, this step will separate the kidney from the adrenal gland superiorly, which may or may not be directly visualized. It should now be confirmed that the only remaining attachments of the kidney are the hilar vessels and the ureter.

Ureteral Ligation

After confirmation that the recipient and transplant surgeon are ready to receive the allograft, the ureter is clipped distally and divided.

Hilar Ligation

The renal artery is now ready for ligation, which may be accomplished with either an endoscopic vascular stapler or with multiple titanium clips. A stapler is typically preferred for ligation of the vein owing to its larger size, and the entire length of the stapler jaws must be visualized to avoid inadvertent ligation of adjacent structures.

Specimen Extraction

The allograft is now ready for removal. It may be placed in an Endo Catch specimen retrieval bag; the surgeon may use a hand placed through the extraction site. A mini–Gibson muscle-splitting incision may be used for this purpose, which can allow the surgery to remain purely retroperitoneal. Alternatives include a mini–flank incision by connecting two of the port-site incisions or creating a mini–Pfannenstiel incision and a small peritonotomy.

LAPAROENDOSCOPIC SINGLE-SITE DONOR NEPHRECTOMY

Periumbilical and Pfannenstiel incisions have both been described in performance of laparoscopic donor nephrectomy. We have used the Pfannenstiel approach because of reduction in postoperative pain and improved cosmesis: the patient will typically not have any visible scars. This approach is more challenging than standard laparoscopy owing to the limited ability to triangulate with the camera and working instruments. Because the safety of the donor patient is the first priority, the threshold to convert to standard laparoscopy should be low if any significant difficulty with dissection is encountered. Conversion is also advised if there is any perceived or real compromise to the allograft itself.

Costs of laparoendoscopic single-site (LESS) donor nephrectomy may be higher, especially if purpose-built surgical devices are used. Developing flaps above the fascia through the Pfannenstiel LESS approach has allowed us to avoid these purpose-built devices because conventional laparoscopic ports may be used and spaced to maintain triangulation. Other disadvantages reported in some series include longer warm ischemia time.

POSTOPERATIVE MANAGEMENT

Pain control for donor patients is initially achieved with a combination of local anesthetic injected at the incision sites at the time of surgery and intravenous medications. Patients are given a patient-controlled anesthesia device overnight after surgery and are transitioned to oral medication the following morning. Early ambulation is strongly encouraged. The Foley catheter is removed the morning after surgery. Incentive spirometry is used to minimize atelectasis and risk of postoperative pneumonia. Deep venous thrombosis prophylaxis is continued, including sequential compression devices until ambulation is adequate and subcutaneous heparin. There is no role for postoperative antibiotics in standard settings.

Dietary management includes allowing patients access to clear liquids on the evening of the surgery. If the patient is nauseated, liquids are held until the morning of postoperative day 1. Bisacodyl suppositories are administered on the morning of surgery to promote flatus and reduce abdominal distention if present. Ketorolac is used for pain control to minimize narcotic requirement and associated constipation. Intravenous fluids are stopped on the morning after surgery, provided liquid intake is adequate. Solid foods are held until the patient is passing flatus.

Discharge typically occurs on either postoperative day 1 or 2. If the patient is not yet passing flatus at discharge, he or she is encouraged to advance the diet at home once this occurs. Follow-up office visits are 3 to 4 weeks after surgery, provided the postoperative course is typical.

COMPLICATIONS

Surgical complications are relatively uncommon in laparoscopic donor nephrectomy relative to other laparoscopic renal surgery. Several factors contribute to the lower complication rate, including normal and undistorted anatomy; overall health of donor patients, who often have few if any medical comorbidities; and surgeon experience—with donor surgeons often among the most experienced laparoscopic surgeons at their institution. Nonetheless, laparoscopic donor surgery is not without risk, and these risks should not be minimized.

Vascular complications are among the most common and can be significant, occasionally requiring the addition of a hand port or open conversion to safely control. The level of dissection required around the hilar vessels, aorta, and vena cava is often more extensive than that with laparoscopic radical or simple nephrectomy owing to the need to preserve vascular length for the recipient. Small vessels may be avulsed from more major vessels during dissection, sometimes resulting in significant blood loss or requiring suture repair. Vascular stapling devices should be used with great care; malfunctions have been reported, with need for rapid conversion to open surgery to control bleeding. Being prepared to handle such bleeding is critical. Hem-o-lok clips have been used in the past to ligate renal hilar vessels, but because of multiple donor patient deaths associated with these cases, the U.S. Food and Drug Administration (FDA) recommends against the use of these clips for renal hilar vessel ligation in donor nephrectomy.

TIPS AND TRICKS

- Maintain posterolateral attachments of the kidney until after the renal hilar vessels are completely skeletonized.
- Anterior traction on the kidney during hilar dissection will facilitate gaining maximum vascular length.
- Minimize skeletonization of the ureter to preserve its blood supply.
- Reinspect the ligated renal hilum, adrenal gland, ureteral stump, and spleen (left side) or liver (right side) completely after specimen extraction to ensure the lack of injury and adequate hemostasis.
- Avoid the use of cautery when performing dissection adjacent to the bowel, especially when mobilizing the duodenum in right-sided donor nephrectomy.
- Be prepared to add a hand port or convert to open surgery if significant bleeding or vascular injury occurs.

21 Laparoscopic Renal Cyst Decortication

Matthew Ziegelmann, Bohyun Kim, Matthew Gettman

INDICATIONS AND CONTRAINDICATIONS

Renal cystic disease is common, with an increasing prevalence likely related to the use of cross-sectional imaging over the last several decades. Renal cysts have been identified in up to one third or more of patients 50 years of age and older. The majority of these cysts are asymptomatic and only incidentally identified during evaluation for alternative indications. The Bosniak classification is used to classify renal cysts based on features more suspicious for malignancy, such as enhancement, septation, calcification, and solid elements (Table 21-1). For asymptomatic simple cysts (Bosniak class I or II), no further evaluation or treatment is necessary. Cysts classified as Bosniak class IIF require ongoing monitoring. Patients with class III or IV cysts should be counseled toward surgery with radical, or ideally partial, nephrectomy because of the higher rate of malignancy (Fig. 21-1). Further discussion regarding management of class III and IV renal cysts is therefore beyond the scope of this chapter.

Symptomatic simple renal cysts can significantly affect a patient's quality of life. Displacement of adjacent renal tissue or spontaneous bleeding into the cyst can result in continuous or intermittent pain episodes, and compression of the collecting system can cause intermittent upper tract obstruction. In addition, fluid within the cyst can become infected, acting as a nidus for recurrent urinary tract infections. Surgical intervention with laparoscopic decortication can be considered in those patients with symptomatic renal cysts, in the absence of imaging findings suspicious for malignancy. Other treatment modalities including percutaneous cyst aspiration with injection of a sclerotic agent can also be considered, although success rates are lower compared with laparoscopic cyst decortication. Notably, patients with symptomatic renal cysts in the setting of polycystic kidney disease are often excellent candidates for decortication. Contraindications include inability to tolerate general anesthesia, untreated infection, history of extensive abdominal or retroperitoneal surgery, and uncorrected bleeding diathesis.

PATIENT PREOPERATIVE EVALUATION AND PREPARATION

Before laparoscopic cyst decortication, patients should undergo a full history and physical examination. Important elements in the history include symptom severity and timing, family history of renal cystic disease or malignancy, current medications, and medical comorbidities. Prior abdominal and urologic procedures should be documented. Physical examination including cardiovascular system, pulmonary system, abdominal or flank area, and genitourinary system should be performed to assess for additional comorbidities. Preoperative laboratory evaluation should include an electrolyte panel, blood urea nitrogen (BUN), creatinine, complete blood count, urinalysis, and urine culture. Ideally, patients should undergo computed tomography (CT) of the abdomen and pelvis with nephrographic and delayed phases to carefully evaluate the renal parenchyma and cystic structures for findings suggestive of malignancy. In patients with medical renal disease or contrast allergies, in whom iodinated contrast is contraindicated, alternative imaging with renal ultrasound or magnetic resonance imaging (MRI) should be considered. After determination of the appropriate candidacy for laparoscopic cyst decortication, a careful discussion regarding patient expectations is important during the informed consent. Patients must understand that, despite appropriate surgical intervention, symptoms may persist.

OPERATING ROOM CONFIGURATION AND PATIENT POSITIONING

Surgical approach (retroperitoneal versus transabdominal) dictates patient positioning. The transabdominal approach is most commonly performed. The retroperitoneal approach can be especially useful for cystic lesions in the posterior aspect of the kidney, although these lesions can often be exposed transabdominally with additional renal mobilization.

TABLE 21-1 Bosniak Classification

Type	Radiologic Findings	Computed Tomography Attenuation and Enhancement	Management
I	No septa, calcification, or solid components	Water attenuation No enhancement	No follow-up
II	Thin hairline septa, fine septal or wall calcifications Possible minimal enhancement of thin septae or wall Hyperdense cyst <3 cm	Water or high attenuation No enhancement	No follow-up
IIF	Increased septae Mild thickening and enhancement of the septae Possible thick nodular calcifications Hyderdense cyst >3 cm	Variable attenuation No or little enhancement	Imaging follow-up
III	Thickened irregular walls or septa with possible enhancement	Variable attenuation Contrast enhancement	Surgery
IV	Solid enhancing component	Variable attenuation Contrast enhancement	Surgery

Modified from Israel GM, Bosniak MA. An update of the Bosniak renal cyst classification system. *Urology*. 2005;66:484-488.

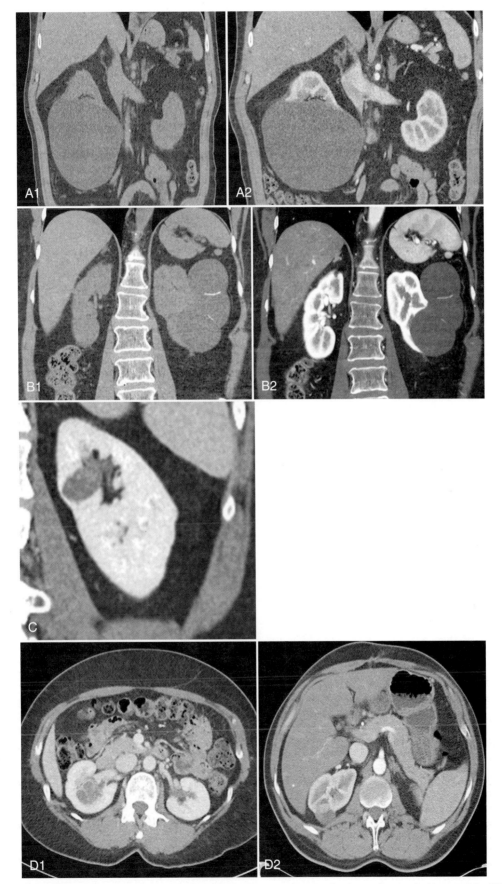

Figure 21-1. Examples of Bosniak cyst classification. **A,** Bosniak type I—coronal contrast-enhanced computed tomography (CT) reconstruction demonstrates no septa, calcification, or solid components within the right renal cystic lesion (**A1,** precontrast; **A2,** postcontrast). **B,** Bosniak type II—coronal noncontrast CT reconstruction demonstrates thin rim calcifications along the fine septae of the left renal cystic lesion (**B1,** precontrast; **B2,** postcontrast). **C,** Bosniak type IIF—coronal CT reconstruction after contrast demonstrates mild thickening and enhancement. **D,** Bosniak types III **(D1)** and IV **(D2)**—transaxial contrast-enhanced CT demonstrates thickened wall and septae of the cystic lesion (type III) and enhancing solid portions (type IV).

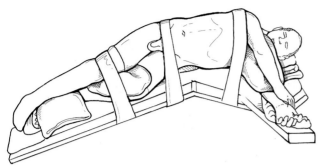

Figure 21-2. Modified 45-degree flank positioning for the transabdominal approach. Care should be taken to ensure that all pressure points are adequately padded, and the patient should be appropriately secured with tape or safety straps. The patient should be positioned such that the operating table can be adequately flexed between the iliac crest and the ribs, allowing for improved exposure during trocar placement. The ipsilateral hip is slightly more posterior compared with a true flank position.

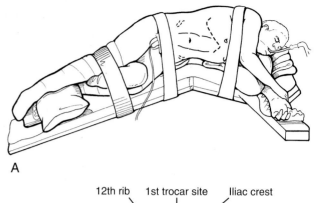

A

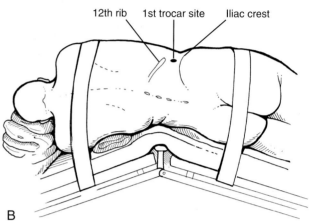

B

Figure 21-3. A, True flank positioning for the retroperitoneal approach. The contralateral (lower) leg is flexed; the ipsilateral leg remains straight. A designated arm supporter or pillow is placed between the outstretched arms. Again, tape or safety straps are used to ensure that the patient is secured to the operating room table. **B,** An axillary roll should be used along with the kidney rest, with the table in flex to open the retroperitoneum.

Patients should receive appropriate perioperative antimicrobial therapy, and this should be discontinued within 24 hours of the procedure in the absence of extenuating circumstances. Routine urinary and gastrointestinal decompression is warranted with placement of an indwelling Foley catheter and orogastric tube (this is removed at the cessation of the procedure, before extubation). If the cyst appears to be in close proximity to the collecting system, a ureteral catheter can be placed to assist with intraoperative collecting system evaluation. This can be converted to an indwelling ureteral stent if necessary. If there is no concern for collecting system injury, the ureteral catheter and indwelling urinary catheter can be removed before hospital discharge. It is also important to ensure that sequential compression devices are in place (unless contraindicated) to prevent lower extremity deep vein thrombosis.

Patient positioning is dictated by approach, with 45-degree flank position for the transabdominal approach (Fig. 21-2) and full flank position for the retroperitoneal approach (Fig. 21-3). An axillary roll is routinely placed to prevent neuromuscular injury. The kidney rest is used with the retroperitoneal approach. With the transabdominal approach, the surgeon and assistant stand on the side contralateral to the lesion (Fig. 21-4, *A*). During the retroperitoneal approach, the surgeon stands posterior to the patient (Fig. 21-4, *B*).

TROCAR PLACEMENT

The surgeon verifies correct patient positioning, taking care to ensure the patient is adequately secured and that pressure points are appropriately padded. The patient should be prepared and draped aseptically. With the transabdominal approach, the surgeon establishes pneumoperitoneum with either a Hassan or Veress needle technique. This step can be facilitated by tilting the patient into a more supine position. After adequate pneumoperitoneum has been achieved, 10/12-mm ports are placed in the midline at the umbilicus and at the midclavicular line just below the level of the umbilicus (just lateral to the rectus margin). A third 5-mm port is placed in the midline halfway between the umbilicus and the xiphoid process (Fig. 21-5, *A*). Triangulation of the working and camera ports can help avoid internal instrument collisions. For obese patients the same trocar configuration is used, but frequently the trocars need to be shifted more laterally toward the target anatomy (Fig. 21-5, *B*). After access, the peritoneal cavity is evaluated for injury or other intra-abdominal pathology.

On the right, an additional 5-mm port placed in the midline just below the xiphoid process can be used for retraction purposes. Locking grasping forceps can then be used to grab the abdominal wall peritoneum lateral to the liver or spleen to aid with visualization. Although this approach has been described for standard laparoscopic techniques, the same configuration can be used for a robotic-assisted approach to cyst decortication. Closure of the 10/12-mm ports is recommended, especially if a cutting-type trocar was used for initial placement.

The retroperitoneal approach is an alternative to the transabdominal approach, especially for posterior-based renal cysts (Fig. 21-6). Initially, identify the 12th rib and make a small incision just inferior to the tip, dissecting down through the lumbodorsal fascia. Blunt dissection is used to develop the plane between the psoas muscle and Gerota fascia. A retroperitoneal dissection balloon can then be used to develop this space while pushing the peritoneum medially. A 10/12-mm trocar is placed, and the laparoscope is used to verify correct positioning. Under direction visualization, an additional 10/12-mm trocar can then be placed in the anterior axillary line. Direct visualization is important to avoid inadvertent puncture of the peritoneum at this point. After this, a 5-mm trocar can then be placed cephalad, in the anterior axillary line.

PROCEDURE (SEE VIDEO 21-1)

If there is concern for communication with the collecting system, an externalized ureteral stent should be placed before

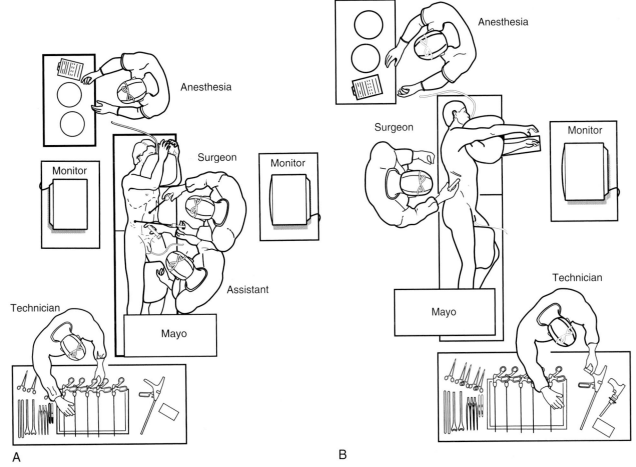

Figure 21-4. Operating room setup. **A,** Transabdominal approach. Patient is placed in the modified 45-degree flank position, with the operating surgeon and assistant standing on the side contralateral to the cystic lesion. **B,** Retroperitoneal approach. Patient is placed in the full-flank position, and the surgeon is positioned posterior to the patient.

the patient is placed in the flank position. The initial maneuver for renal exposure is mobilization of the colon. For a right-sided renal cyst, the ascending colon should be identified and reflected medially along the line of Toldt from the cecum inferiorly to the hepatic flexure superiorly (Fig. 21-7, *A*). Dissection can be carried out with the aid of sharp and blunt dissection. When using electrocautery, take care to avoid inadvertent bowel injury. The duodenum should be identified, and if necessary kocherization can be performed by incising the mesentery along the lateral edge of the duodenum and deflecting it medially (Fig. 21-7, *B*). When approaching a left-sided renal cyst, the descending colon is mobilized along the line of Toldt, from the sigmoid colon inferiorly to the splenic flexure superiorly, including the splenocolic ligament (Fig. 21-8). After splenorenal ligament division, the Gerota fascia is identified.

The renal cyst is often easily discernable at this point when visualizing the Gerota fascia, appearing as a cystic structure arising from the renal parenchyma. If the lesion is not easily identified, intraoperative ultrasound is helpful for cyst identification. Once the cyst has been definitively identified, the surrounding perirenal and pararenal fat should be dissected away. A laparoscopic needle and syringe can be introduced, and the cyst fluid aspirated and sent for analysis (Fig. 21-9). Laparoscopic shears with electrocautery can then be used to excise the cyst at the level of the interface with the normal renal tissue (Fig. 21-10). Despite the low risk of malignancy,

if desired the cyst can be sent for pathologic review. The cyst margin can then be fulgurated with electrocautery. Unless required for hemostasis, extensive cauterization of the cyst base is not recommended.

If a ureteral stent was placed preoperatively owing to concern for proximity of the cyst to the collecting system, methylene blue can be injected to evaluate for collecting system injury. If identified, this should be repaired with absorbable suture. The externalized stent can then be converted to an indwelling double-J stent, and a drain can be left adjacent to the kidney to monitor for urine leak. The pneumoperitoneum should be lowered at this point in the operation to be sure there is excellent hemostasis. Trocars are then removed under direct visualization, and trocar skin incisions are closed with subcuticular absorbable 4-0 suture. Sterile dressings are then applied to each trocar site.

For the retroperitoneal approach, the space is developed and ports are placed as described previously. Again, the cyst of interest is often readily visualized at this time, and the laparoscopic ultrasound device should be available if necessary. The Gerota fascia and surrounding perirenal fat should then be cleared away. The cyst should be aspirated and excised in a fashion similar to that described previously for the transabdominal approach. Again, ensure excellent hemostasis before port removal and close the port sites in standard fashion. On exit from the abdomen, the lumbodorsal fascia is closed with 2-0 absorbable suture.

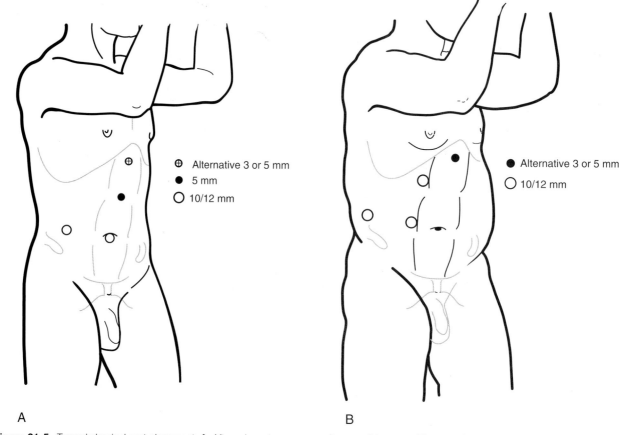

A   B

Figure 21-5. Transabdominal port placement. **A,** After adequate pneumoperitoneum (Hassan or Veress techniques), 10/12-mm ports are placed at the umbilicus and at the midclavicular line, just below the level of the umbilicus (just lateral to the rectus margin). A third 5-mm port is placed in the midline halfway between the umbilicus and the xiphoid process. **B,** In obese patients, the trocars may be shifted laterally toward the target anatomy

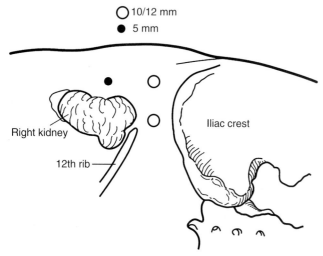

Figure 21-6. Retroperitoneal port placement. Initial 10/12-mm trocar is placed just inferior to the tip of the twelfth rib. A second 10/12-mm trocar can be placed in the anterior axillary line, and a smaller 5-mm trocar placed cephalad to this.

POSTOPERATIVE MANAGEMENT

The orogastric tube is removed before extubation, and the Foley catheter is removed on postoperative day 1, unless there is concern for injury to the urinary tract. Patients routinely receive a single dose of perioperative prophylactic antibiotics per American Urological Association (AUA) recommendations. The majority of patients have adequate pain control with oral analgesics, and the patient should begin ambulating on the evening of the procedure. Mechanical and chemical perioperative thromboembolic prophylaxis should be implemented if indicated. The patient is started on a clear liquid diet immediately, and this is transitioned to a general diet on postoperative day 1. The majority of patients are discharged to home on postoperative day 1. Additional follow-up is not typically required unless the patient has postoperative concerns.

COMPLICATIONS

Please see Chapter 12 for a detailed discussion regarding complications associated with laparoscopic access and exposure of the kidney. Immediate postoperative bleeding from an injured vessel or inadequate cyst wall fulguration can occur, manifesting as hemodynamic instability or grossly sanguineous output from a drain (although drains are rarely left in place with this procedure). Delayed bleeding can also occur as a result of a vascular malformation (pseudoaneurysm or arteriovenous malformation). However, this is much less common than what is seen with partial nephrectomy. Delayed bleeding can be associated with gross hematuria, flank pain, delayed return of bowel function, and failure to thrive. A high index of suspicion for vascular malformation must be considered in the setting of new-onset gross hematuria, and these patients should undergo diagnostic and therapeutic angiography. Patients with delayed bleeding that manifests with retroperitoneal hematoma can

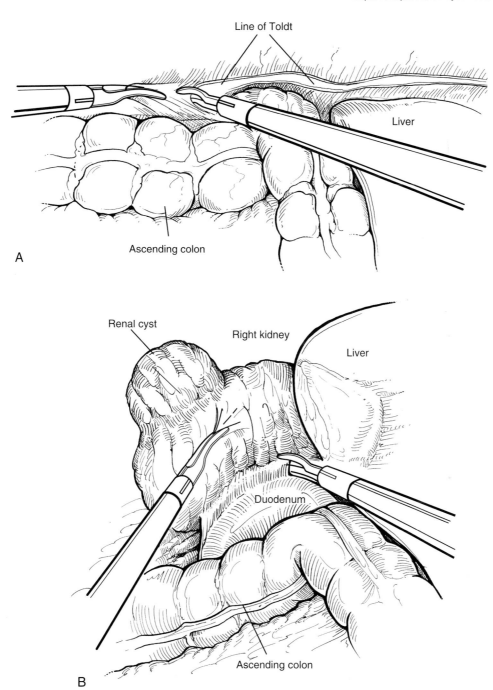

Figure 21-7. Right-sided dissection. **A,** The first step is mobilization of the ascending colon along the line of Toldt. **B,** After taking down the ascending colon, the duodenum can be mobilized medially (Kocher maneuver) to improve exposure to the right kidney.

often be managed conservatively with serial hemoglobins and bed rest. In those patients with cystic lesions adjacent to the renal collecting system, intraoperative collecting system injury may be missed despite careful surgical technique and methylene blue instillation via a retrograde stent at the time of the procedure. These patients again develop nonspecific symptoms including pain, failure to thrive, and delayed return of bowel function. A CT scan with intravenous contrast and delayed images can aid in identification of a collecting system injury. Treatment includes urinary tract decompression with a retrograde double-J stent and Foley catheter. A drain may be required for larger, symptomatic urinomas. Patients who do not respond to urinary tract decompression may require further surgical exploration.

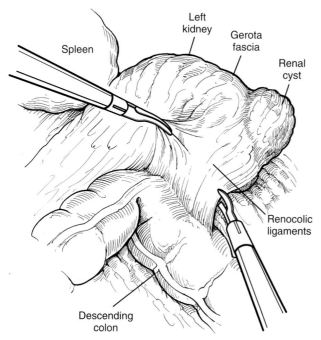

Figure 21-8. Left-sided dissection. Carefully take down the perirenal and pericolic ligamentous attachments to improve exposure for identification of the renal cyst of interest. Take care to avoid excess tension on the bowel and spleen during mobilization.

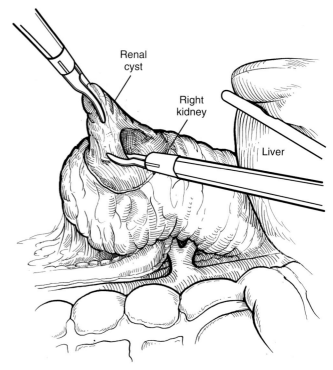

Figure 21-10. Cyst excision is performed with the aid of laparoscopic shears. Despite the low risk of malignancy, the cyst may be sent for pathologic review.

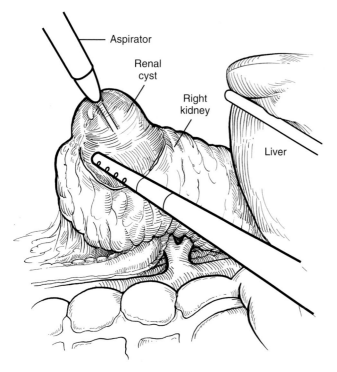

Figure 21-9. Aspiration of the cyst contents via laparoscopic aspiration needle.

TIPS AND TRICKS

- Establishing an accurate diagnosis is the most important consideration.
- Ureteral catheterization and intraoperative methylene blue instillation helps exclude injury to the collecting system.
- Placement of a Jackson-Pratt drain can be helpful when the cyst appears close to the collecting system.
- When excising a large cyst, it is helpful to avoid aspirating the entire cyst contents—this can help prevent cyst collapse and facilitate complete excision.
- Cyst collapse can also be prevented by keeping the aspiration needle in place after sufficient fluid has been removed and further opening the puncture site with the scissors while the cyst wall is tented upward by the laparoscopic needle.
- When performing cyst decortication for patients with autosomal dominant polycystic kidney disease, effort should be made to decorticate as many cysts as possible on all surfaces of the kidney.
- If the kidney is hypermobile after decortication, it can be fixed posteriorly to muscle with absorbable 3-0 Vicryl suture before the abdomen is exited.
- When one encounters suspicious cyst wall features intraoperatively (e.g., thickened cyst wall), the specimen should be sent for frozen section determination before the procedure is concluded.

22 Laparoscopic Renal Biopsy

Jathin Bandari, Stephen V. Jackman

Renal biopsy is a crucial tool in the diagnosis of medical disease of the kidney. Histologic information is pivotal in making treatment decisions and providing prognostic information. Ultrasound-guided percutaneous needle biopsy is the current standard for obtaining renal tissue. It has the advantage of being performed with use of local anesthesia in an outpatient setting. Unfortunately, there is up to a 5% rate of significant hemorrhagic complications.

In instances in which percutaneous biopsy has failed or is considered to pose a high risk, patients are traditionally referred for open renal biopsy. This procedure allows the advantage of obtaining hemostasis and plentiful cortical tissue under direct vision. However, open renal biopsy has the associated morbidity of an incision and general anesthesia. Laparoscopic renal biopsy combines the advantages of open biopsy with the decreased morbidity of a one- or two-port outpatient procedure. General anesthesia is still required.

INDICATIONS AND CONTRAINDICATIONS

The indication for renal biopsy is suspected renal disease, the treatment of which would be influenced by the results of histopathologic tissue analysis. The indications for directly visualized renal biopsy include three categories: failed percutaneous needle biopsy, difficult anatomy, and high risk for bleeding complications.

Anatomic factors that may make a patient unsuitable for percutaneous biopsy include morbid obesity, multiple bilateral cysts, and a body habitus that makes positioning impossible. The risk of hemorrhagic complication may outweigh the advantages of percutaneous biopsy in patients who are receiving long-term anticoagulation, have coexistent coagulopathy, or refuse blood transfusion under any circumstance. Laparoscopic renal biopsy is contraindicated in patients with uncorrected coagulopathy, uncontrolled hypertension, or inability to tolerate general anesthesia.

PATIENT PREOPERATIVE EVALUATION AND PREPARATION

Patients undergo routine screening history, physical examination, and blood analyses, including a complete blood count, basic metabolic panel, coagulation panel, and blood typing with antibody screening. Any problems are evaluated and corrected to the extent possible as determined by the urgency of the biopsy. In addition, patients must be told to refrain from taking aspirin, nonsteroidal anti-inflammatory drugs, and anticoagulants for 5 to 10 days before their procedure. Patients with bleeding disorders need 2 to 4 units of packed red blood cells crossmatched and available before the start of the procedure. Patients on long-term anticoagulation are managed in concert with their primary physician, nephrologist, or cardiologist. Cessation before the procedure and continuation thereafter is dependent on clinical necessity.

Patients with thrombocytopenia, which is common in several renal diseases, can receive platelets 30 minutes before incision to boost their platelet count to greater than 50,000 cells/mm³.

Further platelet transfusion is not necessary in the absence of symptomatic bleeding. Uremic patients may benefit from desmopressin acetate (DDAVP) treatment to improve platelet function.

OPERATING ROOM CONFIGURATION AND PATIENT POSITIONING

The surgeon and assistant both stand at the patient's back. Place the video monitor in front of the patient. Position the scrub nurse or technician in front of the patient, caudad to the monitor (Fig. 22-1). In addition to standard laparoscopic equipment, required tools include an optical trocar (Visiport [Covidien, Norwalk, Conn.]; Optiview [Ethicon Endo-Surgery, Cincinnati, Ohio]; or Kii Optical Separator [Applied Medical, Rancho Santa Margarita, Calif.]), 5-mm two-tooth laparoscopic biopsy forceps, argon beam coagulator, and oxidized regenerated cellulose (Surgicel [Johnson & Johnson, Arlington, Tex.]).

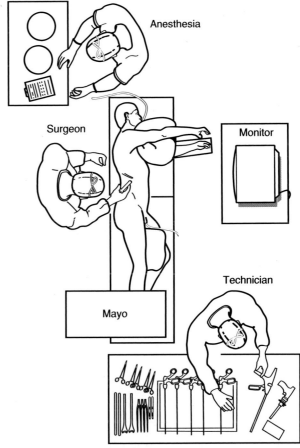

Figure 22-1. The surgeon stands behind the patient, and a single video monitor is placed in front of the patient. The scrub nurse or technician is located in front of the patient caudad to the monitor.

159

Place the patient on the operating table in the supine position, then apply antiembolism stockings and sequential compression devices. Induce general endotracheal anesthesia, then place an orogastric tube and a urethral catheter. Give 1 to 2 g of cefazolin for antimicrobial prophylaxis.

The choice of which kidney should undergo biopsy is primarily based on patient-specific anatomic considerations. In addition, a right-sided procedure may be more comfortable for right-handed surgeons, whereas biopsy of the left kidney may involve better working angles owing to its higher position. The technique is essentially the same regardless of side.

After inducing anesthesia, carefully roll the patient into the full flank position with the umbilicus over the table break. Fully flex the table to increase the space between the iliac crest and the costal margin. Carefully support the head with the headrest, folded sheets, and a head support ring. Align the cervical spine with the thoracic and lumbar spine. Place an axillary roll just below the axilla, and gently extend the arms. Pad the lower elbow with egg crate foam, and place several pillows between the arms.

Securely tape the upper body and arms to the table in position using 3-inch cloth adhesive tape. Use egg crate foam to protect the skin, upper elbow, and nipples from direct contact with the tape. Some skin contact is occasionally necessary to adequately stabilize the patient.

Flex the lower leg at the hip and knee and pad under the ankle. Leave the upper leg straight and separate it from the lower leg with one or two pillows. Place a standard safety strap around the legs and table at a level just below the knees. Securely tape the pelvis in position with more cloth tape, using a towel or egg crate foam over the genitalia for protection. Place grounding pads for electrocautery and the argon beam coagulator on the exposed upper thigh. Prepare and drape the patient in standard surgical fashion (Figs. 22-2 and 22-3).

TROCAR PLACEMENT
Two-Site Approach

Retroperitoneal access is identical for right- and left-sided procedures. Mark the skin midway between the iliac crest and the tip of the 12th rib roughly in the posterior axillary line (Fig. 22-4). Make a 10-mm transverse incision in the skin, and use a small curved hemostat to spread the skin and subcutaneous fat. Place a 0-degree lens focused on the blade of an optical trocar in the incision. Holding the optical trocar perpendicular to the skin and aiming approximately 10 degrees anteriorly, repeatedly fire the blade under direct vision until the retroperitoneum is entered. This requires traversing subcutaneous fat and either the lumbodorsal fascia or the flank musculature (external and internal obliques and the transversus abdominis) (Fig. 22-5). Straying too far anteriorly can result in peritoneal entry or colon injury, whereas posteriorly the quadratus or psoas muscles can be damaged, resulting in excessive bleeding.

Once the retroperitoneum is entered, remove the Visiport, leaving behind the 12-mm port. Begin CO_2 insufflation at a pressure of 15 mm Hg. Use blunt dissection with the laparoscope to develop the retroperitoneal space. Anteriorly, sweep the peritoneum medially with the laparoscope, exposing the underside of the transversalis fascia (Fig. 22-6). Once anterior dissection has mobilized the peritoneum medial to the anterior axillary line, place a 5-mm port under direct vision at the same level as the first port (Fig. 22-7). Then use laparoscopic scissors with electrocautery or a Harmonic Scalpel (Ethicon Endo-Surgery, Cincinnati, Ohio) to assist in completion of retroperitoneal space development. The superior extent of dissection is the Gerota fascia at the level of the lower pole of the kidney.

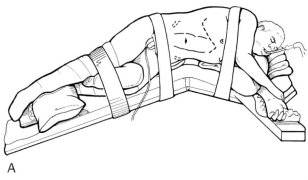

A

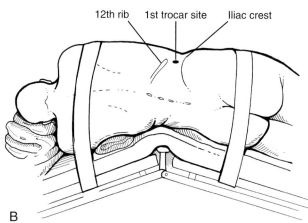

12th rib   1st trocar site   Iliac crest

B

Figure 22-2. A, The patient is placed into a full flank position with the umbilicus over the table break. The table is fully flexed to increase the space between the iliac crest and the costal margin. In addition, the kidney rest may be raised as needed. The head is carefully supported with the headrest, folded sheets, and a head support ring. The lower elbow should be padded with egg crate foam, and several pillows are placed between the arms. The chest, pelvis, thigh, lower leg, and arms are securely taped with 3-inch cloth adhesive tape. **B,** The cervical spine should be aligned with the thoracic and lumbar spine. An axillary roll is placed just below the axilla, and the arms are gently extended.

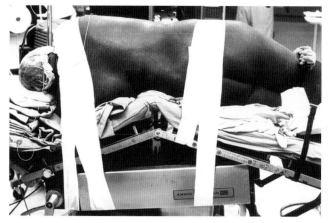

Figure 22-3. Patient positioned for laparoscopic renal biopsy.

Open, Hasson-type entry into the retroperitoneum and balloon dissection is an alternative to the method just described (see Chapter 10). The balloon is best placed inside the Gerota fascia before inflation, if possible, for the most efficient access to the kidney.

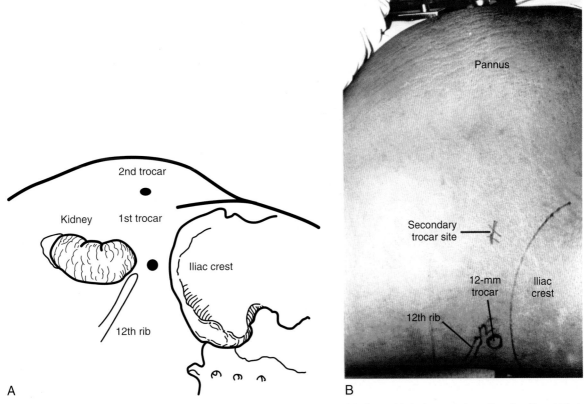

Figure 22-4. The skin is marked midway between the iliac crest and the tip of the 12th rib roughly in the posterior axillary line (**A** and **B**). A 10-mm transverse incision is made in the skin, and a small curved hemostat is used to spread the skin and subcutaneous fat.

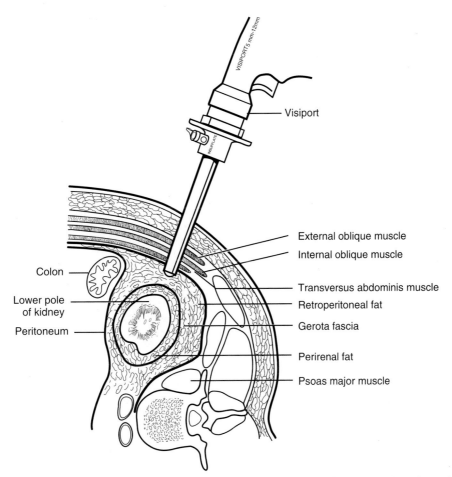

Figure 22-5. Use of an optical trocar such as the Visiport (U.S. Surgical, Norwalk, Conn.) allows the trocar to be advanced through the fascial layers into the retroperitoneum under direct vision.

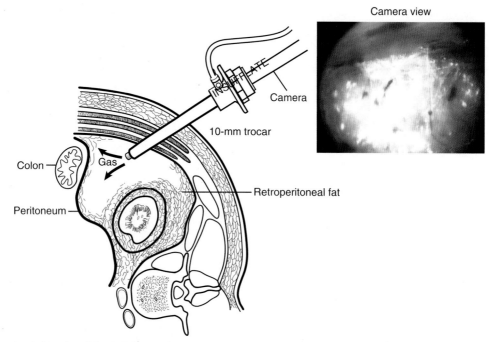

Camera view

Figure 22-6. The visual obturator of the optical trocar is removed and the 0-degree laparoscope is used to bluntly push the peritoneum medially, creating a working space large enough to allow placement of the second trocar. Insufflation will help maintain the space as it is created. During this dissection, the laparoscope is directed medially, toward the peritoneum and abdomen.

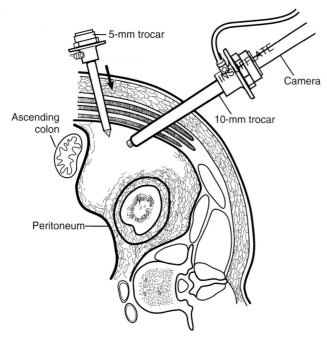

Figure 22-7. A 5-mm trocar is placed under direct vision. The working instruments are passed through this port. The camera can be used to assist with further dissection and is frequently cleaned to maintain visualization.

Single-Site Approach

A 2.5-cm transverse incision is made between the iliac crest and the tip of the 12th rib in the posterior axillary line. Finger dissection followed by balloon dissection of the retroperitoneal space is performed. A single port device of choice is placed. We prefer the GelPoint (Applied Medical, Rancho Santa Margarita, Calif.), which allows the surgeon to change

trocars dynamically if necessary. We begin with a 5- or 12-mm camera port and one or two 5-mm trocars. A standard straight laparoscope and instruments are adequate for visualization and dissection; however, a flexible laparoscope and bent instruments may be useful.

PROCEDURE (SEE VIDEO 22-1)
Kidney Exposure and Biopsy

Once both the camera and working trocar are in position and an adequate working space has been created, direct the instruments away from the midline toward the lower pole of the kidney (Fig. 22-8). Locate the kidney by palpation and sharp dissection through the Gerota fascia. The change to a darker-yellow fat on entry into the Gerota fascia helps identify the kidney (Fig. 22-9). In morbidly obese patients or other difficult situations, preoperative transcutaneous or intraoperative ultrasound may be valuable in localizing the kidney.

Once the Gerota fascia has been incised, sweep the perirenal fat aside to expose an approximately 2-cm × 2-cm area of the lower pole (Fig. 22-10). Use the 5-mm two-tooth biopsy forceps to take two or three good cortical renal biopsy specimens (Fig. 22-11). Place these in saline and transport them immediately to pathology for confirmation that adequate kidney tissue was obtained. Do not place the specimens in formalin; important information will be lost if the specimens are placed in formalin before processing. Frozen section or gross inspection under a dissecting microscope will confirm the presence of renal tissue. The pathologist can then place the tissue in the appropriate fixative for analysis.

Hemostasis and Closure

Obtain hemostasis with the argon beam coagulator. During activation of the argon beam, it is important to vent the increased pressure created in the retroperitoneum by the flow of argon gas (Fig. 22-12). While awaiting pathologic

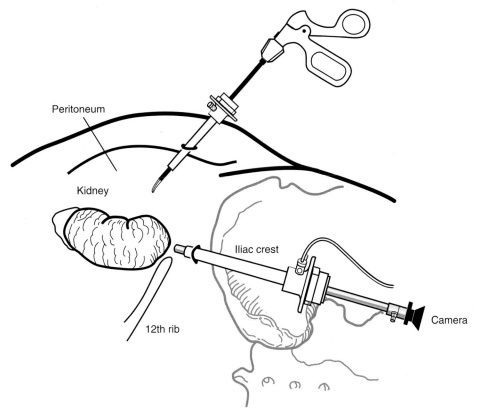

Figure 22-8. Once both trocars are in position, the camera and scissors are turned away from the midline and directed toward the lower pole of the kidney.

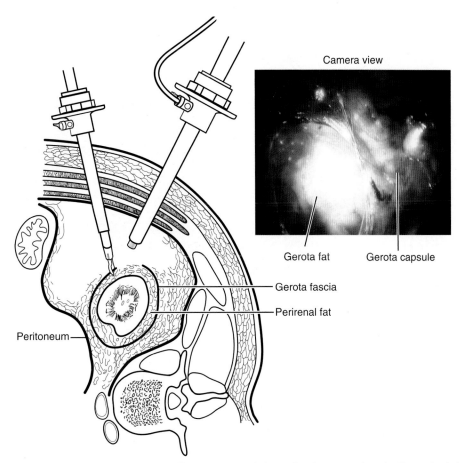

Figure 22-9. The Gerota fascia is opened with the scissors. The change to a darker-yellow fat on entry into the Gerota fascia is helpful in positively identifying the perirenal fat. Placing the camera and instrument in the opening and moving them in opposite directions enlarges the window.

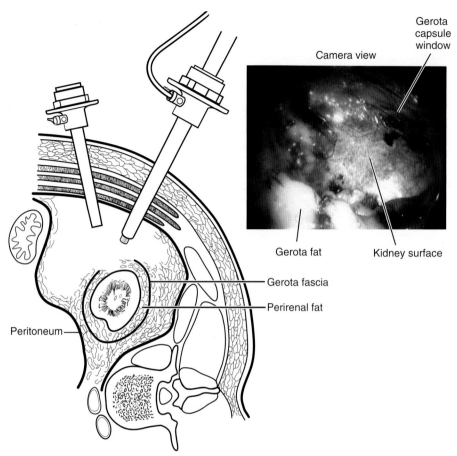

Figure 22-10. The perirenal fat is swept aside to expose the renal parenchyma.

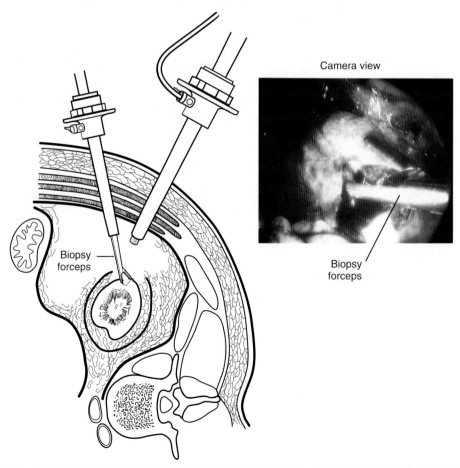

Figure 22-11. A 5-mm two-tooth biopsy forceps is used to take two or three samples from the lower pole of the kidney.

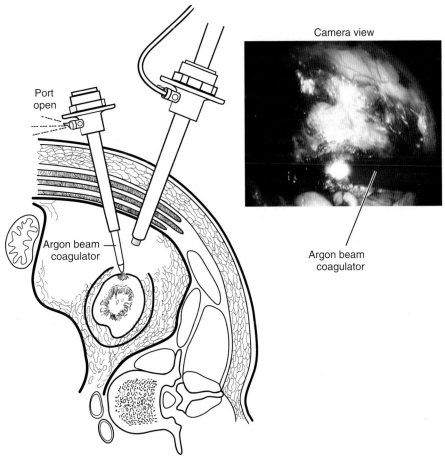

Figure 22-12. The argon beam coagulator is used to obtain hemostasis. The pneumoperitoneum pressure is lowered to 5 mm Hg, and the site of the biopsy is observed for active bleeding, which is re-treated with argon beam coagulation.

confirmation that the specimen is sufficient, lower the insufflation pressure to 5 mm Hg for at least 5 minutes and inspect the entire retroperitoneum for hemostasis. Treat persistent bleeding from the biopsy site with repeated argon beam coagulation. Pack oxidized cellulose (Surgicel) into the biopsy site and apply direct pressure (Fig. 22-13). Other adjuncts to hemostasis are needed rarely; these include various fibrin glues, matrix hemostatic sealant (FloSeal, Baxter Healthcare, Deerfield, Ill.), and surgical adhesives (BioGlue, CryoLife, Kennesaw, Ga.). Clip oozing vessels that are distant from the biopsy site with a 5-mm clip applier instead of electrocautery or argon beam; these may cause a thermal injury to the bowel on the other side of the peritoneum.

After confirming hemostasis under low pressure, discontinue insufflation and remove the 5-mm port under direct vision. Evacuate the gas via the 12-mm port with the assistance of manual flank compression and large-volume breaths given by the anesthesiologist. If the peritoneum has not been perforated, the fascial layers do not require suture closure. In the single-site approach, simply remove the device to desufflate and consider closing the lumbodorsal fascia with a 0 absorbable braided suture. Irrigate the skin incisions, inspect them for hemostasis, and close them with a 4-0 absorbable subcuticular suture. Apply skin glue or sterile skin closure tapes.

POSTOPERATIVE MANAGEMENT

Routine postoperative monitoring is performed based on the patient's health status. Specific attention is given to blood pressure control. Most nonhospitalized patients (i.e., those undergoing biopsy as an outpatient procedure) can be discharged the same day or the next morning. They are given oxycodone with acetaminophen for pain control and are instructed to avoid vigorous activity for 6 to 8 weeks.

COMPLICATIONS

Hemorrhage is the most common major complication. Careful resumption of anticoagulation is mandatory. Evaluate a persistent decline in hematocrit or symptoms of hypovolemia using computed tomography (CT) scan. Colon injury may manifest as fever, ileus, or leukocytosis. Laparoscopic bowel injuries may manifest atypically as only port-site pain and vague constitutional symptoms. Again, CT scan is the initial diagnostic modality of choice.

A review of 74 consecutive patients who underwent laparoscopic renal biopsy reported 96% success in obtaining adequate tissue for histopathologic diagnosis. Mean blood loss was 67 mL, and operative time was 2 hours. Surgical complications included one inadvertent biopsy each of the spleen and liver without consequence, one seromuscular colonic injury, one postoperative hematoma, and two intraoperative bleeds. One patient on high-dose steroids died secondary to a perforated peptic ulcer 7 days after surgery. Forty-three patients (58%) were discharged within 24 hours.

SUMMARY

Laparoscopic renal biopsy is a less invasive alternative to open renal biopsy in centers where the proper equipment and

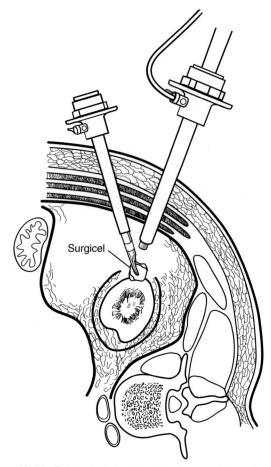

Figure 22-13. Oxidized cellulose (Surgicel) is passed down the 5-mm port and placed over the area of the biopsy.

expertise are available. Many patients can be treated in an outpatient setting. Adequate tissue, rich in glomeruli, is obtained from the cortex of the kidney, and hemostasis is obtained under direct vision before closure.

TIPS AND TRICKS

- Intraoperative ultrasound can be helpful both before and during the procedure to locate the lower pole of the kidney in obese patients.
- The change to a darker-yellow fat color is indicative of entry into Gerota fascia.
- Careful attention to postoperative blood pressure management and anticoagulation is key to the prevention of complications.

SUGGESTED READINGS

Micali S, Zordani A, Galli R, et al. Retroperitoneoscopic single site renal biopsy surgery: right indications for the right technique. *BMC Urol.* 2014;14:80–85.

Shetye KR, Kavoussi LR, Ramakumar S, et al. Laparoscopic renal biopsy: a 9-year experience. *BJU Int.* 2003;91:817–820.

Wickre CG, Golper TA. Complications of percutaneous needle biopsy of the kidney. *Am J Nephrol.* 1982;2:173–178.

23 Laparoscopic and Percutaneous Delivery of Renal Ablative Technology

Ramy Youssef, Kyle J. Weld, Jaime Landman

The incidence of renal tumors and particularly small renal masses (SRMs) has increased significantly, mostly because of increased use of and advances in cross-sectional imaging. Historically, radical nephrectomy (RN) was the standard of care for management of renal masses. Later, partial nephrectomy (PN) was found to be oncologically equivalent, with the added benefit of preserving renal function. In 2009, the American Urological Association (AUA) guidelines described PN as the standard of care for the majority of pT1a tumors. Cryoablation (CA) and radiofrequency ablation (RFA) are recommended as alternative less-invasive treatment modalities, particularly in patients with major comorbidities. Reasons cited have included the following: Local tumor recurrence might be more likely with ablative procedures; measures of success were not defined; and salvage surgical therapy may be difficult. Recent studies have shown that CA can achieve good oncologic outcomes similar to those of PN series for SRMs. Ablation has become more popular as a nephron-sparing or minimally invasive treatment for SRMs, particularly in centers with adequate resources and experience. Despite the concern about difficulty of salvage surgery after ablation, the most commonly used option after failed ablation therapy is repeat ablation.

With the introduction of liquid nitrogen– or argon-cooled probes, targeted renal CA became clinically feasible. Temperatures as low as $-195.8°$ C can be produced, resulting in direct cell injury with intracellular ice crystal formation or secondarily by reperfusion injury during the thawing phase. Histologically, coagulative necrosis is eventually replaced by fibrosis in the targeted tissue. Similarly, coagulative necrosis can also be accomplished by heating soft tissue to temperatures exceeding $60°$ C. RFA achieves temperatures in this range by delivering a monopolar electrical current via a needle electrode. The first attempts at percutaneous cryoablation (PCA) were reported in 1995, and Gill and associates reported their initial series of renal laparoscopic cryoablation (LCA) in 1998. Zlotta and colleagues reported the first percutaneous renal RFA in 1997, and laparoscopic RFA was first used clinically as a hemostatic measure preceding laparoscopic partial nephrectomy (LPN).

INDICATIONS AND CONTRAINDICATIONS

The indications for ablative procedures are similar to the indications for nephron-sparing surgery (NSS) for SRMs in general. Patients who have typically been candidates for RN are not generally considered candidates for ablative therapy. In the modern era, patients with a clinical T1a renal mass should be evaluated with high-quality cross-sectional imaging modalities such as computed tomography (CT) or magnetic resonance imaging (MRI). Renal biopsy, whether ultrasound guided or CT guided, should be discussed. Although pretreatment needle biopsy has been rarely used in the past, we now believe that the vast majority of T1a renal cortical neoplasms should undergo biopsy before management options are discussed with the patient. Indeed, patients with cT1a indolent renal cell carcinoma (RCC) subtypes such as papillary type 1

and chromophobe RCC are optimal candidates for ablative therapies because they can enjoy the benefits of the minimally invasive approach with little risk of disease-related mortality. Similarly, pretreatment renal tumor biopsy has allowed us to almost eliminate the need for any procedure in patients with benign renal cortical neoplasms. The natural history and the relative risk of benign versus malignant pathology should be an essential part of patient counseling. Active surveillance and its role, particularly in the management of SRMs, should be one of the options always discussed. Discussion of radical versus nephron-sparing treatment modalities (PN and ablation) should include a comprehensive discussion about oncologic outcomes, renal function outcomes, possible complications, and potential morbidities. Urologists should discuss the potential advantages of NSS and ablation in imperative and elective settings, including decreasing the risk of chronic kidney disease (CKD), dialysis, and associated cardiovascular (CVS) events.

Patients with a cT1a small (<4 cm) contrast-enhancing renal mass or a complex renal cyst suspicious for RCC and imperative indications for NSS (anatomically or functionally solitary kidney) are good candidates for ablative technologies. Relative indications occur in the presence of diseases that may impair the normal contralateral kidney, such as diabetes mellitus, hypertension, nephrolithiasis, and renal artery stenosis.

Patients with inherited diseases that have a propensity for multifocal and recurrent tumors, such as von Hippel-Lindau disease, are well suited for ablative procedures. In this patient population, recurrent tumors can be treated in a minimally invasive manner on multiple occasions. In our experience, repeated laparoscopic treatment of tumors with CA is feasible because the laparoscopic approach causes minimal scarring. Indeed, a percutaneous ablative approach is even more easily repeated, and, in our experience, offers very little additional challenge over a primary percutaneous ablation.

Patients with a shorter life expectancy, such as older patients with impaired performance status, are more likely to be treated with a less invasive treatment modality such as CA or to choose active surveillance because they may not be fit for surgery. Again, in these patients a preprocedure biopsy allows for more precise decision making because only the most aggressive RCC variants would require active treatment in older patients with multiple comorbidities.

Treatment of patients with centrally located renal tumors or with cystic lesions remains controversial. LPN is particularly challenging in patients with endophytic tumors. Accordingly, ablative technologies, which can be targeted by imaging modalities, are ideally suited for these tumors. In the University of California, Irvine experience, approximately one third of all tumors treated have been endophytic. With short follow-up, we have had excellent results. Management of cystic lesions has been similarly controversial.

Contraindications for laparoscopic ablative procedures include coagulopathy, history of peritonitis or multiple adhesions, and severe obstructive airway disease. Contraindications for percutaneous ablative procedures include the presence of

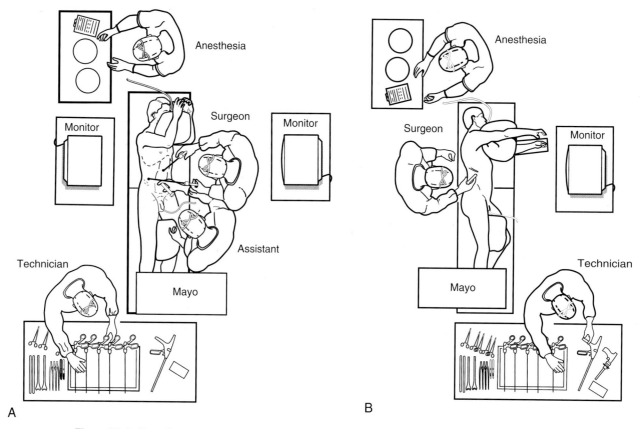

Figure 23-1. Operating room configuration for transperitoneal approach **(A)** and retroperitoneal approach **(B)**.

overlying structures such as bowel, liver, or spleen that interfere with probe placement. In general, tumors within 1 cm of bowel structures, the ureteropelvic junction, or the hilar vasculature are contraindicated. These tumors are more safely approached laparoscopically to allow for mobilization of these sensitive structures to protect them during tumor ablation.

PATIENT PREOPERATIVE EVALUATION AND PREPARATION

Informed consent is gained from the patient after a full discussion of the risks, benefits, and alternatives. Routine serum hematology, chemistries, liver function tests, coagulation studies, and a type and screen are performed. For all ablative renal procedures we require a high-quality and recent (within 3 months) CT scan or MRI with and without intravenous contrast. Exceptions are made for patients with chronic kidney disease who have a bona fide risk from contrast material (e.g., glomerular filtration rate [GFR] <30). For percutaneous procedures, we occasionally require imaging with the patient in the prone position to reveal exact intra-abdominal organ position when probe placement is attempted. Indeed, patients with upper pole tumors near the pleural reflections, and those with tumors close to bowel structures should be considered for prone axial imaging because the anatomic changes associated with the positional changes may result in inability to successfully execute the procedure. A standard metastatic evaluation including a chest radiograph is performed.

For laparoscopic procedures, the selection of transperitoneal or retroperitoneal approach is based on tumor location, the patient's surgical history, and preference. However, the majority of tumors that historically were treated with a retroperitoneal approach are not managed via the less invasive outpatient percutaneous approach.

High-quality and recent (within 3 months) axial imaging is a critically important part of preoperative preparation. For laparoscopic procedures, axial imaging studies can help expedite identification of the tumor. In addition, probe targeting is critically important and is greatly facilitated by high-quality imaging; probe deployment can be optimized by coordinating the gestalt picture of the laparoscopic view, the laparoscopic ultrasound image, and the preoperative imaging.

OPERATING ROOM CONFIGURATION AND PATIENT POSITIONING

For laparoscopic procedures, position the monitor on the opposite side of the patient from the surgeon. The insufflation pressure and CO_2 flow rate should be easily visible by the surgeon. The scrub nurse stands beside the surgeon. The equipment specific to the ablation procedure is best positioned at the feet of the patient, allowing these connections to pass perpendicular and over the top of the cords from the monitor. The same considerations apply for percutaneous procedures. With the patient prone, stand on the same side as the lesion and, ideally, have a straight-line view of the imaging monitor. The anesthesiologist occupies the room at the head of the patient, leaving room at the patient's feet for ablation equipment (Fig. 23-1).

For laparoscopic transperitoneal procedures, position the patient in a 70-degree flank position with the patient's ventral surface aligned with the edge of the operating table. For retroperitoneal procedures, use a 90-degree flank position, typically with the patient centered in the middle of the operative table. With the patient's iliac crest at the break in the table, flex the table. Flex the contralateral knee. Place an axillary roll, and carefully pad all pressure points. Position the arms to prevent brachial plexus tension (Fig. 23-2). After

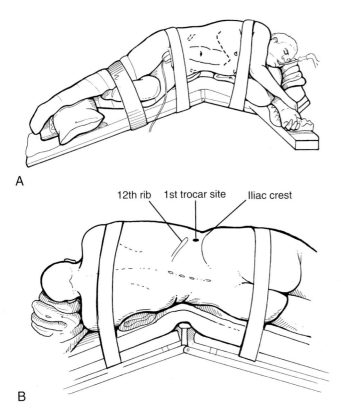

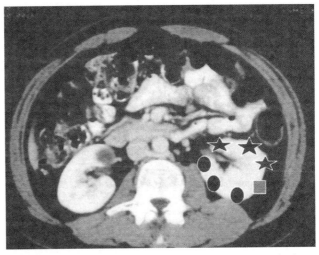

Figure 23-3. Anterior tumors *(stars)* are usually best approached by a transperitoneal approach. Tumors *(circles)* are usually best approached with a retroperitoneal approach. The tumor indicated by a square is in a location that can be treated with either approach.

Figure 23-2. A, Patient positioned for a transperitoneal approach. **B,** Patient positioned for a retroperitoneal approach.

the patient is adequately positioned, secure the patient to the table at the chest, hip, and knee in case rotation of the table is needed during the procedure. For percutaneous procedures, place the patient in the prone position.

TROCAR PLACEMENT

Laparoscopic ablative technology can be applied via a transperitoneal or retroperitoneal approach. Anterior renal tumors are best approached transperitoneally, whereas posterior tumors are accessed retroperitoneally. Preference dictates the approach for lateral tumors. However, imposing the wrong approach results in the need for additional renal mobilization and can result in suboptimal angles of ablation. Whenever possible, treat anterior tumors with a transperitoneal approach and treat posterior tumors with a retroperitoneal approach (Fig. 23-3).

A template for transperitoneal renal surgery trocar positions is presented in Figure 23-4. With no history of abdominal surgery, place a Veress needle, if needed, at the anterior superior iliac spine trocar site to establish a pneumoperitoneum of 15 mm Hg. If the AirSeal insufflation technology (SurgiQuest, Milford, Conn.) is used, after initial access at 15 mm Hg, most procedures are performed at 10 mm Hg. If there has been prior lower abdominal surgery, obtain initial access at the subcostal trocar site. Place the lower trocar approximately 1 inch medial and superior to the anterior superior iliac spine, and place the subcostal trocar in the midclavicular line. Use a visual dilating trocar with a 0-degree lens for optimal initial trocar placement. Subsequently, introduce the remaining trocars under laparoscopic vision via the initial trocar site. Place the third trocar between the two working trocars at the midline or just lateral to the rectus muscle. The third trocar can also be deployed at the umbilicus. This trocar serves as the primary access site for the laparoscope. Place an optional fourth 5-mm trocar at the

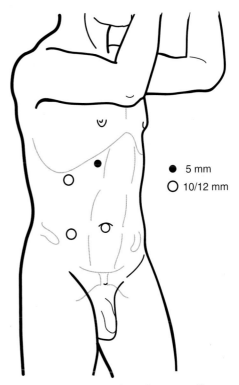

Figure 23-4. Transperitoneal trocar positions.

posterior axillary line, if needed, to optimize tumor position for probe entry or, for right-sided tumors, place the trocar just inferior to the xiphoid to introduce a locking grasper for liver retraction. Shift transperitoneal trocar positions laterally for obese patients or cephalad for upper pole tumors.

Figure 23-5 demonstrates a suggested trocar template for retroperitoneal surgery. Obtain initial access with the Hasson technique at the tip of the 12th rib. Then position a trocar-mounted balloon dissection device posterior to the kidney and inflate it. This device creates a working space to allow placement of the next trocar. Place the second trocar at the lateral border of the erector spinae muscle just below the 12th rib. Place the third trocar at the intersection of the

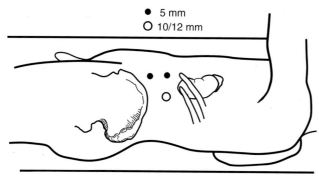

● 5 mm
○ 10/12 mm

Figure 23-5. Retroperitoneal trocar positions.

anterior axillary line and the downward sloping line made by the extension of the first two trocars.

PROCEDURE

Laparoscopic Tumor Exposure

If transperitoneal access has been gained, take a brief survey of the intraperitoneal organs. Inspect the bowel for injury, and look at the liver for evidence of mass lesions. Deflect the colon with gentle medial traction provided by an atraumatic laparoscopic grasper. Incise the thin layer of mesentery lateral to the edge of the colon but medial to the actual line of Toldt to expose the bloodless plane between the mesentery and Gerota fascia. On the right, expose the duodenum and cauterize. These steps provide visualization of the anterior surface of the Gerota fascia overlying the kidney and anterior hilum. For the retroperitoneal approach, the psoas muscle and the pulsations of the renal artery are usually immediately visible and serve as important anatomic landmarks.

Regardless of approach, enter the Gerota fascia 1 to 2 cm away from the tumor. The application of laparoscopic ultrasound with a flexible probe is of extraordinary value in expediting the identification of tumor location and selecting the location for entry through the Gerota fascia. Excise the fat overlying the tumor, and send it for histopathologic examination. If the fat is densely adherent to the area over the tumor, we assume possible fat invasion (T3a disease), and the fat is left over the tumor and ablated with the tumor. Extensively mobilize the kidney within the Gerota fascia. Renal mobilization allows for passage of a flexible laparoscopic ultrasound probe on the surface of the kidney opposite the tumor to optimize imaging and targeting of the tumor. Note the tumor size, margins, vascularity, and proximity to collecting system or hilar structures. Next, if preprocedure biopsy has not been performed, percutaneously pass a biopsy device with a 15-gauge Tru-Cut needle (ASAP Biopsy System, Microvasive; Boston Scientific, Watertown, Mass.) into the tumor and obtain a tissue sample for histopathology.

Laparoscopic Cryoablation

We select the skin site for probe deployment by passing a small-gauge spinal needle. This "finder" needle is minimally traumatic and allows the surgeon to test several sites to achieve optimal skin site selection. Ideally, the CA probes are placed such that the needles are passed perpendicular to the surface of the kidney. Once a skin site has been selected, we percutaneously introduce the probes and visually guide them into the tumor. Because the temperature extremes are realized only at the distal aspect of the probes for CA and RFA, skin complications are rare with the laparoscopic approach. Targeting tumors is the most

challenging component of the procedure and will differentiate success from failure. Intraoperative real-time laparoscopic ultrasound is essential for tumor targeting and, during CA, for monitoring of iceball progression. Depending on tumor size, the number of cryoprobes can vary from one to four. We prefer 1.47-mm IceRod Plus ablation probes (Galil Medical, Plymouth Meeting, Pa.) for the majority of cases. These probes have been characterized to have an ablative diameter of 1.9 cm in an animal model. Typically, a cluster of cryoprobes are positioned 1.5 cm apart in a triangular or quadratic configuration to ensure cryolesion overlap. Alternatively, for a larger ablation zone, we occasionally use 3-mm IceEdge probes (Galil Medical), which result in a larger zone of ablation.

Mobilize the kidney so that the probes enter the renal parenchyma in a perpendicular manner whenever possible. Gently guide the probes with a laparoscopic instrument and insert into the tumor such that they are parallel to one another, thus ensuring proper spacing. Position the flexible laparoscopic ultrasound probe to allow imaging of the deepest margin of the tumor. Introduce the IceRods into the tumor under ultrasound guidance, and advance them just beyond the deepest margin. Next, perform a double freeze cycle, each followed by an active thaw. Continue the first freeze until the iceball extends to a perimeter 1 cm beyond the tumor in every direction. Take care to prevent contact of the iceball with critical structures such as the renal vasculature, ureter, renal pelvis, and bowel structures. Mobilize and retract these structures, as needed, to prevent injury. Freezing intrarenal components of the collecting system does not result in damage or complications. However, freezing the ureteropelvic junction or ureter will result in stricture formation. After an appropriate margin has been achieved, perform an active thaw and deploy a second freeze cycle.

After the second freeze cycle, activate an active thaw and remove the IceRods only when they can be twisted gently without resistance. Exercise care not to apply premature force on the IceRods to avert potential fracture of the iceball from the kidney, which may be associated with significant hemorrhage. After removal of the IceRods, hemostasis is typically good and bleeding has not been a problem with these small-caliber probes. Usually, no hemostatic measures are required, and we no longer use surgical hemostatics (e.g., fibrin glues or FloSeal [Baxter Healthcare, Deerfield, Ill.]). If bleeding does occur, apply gentle pressure for hemostasis.

Laparoscopic Radiofrequency Ablation

Achieve access as described for LCA. Percutaneously introduce the probe and enter the tumor perpendicular to the surface of the kidney. On the basis of tumor size as measured by preoperative CT or MRI and intraoperative ultrasound imaging, deploy the tines to a diameter that ensures ablation of the tumor and a 1-cm margin of normal renal tissue. Multiple impedance-based or temperature-based probes are commercially available. Deploy the probes as per protocols, which are delineated in the manufacturer's recommendations. The size of the ablated area is dependent on the diameter of the deployed tines and the activation time. Typically, activation times range from 3 to 8 minutes, and two cycles are performed with a brief interval between cycles to allow cooling. After the tumor ablation is complete, ablate the probe tract while removing the probe from the kidney. This technique minimizes the risk of bleeding and tumor seeding.

Percutaneous Ablation

Renal PCA is a procedure best performed in a collaborative manner between urologists and interventional radiologists.

TABLE 23-1 Complications of Renal Laparoscopic Cryoablation (LCA) Compared with Laparoscopic Partial Nephrectomy (LPN) and Robotic-Assisted Partial Nephrectomy (RPN)

	Percent LPN or RPN	Percent LCA	Percent Absolute Risk Reduction	Relative Risk	P Value
UROLOGIC					
Bleeding	8.4	4.9	3.5	1.59	.072
Urinary leak	3.0	0.4	2.6	2.51	.046
Injury of adjacent organs	1.1	0.6	0.5	1.10	.855
Pulmonary	3.0	1.9	1.1	1.26	.533
Gastrointestinal	0.9	0.6	0.3	1.11	.831
Conversion	3.0	0.3	2.7	3.74	.002
Other	1.9	1.1	0.8	1.22	.659
NONUROLOGIC					
Cardiac	1.7	0.2	1.5	2.06	.154
Thromboembolic	2.4	0.0	2.4	2.82	.045
Other	2.2	1.1	1.1	1.55	.257

It can be done with the patient under general anesthesia. However, more recently our team has performed the majority of procedures with patients under local anesthesia with conscious sedation (LACS). Position the patient prone in an interventional CT or MRI unit. MRI permits acquisition of sagittal or coronal T1 images to assist in spatial orientation. In our practice, we perform the majority of cases as CT-guided procedures. We recently published our experience at University of California, Irvine comparing 82 patients who underwent PCA under general anesthesia versus 153 patients who had LACS. We could not find a significant difference in immediate treatment failure, recurrences, or treatment-related complications. However, LACS was associated with decreased procedure time and hospital stay. In general, general anesthesia can have potential disadvantages including increased monitoring requirements and recovery time, need to change patient position to prone position, and higher cost.

In an effort to minimize ionizing radiation exposure, we typically do initial skin site determination and access sheath (angiocatheter) placement under ultrasound guidance. Certainly, the amount of targeting that can be performed with ultrasound is a function of physician experience. After the ultrasound-guided initial sheath placement, a 20-gauge needle core biopsy device is deployed just within the renal mass and its position confirmed with CT scanning. In our current practice, needle biopsy is typically performed before the procedure and the procedure is initiated by ultrasound-guided deployment of the IceRod Plus CA probe after the biopsy. Cryoprobes are advanced into the lesion as described for laparoscopic procedures. The number of probes depends on the tumor burden. Obtain repeat scans before ablation to check probe position for adequacy. Routinely, CA protocol consists of two freeze-thaw cycles. Perform ablation as described earlier. After ablation, we allow approximately 20 minutes for iceball thawing and then perform a final CT with half-dose intravenous contrast to assess for enhancement and to evaluate for adequacy of ablation and any hemorrhage. In our experience, a half-dose contrast bolus provides excellent image quality to confirm that the tumor and a margin of normal tissue have been ablated. Alternatively, MRI demonstrates cryolesions as a signal void on T1-weighted images. Pass absorbable hemostatic material through an introducer after removing the probe to assist hemostasis.

POSTOPERATIVE MANAGEMENT

Patients are quickly advanced to a regular diet as tolerated. A hematocrit is checked in the recovery room and the morning after surgery. Percutaneous CA typically permits outpatient care in the majority of cases; otherwise, patients are discharged within 23 hours. As per our protocols, patients have follow-up evaluation 3 months after the procedure with contrast CT or MRI. Then, CT or MRI is performed annually if the tumor has been properly ablated. Complete loss of contrast enhancement on follow-up CT or MRI is considered a sign of complete tissue destruction. Indeed, we have found that 3-month imaging follow-up evaluation is the most accurate in determining the success of ablation. Although each urologist must develop a postoperative follow-up plan, initial postoperative imaging at 3 months is suggested at this time. If there is any suspicion of incomplete ablation, then additional imaging points are added.

COMPLICATIONS AND PERIOPERATIVE OUTCOMES

A recent meta-analysis comparing LCA versus LPN or robotic-assisted partial nephrectomy (RPN) found that patients who underwent LCA were significantly older (weighted mean difference [WMD] 6.1 years), had a higher American Society of Anesthesiologists (ASA) score (odds ratio [OR], 2.65), had smaller tumors (WMD 0.25 cm), and had less frequently proven malignant disease. LCA was associated with shorter operative time (WMD 36 minutes), lower estimated blood loss (EBL; WMD 130 mL), and shorter length of hospital stay (LOS; WMD 1.2 days). Table 23-1 summarizes the complications of LCA compared with LPN or RPN. When compared with LPN or RPN, less technically challenging ablative procedures offer lower complication rates.

In another multi-institutional review of CA and RFA procedures, a comparable overall complication rate of 11.1% was reported (14.4% after CA and 7.6% after RFA). The same authors reported similar complication rates between procedures performed laparoscopically (8.9%) and percutaneously (12.2%). The most common complication reported was pain or paresthesias related to the probe site, which was usually self-limited. RENAL nephrometry score was found to accurately predict outcomes and complications after LCA. However, this was not the case with RFA. We recently evaluated our contemporary multicenter experience from nine U.S. and European academic centers for 176 patients who were treated for SRMs (mean tumor size, 2.6 cm) with LCA or PCA from 2004 to 2007. We did not find a significant difference in perioperative or late complications between LCA (16.9% and 4.35%, respectively) and PCA (13% and 0.8%). However, PCA was associated with significantly shorter procedure times (122 versus 187.5 minutes) and a significant shorter LOS (29 versus 66 hours) compared with LCA (unpublished data, 2016).

TABLE 23-2 Oncological Outcomes of Contemporary Long-Term Renal Cryoablation Studies

Oncologic Outcomes	Percent	Study	Number of Patients	Mean Tumor Size (cm)	Median Follow-Up (mo)	Study Period	Reference
Local recurrence–free survival, 3 and 10 years	98	Mayo Clinic	187	2.8	16	2001-2011	Thompson et al (2015)
	95	Multicenter European	174	2	48	1997-2012	Larcher et al (2015)
Distant metastasis–free survival, 3 and 10 years	100	Mayo Clinic	187	2.8	16	2001-2011	Thompson et al (2015)
	100	Multicenter European	174	2	48	1997-2012	Larcher et al (2015)
Disease-free survival, 5 years	89	Multicenter U.S. and European	176	2.6	69.4	2004-2007	(Unpublished)
	83	Washington University	267	2.5	40	2000-2011	Tanagho et al (2013)
Cancer-specific survival, 5 years	97	Multicenter U.S. and European	176	2.6	69.4	2004-2007	(Unpublished)
	96.4	Washington University	267	2.5	40	2000-2011	Tanagho et al (2013)
Overall survival, 5 years	84	Multicenter U.S. and European	176	2.6	69.4	2004-2007	(Unpublished)
	88	Mayo Clinic	187	2.8	16	2000-2011	Thompson et al (2015)

Larcher A, Fossati N, Mistretta F, et al. Long-term oncologic outcomes of laparoscopic renal cryoablation as primary treatment for small renal masses. *Urol Oncol.* 2015;33:22.e1-22.e9.
Tanagho YS, Bhayani SB, Kim EH, Figenshau RS. Renal cryoablation versus robot-assisted partial nephrectomy: Washington University long-term experience. *J Endourol.* 2013;27:1477-1486.
Thompson RH, Atwell T, Schmit G, et al. Comparison of partial nephrectomy and percutaneous ablation for cT1 renal masses. *Eur Urol.* 2015;67: 252-259.

These findings were consistent with another recently published large single-center experience from Washington University including 145 patients who underwent LCA and 108 patients who underwent PCA in 2000 to 2011.

ONCOLOGICAL OUTCOMES OF LAPAROSCOPIC CRYOABLATION AND PERCUTANEOUS CRYOABLATION: 10- TO 15-YEAR EXPERIENCE

Recent studies have shown that CA can achieve good oncologic outcomes similar to those of PN series for SRMs.

Researchers from the Mayo Clinic published their experience treating more than 1400 patients with CPT1, N0, M0 renal masses with PN (n = 1057), percutaneous RFA (n = 180), and PCA (n = 187) in 2001 to 2011, with median tumor sizes of 2.4 cm, 1.9 cm, and 2.8 cm, respectively. Local recurrence-free survival rates at 3 years for PN, RFA, and PCA were 98%, 98%, and 98%, respectively. This demonstrated that there was no difference in local control. Metastasis-free survival rates at 3 years for PN, RFA, and PCA were 99%, 93%, and 100%, respectively. Overall survival (OS) rates at 3 years for PN, RFA, and PCA were 95%, 82%, and 88%, respectively. The higher OS for PN may reflect selection bias because ablative treatment might be more frequently selected for patients with comorbidities.

Cleveland Clinic evaluated its 15-year experience with LCA (n = 275) versus PCA (n = 137) for SRMs from 1997 to 2012. There were no significant differences in median tumor size (2.5 and 2.2 cm), rates of overall (7.27% and 7.29%) and major complications (0.7% and 3.6%), estimated probability of 5-year OS (89% and 82%), or 5-year disease-free survival (DFS) (79% and 80%) for LCA versus PCA, respectively.

Another large European study retrospectively evaluated 174 consecutive patients who were treated with LCA for SRMs from 2000 to 2013. Median tumor size was 2 cm. Median follow-up was 48 months. Treatment failure–free rate was 98%, 10-year local recurrence–free survival rate was 95%, 10-year metastasis-free rate was 100%, 10-year cancer-specific survival (CSS) was 100%, and OS was 61%.

Another long-term single-center study was published recently comparing 267 patients who underwent LCA and PCA from 2000 to 2011 with 233 patients who underwent RPN from 2007 to 2012 at Washington University. The study showed no difference in complications between CA and RPN, but there was a significant advantage for CA in preserving renal function. The 5-year DFS, CSS, and OS were 83.1%, 96.4%, and 77.1%, respectively, in the CA group versus 100%, 100%, and 91.7% in the RPN group.

We recently evaluated our contemporary multicenter experience from nine U.S. and European academic centers for 176 patients who were treated for SRMs (mean tumor size, 2.6 cm) with LCA or PCA from 2004 to 2007 and had a minimum follow-up of 5 years. The 5-year DFS, CSS, and OS were 89%, 97%, and 83.7%, respectively. Among 176 patients included in the study, 8 (4.5%) died, 20 (11.4%) had local recurrence, and 1 (0.6%) had distant metastasis (Landman group, unpublished data, 2016).

Table 23-2 summarizes oncologic outcomes of contemporary large or long-term single-center and multicenter renal CA studies.

TIPS AND TRICKS

- Tumor location within the kidney and relative to surrounding structures on preoperative imaging indicates whether a laparoscopic or percutaneous approach is prudent.
- Prone or lateral preoperative imaging for percutaneous procedures determines whether intervening structures impede the tract of the ablation probe.
- High-quality recent (within 3 months) axial imaging (CT or MRI) helps facilitate tumor localization and targeting of ablation probes.
- Intraoperative real-time laparoscopic ultrasound is essential for tumor targeting and, during CA, for monitoring of iceball progression.
- Extensive mobilization of the kidney during laparoscopic procedures allows the flexible ultrasound probe to achieve multiple angles of vision of the tumor and ablation probes.
- Both CA and RFA are viable options for the treatment of small renal tumors, less challenging than LPN, and associated with lower complication rates.

SUGGESTED READINGS

Baust JG, Gage AA. The molecular basis of cryosurgery. *BJU Int.* 2005;95:1187–1191.

Camacho JC, Kokabi N, Xing M, Master VA, Pattaras JG, Mittal PK, et al. R.E.N.A.L. (radius, exophytic/endophytic, nearness to collecting system or sinus, anterior/posterior, and location relative to polar lines) nephrometry score predicts early tumor recurrence and complications after percutaneous ablative therapies for renal cell carcinoma: a 5-year experience. *J Vasc Interv Radiol.* 2015;26:686–693.

Campbell SC, Novick AC, Belldegrun A, Blute ML, Chow GK, Derweesh IH, et al. Guideline for management of the clinical T1 renal mass. *J Urol.* 2009;182:1271–1279.

Gettman MT, Bishoff JT, Su LM, Chan D, Kavoussi LR, Jarrett TW, et al. Hemostatic laparoscopic partial nephrectomy: initial experience with the radiofrequency coagulation-assisted technique. *Urology.* 2001;58:8–11.

Gill IS, Novick AC, Soble JJ, Sung GT, Remer EM, Hale J, et al. Laparoscopic renal cryoablation: initial clinical series. *Urology.* 1998;52:543–551.

Hollingsworth JM, Miller DC, Daignault S, Hollenbeck BK. Rising incidence of small renal masses: a need to reassess treatment effect. *J Natl Cancer Inst.* 2006;98:1331–1334.

Huang WC, Levey AS, Serio AM, Snyder M, Vickers AJ, Raj GV, et al. Chronic kidney disease after nephrectomy in patients with renal cortical tumours: a retrospective cohort study. *Lancet Oncol.* 2006;7:735–740.

Johnson DB, Solomon SB, Su LM, Matsumoto ED, Kavoussi LR, Nakada SY, et al. Defining the complications of cryoablation and radio frequency ablation of small renal tumors: a multi-institutional review. *J Urol.* 2004;172:874–877.

Kapoor A, Wang Y, Dishan B, Pautler SE. Update on cryoablation for treatment of small renal mass: oncologic control, renal function preservation, and rate of complications. *Curr Urology Rep.* 2014;15:396.

Karam JA, Wood CG, Compton ZR, Rao P, Vikram R, Ahrar K, et al. Salvage surgery after energy ablation for renal masses. *BJU Int.* 2015;115:74–80.

Kim EH, Tanagho YS, Saad NE, Bhayani SB, Figenshau RS. Comparison of laparoscopic and percutaneous cryoablation for treatment of renal masses. *Urology.* 2014;83:1081–1087.

Larcher A, Fossati N, Mistretta F, Lughezzani G, Lista G, Dell'Oglio P, et al. Long-term oncologic outcomes of laparoscopic renal cryoablation as primary treatment for small renal masses. *Urol Oncol.* 2015;33:22.e1–22.e9.

Lutzeyer W, Lymberopoulos S, Breining H, Langer S. [Experimental cryosurgery of the kidney]. *Langenbecks Arch Chir.* 1968;322:843–847.

Nguyen CT, Lane BR, Kaouk JH, Hegarty N, Gill IS, Novick AC, et al. Surgical salvage of renal cell carcinoma recurrence after thermal ablative therapy. *J Urol.* 2008;180:104–109. discussion 9.

Ogan K, Jacomides L, Dolmatch BL, Rivera FJ, Dellaria MF, Josephs SC, et al. Percutaneous radiofrequency ablation of renal tumors: technique, limitations, and morbidity. *Urology.* 2002;60:954–958.

Okhunov Z, Juncal S, Ordon M, George AK, Lusch A, del Junco M, et al. Comparison of outcomes in patients undergoing percutaneous renal cryoablation with sedation vs general anesthesia. *Urology.* 2015;85:130–134.

Okhunov Z, Shapiro EY, Moreira DM, Lipsky MJ, Hillelsohn J, Badani K, et al. R.E.N.A.L. nephrometry score accurately predicts complications following laparoscopic renal cryoablation. *J Urol.* 2012;188:1796–1800.

Pattaras JG, Moore RG, Landman J, Clayman RV, Janetschek G, McDougall EM, et al. Incidence of postoperative adhesion formation after transperitoneal genitourinary laparoscopic surgery. *Urology.* 2002;59:37–41.

Schmit GD, Thompson RH, Kurup AN, Weisbrod AJ, Boorjian SA, Carter RE, et al. Usefulness of R.E.N.A.L. nephrometry scoring system for predicting outcomes and complications of percutaneous ablation of 751 renal tumors. *J Urol.* 2013;189:30–35.

Seideman CA, Gahan J, Weaver M, Olweny EO, Richter M, Chan D, et al. Renal tumour nephrometry score does not correlate with the risk of radiofrequency ablation complications. *BJU Int.* 2013;112:1121–1124.

Shingleton WB, Sewell Jr PE. Percutaneous renal tumor cryoablation with magnetic resonance imaging guidance. *J Urol.* 2001;165:773–776.

Sivarajan G, Huang WC. Current practice patterns in the surgical management of renal cancer in the United States. *Urol Clin North Am.* 2012;39:149–160, v.

Tanagho YS, Bhayani SB, Kim EH, Figenshau RS. Renal cryoablation versus robot-assisted partial nephrectomy: Washington University long-term experience. *J Endourol.* 2013;27:1477–1486.

Thompson RH, Atwell T, Schmit G, Lohse CM, Kurup AN, Weisbrod A, et al. Comparison of partial nephrectomy and percutaneous ablation for cT1 renal masses. *Eur Urol.* 2015;67:252–259.

Thompson RH, Boorjian SA, Lohse CM, Leibovich BC, Kwon ED, Cheville JC, et al. Radical nephrectomy for pT1a renal masses may be associated with decreased overall survival compared with partial nephrectomy. *J Urol.* 2008;179:468–471.

Uchida M, Imaide Y, Sugimoto K, Uehara H, Watanabe H. Percutaneous cryosurgery for renal tumours. *Br J Urol.* 1995;75:132–136. discussion 6–7.

Zargar H, Samarasekera D, Khalifeh A, Remer EM, O'Malley C, Akca O, et al. Laparoscopic vs percutaneous cryoablation for the small renal mass: 15-year experience at a single center. *Urology.* 2015;85:850–855.

Zlotta AR, Wildschutz T, Raviv G, Peny MO, van Gansbeke D, Noel JC, et al. Radiofrequency interstitial tumor ablation (RITA) is a possible new modality for treatment of renal cancer: ex vivo and in vivo experience. *J Endourol.* 1997;11:251–258.

24 Minimally Invasive Renal Recipient Surgery

Akshay Sood, Wooju Jeong, Mahendra Bhandari, Rajesh Ahlawat, Mani Menon

Minimally invasive surgery (MIS) reduces perioperative morbidity and complications. Indeed, the role of MIS in renal donors has been well established, such that today MIS represents the standard of care for living donor nephrectomies. However, its usefulness for recipient surgery has not been thoroughly evaluated.

Being chronically ill and immunocompromised, kidney transplant (KT) recipients are at greater risk for developing perioperative complications than an average surgical patient. These complications adversely affect both short-term patient recovery and long-term graft and patient survival. Thus, transplant recipients may benefit substantially from MIS. Minimally invasive approaches to KT have been recently described; in 2010 and 2011, Modi and colleagues[1] and Rosales and colleagues[2] described their techniques for laparoscopic kidney transplant (LKT), and Giulianotti and colleagues[3] and Boggi and colleagues[4] described their techniques for robotic-assisted kidney transplant (RKT). These groups noted a slightly slower return of graft function in the postoperative recovery period (compared with open KT); these studies were performed without renal cooling. We hypothesized that warm ischemia might have played a role in the delay noted in the graft function recovery and aimed to develop a technique of RKT that eliminated warm ischemia during recipient intervention. Accordingly, here we describe our novel technique of RKT with regional hypothermia.

INDICATIONS AND CONTRAINDICATIONS

Our indications have expanded over time; currently we consider all patients who are eligible for KT as candidates for RKT with regional hypothermia (assuming that the patient desires MIS), except for patients with multiple previous abdominal surgeries and simultaneous multiorgan transplant. However, during our initial studies we carefully selected patients according to the IDEAL model (idea, development, exploration, assessment, and long-term study) of safe surgical innovation (Balliol Collaboration), to ensure optimal patient outcomes. We recommend that surgeons and institutions seeking to start a minimally invasive KT program should also start by selecting ideal candidates for the initial cases. (In addition, preclinical studies may be performed and surgeons may receive technical mentoring to optimize patient safety.) Our patient selection criteria for the initial studies were as follows.[5]

Inclusion Criteria

- Irreversible chronic renal disease, defined as end-stage renal disease (ESRD) or anticipated ESRD within the next 1 year (preemptive transplant)
- Matched living donor

Exclusion Criteria

- Previous major abdominal surgery with high suspicion for intra-abdominal adhesions
- Significant atherosclerosis of the iliac vessels (>30% blockage)
- Immunologically high risk

- Second transplant
- Simultaneous dual or multiorgan transplant

PATIENT PREOPERATIVE EVALUATION AND PREPARATION

Preoperative Evaluation of Recipient

Preoperative assessment of RKT patients was similar to that of patients undergoing open KT and included gathering information regarding the cause and duration of ESRD and comorbidity status and evaluating ongoing renal replacement therapy. Immunologic compatibility, cardiorespiratory, and serologic evaluations were performed for all patients according to standard transplant protocols.[6]

Immunosuppression Protocol

At our institution (Medanta Hospital), triple immunosuppression therapy is the standard of care for open KT patients. The same protocol was used for patients undergoing RKT. Tacrolimus (0.1 mg/kg) and mycophenolate mofetil (MMF)/sodium (1 g/720 mg twice daily) were started on the day before transplantation and prednisone (40 mg/day) was started on the day of surgery. An induction agent, usually basiliximab or thymoglobulin, was administered after having discussions with the patient regarding human leukocyte antigen (HLA) match status and affordability.[6]

OPERATING ROOM CONFIGURATION AND PATIENT POSITIONING

Operating Room Setup

The ideal operating room setup is shown in Figure 24-1. The setup depicted in the illustration is helpful in promoting good communication among the console surgeon, the bedside assistant, and the anesthesia team.

Patient Position

Patient positioning followed the standard template used for the Vattikuti Institute prostatectomy technique of robotic-assisted radical prostatectomy. Briefly, the patient is placed in lithotomy position with a 15- to 20-degree Trendelenburg tilt (Figs. 24-2 and 24-3). The robot is docked between the legs of the patient. This patient position and robot docking can be used independently of the proposed location for the graft (left versus right iliac fossa). However, the right iliac fossa is the preferred location for renal grafting in general, irrespective of the surgical approach, because the iliac vessels are more superficial and accessible in that location.

INSTRUMENTS

Robotic Instruments and Ports

The following are robotic instruments that are used, including three robotic 8-mm ports: robotic Maryland bipolar

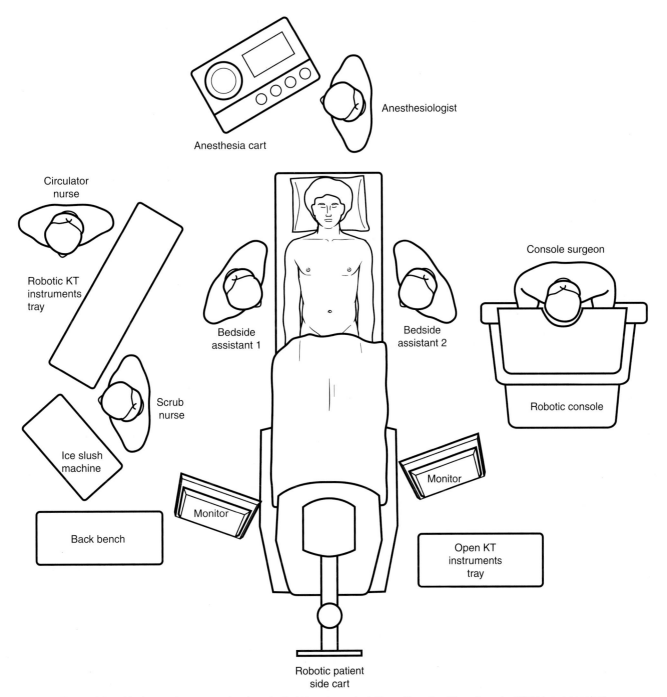

Figure 24-1. Ideal operating room setup for robotic kidney transplantation with regional hypothermia. *KT*, kidney transplant.

grasper; robotic monopolar curved scissors (with cover-tip accessory); robotic Black Diamond Micro Forceps (Intuitive Surgical, Sunnyvale, Calif.); robotic large needle driver; robotic Hem-o-lok applier (Teleflex Medical, Morrisville, N.C.); and robotic ProGrasp Forceps (Intuitive Surgical) (on the fourth arm).

Laparoscopic Instruments

Laparoscopic instruments include MicroFrance laparoscopic grasper (Medtronic, Dublin, Ireland); suture passer; Hem-o-lok applier (5 mm, 10 mm, 12 mm with Weck clips—5 mm, 10 mm, 12 mm) and Reliance Bulldog Clamps with appliers (Scanlan International, Saint Paul, Minn.).

Disposables

Disposables include one GelPoint platform (Applied Medical, Rancho Santa Margarita, Calif.); one 12-mm camera port and one 12-mm assistant port; one 5-French ureteric catheter for flushing; and sutures (5-0 CV-6 ePTFE [Gore-Tex; W. L. Gore & Associates, Flagstaff, Az.] and 4-0 PDS/3-0 V-Loc CV23 6″ [Covidien, New Haven, Conn.]).

Other Equipment

Additional equipment includes an ice-slush machine (Ecolab, St. Paul, Minn.); a slush machine drape (Ecolab); Toomey syringes (modified, nozzle sawed off); and a 3.6-mm aortic punch (Teleflex Medical, Morrisville, N.C.).

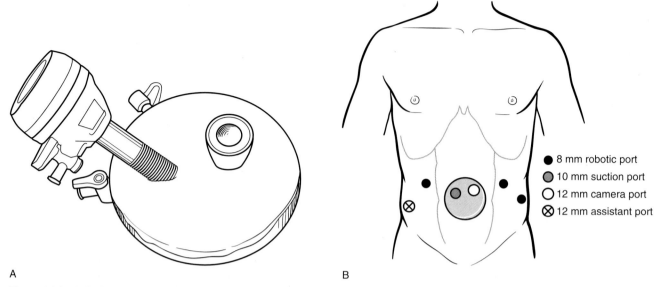

Figure 24-2. A, GelSeal cap with a 12-mm camera-port and a 10-mm assistant port, for the 5-mm suction. **B,** Diagrammatic illustration of port placement for robotic kidney transplantation with regional hypothermia. *(Redrawn from Menon M, Sood A, Bhandari M, et al. Robotic kidney transplantation with regional hypothermia: a step-by-step description of the Vattikuti Urology Institute–Medanta technique [IDEAL phase 2a]. Eur Urol. 2014;65:991-1000.)*

● 8 mm robotic port
● 10 mm suction port
○ 12 mm camera port
⊗ 12 mm assistant port

GelPoint

The GelPoint device is a hand-access platform that allows easy introduction of ice slush and the renal graft. The GelPoint device consists of two components: a GelSeal cap and an access port. A 12-mm camera port and a 5/10-mm suction port are placed into the GelSeal cap ahead of time (see Fig. 24-2, *A*).

TROCAR PLACEMENT

Figures 24-2 and 24-3 depict the GelPoint and trocar placement for RKT with regional hypothermia. With the patient in lithotomy position, a 4- to 5-cm vertical periumbilical incision is made. The access port is inserted through this incision and the prepared GelSeal cap is secured on top of the access port. After the pneumoperitoneum has been established (15-20 mm Hg), the patient is moved to Trendelenburg position. Other ports, including three 8-mm robotic ports and one 12-mm assistant port, are placed as shown, under direct vision (see Fig. 24-2, *B*). The 8-mm robotic ports for the left and right robotic arms are placed along the left and right midclavicular lines just above the level of the umbilicus, respectively. The third 8-mm port for the fourth robotic arm is placed on the patient's left side near the iliac fossa. The 12-mm assistant port is placed near the iliac fossa on the patient's right side as shown in Figure 24-2, *B*.

PROCEDURE (SEE VIDEO 24-1)

We have provided a high-definition video with this chapter to illustrate the surgery steps in a detailed step-by-step manner.

Preparation of Recipient Vascular Bed and Bladder

The procedure starts with identification of external iliac vessels. With the camera lens in a 30-degree upward position, the bladder is taken down with monopolar scissors in the dominant hand and the Maryland bipolar grasper in the nondominant hand. The camera lens is then switched to a 30-degree downward position, and the external iliac vessels are skeletonized (Fig. 24-4). Small vascular and lymphatic offshoots are identified and controlled. Next, a transverse incision is made 2 to 3 cm distal to the cecum, and peritoneal flaps are raised bilaterally over the psoas, to be used later for extraperitonealizing the graft kidney. Then the bladder is distended with 240 mL of normal saline (via Foley catheter) and detrusor flaps are created in preparation for a subsequent modified Lich-Gregoir ureteroneocystostomy (Fig. 24-5).

Preparation of Donor Graft

While the recipient vascular bed and bladder are being prepared, the graft kidney is harvested laparoscopically in an adjacent operating room by a donor team working in tandem with the recipient team. The coordination of donor and recipient surgery is important, especially in the initial RKT cases, in which the recipient operative times may be longer, to optimize overall ischemia times. The donor organ is prepared in a standard manner as for open KT; it is defatted and perfused with cold Ringer's lactate or normal saline. The graft is then wrapped in a gauze jacket filled with ice slush with an opening to allow access to the hilar structures (Fig. 24-6). The upper pole of the kidney may be marked with a long silk-tie tail to aid in graft orientation after graft insertion. The ice jacket serves two important functions: keeping the graft kidney cold and facilitating atraumatic intracorporeal handling during anastomoses.

Introduction of the Graft and Cooling

The pelvic bed is cooled to 18° to 20° C with the introduction of 180 to 240 mL of ice slush (Fig. 24-7) via modified Toomey syringes (Fig. 24-8). The ice slush should be delivered approximately 10 to 15 minutes before introduction of the graft kidney for effective cooling of the pelvic bed. Next, the camera arm and the GelSeal cap are removed and the graft in its ice jacket is introduced effortlessly though the access port (Fig. 24-9). It is important to orient the lower pole toward the feet of the patient and the hilum toward

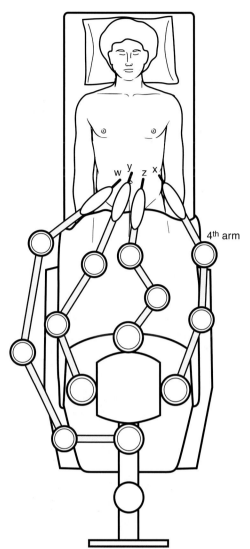

Figure 24-3. Robot docked between the legs of the patient in a manner typical for robotic radical prostatectomy. *(Redrawn from Menon M, Sood A, Bhandari M, et al. Robotic kidney transplantation with regional hypothermia: a step-by-step description of the Vattikuti Urology Institute–Medanta technique [IDEAL phase 2a]. Eur Urol. 2014;65:991-1000.)*

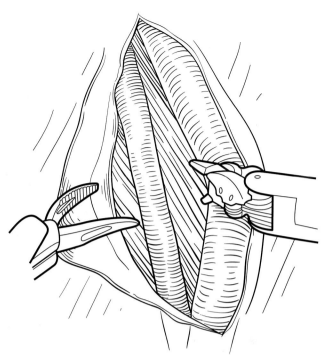

Figure 24-4. Skeletonization of iliac vessel bed. *(Redrawn from Menon M, Sood A, Bhandari M, et al. Robotic kidney transplantation with regional hypothermia: a step-by-step description of the Vattikuti Urology Institute–Medanta technique [IDEAL phase 2a]. Eur Urol. 2014;65:991-1000.)*

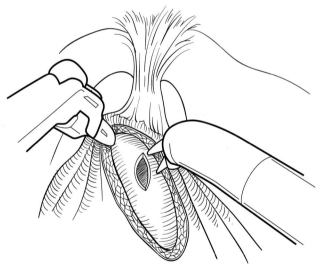

Figure 24-5. Bladder preparation; detrusor flaps are created for ureteroneocystostomy (modified Lich-Gregoir). *(Redrawn from Menon M, Sood A, Bhandari M, et al. Robotic kidney transplantation with regional hypothermia: a step-by-step description of the Vattikuti Urology Institute–Medanta technique [IDEAL phase 2a]. Eur Urol. 2014;65:991-1000.)*

the iliac vessels. More ice slush is added on top of the graft (Fig. 24-10) to achieve uniform and effective regional hypothermia. We have previously shown that by using local hypothermia we were able to overcome the delay in graft function recovery noted by other groups practicing minimally invasive KT.[5]

Venous Anastomosis

The external iliac vein (EIV) is clamped with robotic drop-in bulldog clamps (Fig. 24-11). A venotomy is made with cold monopolar scissors in the dominant hand. Then the scissors are swapped for a large needle driver while Black Diamond Micro Forceps are kept in the nondominant hand. The graft renal vein is anastomosed in a continuous end-to-side manner to the EIV (Fig. 24-12) with Gore-Tex CV-6 suture. The large needle holder is used to pass the stitch, and the Black Diamond Micro Forceps are used to atraumatically hold the vein open and pull the stitch through. Just before completion of the venous anastomosis, the lumen is flushed with heparinized saline via a 5-French ureteric catheter introduced through the 12-mm assistant port. The graft renal vein is occluded with a bulldog clamp, and the EIV is unclamped. Additional ice slush is introduced as and if required (if the venous anastomosis took 20 minutes or longer to complete).

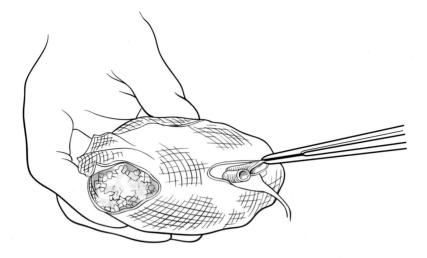

Figure 24-6. Graft kidney wrapped in a gauze jacket filled with ice slush. *(Redrawn from Menon M, Sood A, Bhandari M, et al. Robotic kidney transplantation with regional hypothermia: a step-by-step description of the Vattikuti Urology Institute–Medanta technique [IDEAL phase 2a]. Eur Urol. 2014;65:991-1000.)*

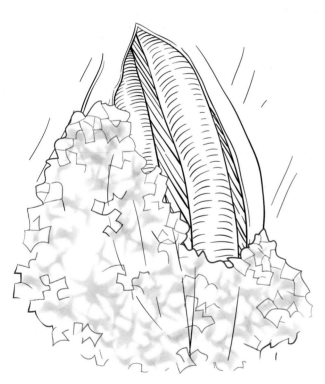

Figure 24-7. Pelvic bed lined with ice slush to achieve pelvic-bed cooling before introduction of the graft kidney. *(Redrawn from Menon M, Sood A, Bhandari M, et al. Robotic kidney transplantation with regional hypothermia: a step-by-step description of the Vattikuti Urology Institute–Medanta technique [IDEAL phase 2a]. Eur Urol. 2014;65:991-1000.)*

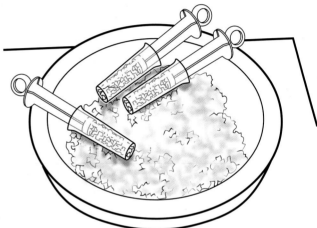

Figure 24-8. Multiple modified Toomey syringes (nozzles cut off) being readied for rapid delivery of ice slush. *(Redrawn from Menon M, Sood A, Bhandari M, et al. Robotic kidney transplantation with regional hypothermia: a step-by-step description of the Vattikuti Urology Institute–Medanta technique [IDEAL phase 2a]. Eur Urol. 2014;65:991-1000.)*

Arterial Anastomosis

Next, the external iliac artery (EIA) is clamped with robotic bulldog clamps. A linear arteriotomy is made with the monopolar scissors or the robotic scalpel (scissors work well; hence, this choice is optional). This is converted to a circular arteriotomy (Fig. 24-13) with a 3.6-mm aortic punch introduced through the GelPoint by the assistant surgeon. The renal artery is anastomosed in a continuous end-to-side fashion to the EIA with Gore-Tex CV-6 suture (Fig. 24-14). After flushing and testing of the anastomotic integrity, the graft renal artery is temporarily clamped and the EIA is unclamped. If the anastomosis appears secure, the renal artery and vein bulldog clamps are removed and the gauze jacket is removed. The graft kidney is visually inspected for color (pink), turgor (taut), and on-table diuresis (grossly visible urine formation). Then the graft kidney is retroperitonealized by approximating the peritoneal flaps prepared earlier (Fig. 24-15). This step ensures against graft torsion (versus leaving the graft intraperitoneal). After unclamping, the pneumoperitoneum pressure is dropped to 8 mm Hg and an intravenous bolus of 100 mg furosemide is given.

Ureteroneocystostomy

With the modified Lich-Gregoir technique, the ureter is apposed to the bladder mucosa in a continuous manner (4-0

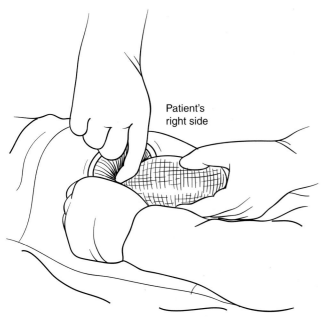

Figure 24-9. Graft kidney being introduced through the access port (GelSeal cap and the camera arm have been removed).

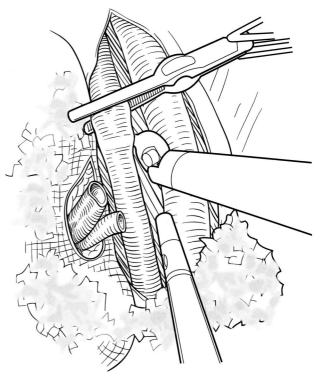

Figure 24-11. External iliac vein clamped with a robotic bulldog clamp. *(Redrawn from Menon M, Sood A, Bhandari M, et al. Robotic kidney transplantation with regional hypothermia: a step-by-step description of the Vattikuti Urology Institute–Medanta technique [IDEAL phase 2a]. Eur Urol. 2014;65:991-1000.)*

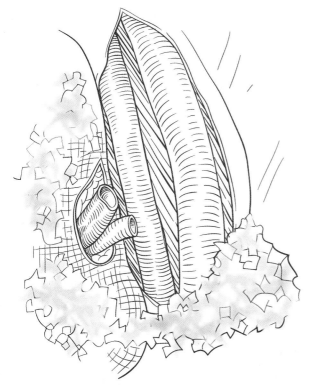

Figure 24-10. Additional ice slush delivered onto the graft kidney immediately after its introduction, to achieve uniform cooling. *(Redrawn from Menon M, Sood A, Bhandari M, et al. Robotic kidney transplantation with regional hypothermia: a step-by-step description of the Vattikuti Urology Institute–Medanta technique [IDEAL phase 2a]. Eur Urol. 2014;65:991-1000.)*

polydioxanone suture). A double-J stent, introduced through the 12-mm assistant port, is inserted into the ureter after completion of the posterior wall of the mucosal ureteroneocystostomy. The detrusor is closed atop in a continuous fashion with the V-Loc suture (Fig. 24-16), and this closure creates

an antirefluxing mechanism. It is important to note that we perform (and strongly recommend) retroperitonealization before ureteroneocystostomy because it gives time to observe the graft vessels for any potential kinking or compression that might have occurred during retroperitonealization. At the end of each case, after fascia-muscle and skin closure in the standard manner, we perform Doppler ultrasound to ensure optimal graft vascularity.

Extra: Accessory Vessels

In 6 of the 79 patients, the graft kidney had an accessory polar artery measuring 1.2 to 1.6 mm in diameter, perfusing more than 10% of the parenchyma. These were considered unsuitable for bench reconstruction. Therefore we decided to anastomose the accessory artery to the recipient inferior epigastric artery (IEA). The recipient IEA is prepared for anastomosis before introduction of the kidney in such cases. A bulldog clamp is used to occlude the stump, and the distal end is secured (Fig. 24-17). The accessory polar artery is anastomosed to the IEA with 7-0 or 6-0 Prolene sutures (Fig. 24-18). This step may be technically challenging for surgeons learning the technique, given the small caliber of the vessels. However, the surgeon may take his or her time because the ischemia clock is not ticking. We use interrupted sutures for this step.

Extra: Nonsurgical Considerations
Anesthesia

Anesthesia in patients undergoing RKT with regional hypothermia is induced, maintained, and monitored in a manner similar to that for open KT. Specifically, patients are

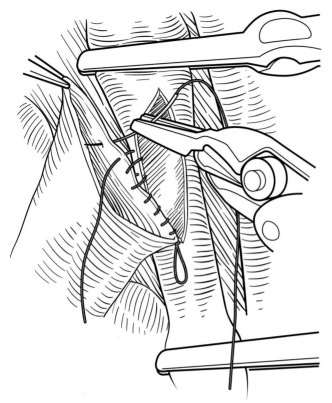

Figure 24-12. End-to-side continuous venous anastomosis. *(Redrawn from Menon M, Sood A, Bhandari M, et al. Robotic kidney transplantation with regional hypothermia: a step-by-step description of the Vattikuti Urology Institute–Medanta technique [IDEAL phase 2a]. Eur Urol. 2014;65:991-1000.)*

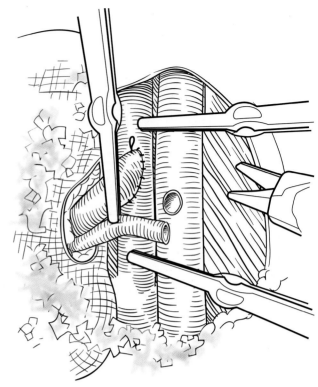

Figure 24-13. External iliac artery clamped with a robotic bulldog clamp and linear arteriotomy converted to circular arteriotomy with a 3.6-mm aortic punch. *(Redrawn from Menon M, Sood A, Bhandari M, et al. Robotic kidney transplantation with regional hypothermia: a step-by-step description of the Vattikuti Urology Institute–Medanta technique [IDEAL phase 2a]. Eur Urol. 2014;65:991-1000.)*

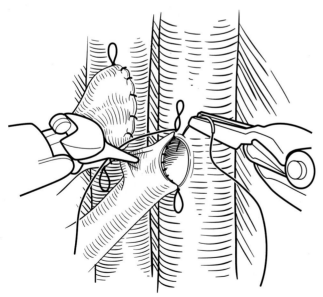

Figure 24-14. End-to-side continuous arterial anastomosis. *(Redrawn from Menon M, Sood A, Bhandari M, et al. Robotic kidney transplantation with regional hypothermia: a step-by-step description of the Vattikuti Urology Institute–Medanta technique [IDEAL phase 2a]. Eur Urol. 2014;65:991-1000.)*

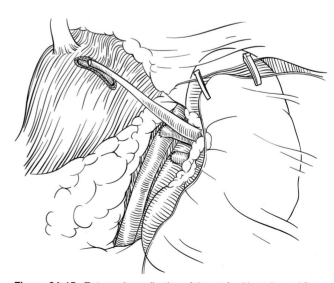

Figure 24-15. Retroperitonealization of the graft with peritoneal flaps prepared earlier during iliac vessel bed dissection.

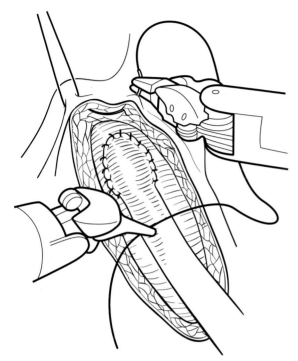

Figure 24-16. Ureteroneocystostomy (modified Lich-Gregoir). *(Redrawn from Menon M, Sood A, Bhandari M, et al. Robotic kidney transplantation with regional hypothermia: a step-by-step description of the Vattikuti Urology Institute–Medanta technique [IDEAL phase 2a]. Eur Urol. 2014;65:991-1000.)*

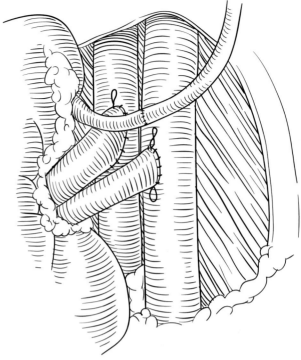

Figure 24-18. Lower-pole accessory artery anastomosis to the inferior epigastric artery with 6-0 Prolene sutures. *(Redrawn from Menon M, Sood A, Bhandari M, et al. Robotic kidney transplantation with regional hypothermia: a step-by-step description of the Vattikuti Urology Institute–Medanta technique [IDEAL phase 2a]. Eur Urol. 2014;65:991-1000.)*

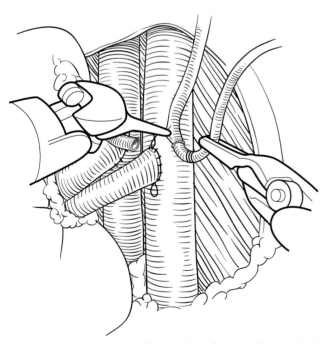

Figure 24-17. Inferior epigastric artery being flushed with heparinized saline using a 5-French ureteric catheter. *(Redrawn from Menon M, Sood A, Bhandari M, et al. Robotic kidney transplantation with regional hypothermia: a step-by-step description of the Vattikuti Urology Institute–Medanta technique [IDEAL phase 2a]. Eur Urol. 2014;65:991-1000.)*

premedicated with intravenous midazolam (1 mg on operating table) and induced with propofol (2 mg/kg), atracurium (0.5 mg/kg), and fentanyl (2 μg/kg). Anesthesia is maintained with a volatile anesthetic agent (e.g., sevoflurane) and an air-oxygen mixture. Intraoperative analgesia is maintained with fentanyl boluses. Patients are kept paralyzed with atracurium (0.25 mg/kg/hr) until the undocking of the robot. A methylprednisone bolus is administered via slow intravenous route just before graft reperfusion, and a bolus injection of furosemide (Lasix) 100 mg is given intravenously soon after.[6]

Intraoperative Fluid Management

Because patients undergoing RKT are in Trendelenburg position (versus supine in open KT), a fluid restriction policy is followed during the initial part of the operation, to avoid pooling of fluid in the dependent areas (head and neck region). RKT recipients receive 10 mL of 0.9% normal saline per kilogram per hour from the start of the procedure until graft reperfusion, whereas patients undergoing open KT are infused at a consistent rate of 30 mL/kg/hr throughout the intervention. Liberal hydration, however, is started in RKT patients after completion of anastomoses, and a total of 2.5 to 3 L of fluid is infused by the time the patient is extubated. The mean arterial pressure is maintained above baseline (approximately 20%), from graft reperfusion onward.[6]

POSTOPERATIVE MANAGEMENT

Postoperatively, patients are admitted to a dedicated transplant intensive care unit for the first 4 days and monitored for hemodynamic status including heart rate, blood pressure, central venous pressure (CVP), oxygen saturation, and urine output (same as for open KT patients). Serum laboratory tests are repeated twice daily for the first 2 days, and daily thereafter until discharge. A follow-up graft Doppler ultrasound is performed on postoperative day 1 and a note of flow velocities and resistive indices is made. Postoperative pain is comfortably managed by continuous infusion of fentanyl (0.5 μg/kg/hr) with morphine as rescue (patient-controlled analgesia [PCA]). The pain management is much less aggressive than for patients undergoing open KT, who often require central neuraxial pain therapy. Postoperative fluid management is identical to that for open KT. Patients are kept well hydrated and have a CVP line for the first 48 hours. Specifically, for the first 24 hours, we administer 90% to 100% normal saline or half–normal saline replacement per the previous hours' urine output, which is reduced to 70% to 80% replacement over the next 24 hours. Abdominal drains are removed on postoperative day 2 or 3, once the drain output turns serous and fluid creatinine is normal. The Foley catheter is removed on postoperative day 4. The ureteral stent is removed 3 weeks after transplantation.[6]

COMPLICATIONS AND INDICATIONS TO CONVERT TO OPEN SURGERY

Complications

The most common complications in RKT are the same as those in open KT and are either immunologic or infectious in nature. The chief surgical complications are bleeding and vessel kinking. However, twice-daily hemoglobin and Doppler ultrasound at time of skin closure and on postoperative day 1 provide reasonable confidence against the presence of these complications (as well as against graft vessel thrombosis or stenosis), if the test results are negative. In contrast to open KT, the risk of surgical site infections is significantly decreased in RKT patients[7]; nonetheless, routine port site inspection is good practice. On the other hand, certain complications are unique to RKT, including facial and eye edema and subcutaneous emphysema caused by use of the Trendelenburg position and GelPoint, respectively. The surgeon should be aware of these complications. In our experience, none of the 54 patients developed subcutaneous emphysema, whereas 3 of the 54 (5.6%) developed facial or neck edema. In all patients the edema was self-limiting and resolved by postoperative day 2 without any intervention; nonetheless, we now routinely counsel patients about this side effect, follow a fluid infusion restriction policy, and monitor patients for neurologic deficits if facial or neck edema develops.[6]

Indications to Convert to Open Surgery

Patient safety should be the foremost concern. Open conversion should not be considered a failure and must not be delayed if the situation demands it. Indications for an open conversion may include failure to progress, inability to maintain graft hypothermia, poor quality of vascular anastomoses, and concerns regarding safety and quality. However, it must be noted that in our experience, only 1 surgery of 79 required conversion to an open setting, secondary to a small inadvertent instrumental injury to the graft during retroperitonealization. In this case, we extended the midline incision to make sure that the graft was satisfactory.

TIPS AND TRICKS

- Be sure that the patient is positioned properly and well secured before the beginning of the procedure.
- The operating room should be set up in a way that allows effective communication among the console surgeon, the assistant surgeon, and the anesthesia team.
- The coordination of donor and recipient surgery is important, especially in the initial RKT cases, in which the recipient operative times may be longer, to optimize overall ischemia times.
- A gauze jacket filled with ice slush should be used because it allows cooling of the graft as well as atraumatic handling. A silk tie may be used to mark the upper pole of the graft to aid in intracorporeal orientation.
- An aortic punch should be used to convert linear arteriotomy to circular arteriotomy.
- The pneumoperitoneum should be dropped from 15 to 20 mm Hg to 8 mm Hg after completion of vascular anastomoses and revascularization, to minimize the effect of pneumatic compression on vessels and graft blood flow.
- The graft should be retroperitonealized to prevent delayed graft torsion.
- The graft should be retroperitonealized before ureteroneocystostomy because it provides a window of time to observe any kinking or compression of the graft vessels that might have occurred during retroperitonealization.
- Intraoperative fluid restriction protocols should be used for RKT patients, to decrease the risk of facial or eye edema secondary to Trendelenburg positioning.
- An on-table Doppler ultrasound should be performed immediately after skin closure, particularly in the initial cases, to ensure adequate graft vascularization.

REFERENCES

1. Modi P, Rizvi J, Pal B, Bharadwaj R, et al. Laparoscopic kidney transplantation: an initial experience. *Am J Transplant.* 2011;11:1320–1324.
2. Rosales A, Salvador JT, Urdaneta G, et al. Laparoscopic kidney transplantation. *Eur Urol.* 2010;57:164–167.
3. Giulianotti P, Gorodner V, Sbrana F, et al. Robotic transabdominal kidney transplantation in a morbidly obese patient. *Am J Transplant.* 2010;10. 147814–82.
4. Boggi U, Vistoli F, Signori S, et al. Robotic renal transplantation: first European case. *Transpl Int.* 2011;24:213–218.
5. Menon M, Sood A, Bhandari M, et al. Robotic kidney transplantation with regional hypothermia: a step-by-step description of the Vattikuti Urology Institute–Medanta technique (IDEAL phase 2a). *Eur Urol.* 2014;65:991–1000.
6. Sood A, Ghosh P, Jeong W, et al. Minimally invasive kidney transplantation: perioperative considerations and key 6-month outcomes. *Transplantation.* 2015;99:316–323.
7. Oberholzer J, Giulianotti P, Danielson KK, et al. Minimally invasive robotic kidney transplantation for obese patients previously denied access to transplantation. *Am J Transplant.* 2013;13:721–728.

25 Laparoscopic Pyeloplasty

Aaron M. Potretzke, Sam B. Bhayani

Laparoscopic pyeloplasty has evolved into a new standard of care for the treatment of ureteropelvic junction (UPJ) obstruction. Since it was introduced in the early 1990s, the laparoscopic approach has maintained the high efficacy of open surgery without the coincident morbidity of the open incision. In addition, the approach is favored over endopyelotomy because complex reconstruction can be performed, even in the presence of aberrant crossing vessels. The surgery does require intracorporeal suturing skills, which may be perfected in an inanimate trainer before operative intervention.

INDICATIONS AND CONTRAINDICATIONS

The indications for laparoscopic pyeloplasty include documented UPJ obstruction. Preoperative three-dimensional computed tomography (CT) reconstruction of the UPJ may allow visualization of crossing vessels but is not necessary in all patients. There are few contraindications to laparoscopic pyeloplasty. With the exception of routine surgical contraindications (medical comorbidities, multiple surgeries or infections, renal or ureteral adhesions, uncorrected coagulopathies), the operation may be performed in patients of virtually any age and with any anatomic abnormality. Crossing vessels, renal stones, and duplicated collecting systems can all be addressed laparoscopically. Laparoscopic pyeloplasty may also be performed after failed endopyelotomy, failed open pyeloplasty, or even failed laparoscopic pyeloplasty.

PATIENT PREOPERATIVE EVALUATION AND PREPARATION

In assessing the degree of obstruction, a diuretic renal scan may help quantify blockage and residual function. An intravenous urogram or retrograde pyelogram may help define anatomic considerations before reconstruction. A CT angiogram or three-dimensional reconstruction of the UPJ may reveal anterior crossing arteries or veins that will require dismembered pyeloplasty and transposition of the vessels. None of these studies, however, is absolutely compulsory because none of them is likely to change the need for surgical intervention. Nevertheless, the studies may produce a surgical map of the field, thus allowing for less intraoperative speculation.

Obtain informed consent from the patient and discuss major risks, benefits, and alternatives. Discuss general surgical risks and other risks more germane to the procedure, including the possibility of urine leak, injury to surrounding structures, failure of surgery, migration of stents and drains, open conversion, bleeding, loss of kidney function, and nephrectomy.

Patients may have existing indwelling stents from the diagnosis of obstruction and pain. Typically, indwelling stents may cause ureteral edema and thickening, and identification of the UPJ may be difficult. Consider removing the stent 1 week before surgery if the patient can tolerate this intervention.

Give the patient a bottle of magnesium citrate and clear liquids the day before surgery. This bowel preparation, although not completely necessary, allows decompression of the intestines and may help in visualization during dissection. A negative urine culture is needed, or antibiotics are given at the time of surgery. After induction of general anesthesia, place an orogastric tube. Perform flexible or rigid cystoscopy and place a stent into the affected kidney. Use a long stent (7 French × 28 cm) so that it does not migrate out of the bladder during reconstruction. Perform a retrograde pyelogram if it is indicated. Place a urethral catheter, and reposition the patient for the pyeloplasty.

OPERATING ROOM CONFIGURATION AND PATIENT POSITIONING

The operating room is configured so that the surgeon and staff have excellent views of the laparoscopic surgical monitors (Fig. 25-1).

Positioning can be performed in a variety of methods. If a difficult dissection is anticipated, position the patient over the break in the table in case open conversion is needed. Place the patient into the full flank position (90 degrees) or the modified flank position (60 degrees, supported by a gel roll). Place the arms high so that they do not interfere with suturing (Fig. 25-2). No flexion is necessary in most cases. Consider adding an axillary roll and ensure that adequate padding is used.

TROCAR PLACEMENT

Insert a Veress needle and establish a pneumoperitoneum. Place a 10/12-mm trocar at the umbilicus, a 5-mm trocar 6 to 8 cm superior to the umbilicus, and a 10/12-mm trocar 6 to 8 cm below the umbilical trocar. Place all trocars in the midline; this positioning facilitates ergonomic suturing (Fig. 25-3).

PROCEDURE (SEE VIDEO 25-1)

Use a 30-degree lens throughout the operation. Deflect the colon using standard laparoscopic techniques, similar to a radical nephrectomy, and identify the ureter. Take care not to mobilize the ureter aggressively because it is necessary to preserve the periureteric blood supply.

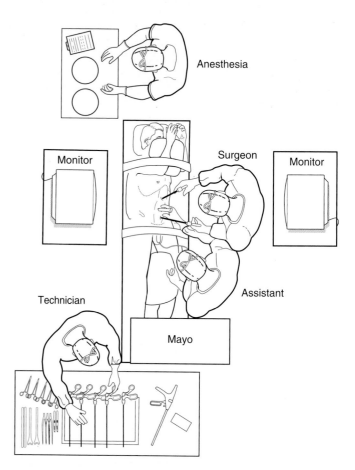

Figure 25-1. To allow visualization of the procedure by all members of the surgical team, the surgeon and assistant stand on the side contralateral to the pathology. The scrub nurse or technician stands on the opposite side to help with management of instrumentation.

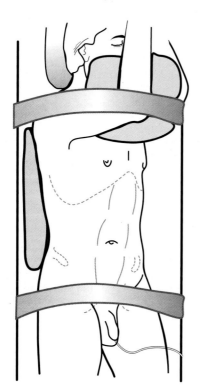

Figure 25-2. The umbilicus should be centered at the table break in the event that an open repair would be performed. An axillary roll is placed under the lower arm, which is brought out perpendicular to the patient. The arms are then positioned in a "praying position" near the patient's head and separated by a small pillow. The contralateral lower knee is bent at a 90-degree position and the ipsilateral leg is kept straight with pillows or foam placed between them. Wide cloth tape is placed across the upper shoulder and arm and the hip and secured to the operative table.

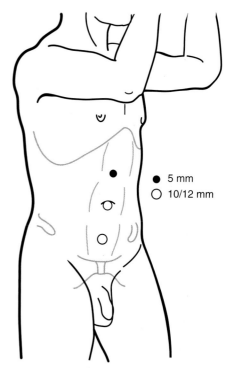

Figure 25-3. Trocar placement includes three midline trocars. A 10/12-mm trocar is placed at the umbilicus. The second port (5 mm) is placed midway between the xiphoid process and the umbilicus. A third trocar is located midway between the umbilicus and the symphysis pubis.

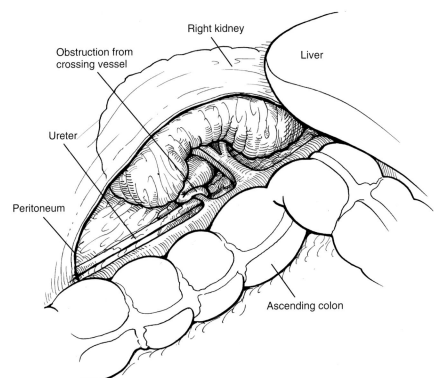

Right kidney

Obstruction from
crossing vessel

Liver

Ureter

Peritoneum

Ascending colon

Figure 25-4. After the colon is deflected, the ureter is identified at the lower pole of the kidney. A crossing vessel is identified causing obstruction at the level of the ureteropelvic junction.

Expose the ureter only at the UPJ. The area can be easily found because the pelvis is typically hydronephrotic and the stented ureter can be felt with laparoscopic graspers. The gonadal vein may be mistaken for the ureter, and palpation of the structure may clarify the structure's identity. Take care in dissection of the UPJ because a crossing vessel may be present (Fig. 25-4). Once the UPJ has been identified and crossing vessels have been recognized, free the renal pelvis from its peripelvic attachments near the UPJ. This allows mobilization of the pelvis and proximal ureter for the anastomosis. Important, during the dissection of the UPJ, avoid clips because they could erode into the repair. Control bleeding with energy sources (e.g., ultrasonic shears, bipolar cautery, monopolar cautery), but avoid direct use of energy on the ureter. Control oozing at the cut edge with the sutures during repair.

Hynes-Anderson Dismembered Pyeloplasty

Once a crossing vessel is suspected during preoperative imaging or observed during the procedure itself, a Hynes-Anderson dismembered pyeloplasty is the treatment of choice. This approach can also be used in virtually any UPJ obstruction.

A segmental renal vessel can be identified in close proximity to the UPJ in up to 60% of patients, and its anterior position may be the cause of the obstruction. Perform the anastomosis between the ureter and the renal pelvis anterior to the vascular obstructing component.

When the renal pelvis is identified, mobilize it along with a small portion of the proximal ureter. Take care not to damage the small vessels supplying the pelvis; theoretically this could provide better viability of the anastomosis.

Make a circumferential incision over the renal pelvis above the anastomotic area (Fig. 25-5) and insert the stent.

Complete the incision around the stent and along the renal pelvis wall. Take down redundant tissue to enable better approximation and technical results. Distally transect the UPJ using laparoscopic scissors and either remove the ring of ureteral obstructing tissue or incorporate it in the spatulation. Take care not to damage the ureteral stent during this manipulation. Make a 1-cm spatulation incision along the lateral or posterior wall of the proximal ureter. Spatulate the renal pelvis, if needed. Place a 4-0 polyglactin stitch at the tip of the spatulated ureter and then through the renal pelvis.

Once this knot has been tied or secured with a Vicryl clip, use this stay suture to assist in applying interrupted sutures along the posterior pyelotomy, tying each knot outside of the urinary tract. These 4-0 sutures can also be placed with the EndoStitch laparoscopic suturing device (Covidien, Minneapolis, Minn.) (Figs. 25-6 and 25-7). Once the posterior wall is completed, insert the stent inside the renal pelvis and tailor the anterior portion of the renal pelvis to the spatulated ureter with interrupted 4-0 sutures.

Another method for the pyelotomy closure that is used today is a continuous closure with a double-armed, knotted suture. Tie the sutures at their free end with a simple knot and drive each needle outside-in on the renal pelvis. One suture runs along the posterior wall continuously and the other runs over the anterior wall. Tie them together at the end, outside of the system, with a knot or a Lapra-Ty Vicryl clip (Ethicon, Cincinnati, Ohio) (Fig. 25-8).

Foley Y-V Pyeloplasty

Foley Y-V pyeloplasty is used in a small renal pelvis with a high inserted ureter and no crossing vessels. Make a wide-based V-shaped incision over the anterior aspect of the renal pelvis with the laparoscopic scissors (Fig. 25-9).

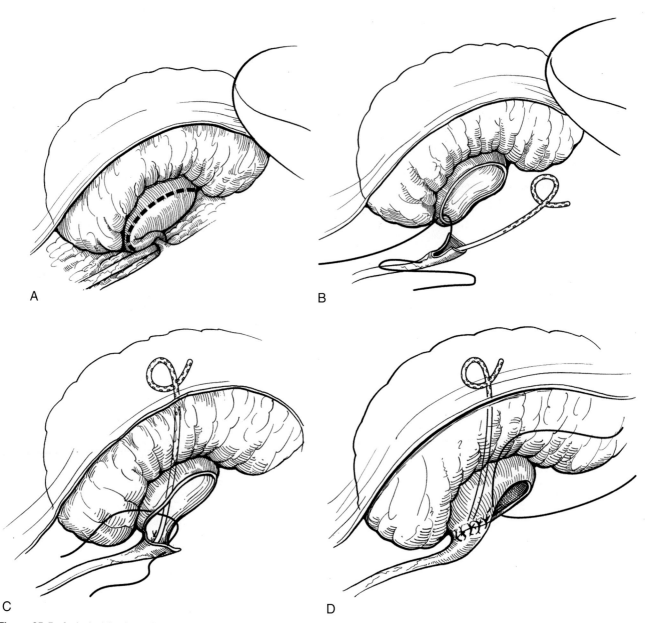

Figure 25-5. A, An incision is made on the dilated pelvis to transect the ureteropelvic junction. Care is taken to avoid cutting the stent. **B,** The ureter and pelvis are placed anterior to the crossing vessel. The redundant pelvis and stenotic ureteropelvic junction have been excised and the proximal ureter spatulated. The first suture has been placed from the apex of the spatulated ureter to the most dependent portion of the renal pelvis. **C,** The ureteral stent is positioned in the pelvis and the top of the ureter is sutured to the pelvis. **D,** Interrupted sutures are placed to complete the repair, and the reduction pyeloplasty is closed.

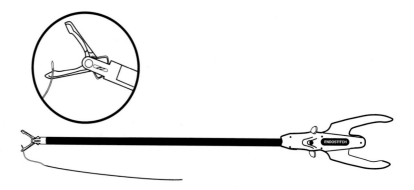

Figure 25-6. The EndoStitch device (Covidien, Minneapolis, Minn.) allows the needle to be passed from one jaw of the instrument to the other by switching the toggle on the handle.

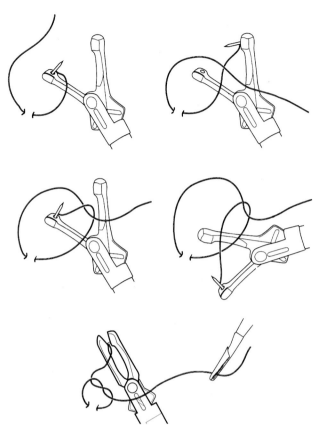

Figure 25-7. Suture pattern with the EndoStitch (Covidien, Minneapolis, Minn.), which allows rapid intracorporeal knot tying.

Continue with a vertical incision through the anterior proximal ureter, as low as 1 cm below the obstructed area. Using a 4-0 polyglactin suture, approximate the tip of the V shape to the apex of the proximal ureter incision. First, suture the medial arm of the V shape with interrupted 4-0 sutures using EndoStitch or standard knots, then insert the ureteral stent into the renal pelvis and close the anterior arm of the V shape with interrupted suturing.

Fenger Nondismembered Pyeloplasty

Fenger nondismembered pyeloplasty is used with a small renal pelvis and no crossing vessels. The procedure uses the Heineke-Mikulicz principle of a longitudinal incision closed in a transverse fashion. Compared with the procedures previously described, less suturing is needed and thus a shorter operative time is required.

Make one long incision with laparoscopic scissors along the anterior renal pelvis and proximal ureter (Fig. 25-10), ending about 1 cm below the obstructed area. Place a 4-0 polyglactin suture from the superior apex of the incision on the renal pelvis, and approach to the inferior apex of the incision on the proximal ureter. Then use three or four interrupted sutures on each side for the transverse closure of the incision.

Take care not to damage the internal ureteral stent with the closure of the incision. With this approach there is no need to free the stent outside the renal pelvis.

There is some debate as to whether this approach is as efficacious as a dismembered pyeloplasty.

Drain Placement

Leave a closed bulb suction drain in close proximity to the anastomotic area, preferably in a posterior position. A 7-French or 10-French Jackson-Pratt drain is commonly used.

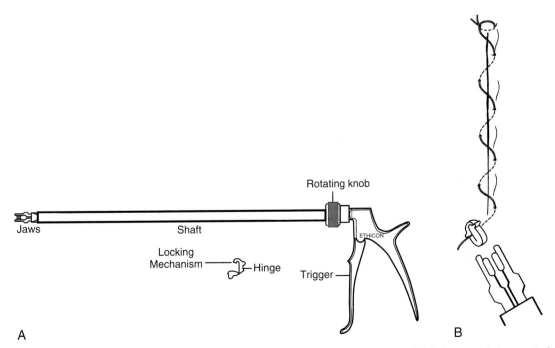

Rotating knob

Jaws

Shaft

Locking Mechanism — Hinge

Trigger —

ETHICON

A

B

Figure 25-8. A, The Lapra-Ty 5-mm-shaft, single-use clip applier (Ethicon Endo-Surgery, Cincinnati, Ohio) allows rapid placement of an absorbable, locking clip. **B,** The clip can be placed on the end of the suture to secure the end without having to tie a knot.

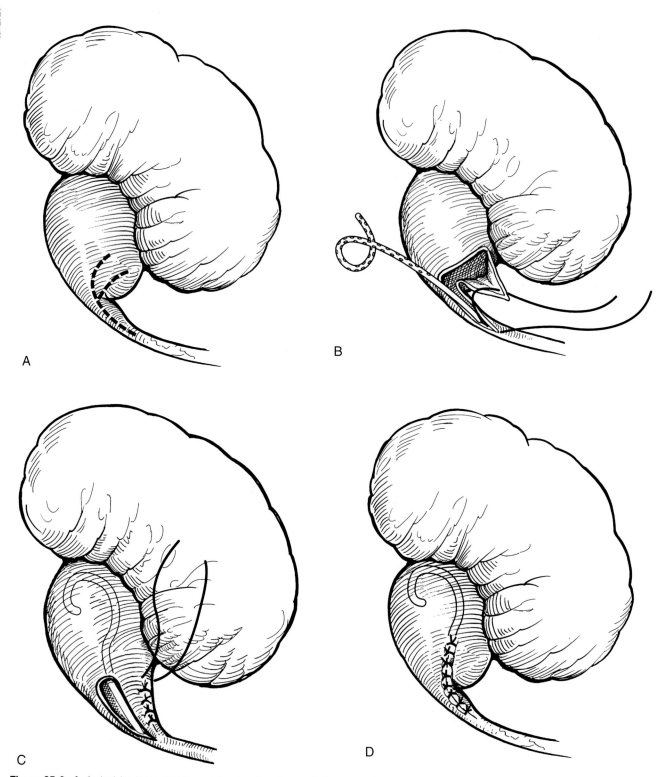

A

B

C

D

Figure 25-9. A, An incision is made in the pelvis extending down onto the ureter through its insertion into the pelvis. A V is formed with arms equal in length to the incision over the ureter. **B,** A 4-0 absorbable suture is passed with the EndoStitch (Covidien, Minneapolis, Minn.) through the apex of the V and the apex of the ureteral incision. **C,** The inside of the V incision is closed with a running suture. **D,** The anterior incision is closed with 4-0 absorbable suture in an interrupted or running fashion to complete the repair.

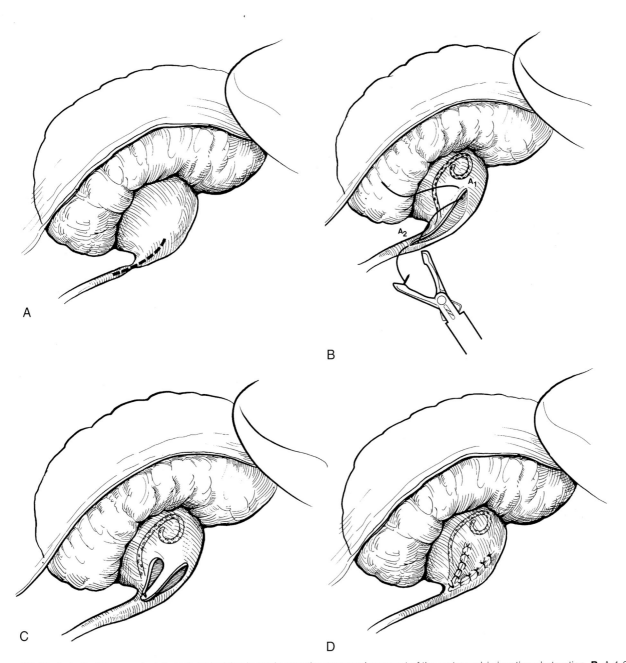

Figure 25-10. A, In the "Fenger-plasty" repair an incision is made over the narrowed segment of the ureteropelvic junction obstruction. **B,** A 4-0 absorbable suture is placed at the superior and inferior apex of the incision A1-A2. **C,** The superior and inferior limits of the incision are approximated. **D,** The pelvis is closed with interrupted suture.

Introduce the drain intra-abdominally through one of the laparoscopic ports (Fig. 25-11). Then make a new stab incision at the lateral abdominal wall and extract the drain outside the abdomen using a small hemostat. Alternatively, pass a drain with a sharpened spike into the retroperitoneum under direct vision, toward a trocar advanced deep into the abdomen, and toward the sharpened spike; pull the drain into the trocar with spoon forceps. A retroperitoneal position for the drain is preferred because urinomas can drain posteriorly when the patient is recovering in the supine position. Use a nonabsorbable skin stitch to secure the drain.

POSTOPERATIVE MANAGEMENT

A 48-hour admission is typical. However, because urine leaks into the peritoneal cavity during the reconstruction, bowel may be irritated. As a result, the patient may have a slower return of normal bowel function and more postoperative pain compared with laparoscopic nephrectomy patients. Remove the orogastric tube at the end of the procedure. Give clear liquids the night of surgery and advance diet as tolerated.

Some surgeons give oral antibiotics throughout the stented period, but most give oral antibiotics only 2 to 3 days before stent removal. Take out the urethral catheter after 48 hours.

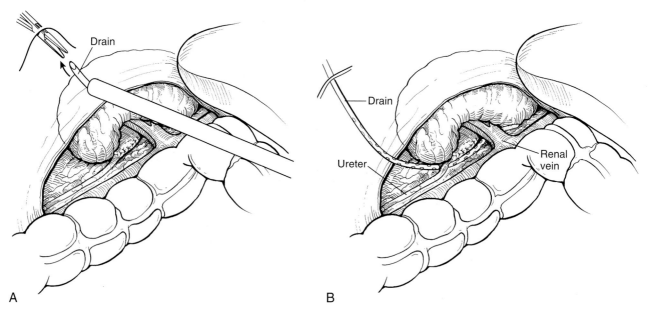

A

B

Figure 25-11. A, A hemostat is advanced through a small stab incision in the flank. The hemostat passes under the incised edge of the perito-neum. The drain is passed through one of the trocars, which had been advanced into the abdomen as far as possible and aids in directing the drain to the hemostat. **B,** The hemostat pulls the drain out of the flank incision and can then be trimmed to the appropriate length and placed under the ureteropelvic junction.

It is mandatory to closely measure the drain output once the urinary catheter has been removed. If this output does not increase in the 8 to 12 hours after catheter removal, remove the drain and discharge the patient.

Suspect anastomotic leak if an increased amount of urine (creatinine level of the drain fluid is higher than the plasma creatinine) is measured in the retroperitoneal drain after uri-nary catheter removal. Reinsert the catheter into the bladder until the drain output no longer contains urine. This may take 1 to 2 weeks. Consider the possibility of an obstructed or mal-positioned stent if drain output is high with the catheter in place. A CT scan can help in assessment of stent positioning.

Leave the stent in place for 3 to 4 weeks. Consider a diuretic renal scan 6 weeks after surgery and every 4 to 6 months for 2 years. Failures usually occur within the first year postoperatively.

COMPLICATIONS

Anastomotic urinary leakage and formation of a retroperito-neal urinoma are uncommon complications of this procedure. Attempt conservative approach with urinary bladder catheter-ization and continued suction drainage. Place the drain to allow gravity to promote drainage through the collecting sys-tem. Usually, catheterization results in decreased drain output and the anastomosis heals.

Laparoscopic exploration and repositioning of the drain may be needed with large-volume urinomas or irritative peritoneal signs. Consider an evaluation including CT scan because it may indicate stent position, undrained fluid collec-tions, or coincident pathology such as trocar hernias.

Postoperative adynamic ileus is common and usually responds to readmission and conservative treatment with intravenous fluids. Bleeding is a rare complication and is usu-ally managed conservatively, but bleeding may necessitate administration of blood products.

Procedure failure with recurrence of the UPJ obstruction (radiologically or according to a follow-up diuretic renal scan)

is more common after secondary procedures and is reported in up to 15% of secondary procedures compared with less than 5% of primary procedures. Treatment of the failed lapa-roscopic pyeloplasty has not been extensively studied, but endoscopic, laparoscopic, and open management have been described to be successful.

ROBOTIC-ASSISTED LAPAROSCOPIC PYELOPLASTY

The advent of robotic technology has provided a more facile platform with which to perform minimally invasive pyelo-plasty. The robotic approach has garnered attention owing to its shorter learning curve, increased dexterity, and improved vision. With the exception of highly experienced laparoscopic sur-geons, most find greater ease of suturing with robotic assistance.

The room setup differs from a laparoscopic procedure only in that the robot will approach the patient posteriorly, in the position of the monitor shown in Figure 25-1. Patient posi-tioning is identical to that of laparoscopic pyeloplasty.

Robotic trocar placement is variable and depends on sur-geon preference. Patients of greater abdominal girth should have the trocars lateralized slightly. One possibility of trocar placement is depicted in Figure 25-12. The procedure is most often approached transperitoneally. Either three or four arms can be used in the technique. The fourth arm can be used for additional retraction. For example, the first suture placed dur-ing creation of the anastomosis can be held with the fourth arm to rotate the pelvis for better suturing angles.

The operation begins with robotic scissors held in the sur-geon's right hand and a ProGrasp instrument (Intuitive Surgical, Sunnyvale, Calif.) in the left. Suturing is performed with either two robotic needle drivers or a needle driver and the ProGrasp. The operation otherwise proceeds in identical fashion to that previously described for laparoscopic pyeloplasty. The anasto-mosis can be constructed with either interrupted sutures or two running sutures—one each for the posterior and anterior aspects.

The experience of robotic pyeloplasty is becoming more commonplace. The benefits of laparoscopic pyeloplasty when

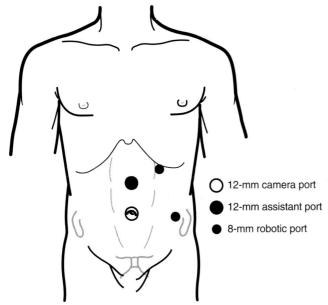

Figure 25-12. Positioning and trocar placement for a left pyeloplasty. The camera trocar is placed at or just lateral to the umbilicus. The left robotic arm is placed subcostally, and the right is placed approximately 4 cm cephalad to the anterior superior iliac spine. A 12-mm assistant port is placed approximately 9 cm cephalad to the camera trocar.

○ 12-mm camera port

● 12-mm assistant port

● 8-mm robotic port

compared with open pyeloplasty (e.g., shorter hospital stay, faster convalescence, and improved cosmesis) are preserved with robotic pyeloplasty. Most robotic pyeloplasty series report success rates of 94% to 100%. Reported complication rates are variable but mirror those of laparoscopic pyeloplasty.

TIPS AND TRICKS

- A high-resolution CT scan can aid in identifying crossing vessels before the operation.
- Removing a stent 1 week before the procedure may decrease ureteral edema.
- Use a long stent (7 French × 28 cm) so that the stent does not migrate cephalad during the reconstruction.
- If visualization is poor (obese patients), add an extra trocar for retraction.
- Vicryl clips can assist with laparoscopic knot tying.
- If anastomotic leak is suspected, check the creatinine level in the drain fluid.
- Failures occur most commonly in the first year after the procedure.

SUGGESTED READINGS

Autorino R, Eden C, El-Ghoneimi A, et al. Robot-assisted and laparoscopic repair of ureteropelvic junction obstruction: a systematic review and meta-analysis. *Eur Urol.* 2014;65:430–452.

Baldwin DD, Dunbar JA, Wells N, McDougall EM. Single-center comparison of laparoscopic pyeloplasty, Acucise endopyelotomy, and open pyeloplasty. *J Endourol.* 2003;17:155–160.

Bove P, Ong AM, Rha KH, Pinto P, Jarrett TW, Kavoussi LR. Laparoscopic management of ureteropelvic junction obstruction in patients with upper urinary tract anomalies. *J Urol.* 2004;171:77–79.

Chen RN, Moore RG, Kavoussi LR. Laparoscopic pyeloplasty. Indications, technique, and long-term outcome. *Urol Clin North Am.* 1998; 25:323–330.

Desai MM, Desai MR, Gill IS. Endopyeloplasty versus endopyelotomy versus laparoscopic pyeloplasty for primary ureteropelvic junction obstruction. *Urology.* 2004;64:16–21. discussion 21.

Eichel L, Khonsari S, Lee DI, et al. One-knot pyeloplasty. *J Endourol.* 2004;18:201–204. discussion 204.

Inagaki T, Rha KH, Ong AM, Kavoussi LR, Jarrett TW. Laparoscopic pyeloplasty: current status. *BJU Int.* 2005;95(Suppl 2):102–105.

Kavoussi LR, Peters CA. Laparoscopic pyeloplasty. *J Urol.* 1993;150: 1891–1894.

Khaira HS, Platt JF, Cohan RH, Wolf JS, Faerber GJ. Helical computed tomography for identification of crossing vessels in ureteropelvic junction obstruction—comparison with operative findings. *Urology.* 2003;62:35–39.

Lucas SM, Sundaram CP. Transperitoneal robot-assisted laparoscopic pyeloplasty. *J Endourol.* 2011;25:167–172.

McDougall EM, Elashry OM, Clayman RV, Humphrey PA, Rayala HJ. Laparoscopic pyeloplasty in the animal model. *JSLS.* 1997;1:113–118.

Peters CA. Pediatric robot-assisted pyeloplasty. *J Endourol.* 2011;25: 179–185.

Rabah D, Soderdahl DW, McAdams PD, et al. Ureteropelvic junction obstruction: does CT angiography allow better selection of therapeutic modalities and better patient outcome? *J Endourol.* 2004; 18:427–430.

Schuessler WW, Grune MT, Tecuanhuey LV, Preminger GM. Laparoscopic dismembered pyeloplasty. *J Urol.* 1993;150:1795–1799.

Sundaram CP, Grubb RL 3rd, Rehman J, et al. Laparoscopic pyeloplasty for secondary ureteropelvic junction obstruction. *J Urol.* 2003;169:2037–2040.

Teber D, Dekel Y, Frede T, Klein J, Rassweiler J. The Heilbronn laparoscopic training program for laparoscopic suturing: concept and validation. *J Endourol.* 2005;19:230–238.

Turk IA, Davis JW, Winkelmann B, et al. Laparoscopic dismembered pyeloplasty—the method of choice in the presence of an enlarged renal pelvis and crossing vessels. *Eur Urol.* 2002;42:268–275.

Uberoi J, Disick GI, Munver R. Minimally invasive surgical management of pelvic-ureteric junction obstruction: update on the current status of robotic-assisted pyeloplasty. *BJU Int.* 2009;104: 1722–1729.

Varkarakis IM, Bhayani SB, Allaf ME, et al. Management of secondary ureteropelvic junction obstruction after failed primary laparoscopic pyeloplasty. *J Urol.* 2004;172:180–182.

26 Ureterolysis

Michael C. Ost, Jeremy N. Reese

Ureterolysis is performed to relieve ureteral obstruction caused by extrinsic compression. Retroperitoneal fibrosis (RPF) is a rare (1 in 200,000-500,000) chronic process characterized by inflammation and mononuclear infiltration that is idiopathic in about two thirds of patients. Secondary causes include certain malignancies, infections, prior radiation, previous surgeries, autoimmune disorders, and certain drugs. Patients typically have flank or abdominal pain, azotemia, and hydronephrosis from ureteral involvement, which is present in 60% to 100% of cases. The aorta and vena cava are also frequently involved; this may result in lower extremity edema, claudication, or testicular pain. Medical treatment with glucocorticoids can be effective, but the dose and duration of treatment have not been well established.

Open ureterolysis has been associated with a success rate exceeding 90% in long-term resolution of ureteral obstruction. In 1992, Kauvoussi and colleagues[1] first described laparoscopic ureterolysis. Since that time, multiple authors have reproduced these techniques with success rates similar to the open approach. In 2006, Mufarrij and Stifelman[2] reported the first successful robotic-assisted laparoscopic ureterolysis. They described improved visibility and dexterity and decreased surgeon fatigue. This chapter focuses on both purely laparoscopic and robotic-assisted laparoscopic ureterolysis, although hand-assisted techniques have also been described.

INDICATIONS AND CONTRAINDICATIONS

No current consensus exists on whether patients should undergo primary ureterolysis or steroid treatment for RPF after renal obstruction is relieved either through ureteral stenting or placement of a nephrostomy tube. There are several reports of a vigorous response to a course of high-dose prednisone, often in combination with azathioprine, tamoxifen, or mycophenolate mofetil. Unfortunately, the optimum dose and duration are not well established and some cases are refractory to these treatments.

Indications for surgical intervention include failure of or intolerance to medical treatments (e.g., diabetes) or recurrent RPF. Arguments for "up-front" surgery have been made, especially when tissue diagnosis is needed, which often requires deep tissue samples that are not readily obtained through percutaneous sampling. Surgical treatment is contraindicated when extrinsic compression is known to be from malignancy (e.g., lymphoma or metastatic disease) or other treatable conditions such as endometriosis.

PATIENT PREOPERATIVE EVALUATION AND PREPARATION

Initial workup for RPF includes a detailed history and physical examination. Serum laboratory values are obtained, including complete blood count with differential, metabolic panel with creatinine, erythrocyte sedimentation rate, and C-reactive protein. If there is any reason to suspect an underlying malignancy or autoimmune disease, appropriate consultations with oncologists and rheumatologists, respectively, are undertaken. Computed tomography (CT) or magnetic resonance imaging (MRI) is performed to assess for burden of disease

and evidence of hydronephrosis or renal atrophy. If there is evidence of long-standing obstruction, a diuretic renal scan is performed. Contrast-enhanced images of the ureters are obtained through CT or MRI urography if there is no planned ureteral decompression but are otherwise obtained with pyelography at the time of stent or nephrostomy tube placement. Images of the affected ureter typically reveal a classic triad of medial deviation, extrinsic compression, and hydronephrosis (Fig. 26-1).

After confirmed diagnosis and ureteral decompression, it is our current practice to offer patients a choice between a trial of medical therapy or up-front robotic-assisted ureterolysis. Medical therapy is guided by rheumatologic or oncologic consultation. If patients are intolerant of medical therapy or improvement does not occur after 4 to 8 weeks of medical therapy, we recommend robotic-assisted ureterolysis. Before informed consent is given, all patients are counseled regarding the possibility of neoureterocystostomy with or without Boari flap or psoas hitch, ileal ureter, nephrectomy, or conversion to open surgery.

OPERATING ROOM CONFIGURATION AND PATIENT POSITIONING

We use an operative table that is fluoroscopy compatible, can be slid toward the head and foot, and has a removable foot to accommodate lithotomy positioning for the endoscopic portion of the procedure. The operating room scrub and equipment tables are placed opposite the operative side (e.g., on the patient's right if the left ureter is being lysed), as shown in Figure 26-2. This will also be the location of the assistant during a robotic-assisted procedure or both surgeon and assistant during a pure laparoscopic procedure. A monitor is placed opposite the assistant. The table is padded with either gel or foam before the patient is transferred.

After induction of general anesthesia, an orogastric tube is placed and the patient is completely paralyzed. The patient is initially placed in lithotomy position. Bilateral retrograde pyelograms are obtained to localize the affected area of the ureter(s) and ensure there is no contralateral involvement when unilateral disease is suspected. A new ureteral stent is placed and a Foley catheter is inserted. The patient's midline is then marked and marks are made for the anticipated location of the ports, as described later. The patient is left in stirrups and placed in a modified lateral decubitus position with the affected side up (Fig. 26-3). Keeping the patient in stirrups allows for access to the urethra should the stent need to be manipulated or for performance of simultaneous ureteroscopy. A large gel roll is placed under the scapula of the operative side. A small gel roll is used for an axillary roll to prevent a brachial plexus injury. The dependent arm is secured on an arm board and protected with thick egg crate foam. The other arm is placed caudally, with the wrist resting over the iliac crest. Foam is used above and below the arm, and the elbow is subtly flexed to protect the ulnar nerve. The patient's chest is secured with 3-inch cloth tape that is wrapped across the upper shoulder, coming just under the patient's nipples and then around the table two times. The nipples and chest skin are protected with foam. The hip is secured similarly,

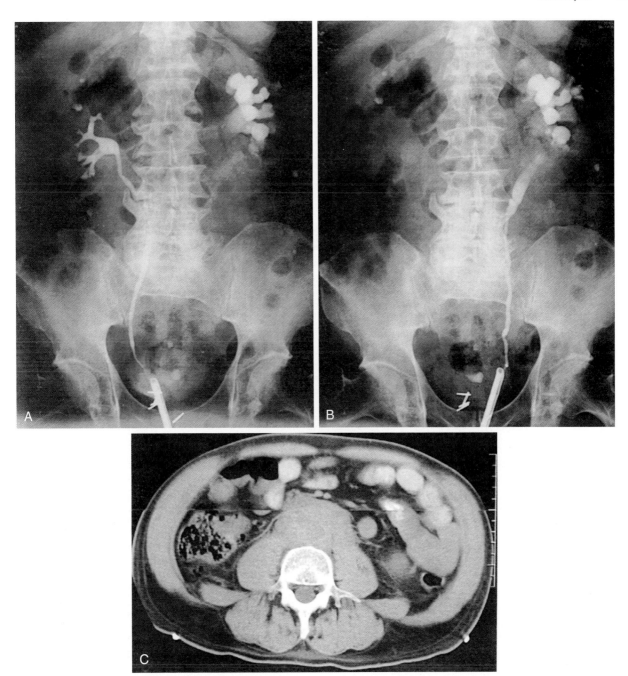

Figure 26-1. Retroperitoneal fibrosis. **A,** Right-sided retrograde ureterogram shows medial displacement of the midureteral segment. **B,** Left-sided retrograde ureterogram shows medial displacement of the ureter in the same area as the right side. **C,** A computed tomography scan demonstrates the area of dense fibrosis causing ureteral obstruction.

crossing the pubic bone and securing the Foley catheter. The patient is test rolled in each direction to ensure that the patient is secure and all pressure points are amply padded. Often the anesthesia provider must secure the head with additional towels or foam and a piece of thin tape to prevent movement. An alcohol-based preparation is used over the entire abdomen in case open conversion is necessary, and the patient is draped. An open tray should be in the room for the duration of the procedure.

For secondary RPF that is thought to be isolated to the pelvis, the patient is secured in lithotomy position to permit ready access to the distal ureters bilaterally. This approach also allows for bladder mobilization or creation of a Boari flap or a psoas hitch if ureteral reimplantation is required.

TROCAR PLACEMENT

We use a Veress needle to establish intraperitoneal access and insufflation. We enter at a site that is superior and lateral on the abdomen to avoid as much abdominal fat as possible. After insertion, aspirate to ensure that no blood or bowel contents are present, and perform a drop test with saline and reaspirate. Insufflation is done on low flow to witness low opening pressures before increasing the flow rate to a maximum pressure of 15 mm Hg. A 12-mm camera port is placed through the umbilicus with the assistance of a 12-mm Visiport (Covidien, Norwalk, Conn.) or a 12-mm bladeless trocar dilator such as the Endopath Xcel (Ethicon Endo-Surgery, Cincinnati, Ohio). A 30-degree laparoscopic camera is immediately inserted

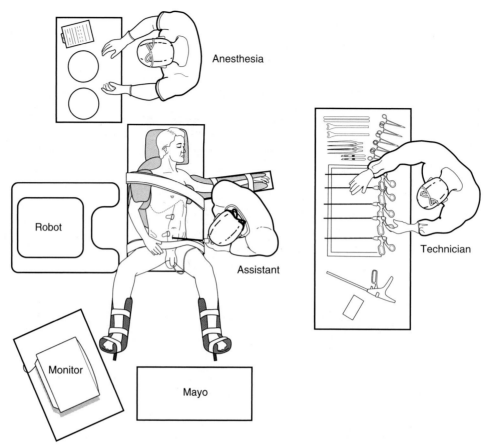

Figure 26-2. The robot is docked perpendicular to the operative table. A monitor is placed within clear view of the assistant. The surgical technician and table are behind the assistant.

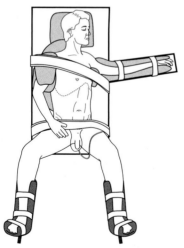

Figure 26-3. The patient is placed in modified lateral decubitus position with the legs in stirrups to allow urethral access during surgery. Wide tape is used over the shoulders and hips to secure the patient during table rotation.

to confirm intra-abdominal placement and to check the structures surrounding the Veress needle insertion site. On a line 8 cm lateral to the midline in the direction of the affected ureter, measuring one handbreadth both above and below the umbilicus, 8-mm robotic ports are inserted. A 5-mm assistant port is placed on the midline below the caudal robotic port (Fig. 26-4, *A*). If a pure laparoscopic approach is planned, we do

not place an assistant port, and we use 5-mm trocars in lieu of the robotic ports. The cephalad trocar is kept on the midline between the umbilicus and the xiphoid process, and the caudal port is placed on a line between the ipsilateral anterior superior iliac crest and the umbilicus (Fig. 26-4, *B*).

For RPF isolated to the pelvis that we plan to address robotically, the trocar arrangement includes a 12-mm camera port in the midline, midway between the umbilicus and the xiphoid process; 8-mm robotic ports are placed at least 8 cm from the midline in each respective hemiabdomen. Assistant ports may be placed in any quadrant (e.g., 5-mm port in left lower quadrant and 5-mm port in left upper quadrant) (Fig. 26-4, *C*).

PROCEDURE (SEE VIDEO 26-1)

After satisfactory trocar placement, the table and the patient are rotated maximally toward the surgeon. We dock the robot perpendicular to the table and use monopolar scissors in the right hand and either ProGrasp forceps (Intuitive Surgical, Sunnyvale, Calif.) or a Maryland bipolar grasper in the left hand. The assistant uses a suction irrigator to provide countertraction and to assist with tactile blunt dissection. For pure laparoscopy, monopolar scissors are used in the right hand and an atraumatic grasper in the left hand.

Mobilize the Colon

With the patient in a lateral position, gravity is used to assist in medial reflection of the colon. A combination of sharp dissection and electrocautery is used to incise along the white line of Toldt. The colon is medialized to the aorta from the spleen to

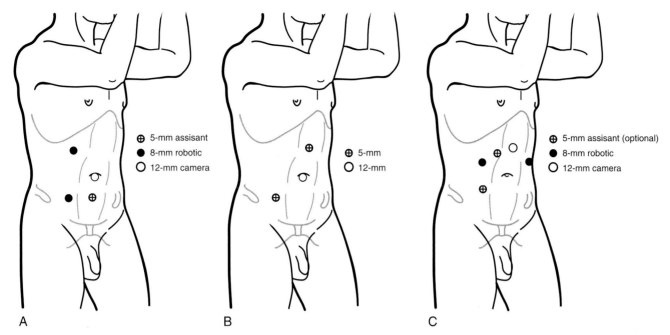

Figure 26-4. Trocar placement for traditional robotic ureterolysis **(A)**, pure laparoscopic ureterolysis **(B)**, and robotic-assisted ureterolysis limited to the pelvis **(C)**.

the iliac vessels on the left and to the vena cava from the liver to the iliac vessels on the right; keep in mind that the duodenum must be kocherized on the right. Dissection caudal to the iliac vessels is typically unnecessary unless there is known disease in the pelvic ureter—this is rare for primary RPF. Whether dissecting on the right or the left side, the respective colorenal ligaments are incised to expose the retroperitoneum. As the colon is deflected, the mesenteric fat can be distinguished from the retroperitoneal fat by lifting up on the Gerota fascia, which can be used as a backboard to bluntly sweep the mesenteric fat and colon medial to the level of the aorta or vena cava. It is often difficult to deflect the colon over the area of fibrosis.

Expose the Ureter

Using the information obtained from prior imaging and the retrograde pyelograms performed at the beginning of the procedure, we first expose healthy ureteral segments both inferiorly and superiorly to the entrapped area (Fig. 26-5). In patients with extensive disease this can be very difficult, and intraoperative ultrasound can help identify the stents to localize the ureters. We typically use monopolar scissors in the right hand and a bipolar Maryland grasper in the left hand. The unaffected portion of the ureter is dissected circumferentially and marked with vessel loops that are shortened and secured with metal clips. Sharp dissection continues with the bipolar Maryland graspers and countertraction from the assistant on the vessel loop until the dense fibrotic tissue encasing the ureter is encountered. At this point a biopsy sample of the tissue is taken and sent for both frozen and permanent specimens. Care must be taken not to perform biopsy on a concealed major vessel or ureter. If no malignancy (e.g., lymphoma) is identified on the frozen section, we proceed with the ureteral dissection.

Ureterolysis

With use of robotic monopolar scissors in the right hand, bipolar Maryland forceps in the left, and countertraction by the assistant on the vessel loop, the fibrotic tissue is split and

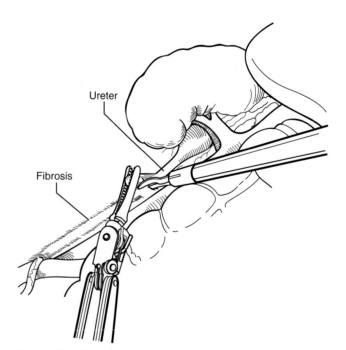

Figure 26-5. Once the colon has been deflected, the healthy portion of the ureter is dissected free circumferentially above and below the area of fibrosis.

circumferentially freed over the ureter, with every attempt made to stay just outside the adventitial layer (Fig. 26-6). A laparoscopic right angle is used when performing the procedure purely laparoscopically. Electrocautery is used sparingly during the periureteral dissection to avoid thermal injuries. When healthy tissue is encountered, a thorough inspection of the ureter is performed. Ureterotomies are often unavoidable and should be primarily repaired with absorbable suture; we use 4-0 polyglactin suture.

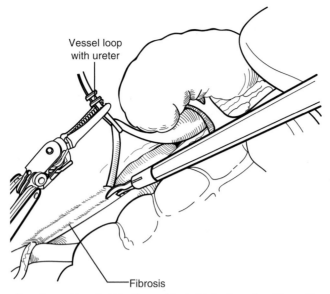

Figure 26-6. Countertraction from a clipped vessel loop held by the assistant aids in dissection. Sharp dissection is used to free the ureter from the surrounding fibrosis.

Omental Wrapping

Omental wrapping is indicated when the ureter has undergone significant thinning through extensive dissection. Because of this, there is an increased risk for urine leak and recurrent fibrosis. Using a ProGrasp in the left hand and bipolar Maryland forceps in the right, locate the omentum and evaluate whether there is sufficient length to pass under and then back over the ureter to completely cover the affected segment of ureter. This is secured in place with a running 4-0 polyglactin suture, Weck Hem-o-lok clips (Teleflex, Morrisville, N.C.), or an Endo Stitch device (Covidien, Norwalk, Conn.) laparoscopically. When there is insufficient length, a LigaSure (Valleylab, Boulder, Colo.) or Harmonic Scalpel (Ethicon Endo-Surgery, Cincinnati, Ohio) can be used to create an omental flap. When creating an omental flap it is important to remember that the arterial blood supply comes from the right and left gastroepiploic arteries. One of these must be spared as the omentum is separated from the stomach and the short gastric arteries are divided. The most distal aspect of the flap is brought under the ureter from medial to lateral and is secured to the side wall with either Weck Hem-o-lok clips or 2-0 polyglactin suture. If there is sufficient length, the distal edge of the omentum is then brought over the ureter and similarly fastened to itself (Fig. 26-7). An omental wrap serves to both lateralize and intraperitonealize the ureter.

Closing

After inspecting the abdomen for any bleeding or injuries, the robot is undocked. Under direct vision a sharp-tipped laparoscopic grasper is inserted laterally into the abdomen. The grasper is guided out of the inferior trocar protected by the suction irrigator. A No. 10 flat Jackson-Pratt (JP) drain is then grasped and pulled out through the new stab incision. The drain is placed in the lateral gutter with laparoscopic DeBakey forceps. The fasciae for all 12-mm and 10-mm port sites are closed with interrupted 2-0 polyglactin under direct vision with a Carter-Thomason or a Weck EFx fascial closure device (Teleflex Medical, Morrisville, N.C.). The abdomen is desufflated and the skin is closed with 4-0 polyglactin.

POSTOPERATIVE MANAGEMENT

The orogastric tube is removed at the time of extubation. Patients are given a clear liquid diet on postoperative day 0. The Foley catheter is removed on postoperative day 1 and the diet is advanced. If there is no increase in JP drainage output, the drain is removed on postoperative day 2. If drain output is high, a drain creatinine level is confirmed to be equal to or less than serum levels before removal. Care must be taken to ensure there is no evidence of a lymphatic leak, which is characterized by a large volume of turbid or milky fluid. Chylous leaks are confirmed by sending fluid for triglyceride or chylomicron levels. For pain, patients are given oral acetaminophen and oxycodone with ketorolac as needed if there is no concern for bleeding or known renal disease. Patients are typically discharged home on postoperative day 2. Follow-up is in 4 to 6 weeks for stent removal and then again 4 to 6 weeks later with a renal ultrasound and electrolyte panel. Many institutions initiate a course of steroids at this time, although that is not our current practice. We see patients again in 6 months, and another ultrasound or CT scan is performed. Any increase in hydronephrosis prompts a diuretic renal scan. Patients are otherwise followed annually at this point, with a renal ultrasound and basic metabolic panel before each clinic appointment.

COMPLICATIONS

The complications related to laparoscopic access are well described elsewhere in this text. Intraoperative complications that are unique to ureterolysis include ureteral injury, vascular injury, and bowel injury. Postoperatively, complications may include urine leak, lymphatic leak, ileus, and reobstruction in the long term. Ureteral injuries are common owing to the difficult nature of the operation. When recognized intraoperatively, they should be repaired primarily. If this is not possible, a neoureterocytostomy with or without Boari flap or psoas hitch, ileal ureter, or nephrectomy may be necessary depending on the patient's comorbidities and information obtained during preoperative counseling. Injuries to the major vessels or bowel should be addressed by the appropriate surgical subspecialist.

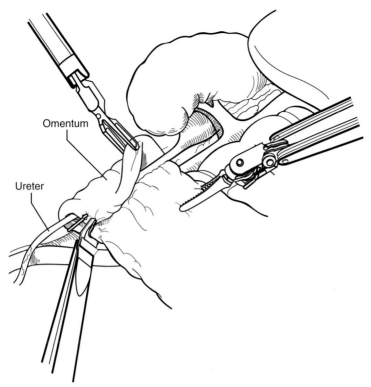

Figure 26-7. A flap of omentum can be placed under and then around the ureter to secure it in an intraperitoneal location to reduce the chance of recurrence.

TIPS AND TRICKS

- Intraoperative ultrasound and ureteroscopy can be helpful in locating and identifying the entrapped areas of the ureter.
- Place vessel loops around liberated portions of the ureter to increase countertension and aid with dissection.
- There is no documented benefit to prophylactic ureterolysis of the unaffected ureter.
- Conversion to hand assistance before opening may give better tactile feedback to avoid the larger incision and increased morbidity of open surgery.
- Robotic-assisted, pure laparoscopic, and hand-assisted ureterolysis procedures have similar outcomes; the surgeon should perform the procedure with which he or she is most comfortable and experienced.

REFERENCES

1. Kavoussi LR, Clayman RV, Brunt LM, Soper NJ. Laparoscopic ureterolysis. *J Urol.* 1992;147:426–429.
2. Mufarrij PW, Stifelman MD. Robotic ureterolysis, retroperitoneal biopsy, and omental wrap for the treatment of ureteral obstruction due to idiopathic retroperitoneal fibrosis. *Rev Urol.* 2006;8:226–230.

27 Laparoscopic and Robotic-Assisted Ureteral Reimplantation

Nicholas Kavoussi, Monica S.C. Morgan

INDICATIONS AND CONTRAINDICATIONS

Traditionally, ureteral reimplantation has been performed through an open midline or Pfannenstiel incision. Fortunately, surgical and technologic advancements have permitted minimally invasive techniques, both laparoscopic and robotic-assisted, to become increasingly used. Minimally invasive surgery (MIS) offers a shorter hospital stay, less postoperative pain, and improved cosmesis. Whereas a laparoscopic approach requires advanced intracorporeal suturing skills and substantial laparoscopic proficiency, robotic-assisted ureteroneocystostomy offers simplified suturing with equivalent benefits.

Ureteral obstruction can be attributed to inflammatory, infectious, iatrogenic, or traumatic causes, as well as stone disease and mass lesions (either benign or malignant). In certain cases, a medical or endoscopic approach may be initially considered. However, when conservative management is unsuccessful or deemed unsuitable for a certain pathology, ureteral reimplantation is indicated. Ureteral reimplantation may be performed in any patient with obstruction or trauma affecting the distal third ureter, provided a tension-free anastomosis can be performed. In children, ureteral reimplantation is commonly performed in the setting of vesicoureteral reflux. Further evaluation and surgical nonrefluxing techniques in the setting of vesicoureteral reflux are beyond the scope of this chapter.

Alternative surgical strategies should be considered for lesions that involve the midureter or proximal ureter, multiple malignant masses throughout the urinary tract, or a poorly functioning ipsilateral kidney.

PATIENT PREOPERATIVE EVALUATION AND PREPARATION

A surgical approach for the treatment of ureteral pathology necessitates adequate antegrade and retrograde imaging to define the length and location of the segment of abnormal ureter, as well as the surrounding pelvic anatomy. Planning should also include a detailed discussion with the patient regarding prior pelvic radiation, trauma, and abdominal or pelvic surgeries. Computed tomographic urography is useful in the assessment of a patient's anatomy. If there is concern regarding renal function, a nuclear medicine renal scan can also be performed. A nephrostomy tube is often indicated to allow for drainage of the kidney while surgical planning takes place. Routine preoperative evaluation including laboratory testing is also recommended.

With this information, the benefits and risks of open and laparoscopic or robotic-assisted repairs should be discussed with the patient. Furthermore, patients should be counseled about the possibility of performing alternative techniques for ureteral reconstruction such as a psoas hitch, Boari flap, or ileal ureter. Although extraperitoneal approaches do not traditionally warrant a bowel preparation, transperitoneal approaches and the potential use of the bowel in reconstruction certainly do.

OPERATING ROOM CONFIGURATION AND PATIENT POSITIONING

The operating room is ergonomically configured, allowing enough space and adequate visualization of the procedure for all involved personnel. After general anesthesia and endotracheal intubation, an orogastric tube is placed for decompression of the stomach. Compression boots are also applied for lower extremity thrombosis prophylaxis. The patient is positioned supine with arms tucked at the sides and the legs placed on spreader bars or stirrups. Padding is placed around the elbows to protect the ulnar nerve from injury, and around the lateral knees to protect the common peroneal nerve (if the patient is placed in stirrups). Aligning the hips with the break in the table maximizes ease of access to the pelvis. Security belts and tape are applied across the chest to provide support and safe positioning. The entire abdomen and genitalia are prepared in a sterile manner and draped. A urethral catheter is placed within the sterile field to allow for access during the surgical procedure. Angling the table approximately 15 degrees in Trendelenburg while simultaneously tilting the contralateral side of the table downward maximizes exposure for the procedure (Fig. 27-1).

TROCAR PLACEMENT

A Veress needle is inserted at the base of the umbilicus to achieve insufflation of the abdomen. A supraumbilical 12-mm incision is made for placement of an optical trocar. An 8-mm robotic port is placed at the level of the iliac crest, just lateral to the rectus muscle on the contralateral side to the affected ureter. A second 8-mm robotic port is placed on the ipsilateral side of the affected ureter one to two fingerbreadths inferior to the supraumbilical optical port and lateral to the rectus muscle. A 12-mm assistant port is triangulated laterally to the optical port and superiorly to the contralateral robotic port. Laparoscopic trocar placement is similar, with each working trocar at the level of the iliac crest (Fig. 27-2).

PROCEDURE (SEE VIDEO 27-1)

After achieving insufflation with a Veress needle and placing the trocars, deflect the colon medially by mobilizing it along the white line of Toldt (from the liver on the right and the spleen on the left). Create a peritoneal window and identify the ureter crossing the iliac vessels (Fig 27-3). In men, the ureter can also be found crossing posteriorly to the vas deferens; in women, it can be found deep in the peritoneal fold between the uterus and the bladder in the area of the trigone. Mobilize the ureter cranially and caudally while carefully preserving the adventitial tissue to maintain vascularization. A vessel loop can be placed around the ureter to aide in manipulation during dissection (Fig. 27-4, A).

Spatulate the distal end of the healthy ureter (i.e., proximal to the stricture) on its medial-posterior surface for approximately

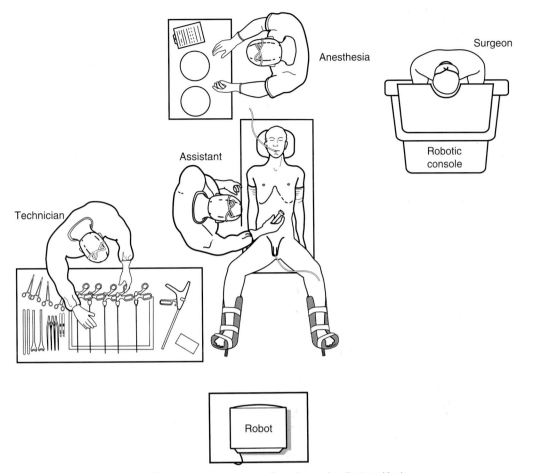

Figure 27-1. Operating room configuration and patient positioning.

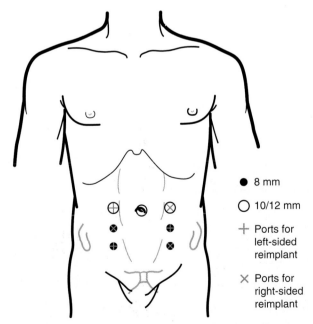

Figure 27-2. Trocar placement. A 12-mm robotic port is placed at the umbilicus. The 8-mm robotic ports are placed as shown. A left-sided reimplant would use the + ports for placement, and a right-sided reimplant would use the x ports. The camera is placed at the umbilicus through a 10/12-mm trocar, and two additional trocars are placed at the level of the anterior superior iliac crest, lateral to the rectus muscles.

- ● 8 mm
- ○ 10/12 mm
- + Ports for left-sided reimplant
- × Ports for right-sided reimplant

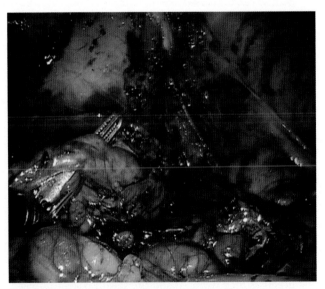

Figure 27-3. A peritoneal window is created and the ureter is exposed. The adventitia should remain in place, so as to not disrupt the vascularization of the distal ureter.

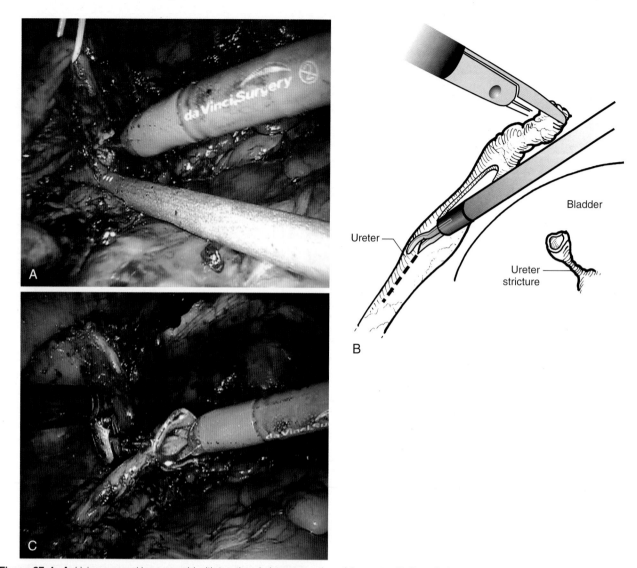

Figure 27-4. **A,** Using a vessel loop can aid with traction during transection of the ureter. **B,** Spatulation can occur before or after the ureter is transected. The diseased part of the ureter can also be transected and grasped without concern for compromising the tissue. **C,** The ureter should be spatulated approximately 1.5 cm on the posteromedial surface.

1.5 cm (Fig. 27-4, *B* and *C*). Refraining from complete transection at this time may help with stent placement later in the procedure.

Distend the bladder with approximately 200 mL of saline and mobilize the bladder by dissecting off the anterior, posterior, and lateral aspects of the peritoneum (Fig. 27-5). The urachus should be clipped and transected. Occasionally, the contralateral superior and middle vesical arteries need to be divided for additional mobility, ensuring a tension-free anastomosis. If greater bladder mobility is required, a psoas hitch may be performed by suturing the dome of the bladder to the ipsilateral psoas muscle with a 2-0 absorbable suture and wet clips.

At this point, place a 14-gauge hypodermic needle approximately two fingerbreadths superior to the pubic symphysis. The needle is then removed and the sheath is kept in place. Under direct vision, advance a 0.035 stiff-shaft guidewire through the sheath, and then advance a 5-French angiographic catheter over the guidewire to ensure it reaches the renal pelvis. Use a nontraumatic grasper and gently hold the adventitia of the ureter under mild tension to ease advancement of the guidewire and angiographic catheter (Fig. 27-6).

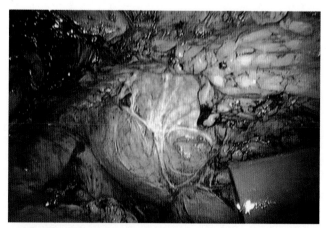

Figure 27-5. The peritoneum is dissected off the bladder completely, and a clean area, fit for the anastomosis, is ensured.

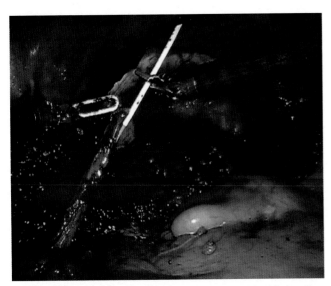

Figure 27-6. A wire is percutaneously introduced and guided up the ureter. A stent can then be advanced over the wire.

If the ureter is not fully transected yet, the diseased end of the ureter may be fully grasped because it will not be part of the ureteroneocystostomy. After the floppy end of the guidewire is in the kidney, remove the 5-French angiographic catheter and place an appropriately sized 6-French double-J stent up the ureter to the kidney. This may also be done later in the case but should be performed before the completion of the anastomosis. The ureter should be fully transected at this point.

The ureter should be anastomosed to the ipsilateral region of the bladder dome. Carefully incise the detrusor approximately 3 cm in length down to the mucosa, creating a trough (Fig. 27-7, *A* and *B*). The mucosa should be easily identified and should protrude out between the edges of the detrusor muscle. A 3-0 absorbable suture can be placed through the trough to aide in traction when entering through the mucosa (Fig. 27-7, *C*). Enter the mucosa in the distal trough; 3-0 absorbable sutures on a round-body needle are used to perform the anastomosis. Ensure that the ureter is not twisted and can be reapproximated without tension. Place the first stitch through the proximal incision of the open mucosa and the apex of the spatulated ureter (Fig. 27-8). The distal end of the

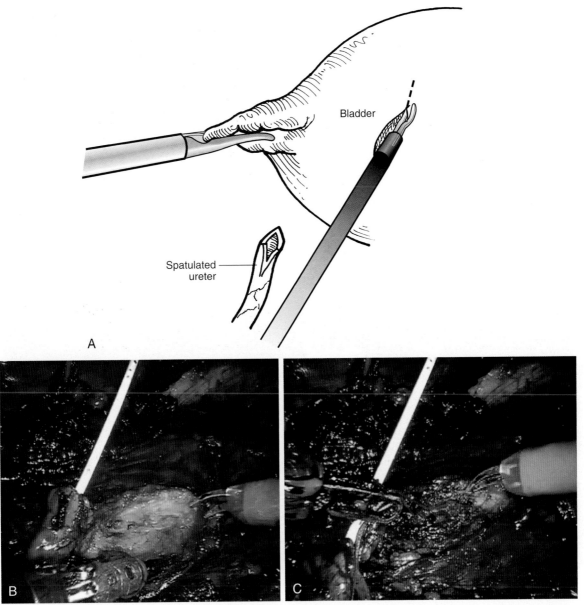

Figure 27-7. A, A trough is created on the dome of the bladder by dissecting down to the deep side of the urothelium through the detrusor. **B,** Entry into the bladder at this stage leads to decompression. **C,** A suture can be placed at the proximal end of the trough to help with traction and dissection. This suture can also be used to begin the anastomosis.

stent can then be placed in the bladder. Run the initial stitch distally, approximating the lateral, spatulated ureter to the lateral bladder mucosa incision. A second suture can be run in a similar fashion on the medial side (Fig. 27-9).

Test the integrity of the anastomosis and evaluate for leakage by filling the bladder with approximately 200 to 300 mL of normal saline, via the urethral catheter. Place a closed 19-French suction drain behind the anastomosis. Evaluate for visceral injury and bleeding in the peritoneal cavity before removing the trocars. Remove the trocars under direct vision to evaluate for abdominal wall bleeding that needs to be ligated. Fascial defects and skin should be appropriately closed.

POSTOPERATIVE MANAGEMENT

Maintain a urethral catheter and drain after the procedure. The nephrostomy tube may be removed the day after the surgery. The following day, send drain fluid to the laboratory and assess for urine. The drain can be removed, provided the fluid is serous. The urethral catheter should be maintained for 7 to 10 days and removed in the office. Cystography may be performed before removal of the catheter to verify the integrity of the anastomosis. Remove the ureteral stent cystoscopically at 4 to 6 weeks postoperatively. Upper tract imaging is routinely performed in all patients to evaluate for obstruction postoperatively with either an intravenous pyelogram or a nuclear

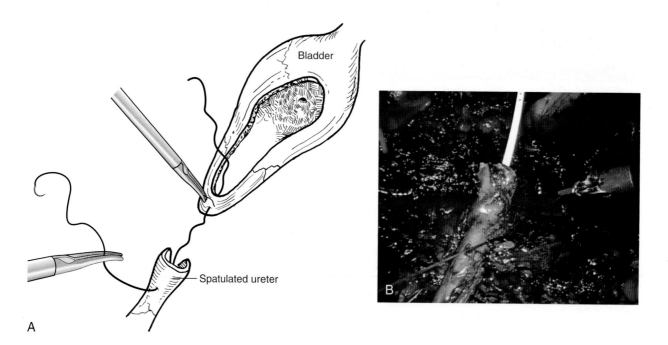

Figure 27-8. A, The proximal edge of the cystotomy is sutured to the apex of the spatulated ureter. **B,** The stent can be placed in the bladder after the apex has been approximated with cystotomy.

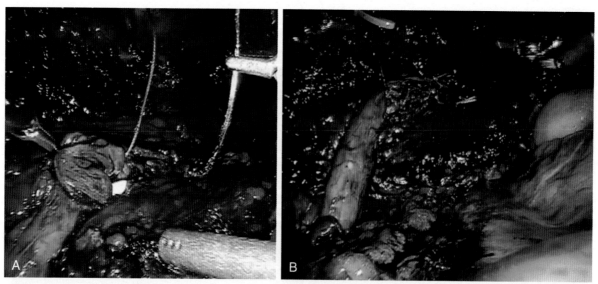

Figure 27-9. A, Suture can be run between the bladder and each spatulated edge of the ureter. **B,** The bladder should be filled with 200 to 300 mL of normal saline to test the anastomosis.

medicine renal scan at 6 months and again at 1 year. Patients may undergo follow-up as needed after that.

COMPLICATIONS

Urine leak at the site of reimplantation, manifesting as prolonged urinary drainage from the drain, may occur in some patients. Optimizing drainage of the urinary tract with a stent and a urethral catheter will usually aid in resolution. In this situation, radiologic studies to ensure proper stent position are necessary.

After removal of the stent, obstruction may occur. This can be caused by narrowing at the anastomotic site or iatrogenic injury to the ureter intraoperatively. A nuclear medicine renal scan is helpful to confirm obstruction. Endoscopic balloon dilation of the narrowing may effectively relieve obstruction. If obstruction persists, revision of the reimplant is recommended.

TIPS AND TRICKS

- Carefully review films, anatomy, and length of the lesion for surgical planning.
- A retrograde pyelogram can be performed intraoperatively before reimplantation to confirm anatomy of the obstruction.
- The vessel loop can help hold the ureter under gentle tension while it is dissected cranially and caudally.
- Spatulation of the ureter and percutaneous stent placement before complete transection of the ureter may facilitate these surgical steps.
- Division of the superior and middle vesical arteries allows for additional mobilization of the bladder.
- Use a 14-gauge needle for percutaneous placement of the stent.
- Test the anastomosis intraoperatively by filling the bladder.

28 Laparoscopic/Robotic Boari Flap Ureteral Reimplantation

Koon Ho Rha, Dae Keun Kim

Reconstructive management of the ureter is a challenging procedure and represents an evolving field in urology, especially in minimally invasive techniques. Treatment of ureteral defects, such as ureteral stricture, fistula, and urothelial cancer, requires ureteral reconstruction to obtain normal urinary drainage. The laparoscopic technique for creation of a Boari flap was initially described in 2001 by Fugita and colleagues. With the technologic developments in minimally invasive surgery, Schimpf and colleagues performed the first Boari flap procedure using a robotic platform. Robotic assistance offers the advantages of instrument flexibility during reconstruction and magnified vision. However, because of the limited number of cases and its technical novelty, clinical experience with laparoscopic and robotic Boari flap creation is still limited.

INDICATIONS AND CONTRAINDICATIONS

The indications for a Boari flap include iatrogenic ureteral injury, ureteral strictures, ureterovaginal fistula, and urothelial tumor located in the ureter. However, use of the Boari flap is contraindicated in cases of small-capacity irradiated bladder. The psoas hitch is an effective procedure to bridge a defect of the lower third of the ureter. Ureteral defects proximal to the pelvic brim usually require more than a simple psoas hitch alone. A psoas hitch can provide an additional 5 cm of length compared with ureteral reimplantation alone. Its advantages over a Boari flap include simplicity, improved vascularity, ease of endoscopic surveillance, and minimal voiding difficulties. Midureteral defects present a particular surgical challenge because this area has a tenuous blood supply and there are potential problems achieving a tension-free repair. When the diseased segment is too long or ureteral mobility is too limited for a primary ureteral reimplantation or psoas hitch, a laparoscopic or robotic Boari flap procedure may be a useful alternative. A Boari flap procedure can be performed to bridge defects up to 12 to 15 cm, and spiraled bladder flaps can reach to the renal pelvis in some patients. As with a psoas hitch, preoperative complete visualization of the ureter and evaluation of the bladder function are mandatory. Preoperatively address bladder outlet obstruction and neurogenic dysfunction, and realize that a small bladder capacity predicts poor postoperative outcome. The benefits of a laparoscopic or robotic approach for Boari flap surgery for patients with multiple medical comorbidities include less postoperative pain, less blood loss, and shorter hospital stay; however, with regard to technical feasibility, laparoscopic or robotic Boari flap surgery in patients with morbid obesity and major surgical history is challenging. Increased abdominal girth disturbs the range of motion of laparoscopic instruments and robotic arms. In addition, the surgeon must ensure that trocars and instruments are of the appropriate length to gain access to the target anatomy.

Although the psoas hitch and Boari flap have conventionally been performed by open surgery, the advantages of the laparoscopic or robotic technique have rapidly come into the limelight. With robotic assistance, instrument flexibility during reconstruction and magnified vision are the additional advantages over laparoscopic reconstructive surgery.

PATIENT PREOPERATIVE EVALUATION AND PREPARATION

Preoperative evaluation of patients who will undergo laparoscopic or robotic Boari flap surgery may depend on the reason for surgery. However, urine study and basic imaging are imperative.

Patients should be initially evaluated with urinalysis, urine culture and serum creatinine, and electrolytes. Basic imaging, including renal ultrasound and computed tomography (CT) urograms with delayed images, will demonstrate ureteral defects or obstruction.

Technetium 99m mercaptoacetyltriglycine (MAG3) renography is of benefit in assessing the degree of preoperative obstruction and in postoperative follow-up for assessment of obstruction. Also, MAG3 renography confirms preoperative renal function. Concomitant antegrade and retrograde pyelography could provide exact information regarding the length and location of stricture ("up and down–o–gram") and aid in preoperative planning. In patients in whom urothelial malignancy is suspected, ureteroscopic evaluation with washing cytology and biopsy is needed before surgery. In assessing for reconstruction of the ureter, for defects of 6 to 10 cm, a psoas hitch would be appropriate; for longer defects—12 cm to 15 cm—a Boari flap procedure should be performed. After thorough review of all options, including psoas hitch and other endoscopic methods, if the laparoscopic or robotic Boari flap procedure is selected, evaluation of the bladder volume is needed. Review previous radiation or injury to the bladder. Carefully review previous pelvic surgeries to plan the laparoscopic or robotic Boari flap procedure.

Patient preparation starts with informed consent. Inform the patient of possible postoperative complications such as obstruction, urine leakage, postoperative voiding symptoms, and the potential for open procedure conversion. Bowel preparation is usually not necessary; however, some centers perform bowel preparation using sodium phosphate or bisacodyl to decompress the colon during the transperitoneal approach. Administer a broad-spectrum antibiotic before the operation.

OPERATING ROOM CONFIGURATION AND PATIENT POSITIONING

For patient positioning for the laparoscopic Boari flap procedure, the operating room is configured so that the entire team can view the procedure on the monitor. After the induction of general anesthesia and intubation, prepare the patient in a supine position and carefully secure the patient to the table

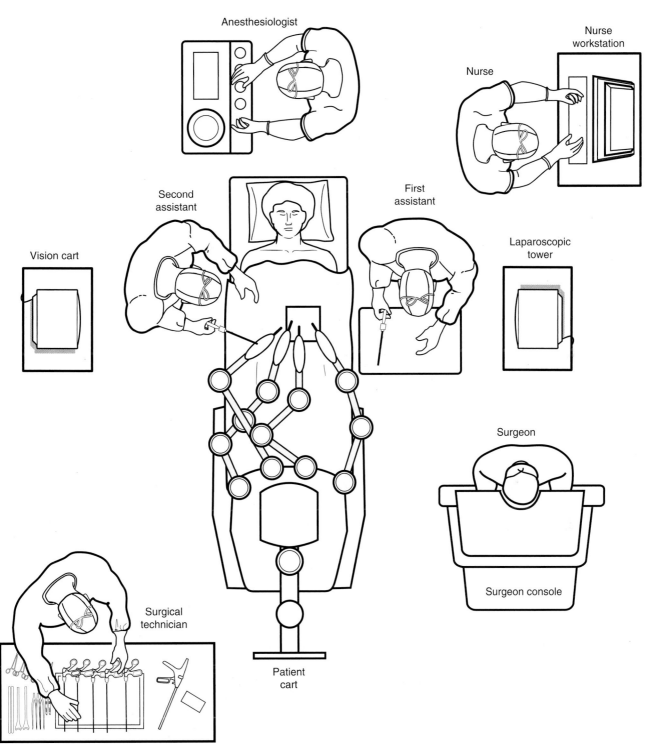

Figure 28-1. Operating room setup and surgical team for robotic Boari flap surgery. *(Redrawn from Higuchi TT, Gettman MT. Robotic instrumentation, personnel and operating room setup. In: Su LM, ed.* Atlas of Robotic Urologic Surgery. *New York: Humana Press; 2011.)*

for use of the Trendelenburg position with the operative site elevated at a 45-degree angle, which can be used to move the bowel contents away from the bladder. Surgically prepare the skin from the xiphoid process to the upper thigh, including the genitalia. An 18 French Foley catheter is inserted.

For patient positioning for robotic Boari flap surgery, prepare the patient in a lithotomy position and carefully secure the patient with a chest band to the table so that a steep Trendelenburg position can be used. The patient is positioned with the legs abducted 60 degrees and slightly flexed at the knee (Figs. 28-1 and 28-2). Surgically prepare the skin from the xiphoid process to the upper thigh, including the genitalia; an 18-French Foley catheter is inserted after draping. The robot is docked between the patient's legs.

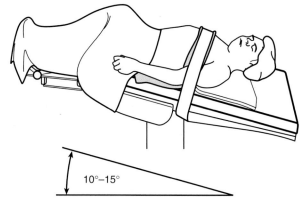

Figure 28-2. Patient position for docking procedure of robotic system in robotic Boari flap surgery.

TROCAR PLACEMENT

Insert the initial trocar at the supraumbilicus using a Veress needle technique with insufflation with CO_2 to access the intraperitoneal cavity via a 12-mm supraumbilical port for the camera. Use CO_2 insufflation pressure up to 20 mm Hg to ensure tense pneumoperitoneum during port placement. Place the first 12-mm camera port on the supraumbilical site using a Visiport Plus Optical Trocar (Covidien, Minneapolis, Minn.), which permits visualization while the initial trocar is introduced. The camera port trocar is secured with a 1-0 silk suture to prevent inadvertent withdrawal during surgery. The abdomen is inspected with the 30-degree downward lens, and additional ports are placed under direct vision. For a laparoscopic Boari flap procedure, place two additional 5-mm working trocars under direct vision at the level of the iliac crest along the lateral edge of the rectus muscle, triangulating these with the camera port. An additional 5-mm assistant port is placed on the cranial side on the line of the lateral edge of the rectus muscle (Fig. 28-3).

For robotic Boari flap surgery, trocar placement through the introduction of the initial endoscopic (camera) port is similar to that for laparoscopic technique. After the initial endoscopic port has been introduced, the trocar positioning is as follows: two 8-mm robotic ports are placed bilaterally at each side 8 cm lateral to the midline camera port at the level of the umbilicus; a fourth 8-mm robotic port is placed on the contralateral side of the pathologic ureter 8 cm lateral to the ipsilateral 8-mm robotic port at a level 3 cm above iliac crest; a 5-mm assistant port is placed between the camera port and the 8-mm robotic port; a 12-mm assistant port is placed on the contralateral side of the fourth arm at a level 3 cm above the iliac crest; and 5-mm and 12-mm assistant ports are placed contralateral to the target side (Fig. 28-4). The robotic arm is docked to the patient; bipolar Maryland forceps are placed on the nondominant hand, and monopolar scissors are placed on the dominant hand. The ProGrasp instrument (Intuitive Surgical, Sunnyvale, Calif.) is placed on the fourth robotic arm.

PROCEDURE (SEE VIDEOS 28-1 AND 28-2)

After placement of ports and completion of the docking procedure, laparoscopic or robotic Boari flap surgery requires the following steps:

1. Adhesiolysis of any intra-abdominal adhesions.
2. Incision of the white line of Toldt and medial mobilization of the colon.
3. Ureteral identification and free dissection from its surrounding attachment with preservation of ureteral vascularity to maximize ureteral blood supply.

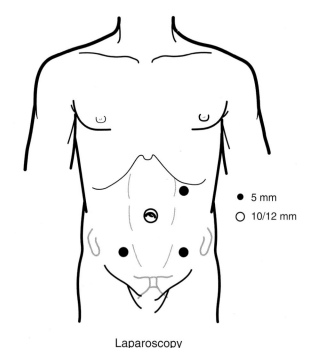

● 5 mm
○ 10/12 mm

Laparoscopy

Figure 28-3. In the laparoscopic Boari flap procedure, a 12-mm trocar is placed at the supraumbilicus for the camera. Two additional trocars are placed at the level of the anterior superior iliac crest lateral to the rectus muscles. The 5-mm port is placed cranial to the umbilicus and lateral to the rectus muscle. In the robotic Boari flap procedure, a midline, periumbilical point 15 cm from the pubic symphysis is marked. The two medial robotic trocars are placed 15 cm from the pubic symphysis and 8 cm from the periumbilical mark. The two lateral trocars are placed in a straight line 8 cm lateral from the medial trocars. The camera is placed in a 12-mm trocar superior to the umbilicus. A 5-mm assistant port is placed 8 cm cranially from the camera port.

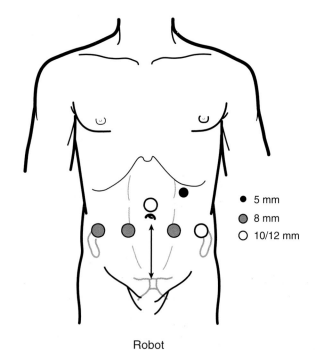

● 5 mm
● 8 mm
○ 10/12 mm

Robot

Figure 28-4. Trocar placement for robotic Boari flap ureteral reimplantation.

4. Identification of the pathologic area of the ureter.
5. Mobilization of the bladder with preservation of blood supply.
6. Fixation of the bladder on the psoas muscle.
7. Creation of the L-shaped bladder flap while preventing flap ischemia.
8. Ureteral spatulation and anastomosis with bladder flap.
9. Observation for hemostasis and drain placement.
10. Closure of the trocar sites.

The main principle of the Boari flap is to close the large gap with a tubularized L-shaped bladder flap; the bladder is mobilized to the pathologic area, with an anterior bladder flap of

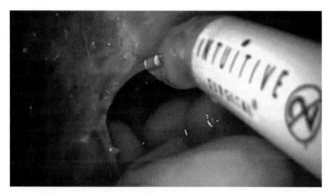

Figure 28-5. Mobilization of sigmoid colon for exposure of the ureter. *(From the video Robotic Boari Flap for Ureteral Stricture. Presented at the European Robotic Urology Symposium [ERUS], London, 2012. Courtesy Michael Stifelman, MD, New York University, Robotic Surgery Center, New York, N.Y.)*

2 cm and a base of 4 cm created and extended to the ipsilateral posterior dome. The ratio of bladder flap length to base width should be within 3:1 to prevent flap ischemia.

For long ureteral defects from 12 to 15 cm in length, a Boari flap technique should be performed in addition to a psoas hitch procedure.

Mobilizing the Colon

The technique of laparoscopic and robotic Boari flap is practically a replication of the open Boari flap technique. The cecum or sigmoid colon is initially mobilized depending on the side of the pathology (Fig. 28-5). Deflect the colon medially by incising the line of Toldt from the liver on the right side and spleen on the left side to the medial umbilical ligament. Then, extend the incision medial to the umbilical ligament on the anterior abdominal wall.

Identifying and Securing the Ureter

In female patients, make the initial dissection in the peritoneal fold between the bladder and uterus to gain access to the ureters in the region of the trigone. In male patients, the ureter can be seen as it crosses posterior to the vas deferens. Create a peritoneal window, and free and elevate the ureter inferior to the vas deferens.

After the mobilization of the sigmoid colon or the caecum, the ureter is identified. The ureter is dissected while preserving vascularity, and the fourth robotic arm is used for traction of the ureter caudally to the pathologic segment. Transect the normal ureter above the pathologic area and spatulate it posteriorly on the normal ureter proximal end (Figs. 28-6, 28-7, and 28-8).

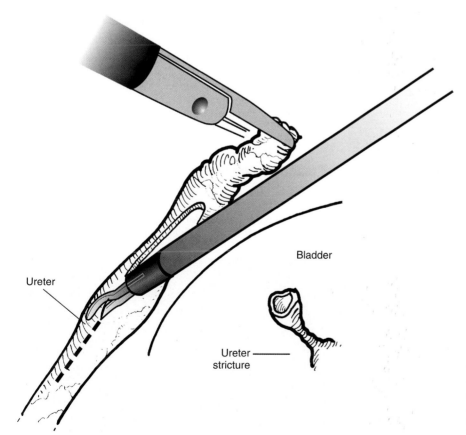

Ureter

Bladder

Ureter stricture

Figure 28-6. A peritoneal window is created and the ureter identified. It can be difficult to locate the precise area of ureteral stricture. An opened catheter can be advanced to the level of the stricture during the procedure with a flexible scope in the male patient or at the start of the procedure in a female patient. Once the stricture has been identified, the ureter is incised. It is helpful to spatulate the ureter before complete transection.

Mobilization of the Bladder

The ureter is transected and the bladder is mobilized as far as possible without ligation of the contralateral superior vesical pedicle. Then, the bladder is mobilized as distal as possible ipsilaterally to the structured ureter (Fig. 28-9). It is very important not to transect the vascular supply of the bladder. Saline was used to fill the bladder, and the surgeon could choose to perform a Boari flap ureteral implantation.

Psoas Hitch

Use 2-0 Vicryl on a round-body needle. Make the first pass into the posterior bladder muscle, then pass the needle into

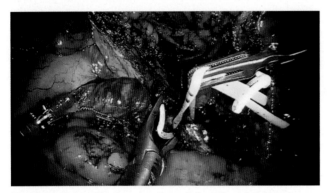

Figure 28-7. Identification of ureter and dissection of pathologic ureter by robotic instruments and VessiLoop. *(From the video Robotic Boari Flap. Courtesy Alejandro R. Rodriguez, Samaritan Urology Center, Samaritan Medical Center, Watertown, N.Y.)*

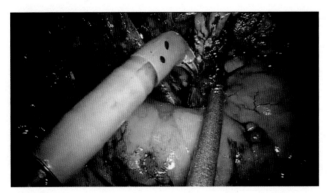

Figure 28-8. Spatulation of proximal ureter by robotic monopolar scissors. *(From the video Robotic Boari Flap. Courtesy Alejandro R. Rodriguez, Samaritan Urology Center, Samaritan Medical Center, Watertown, N.Y.)*

the psoas muscle longitudinally, taking care not to injure any other structure, including the genitofemoral and femoral nerves (Fig. 28-10). Take a second suture lateral to the first to support the hitch.

Creation of the L-Shaped Bladder Flap

If a Boari flap is necessary, fill the bladder with 150 to 200 mL of saline and incise the overlying anterior and contralateral peritoneum. Ligate and transect the urachus with clips. With blunt dissection, free the bladder anteriorly, into the Retzius space. Create an anterior bladder flap with an apex of approximately 2 cm and a base of 4 cm, beginning about 2 cm distal from the bladder neck and extending to the ipsilateral posterior dome (Figs. 28-11 and 28-12).

The flap, fashioned from an anterior cystotomy of 2 cm proximal to bladder neck with a length-to-width ratio of 2:1, is carried toward the bladder dome, assuming that the base of the flap remains wide enough for vascular supply. Fugita and colleagues determined that the apical flap width of 2 cm with a base flap width of 4 cm results in an appropriate vascular supply. The apex of the flap is anastomosed to the distal ureter with 4-0 Vicryl suture (Figs. 28-13 and 28-14). After ureteral anastomosis, the cystotomy is closed in a two-layer fashion with 4-0 Vicryl for the mucosa and submucosa layer and 2-0 Vicryl for the muscle and serosa layer. Bladder flap size varies according to the length of the ureteral defect to be spanned (Fig. 28-15). After completion of the posterior anastomosis, pass the double-J stent up the ureter and renal pelvis under laparoscopic or robotic camera and fluoroscopic guidance by first advancing a guidewire. Advance the stent over the wire, and subsequently remove the wire (Figs. 28-16 and 28-17). Place the double-J stent in the bladder, and use an interrupted 4-0 Vicryl suture to close the anterior flap. Close the cystotomy with running 4-0 Vicryl and 2-0 Vicryl suture to form a watertight seal (Figs. 28-18 and 28-19). Confirm the integrity of the closure by filling the bladder with 250 to 300 mL of saline and reinforcing it with interrupted 2-0 Vicryl suture if any irrigant leaks. The bladder is then filled with 200 mL of saline to exclude any extravasation. Retroperitonealize with the peritoneum using Hem-o-lok clips (Weck Closure Systems, Research Triangle Park, N.C.) (Fig. 28-20). The drain is inserted through the 5-mm assistance port.

Creation of the Submucosal Tunnel

Although it is not mandatory to access the submucosal tunnel for creation of a nonrefluxing ureteral anastomosis, some surgeons have performed a submucosal tunnel procedure in the wall of the bladder for prevention of urine reflux.

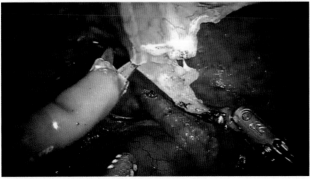
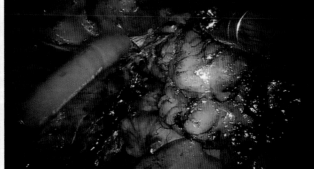

Figure 28-9. Bladder mobilization by incision of medial umbilical ligament with preservation of vascular supply. *(From the video Robotic Boari Flap. Courtesy Alejandro R. Rodriguez, Samaritan Urology Center, Samaritan Medical Center, Watertown, N.Y.)*

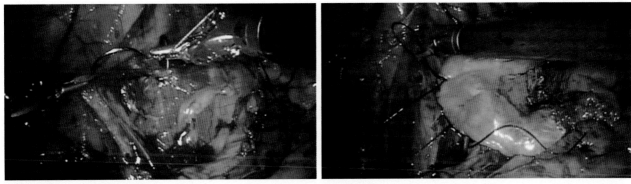

Figure 28-10. Robotic psoas hitch procedure. *(From the video Robotic Boari Flap for Ureteral Stricture. Presented at the European Robotic Urology Symposium [ERUS], London, 2012. Courtesy Michael Stifelman, MD, New York University, Robotic Surgery Center, New York, N.Y.)*

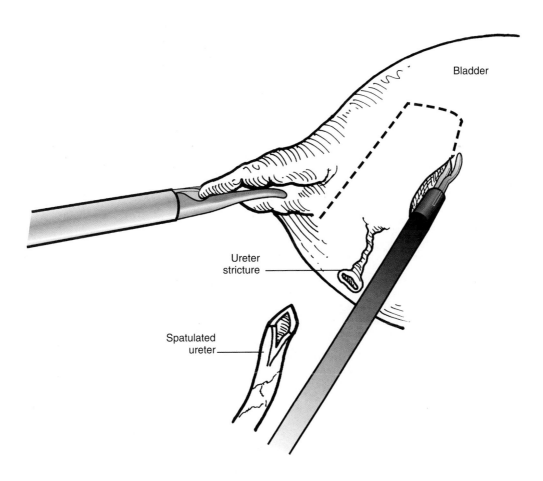

Bladder

Ureter
stricture

Spatulated
ureter

Figure 28-11. For a laparoscopic Boari flap procedure with a bladder catheter, the bladder is distended and the peritoneum opened from the lateral, anterior, and posterior aspects. The surface is cleared, and the bladder is mobilized. The anticipated area of insertion is identified with the bladder distended.

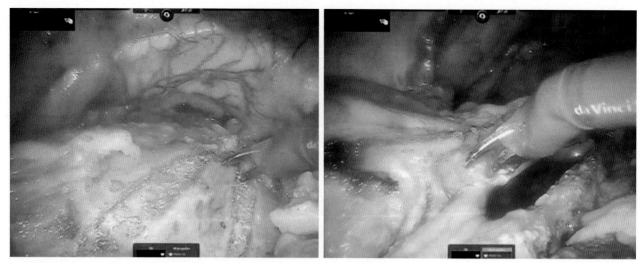

Figure 28-12. Scoring of the Boari flap with robotic monopolar scissors and incision of the flap toward the bladder dome with consideration of the vascular supply. *(From the video Robotic Boari Flap for Ureteral Stricture. Presented at the European Robotic Urology Symposium [ERUS], London, 2012. Courtesy Michael Stifelman, MD, New York University, Robotic Surgery Center, New York, N.Y.)*

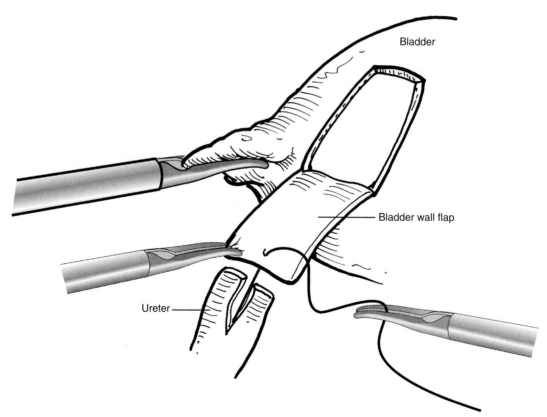

Figure 28-13. For a laparoscopic Boari flap procedure, 4-0 Vicryl suture is placed in the end of the spatulated ureter. The bladder flap is pulled down to ensure a tension-free anastomosis, and the bladder entry site is chosen in an inferior and medial location. The apex suture is placed in the bladder.

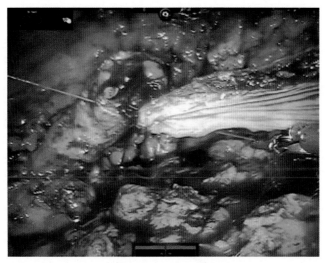

Figure 28-14. The apex of the flap is anastomosed to the distal ureter with interrupted 4-0 Vicryl suture.

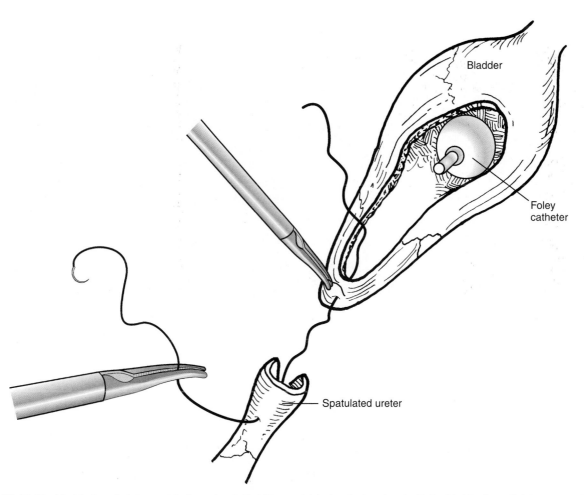

Figure 28-15. The bladder is pulled down while the suture is tied. The spatulated ureter is sutured with the bladder flap with intracorporeal techniques, and a double-J stent is introduced into the bladder.

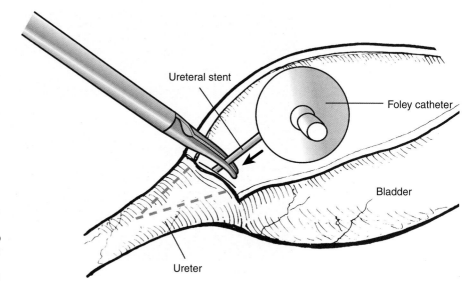

Figure 28-16. The double-J stent is pulled into the bladder and advanced up the ureter over a wire. A grasper is used to gently advance the double-J stent into position. A long stent is chosen so that it can be advanced to the kidney and also be in a dependent portion of the bladder.

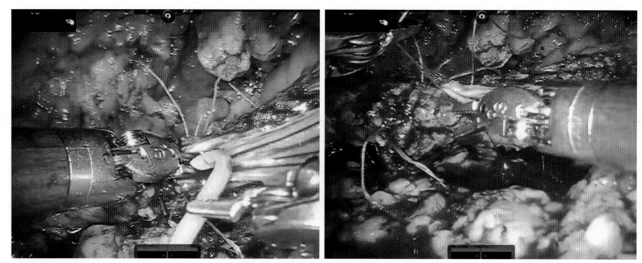

Figure 28-17. After completion of the posterior anastomosis, pass the double-J stent up the ureter and renal pelvis under laparoscopic or robotic camera and fluoroscopic guidance by first advancing a guidewire. Advance the stent over the wire, and subsequently remove the wire. *(From the video Robotic Boari Flap for Ureteral Stricture. Presented at the European Robotic Urology Symposium [ERUS], London, 2012. Courtesy Michael Stifelman, MD, New York University, Robotic Surgery Center, New York, N.Y.)*

This procedure is challenging with a laparoscopic approach in most cases due to the specific angle to the tissue that often cannot be approached by rigid laparoscopic instruments. On the robotic approach, the instruments of 7 degree freedom allows specific angle on submucosal tunnel and suture of ureter and bladder. After creation of submucosal tunneling (Fig. 28-21), the distal end of the ureter is pulled through the tunnel and sutured in the same manner (Fig. 28-22).

Observation for Hemostasis and Injury

After the repair is complete, inspect the bowel and retroperitoneum for potential visceral injury or bleeding at 5 mm Hg pressure, and remove instruments and trocars under direct laparoscopic or robotic vision.

Closure

Close the incision after removing the pneumoperitoneum completely. Place subcutaneous closure sutures at each 8-mm and 5-mm trocar site with absorbable sutures. Close the skin at all port sites in standard fashion.

Laparoendoscopic Single-Site Reconstructive Surgery

Recently, focused on a development of laparoscopy, we have made the transition from multiple-port to single-port access: laparoendoscopic single-site surgery (LESS) (Fig. 28-23). LESS has become attractive for multiple urologic procedures, and nearly entire clinical series of urologic

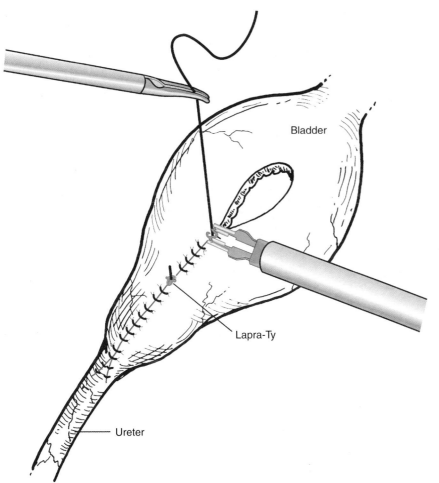

Bladder

Lapra-Ty

Ureter

Figure 28-18. The Lapra-Ty instrument (Ethicon, Cincinnati, Ohio) is useful when closing a long suture line because shorter sutures are usually easier to work with during laparoscopy. The Lapra-Ty is being applied to the first suture closing the bladder. When the anastomosis is complete, the last tie can be replaced with a Lapra-Ty, making the suture line watertight.

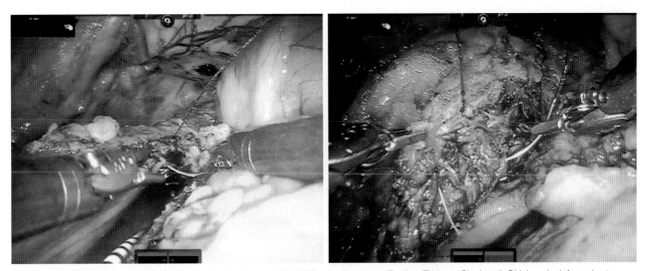

Figure 28-19. Distal closure of the bladder flap in two layers with 4-0 Vicryl using Lapra-Ty clips (Ethicon, Cincinnati, Ohio) and reinforced suture with 2-0 Vicryl. *(From the video Robotic Boari Flap for Ureteral Stricture. Presented at the European Robotic Urology Symposium [ERUS], London, 2012. Courtesy Michael Stifelman, MD, New York University, Robotic Surgery Center, New York, N.Y.)*

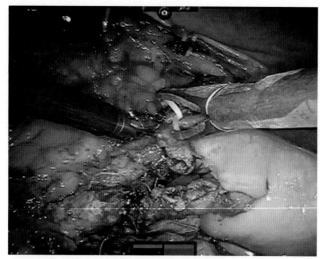

Figure 28-20. Retroperitonealization with the peritoneum using a Hem-o-lok clip (Weck Closure Systems, Research Triangle Park, N.C.) *(From the video Robotic Boari Flap for Ureteral Stricture. Presented at the European Robotic Urology Symposium [ERUS], London, 2012. Courtesy Michael Stifelman, MD, New York University, Robotic Surgery Center, New York, N.Y.)*

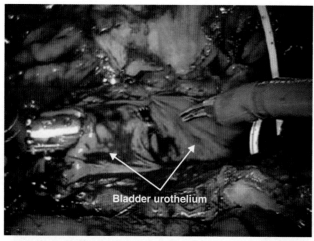

Figure 28-21. Creation of submucosal tunnel in a robotic Boari flap procedure. *(From Do M, Kallidonis P, Qazi H, et al. Robot-assisted technique for Boari flap ureteral reimplantation: is robot assistance beneficial? J Endourol. 2014;28:679-685.)*

procedures have been reported. LESS with a single, hidden incision allows scar-free surgery. However, because of the technical novelty and rarity of cases, there are just a few reports of urologic reconstructive LESS. LESS technique for reconstructive urologic surgery decreased port site complications, scarring, and intermediated levels of discomfort. However, challenges encountered with LESS include difficulty with suturing and clashing of instruments that results from limited triangulation and limitation of retraction. These difficulties are especially problematic during reconstructive urologic procedures in which advanced suturing

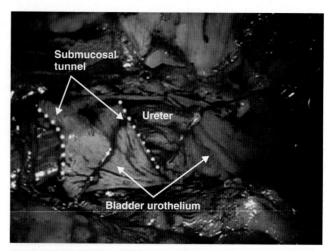

Figure 28-22. Passage of spatulated ureter through the submucosal tunnel. *(From Do M, Kallidonis P, Qazi H, et al. Robot-assisted technique for Boari flap ureteral reimplantation: is robot assistance beneficial? J Endourol. 2014;28:679-685.)*

is required. Accordingly, accessory instrumentation, novel platforms, and robotic LESS have been evaluated to help reduce the level of difficulty. Reports on LESS Boari flap procedures are lacking because of the rarity of diseases and the difficulty of the multiple-suture technique. Further development of technology for reconstructive LESS is required.

POSTOPERATIVE MANAGEMENT

The Jackson-Pratt drain through fourth robotic port is left in the pelvis and is typically removed at 48 hours when the drain creatinine level suggests no urine leakage.

The patient is allowed to start on a clear liquid diet after the surgery, proceeding to a soft diet and then a regular diet as tolerated. The patient ambulates on the first postoperative morning. Pain is controlled with a patient-controlled device administering narcotics or with oral nonsteroidal anti-inflammatory drugs. Anticholinergics are prescribed as an adjunct to postoperative pain medication to decrease bladder spasm or stent-related discomfort. The Foley catheter is typically left in place for 5 to 10 days depending on cystotomy size and the quality of the bladder repair; depending on surgeon preference, cystography may be performed. The rationale for the use of ureteral stents is to prevent urine leakage, promote ureteral healing, and prevent ureter stricture. However, a long duration of ureteral stenting could cause inadequate healing and scar tissue formation. Kerbl and colleagues found no significant difference in the healing of the ureter based on period of stenting. However, most centers recommend that the ureteral stent remain in place for 4 to 6 weeks postoperatively for healing of the ureteral anastomosis site. Recurrent stricture of the ureter could be managed by balloon dilation, endoureterotomy, and surgical revision of the ureter.

COMPLICATIONS

The complications after laparoscopic or robotic Boari flap surgery have been reviewed and are few. Comparison of

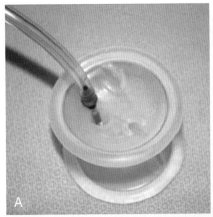
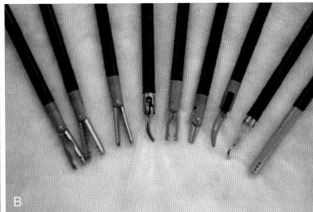
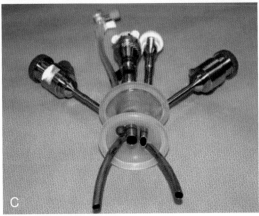

Figure 28-23. The da Vinci system (Intuitive Surgical, Sunnyvale, Calif.) single-site instrumentation. **A,** Multichannel port. **B,** Instruments. **C,** Setup, including the 8.5-mm camera, the two 5-mm robotic instruments through the curved cannulas, and the 5- or 10-mm assistant port. *(From Kaouk JH, Autorino R, Laydner H, et al. Robotic single-site kidney surgery: evaluation of second-generation instruments in a cadaver model. Urology. 2012;79:975-979.)*

complication rates in laparoscopic versus robotic Boari flap procedures has not been studied owing to the small number of patients requiring this surgery. The most common complication is ureteral stricture at the surgical site. A diuretic renogram is helpful in determining actual obstruction. If the obstruction is present, balloon dilation or chronic stent changes may relieve the obstruction. Prolonged urinary drainage through the drain may occur. If the ureteral stent or catheter is well placed, the condition is usually temporary. Review the surgical repair and suturing of the flap, and confirm the position of the ureteral stent or catheter. Hemorrhage, ileus, infection, injury to a major vessel, and bowel injury are possible complications after laparoscopic or robotic Boari flap procedures. The surgical team must be prepared for conversion to an open procedure in an emergent situation; therefore, a general laparotomy set and vascular clamps must be prepared for every procedure.

TIPS AND TRICKS

- Exact information regarding the length and location of the stricture will aid in preoperative planning.
- Check for the appropriate Trendelenburg position and security of the patient before beginning the procedure.
- The tips of the scissors must be visible during electrocautery to avoid inadvertent bowel injury.
- Adequate dissection of the ureter without traumatic manipulation is necessary to preserve vascularity.
- Gentle handling of the bladder will reduce bladder spasm and hematuria.
- The ratio of bladder flap length to base width should be within 3:1 to prevent flap ischemia.
- Meticulous watertight closure of the bladder and ureter should be performed, with adequate postoperative drainage.

SUGGESTED READINGS

Autorino R, Stein RJ, Lima E, Damiano R, Khanna R, Haber GP, et al. Current status and future perspectives in laparoendoscopic single-site and natural orifice transluminal endoscopic urological surgery. *Int J Urol*. 2010;17:410–431.

Baldie K, Angell J, Ogan K, Hood N, Pattaras JG. Robotic management of benign mid and distal ureteral strictures and comparison with laparoscopic approaches at a single institution. *Urology*. 2012;80:596–601.

Desai MM, Stein R, Rao P, Canes D, Aron M, Rao PP, et al. Embryonic natural orifice transumbilical endoscopic surgery (E-NOTES) for advanced reconstruction: initial experience. *Urology*. 2009;73:182–187.

Do M, Kallidonis P, Qazi H, Liatsikos E, Ho Thi P, Dietel A, et al. Robot-assisted technique for Boari flap ureteral reimplantation: is robot assistance beneficial? *J Endourol*. 2014;28:679–685.

Fugita OE, Dinlenc C, Kavoussi L. The laparoscopic Boari flap. *J Urol*. 2001;166:51–53.

Fugita OE, Kavoussi L. Laparoscopic ureteral reimplantation for ureteral lesion secondary to transvaginal ultrasonography for oocyte retrieval. *Urology*. 2001;58:281.

Kerbl K, Chandhoke PS, Figenshau RS, Stone AM, Clayman RV. Effect of stent duration on ureteral healing following endoureterotomy in an animal model. *J Urol*. 1993;150:1302–1305.

Khanna R, Isac W, Laydner H, Autorino R, White MA, Hillyer S, et al. Laparoendoscopic single site reconstructive procedures in urology: medium term results. *J Urol*. 2012;187:1702–1706.

Kimchi D, Wiesenfeld A. Injuries to the lower third of ureter treated by bladder flap plasty: Boari-Kuss technique; report of two cases. *J Urol*. 1963;89:800–803.

Komninos C, Koo KC, Rha KH. Laparoendoscopic management of midureteral strictures. *Korean J Urol*. 2014;55:2–8.

Novick AC, Jones JS, Gill IS, eds. *Operative Urology at the Cleveland Clinic*. Totowa, NJ: Humana Press; 2006.

Phillips EA, Wang DS. Current status of robot-assisted laparoscopic ureteral reimplantation and reconstruction. *Curr Urol Rep*. 2012;13:190–194.

Schimpf MO, Wagner JR. Robot-assisted laparoscopic Boari flap ureteral reimplantation. *J Endourol*. 2008:222691–222694.

Windsperger AP, Duchene DA. Robotic reconstruction of lower ureteral strictures. *Urol Clin North Am*. 2013;40:363–370.

29 Laparoscopic Appendiceal Onlay Flap and Bowel Reconfiguration for Complex Ureteral Stricture Reconstruction

Brian D. Duty

A variety of pathologic conditions may result in ureteral stricture disease. These include urolithiasis, genitourinary infection, retroperitoneal fibrosis, radiation therapy, external trauma, and iatrogenic injury. Strictures below the pelvic brim can usually be managed effectively by ureteral reimplantation with or without bladder advancement. Proximal and midureteral strictures are more difficult to reconstruct. Treatment options include pyeloplasty, ureteroureterostomy, transureteroureterostomy, and ureteral reimplantation with Boari flap and renal mobilization. Long strictures frequently require ileal interposition, autotransplantation, or nephrectomy.

Potential complications of ileal interposition include metabolic acidosis, vitamin B_{12} deficiency, short gut syndrome, hyperoxaluria, small bowel anastomotic stricture, and enterocutaneous fistula. Although autotransplantation avoids potential metabolic and bowel complications, graft loss from perioperative complications has been reported in up to 40% of cases.

Melnikoff first reported using the appendix to treat ureteral stricture disease in 1912. Multiple case reports and small case series have subsequently been published. Appendiceal interposition eliminates the risk of small bowel and vascular complications and decreases the likelihood of metabolic derangements. However, the narrow caliber of the appendix makes performing the anastomosis challenging and increases the risk of ureteroappendiceal anastomotic stricture. Using the appendix as a detubularized onlay flap maintains the potential advantages of interposition and decreases the aforementioned risks.

Reggio and colleagues reported the first laparoscopic appendiceal onlay flap ureteroplasty in 2009. The same institution subsequently published the results from a series of six patients undergoing the laparoscopic onlay procedure with subjective and objective success rates of 66% and 100%, respectively. No perioperative complications were encountered.

Alternatives to the appendiceal onlay procedure include small intestine (Yang-Monti) and colon transverse tubular reconfiguration with end-to-end anastomosis. Both procedures are associated with decreased risk of metabolic complications compared with ileal ureter reconstruction, but the potential for bowel leak and obstruction remain. As with appendiceal interposition, the narrow lumen of the reconfigured bowel segment makes performing the ureteral anastomosis difficult and may carry a higher risk of postoperative stricture.

INDICATIONS AND CONTRAINDICATIONS

Laparoscopic appendiceal onlay flap ureteroplasty should be considered for patients with right proximal or midureteral strictures longer than 1.5 cm. Individuals with shorter, nonischemic strictures may benefit from an initial attempt at endoureterotomy, given its decreased invasiveness and because failure does not preclude future reconstruction.

Patients having undergone an appendectomy are not candidates for the onlay flap procedure. Transverse tubular reconfiguration of the small intestines or colon is a feasible alternative in these patients or those with left-sided strictures.

The absolute contraindications are no different than for most laparoscopic procedures: uncorrected coagulopathy and untreated infection or sepsis. Relative contraindications include morbid obesity, prior abdominal surgery, and retroperitoneal radiotherapy.

PATIENT PREOPERATIVE EVALUATION AND PREPARATION

It is imperative to completely assess stricture location, length, and severity to counsel patients regarding the potential reconstructive options and their associated risks. Various diagnostic tools are available to characterize ureteral strictures, including excretory urography (computed tomography urography, intravenous pyelography) and antegrade and retrograde pyelography.

Patients referred with a ureteral stent can pose a diagnostic challenge if their stricture has not been fully worked up. It is prudent to delay reconstructive surgery because the stent can obscure the true extent of the stricture intraoperatively. Patients with normal renal function and no symptoms before stent placement should have the stent removed and should undergo urography 2 to 4 weeks later. If the patient had renal insufficiency or flank pain before stenting, then stent removal with nephrostomy tube placement should be considered.

A preoperative nuclear medicine scan should be performed in patients with long-standing obstruction and evidence of parenchymal atrophy on anatomic imaging. Patients with ipsilateral renal function less than 20% may be better served by a simple nephrectomy rather than a complex reconstructive procedure.

OPERATING ROOM CONFIGURATION AND PATIENT POSITIONING FOR THE APPENDICEAL ONLAY PROCEDURE

The primary surgeon and assistant stand to the left of the patient facing the abdomen. The scrub nurse stands on the opposite side of the patient. A minimum of two monitors should be available. One monitor is located across from the primary surgeon at chest level. The second monitor provides visualization for the scrub nurse and is positioned at the midabdomen behind the surgeon and assistant (Fig. 29-1).

After induction of general anesthesia and intubation, an orogastric tube is placed by the anesthesia provider. The abdomen is then shaved if needed. The patient is placed in the modified decubitus position with the right flank elevated 30 degrees. The chest and pelvis are secured to the operating

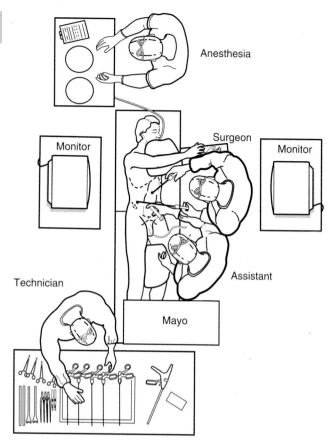

Figure 29-1. Operating room configuration. The surgeon and assistant stand to the left of the patient. The scrub nurse stands to the patient's right side. Monitors are placed on both sides of the patient to allow visualization by all team members.

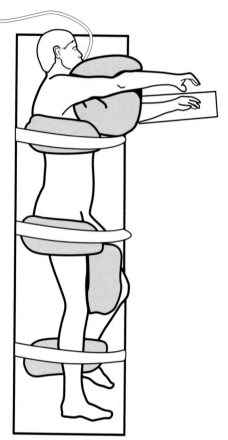

Figure 29-2. Patient positioning. The patient is placed in the modified decubitus position with the right flank elevated 30 degrees. The chest and hips are fixed to the operating room table with wide cloth tape. The right arm is draped over the chest, padded, and loosely secured to the table.

room table with wide cloth tape, and the right arm is draped over the chest and gently secured into place. Foam padding is used to prevent brachial plexus injury. A pillow is placed under the knees (Fig. 29-2). A test roll is then performed by rotating the operating room table to the left to ensure that the patient is adequately secured. The patient is then prepared in a sterile fashion from the nipples to the genitalia.

URETERAL STENT PLACEMENT

Ureteral stent placement can be performed in a retrograde or antegrade fashion. It is my preference to place the stent at the beginning of the procedure. A flexible cystoscope is inserted into the bladder. The right ureteral orifice is cannulated with a guidewire over which a 7-French stent is placed. If fluoroscopy is not used, then the stent should be 2 cm longer than usual. Alternatively, a multilength stent can be placed. In women the stent can be deployed freehand. In men the pusher device will need to be used, either with fluoroscopic guidance or under direct visualization with the flexible cystoscope located within the posterior urethra adjacent to the stent as it is being deployed. After stent placement, a 16-French bladder catheter is inserted.

TROCAR PLACEMENT

Once the stent and bladder catheter have been placed, the operating room table is rotated to the right away from the surgeon. While establishing the pneumoperitoneum, the assistant

typically stands opposite the primary surgeon to the right of the patient. Either the Veress needle or Hasson technique is used to obtain peritoneal access at the level of the umbilicus. Pneumoperitoneum is initially established at 20 mm Hg to provide maximum abdominal distention. The first trocar placed is a 10-mm periumbilical port. Once the initial trocar has been placed, the intra-abdominal contents are inspected to ensure no vascular or bowel injury has occurred. The remaining ports are placed under direct visualization. These include a 12-mm port located along the right midclavicular line halfway between the periumbilical trocar and anterior superior iliac spine and a 5-mm subxiphoid trocar (Fig. 29-3). The pneumoperitoneum is then decreased to 15 mm Hg. The operative table is then rotated to the left to facilitate passive retraction of the intra-abdominal contents by gravity.

PROCEDURE (SEE VIDEO 29-1)
Retroperitoneal Exposure

Once the ports have been placed, the retroperitoneum is exposed by incising the line of Toldt along the right pericolic gutter with either electrosurgical scissors or ultrasonic dissection (Fig. 29-4). The lateral colonic peritoneal reflection is incised from below the right common iliac vessels to the hepatic flexure, which usually rests on the anterior aspect of the lower pole of the kidney (Fig. 29-5). The peritoneum overlying the upper pole of the kidney need not be divided.

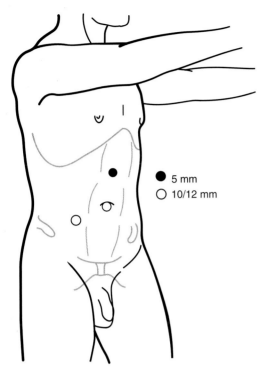

Figure 29-3. Trocar configuration. A 10/12-mm periumbilical camera port and a 10/12-mm right lower quadrant working port are used. A 5-mm subxiphoid trocar is used for the second working port. If required, a liver retractor is placed via an additional 5-mm port cranial and left of the subxiphoid port.

● 5 mm
○ 10/12 mm

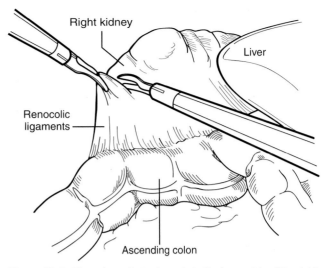

Figure 29-5. The colorenal attachments to the lower pole of the right kidney are divided, allowing for medial mobilization of the hepatic flexure.

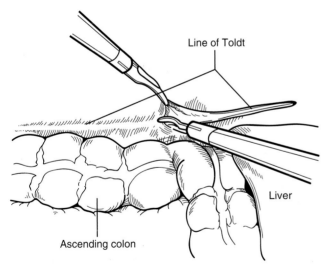

Figure 29-4. The line of Toldt along the right pericolic gutter is incised and the colon is mobilized medially.

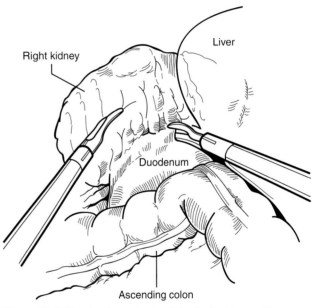

Figure 29-6. The duodenum is sharply kocherized to provide exposure to the proximal ureter.

is mobilized until the anterior aspect of the vena cava is clearly visible.

Identification and Preparation of the Ureter

After exposure of the retroperitoneum, the right ureter is identified. The midureter rests medial to the psoas muscle within the retroperitoneal fat. Near the iliac vessels the right ureter is usually lateral and deep to the gonadal vessels. Ureteral stent placement at the beginning of the procedure helps facilitate ureteral identification. Once the ureter has been located, the gonadal vessels are mobilized medially away from the ureter. If necessary, the gonadal vessels can be divided with bipolar electrocautery or with metal clips.

The ureter proximal and distal to the stenosed segment is completely mobilized. Mobilization should be performed sharply to prevent thermal injury (Fig. 29-7). Bipolar rather than monopolar electrocautery, if needed, should be used to

If the stricture involves the proximal ureter, then the liver will often need to be retracted anteriorly. An additional 5 mm trocar can be placed cranial and to the left of the subxiphoid port. A self-retraining grasper is secured to the right lateral body wall to elevate the liver. Care must be taken to not puncture the diaphragm when securing the grasper.

Proximal ureteral strictures also frequently require the duodenum to be kocherized for optimal exposure. Medial mobilization of the duodenum should be performed sharply and with gentle traction to avoid thermal injury and disruption of the serosa (Fig. 29-6). The duodenum

facilitate hemostasis. Dissection posterior to the strictured ureter is avoided to minimize devascularization of the ureteral flap bed.

Once the strictured segment has been isolated, the anterior wall of the narrowed ureter is opened longitudinally with cold scissors (Fig. 29-8). The incision is carried through to healthy ureter proximally and distally. Care is taken to not transect the ureteral stent.

Harvesting the Appendix

Once the ureter has been prepared, attention is turned to harvesting the appendiceal flap. The appendix is identified and surrounded with laparotomy pads to minimize the risk of contamination of adjacent structures. The length and caliber of the appendix are assessed to ensure it is suitable for the onlay flap. If not sufficient, then an alternative reconstruction

procedure is performed as previously discussed with the patient.

If appropriate for use, then a plane is created between the mesoappendix and the base of the appendix, with care being taken to not damage the appendiceal artery (Fig. 29-9). The base of the appendix is detached from the cecum using an Endo GIA stapling device (Covidien, Minneapolis, Minn.) with 2.5-mm staples (Fig. 29-10). The tip of the appendix is removed and the appendiceal lumen is flushed with a suction-irrigator device. The appendix is then detubularized along its antimesenteric border, and the laparotomy pads are removed from the abdomen (Fig. 29-11).

Performing the Onlay Procedure

After the appendiceal onlay flap has been prepared, the anastomosis is performed. The flap is sutured with 4-0 Vicryl to the

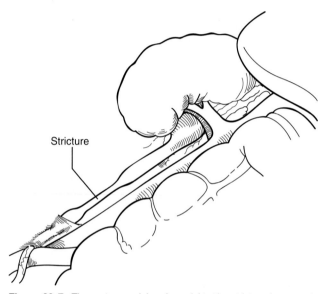

Figure 29-7. The ureter cranial and caudal to the strictured segment is mobilized circumferentially. Dissection is not performed posterior to the ureteral stricture, to maintain blood supply to the onlay bed.

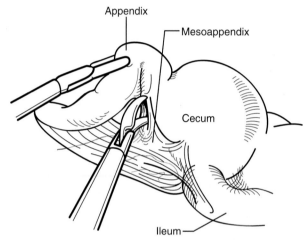

Figure 29-9. A window is created between the mesoappendix and base of the appendix. Care is taken to not damage the appendiceal artery. *(Redrawn from Fischer JE, Jones DB, Pomposelli FB, Upchurch GR Jr, eds.* Fischer's Mastery of Surgery, *6th ed. Philadelphia: Lippincott Williams & Wilkins; 2011.)*

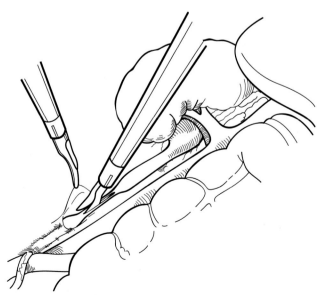

Figure 29-8. The strictured ureter is sharply opened anteriorly. The incision should be carried through to healthy ureter both proximally and distally.

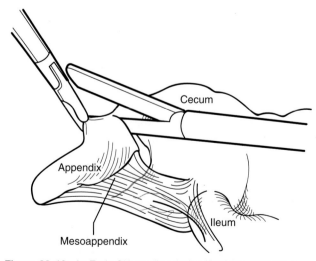

Figure 29-10. An Endo GIA stapling device (Covidien, Minneapolis, Minn.) with 2.5-mm staples is used to detach the base of the appendix from the cecum. *(Redrawn from Fischer JE, Jones DB, Pomposelli FB, Upchurch GR Jr, eds.* Fischer's Mastery of Surgery, *6th ed. Philadelphia: Lippincott Williams & Wilkins; 2011.)*

posterior wall of the longitudinally opened ureter. The medial and lateral walls are sewn individually, with care taken to not entrap the stent in the suture (Fig. 29-12).

Drain Placement and Closure

Once the anastomosis has been performed, hemostasis is obtained and the surgical bed is copiously irrigated. The cecum is once again inspected to ensure the staple line is intact. The liver retractor is removed. Fascial closure sutures (2-0 Vicryl) are preplaced through the periumbilical and right lower quadrant trocar sites with the Carter-Thomason closure device (CooperSurgical, Trumbull, Conn.).

A closed suction drain is then placed through the right lower quadrant port and positioned adjacent to the onlay anastomosis. The port is removed and the preplaced fascial suture is tied around the drain tightly enough to prevent loss of pneumoperitoneum but not so tightly that it prevents drain removal. The drain is secured to the skin with a 3-0 nylon suture.

The pneumoperitoneum is decreased to 5 mm Hg. The abdomen is inspected one last time for bleeding. If there are no concerns, then the pneumoperitoneum is evacuated and

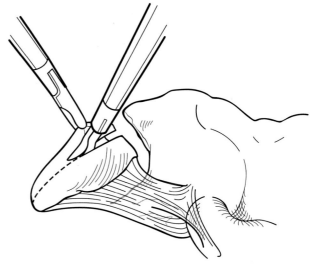

Figure 29-11. The entire length of the appendix is sharply opened along its antimesenteric border.

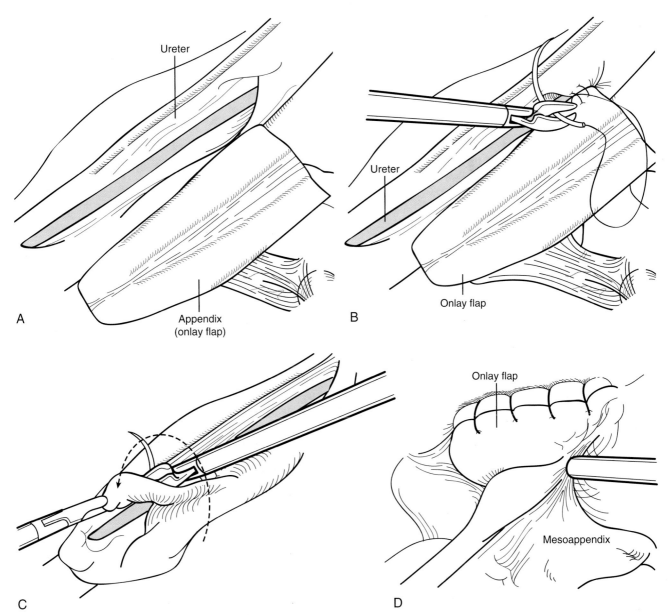

Figure 29-12. The detubularized appendix is anastomosed to the ureteral onlay bed with 2-0 Vicryl suture. **A,** Suturing the appendiceal onlay flap to the proximal end of the incised ureter. **B,** Closure of the medial aspect of the flap. **C,** Lateral closure. **D,** Completed onlay flap.

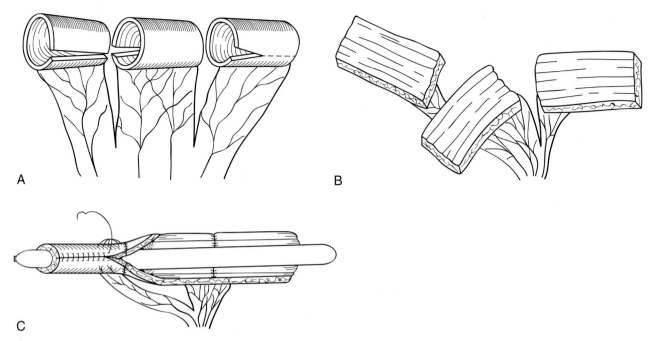

Figure 29-13. A, The ileum is divided into three equal segments, preserving the blood supply to each. **B,** Each segment is opened along its antimesenteric border. **C,** The segments are sewn together and then closed longitudinally over a red rubber catheter. *(Redrawn from Ali-el-Dein B, Ghoneim MA. Bridging long ureteral defects using the Yang-Monti principle.* J Urol. *2003;169:1074.)*

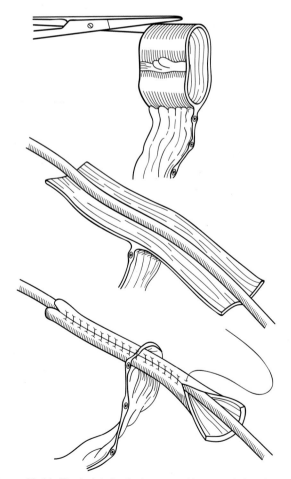

Figure 29-14. The isolated colonic segment is opened along its antimesenteric border and then reconfigured into a long flap, which is closed in a running fashion over a red rubber catheter. *(Redrawn from Lazica DA, Ubrig B, Brandt AS, et al. Ureteral substitution with reconfigured colon: long-term followup.* J Urol. *2012;187:542-548.)*

the remaining trocars are removed. The periumbilical fascial suture is tied down. The remaining incisions are closed in standard fashion.

Small Intestine Transverse Tubular Reconfiguration with Interposition

Preoperative evaluation, operating room setup, patient positioning, and trocar placement are identical to the appendiceal onlay procedure. Approximately 5 cm of terminal ileum is isolated with an Endo GIA stapling device. The exact length varies based on the length of the ureteral defect. Bowel continuity is restored with the Endo GIA device, and the isolated ileal segment is then subdivided into two or three equal 2.5-cm segments (Fig. 29-13). It is imperative to ensure that the individual blood supply to each segment is preserved. The segments are then sharply opened along their antimesenteric borders. The adjacent edges are sewn to each other with 4-0 Vicryl suture. The opened ileal plate is then reconfigured and tubularized over a 16-French red rubber catheter in a running fashion with 4-0 Vicryl suture. The catheter is removed and the proximal ureteral anastomosis is performed in an interrupted fashion. Attention is turned to the distal anastomosis. Once half the anastomosis has been completed, a ureteral stent is placed. The remainder of the anastomosis is completed. A closed suction drain is placed and the surgical site is inspected one last time before the port sites are closed and the abdomen is exited.

Colonic Transverse Tubular Reconfiguration with Interposition

Once the ureteral stricture has been identified, a 3-cm segment of adjacent colon is isolated with the Endo GIA device. Once bowel continuity has been restored, the colonic segment is opened along its antimesenteric border. In contrast to the small intestine procedure, only a single segment of colon is usually required, thereby obviating the need to sew adjacent bowel segments to each other. The colonic segment is then reconfigured creating a long flap, which is once again closed in a running fashion over a 16-French red rubber catheter (Fig. 29-14).

The ureteral anastomoses are then performed in a similar fashion to the small intestine tubularization procedure.

POSTOPERATIVE MANAGEMENT

Most patients spend 1 or 2 nights in the hospital after surgery. They are placed on a clear liquid diet the evening of surgery and advanced to a regular diet on postoperative day 1 in the absence of nausea and vomiting or abdominal distention.

The bladder catheter is removed on postoperative day 2. If the drain output does not significantly increase after catheter removal and has been less than 50 mL for the last 24 hours, then the drain is removed. If the output increases or is greater than 50 mL/day, then the drain fluid is sent for creatinine testing. Urine leak management is detailed later. The ureteral stent is removed in the office 4 to 6 weeks after surgery.

Six weeks after stent removal, renal ultrasound and nuclear medicine scanning are performed. If these studies show no evidence of obstruction, then repeat ultrasonography is performed 6 months after surgery and then annually for 3 years. Additional imaging studies are performed for signs or symptoms of recurrent obstruction such as pain and pyelonephritis.

COMPLICATIONS

General complications associated with laparoscopic surgery to the right upper urinary tract include incisional and internal hernias, abdominal wall hematoma and infection, colon and duodenal injury, liver laceration, and diaphragmatic injury with associated pneumothorax. Standard postoperative complications include prolonged ileus, deep venous thrombosis with or without pulmonary embolism, brachial plexus injury, atrial fibrillation, myocardial infarction, congestive heart failure, and stroke.

Complications specific to the onlay procedure include urinary tract infection, cecal leak, intra-abdominal abscess, urine leak with or without urinoma formation, ureteral obstruction from mucus, and recurrent ureteral stenosis. Urine leak typically manifests with increased drain output and prolonged ileus. Once this has been confirmed by an elevated drain creatinine level, the bladder catheter should be replaced. If the leak persists, the drain should be taken off suction. The drain can also be repositioned by withdrawing a small amount from the incision and resecuring it to the skin. Large-volume urinomas should be drained percutaneously. In rare instances the patient will need to be taken back to the operating room for laparoscopic drainage, urine leak repair, and drain repositioning.

Long-term success rates with the onlay procedure are unknown, given the low number of cases reported in the literature. However, failure rates of 5% to 15% can be expected. Depending on the length and severity of the recurrent stricture, treatment options include chronic ureteral stenting, endoureterotomy, open reconstruction (e.g., ileal ureter, autotransplantation), or nephrectomy.

> **TIPS AND TRICKS**
>
> - Fully characterize the length and severity of the stricture before surgery.
> - If the patient is referred with a ureteral stent and it is feasible to do so, remove the stent 2 to 4 weeks before surgery to reduce ureteral edema and help identify stricture boundaries intraoperatively.
> - Place a multilength stent or a stent 2 cm longer than usual at the beginning of the procedure.
> - Do not mobilize the ureter posterior to the stricture, to maintain blood supply to the onlay bed.
> - Check the drain creatinine level if drain output exceeds 50 mL/day or if the patient has prolonged ileus or signs of peritoneal irritation.

SUGGESTED READINGS

Ali-el-Dein B, Ghoneim MA. Bridging long ureteral defects using the Yang-Monti principle. *J Urol.* 2003;169:1074–1077.

Dagash H, Sen S, Chacko J, et al. The appendix as ureteral substitute: a report of 10 cases. *J Pediatr Urol.* 2008;4:14–19.

Duty BD, Kreshover JE, Richstone L, et al. Review of appendiceal on-lay flap in the management of complex ureteric strictures in six patients. *BJU Int.* 2015;115:282–287.

Lazica DA, Ubrig B, Brandt AS, et al. Ureteral substitution with reconfigured colon: long-term followup. *J Urol.* 2012;187:542–548.

Melnikoff AE. Sur le replacement de l'uretere par anse isolee de l'intestine grele. *Rev Clin Urol.* 1912;1:600–601.

Mesrobian HG, Azizkhan RG. Pyeloureterostomy with appendiceal interposition. *J Urol.* 1989;142:1288–1289.

Reggio E, Richstone L, Okeke Z, et al. Laparoscopic ureteroplasty using on-lay appendix graft. *Urology.* 2009;73:928e7–928e10.

Richter F, Stock JA, Hanna MK. The appendix as right ureteral substitute in children. *J Urol.* 2000;163:1908–1912.

Weinberg RW. Appendix ureteroplasty. *Br J Urol.* 1976;48:234.

Wotkowicz C, Libertino JA. Renal autotransplantation. *BJU Int.* 2004;93:253–257.

30 Buccal Mucosa Graft for Ureteral Strictures

Yuka Yamaguchi, Michael D. Stifelman, Lee C. Zhao

Complex proximal ureteral strictures can be challenging to manage. Whereas distal ureteral to midureteral strictures can be successfully managed with ureteral reimplantation with psoas hitch or Boari flap, proximal ureteral strictures are often managed with ureteroureterostomy. However, when the affected ureteral segment is long, adequate mobilization to bridge the gap between healthy distal and proximal ureteral mucosa to allow for ureteroureterostomy may not be possible. Long or multifocal proximal ureteral strictures may require ileal substitution or autotransplantation of the kidney, options that are associated significant potential morbidity from bowel and vascular complications.

The use of buccal mucosa grafts (BMGs) as an alternative to ileal ureter or autotransplantation has been reported in several case series but has not gained widespread use, perhaps because of the need for an open approach and the relative unfamiliarity of urologists with BMG harvest. However, for reconstructive urologists, BMGs have been a mainstay of treatment for urethral strictures since the 1990s owing to particular characteristics that make it ideal for the urinary tract. It has a panlaminar vascular plexus ideal for engraftment and a thick nonkeratinized epithelium compatible with a wet environment. It is a graft material that has proven to be durable in the urinary tract without the risk of metabolic complications associated with use of bowel interposition. The application of robotic technology with its magnification, three-dimensional visualization, and articulated instruments to facilitate delicate suturing now allows buccal ureteroplasty to be performed in a minimally invasive fashion, which may result in more widespread adoption of this technique.

INDICATIONS AND CONTRAINDICATIONS

Buccal ureteroplasty should be considered in patients who have long or multifocal proximal ureteral strictures that are not amenable to ureteroureterostomy and are being considered for autotransplantation or ileal ureter. Ureteral injury may have various causes such as trauma, iatrogenic injury from ureteroscopy or failed prior reconstructive surgery, or long-standing nephrolithiasis. Renal scan should be performed to demonstrate obstruction and to assess adequate function in the affected kidney. Contraindications to buccal ureteroplasty include any oral diseases that prevent harvest of oral mucosa.

PATIENT PREOPERATIVE EVALUATION AND PREPARATION

Diuretic renography should be considered to determine degree of obstruction and differential renal function. If there is minimal function remaining in the affected kidney, then nephrectomy may be a better option.

The length of the defect in the affected ureter must be evaluated. An antegrade or retrograde radiographic evaluation may be performed depending on whether the patient has a nephrostomy tube. If the degree of stenosis does not allow flow of contrast past the stricture on evaluation, simultaneous antegrade radiography and retrograde radiography or ureteroscopy may be necessary to evaluate stricture length (Fig. 30-1).

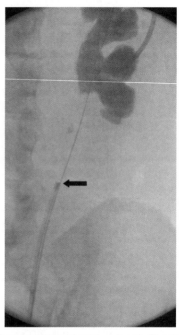

Figure 30-1. Demonstration of stricture length. The tip of the flexible ureteroscope is seen at the distal extent of the stricture *(arrow)*, and antegrade nephrostogram via the nephrostomy tube demonstrates the proximal extent of the stricture. A wire is seen traversing the stricture.

If the patient has a ureteral stent in place, we prefer to remove the stent, and place a nephrostomy tube to allow for accurate evaluation of the affected ureter.

Evaluation for BMG harvest includes careful review of any history of oral diseases such as leukoplakia, which may preclude harvest of oral mucosa.

OPERATING ROOM CONFIGURATION AND PATIENT POSITIONING

Careful consideration must be given to operating room configuration owing to the varied components of the procedure, including the robotic-assisted laparoscopic approach, the ureteroscopic evaluation, and the BMG harvest (Fig. 30-2). Patient positioning must allow adequate access to the patient's mouth for buccal graft harvest as well as optimal configuration for the use of the robot. Practical considerations include positioning of the screens for the cystoscopic tower as well as the video tower for the robot.

The anesthesia machine is at the head of the bed. The patient is positioned in a modified lateral decubitus position with the side of the affected ureter up. If the patient is female, a modified lateral decubitus lithotomy position with the legs secured in Allen stirrups is used to allow for access to the bladder (Fig. 30-3). The upper arm is padded and secured to the patient's side. All pressure points are padded. The genitalia are prepared into the field to allow for intraoperative ureteroscopic

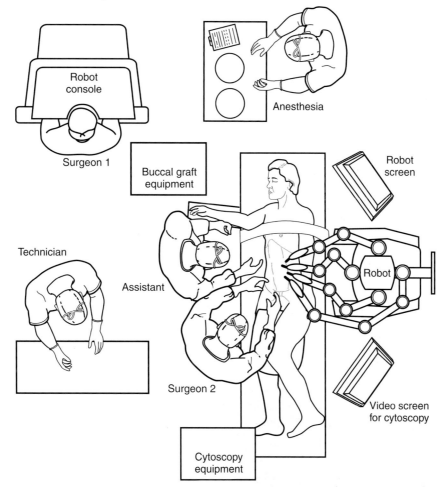

Figure 30-2. Operating room configuration and patient positioning. Patient is positioned in modified right lateral decubitus lithotomy position for left-sided repair. The mouth is draped separately from the abdominal field for buccal mucosa graft harvest.

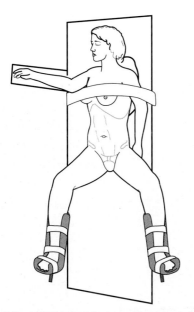

Figure 30-3. If the patient is female, a modified lateral decubitus lithotomy position, with legs secured in Allen stirrups, is used to allow access to the bladder.

evaluation. The endotracheal tube is secured on the dependent side of the mouth to allow for buccal mucosa harvest from the contralateral cheek. The mouth is prepared and draped separately from the rest of the surgical field.

The bedside assistant stands contralateral to the affected ureter and the robot is docked at a right angle to the patient's back. The screen for the robot is placed cephalad to the robot, and the cystoscope tower is placed caudad to the robot to allow both the bedside assistant and the surgeon performing the ureteroscopy to see their respective screens. The scrub nurse stands by the bedside assistant to allow the passage of instruments. A stand with the cystoscopic equipment is at the foot of the bed, and a stand with the equipment for the BMG harvest is placed at the head of the bed.

TROCAR PLACEMENT

The initial incision for the camera port is made cephalad to the umbilicus at the lateral border of the rectus (Fig. 30-4). Three robotic ports are placed—one at the costal margin, another infraumbilical at the lateral border of the rectus, and the last between the umbilicus and anterior superior iliac spine—to allow for adequate spacing of all ports. An assistant port is placed between the camera port and the inferior robotic port. Ports are placed 8 to 10 cm apart as allowed by the patient's size. An additional 5-mm trocar may be necessary for retraction of the liver for a right-sided dissection.

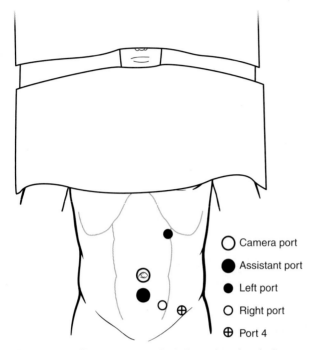

Figure 30-4. Trocar placement is similar to that of pyeloplasty.

- ○ Camera port
- ● Assistant port
- ● Left port
- ○ Right port
- ⊕ Port 4

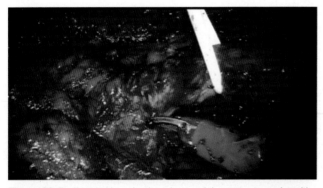

Figure 30-5. A vessel loop is placed around the ureter to assist with retraction as the ureter is dissected.

PROCEDURE (SEE VIDEO 30-1)

A transperitoneal approach is used. Initial camera port placement is achieved with the open Hasson technique, and pneumoperitoneum is achieved. The camera is inserted and the other ports are placed under vision. Once all ports have been placed, the robot is docked at a right angle to the patient, and the colon is deflected along the white line of Toldt. The plane between the Gerota fascia and the colon is developed. The psoas muscle is exposed and the overlying ureter is identified. The ureter is dissected, with care taken to preserve periureteral tissues, and is traced up to the renal pelvis (Fig. 30-5). The presence of two surgical teams allows for simultaneous ureteroscopy during ureterolysis as well as buccal mucosa harvest during preparation of the ureter for graft placement.

Once adequate dissection of the ureter has been performed, ureteroscopy is performed to identify the distal extent of stricture. The near infrared fluorescence modality of the da Vinci Si system (Intuitive Surgical, Sunnyvale, Calif.) allows visualization of the light of the ureteroscope, enabling the surgeon to accurately identify the extent of the stricture (Fig. 30-6). If the ureteroscope can be maneuvered through the stricture, ureteroscopy can also allow the surgeon to identify the proximal extent of stricture. If the strictured segment is too narrow, indocyanine green dye (ICG) can be injected intravenously, and near infrared fluorescence imaging can be used to evaluate ureteral perfusion to confirm the proximal margin of healthy tissue. After administration of ICG, well-perfused ureteral tissue appears green under fluorescence imaging whereas poorly perfused scar appears dark (Fig. 30-7). Both the proximal and distal ends of the ureteral stricture are marked with a stay suture.

The length of stricture is determined. A second surgical team harvests the BMG as specified by the length of stricture. BMG harvest is performed from the ipsilateral cheek. A self-retaining oral retractor and a tongue retractor are placed to maintain exposure of the cheek (Fig. 30-8). Retraction sutures of 2-0 silk are placed inside the vermilion border, away from the lip, and are lifted by an assistant to gain exposure to the harvest site. The intended graft site is marked with a marking pen, taking care to stay away from the Stensen duct near the second upper molar. The base of the site is infiltrated with 1% lidocaine with epinephrine for hydrodissection and hemostasis. The borders of the graft are incised, and the graft is raised

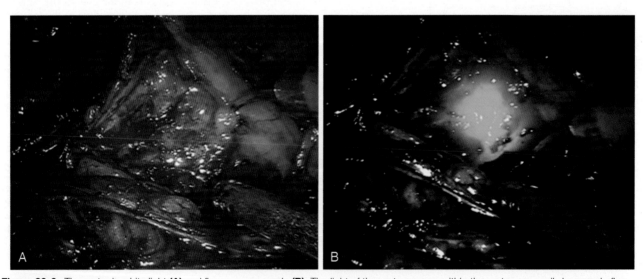

Figure 30-6. The ureter in white light **(A)** and fluorescence mode **(B).** The light of the ureteroscope within the ureter can easily be seen in fluorescence mode.

using Dean or tenotomy scissors, with care taken to leave the underlying tissue intact. A stay suture may be placed on the corners of the BMG to assist with retraction. A Yankauer suction instrument is used to provide upward countertraction as the BMG is dissected down off the cheek. Once the BMG has been harvested, the graft is thinned by removing the submucosal layer. The graft is tailored to the length of the ureteral stricture and 1 to 1.5 cm in width and then placed in normal saline until the recipient site is prepared. Gauze is soaked with the 1% lidocaine with epinephrine and placed into the cheek to assist with hemostasis. Before the end of the procedure, the BMG harvest site is evaluated, and minimal cautery is used for hemostasis as needed.

Although we consider simultaneous harvest of the BMG and robotic preparation of the recipient site to be a time-saving maneuver, the patient may also be repositioned to allow for standard harvest of the buccal graft, usually done with the patient facing upward. The harvest may also be performed before the robot is docked, with the preoperative imaging scans to estimate graft length.

The graft site is prepared by making a ureterotomy lengthwise through the previously demarcated stricture until healthy-appearing, normal-caliber ureter is reached proximally and distally (Fig. 30-9). We have performed both dorsal and ventral ureterotomies for buccal ureteroplasty; both techniques have been successful thus far, and further studies will need to be performed to determine whether one approach is advantageous over the other.

Consideration must be given to the blood supply to the graft. Graft survival is dependent on good apposition to a well-vascularized graft bed to allow engraftment to occur. In patients with dorsal placement of the graft, an omental wrap is sutured in place dorsally, underlying the ureterotomy (Fig. 30-10). In those with ventral grafts, omentum or perirenal fat is sutured in placed over the graft after the graft has been secured in the ureterotomy.

Once the graft site has been prepared, the BMG is then introduced into the abdomen through the assistant port and sutured onto the ureterotomy as an onlay graft (Fig. 30-11). The edges are sutured in running fashion with 4-0 polyglactin

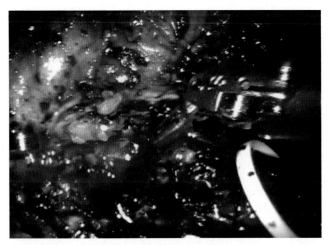

Figure 30-7. After administration of indocyanine green dye, well-perfused ureteral tissue appears green under fluorescence imaging whereas poorly perfused scar appears dark.

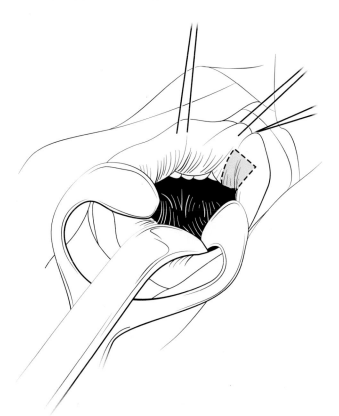

Figure. 30-8. . A self-retaining oral retractor, tongue retractor, and retraction sutures of 2-0 silk are placed inside the vermilion border. Dashed line represents potential graft harvest site.

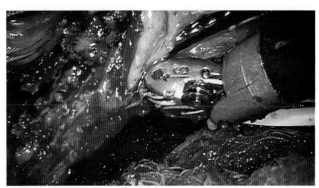

Figure 30-9. The graft site is prepared by making an ureterotomy lengthwise through the previously demarcated stricture until healthy appearing, normal-caliber ureter is reached proximally and distally. The ureteroscope is left in the lumen to identify the ends of the strictured segment.

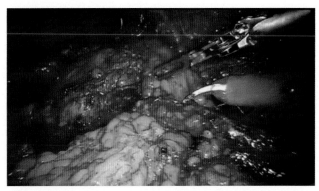

Figure 30-10. An omental wrap is sutured in place dorsally to provide a vascular bed under a dorsal ureterotomy for buccal mucosa graft engraftment.

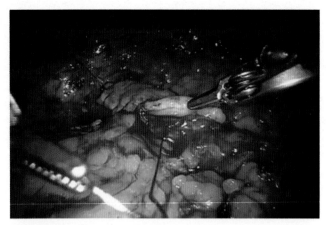

Figure 30-11. The edges of the buccal mucosa graft are sutured in running fashion with 4-0 polyglactin suture onto this ventral ureterotomy.

suture. The graft is also sutured to the omentum or perirenal fat to facilitate graft incorporation. Evaluation with the flexible ureteroscope allows visualization of the anastomosis from the ureteral lumen and allows for early recognition of misplacement of the suture into the back wall of the ureter. Once the anastomosis is complete, ureteroscopy confirms a patent and watertight anastomosis. A guidewire is left in place in the ureter, and a double-J ureteral stent is placed in retrograde fashion. A Foley catheter is placed. A closed suction drain is placed adjacent to the anastomosis once omental or perirenal fat coverage is complete. Instruments and trocars are removed, and the port sites are closed with absorbable suture. The epinephrine-soaked sponge is removed from the mouth, and the BMG harvest site is reevaluated to ensure hemostasis.

POSTOPERATIVE MANAGEMENT

An antiseptic mouthwash is administered postoperatively for improved donor site hygiene. Oral lidocaine gel is used for analgesia of the buccal mucosa harvest site. The patient's diet is advanced as tolerated. We typically leave the Foley catheter for drainage for 24 to 36 hours. If a nephrostomy tube is in place, it is left for drainage as well. The nephrostomy tube is then capped after 36 hours. The drain creatinine level is checked, and if this is consistent with the serum level, the

Foley catheter is removed. A repeat drain creatinine level is checked after removal of the Foley catheter, and if it is consistent with the serum level, the Jackson-Pratt drain is removed before the patient's discharge home, typically on postoperative day 2.

At 6 weeks after surgery, retrograde or antegrade pyelogram is performed to confirm that there is no leak at the graft site before stent and nephrostomy tube removal. Subsequent surveillance includes renal ultrasound to evaluate for hydronephrosis after stent removal and diuretic renography at approximately 3 months postoperatively to ensure the absence of obstruction.

COMPLICATIONS

One complication is urinary leakage from the anastomosis and the subsequent formation of urinoma. This may be managed with prolonged stent drainage and replacement of the Foley catheter to promote drainage through the ureter. A closed suction drain may also be used to drain urine.

Morbidity from BMG is minor and is reported to occur in 4% to 30% of patients. Complications specific to BMG harvest include donor site scarring and contracture with associated jaw opening impairment, perioral sensory defect, and changes in salivary function. Jaw opening limitation in the majority of patients resolves within 3 to 4 weeks. Long-term perioral sensory defects have been observed, but these defects are rarely noticeable to the patient.

TIPS AND TRICKS

- Once the ureter has been isolated, a vessel loop can be placed around the ureter to assist with manipulation.
- The light of the flexible ureteroscope is very useful for identification of the ureter in fibrosis.
- Holding stitches can be used to mark the proximal and distal extent of the stricture. By manipulating the ureter using the holding stitches, one can avoid trauma to the ureter from grasping with robotic instruments.
- For the BMG harvest, a 22-gauge angiocatheter can be placed into the Stensen duct to assist with identification.
- The anastomosis can be performed with the ureteroscope within the ureter to ensure that the surgeon does not inadvertently place sutures that occlude the lumen of the ureter.
- Irrigation applied through the ureteroscope allows for evaluation of urine leakage from the anastomosis.
- A pyelostomy may be formed to help confirm stent placement.

31 Pyelolithotomy and Ureterolithotomy

Justin I. Friedlander

INDICATIONS AND CONTRAINDICATIONS

With the use of shock wave lithotripsy (SWL) and advances in endoscopic technology and instrumentation, open surgery, once the mainstay treatment for ureteral stones, is now uncommon. Currently, open surgery is reserved for impacted stones for which these techniques have failed or in situations in which endoscopic equipment and SWL are unavailable. In the rare instance in which multiple minimally invasive treatments may be required, patients may opt for open surgery if it will ensure a single treatment session. In addition, open surgery may be indicated in the management of urolithiasis associated with anatomic abnormalities such as primary obstructive megaureter and ureteropelvic junction obstruction (UPJO). It also has a small role in the management of large staghorn calculi in patients with morbid obesity or unfavorable collecting system anatomy. Laparoscopic or robotic-assisted pyelolithotomy or ureterolithotomy is an alternative to open treatment and has exactly the same indications. From the first laparoscopic ureterolithotomy reported in 1992 to early reports of robotic-assisted pyelolithotomy in the mid-2000s, these techniques have been shown to be safe and effective. Most reports have been limited to case series with relatively small numbers compared with more conventional options, but this is a reflection of the number of patients (<5%) for whom endoscopic management of urolithiasis fails.

PATIENT PREOPERATIVE EVALUATION AND PREPARATION

Noncontrast computed tomography (CT) provides detailed information about stone size and position, renal pelvis anatomy, and proximity of adjacent organs and blood vessels. If CT is unavailable, kidney, ureter, and bladder x-ray studies in combination with intravenous pyelography will identify stone location, suggest stone consistency, and detail renal calyceal and ureteral anatomy. If a ureteral stricture is suspected, retrograde pyelogram (or antegrade if a percutaneous nephrostomy is in place) can be performed. Midstream urine culture should be performed for all patients before surgery, and culture-specific antibiotics should be given if infection is present.

LAPAROSCOPIC SURGERY (VIDEO 31-1)
Operating Room Configuration and Patient Positioning

The operating room is configured for ready instrument accessibility and visualization of the procedure by the entire surgical team (Fig. 31-1). For the transperitoneal approach, the patient is placed in a lateral position for proximal and midureteral stones. For stones located in the distal ureter, the patient is positioned supine with slight contralateral rotation. For the retroperitoneal approach, the patient is placed in the flank position.

Trocar Placement
Transperitoneal Approach

For midureteral and proximal ureteral stones, three trocars are placed in line: a 10/12-mm umbilical port for the laparoscopic camera, a 10/12-mm port in the midline between the umbilicus and the pubis, and a 5-mm port in the midline between the xiphoid and the camera port (Fig. 31-2). An alternate option for instrument ports is to place them ipsilateral to the stone on the midclavicular line (one subcostal and one lower quadrant). A fourth trocar can be placed on the ipsilateral anterior axillary line, forming a diamond-shaped configuration with the other three ports, if necessary. For distal ureteral stones, use four trocars: one umbilical, one ipsilateral to the stone supraumbilically at the midclavicular line, and two contralateral on the midclavicular line (one in the lower quadrant and the other in line with the umbilicus). If necessary, a fifth trocar can be placed in the suprapubic area.

Retroperitoneal Approach

A small incision is made at the tip of the 12th rib to allow balloon dissection of the retroperitoneal space. If the stone is distal, reposition the balloon dissector so that dissection proceeds more distally. Place the first port through this incision. Place two or three more ports with a combination of manual guidance and direct vision. Place one 5- to 10-mm trocar at the superior edge of the iliac crest, and place another 10-mm port one palm breadth superior to the previous one and over a line that passes over the standard subcostal incision. Place the last 5-mm port on the same vertical line as previously, but one palm breadth cranial (Fig. 31-3).

Procedure

For both the retroperitoneal and transperitoneal approaches, place a ureteral stent at the beginning of the operation to help locate the ureter, if a stent is not already present. This is not always necessary, especially if a bulge caused by the stone itself can be used to identify the ureter. Another option is to leave a guidewire at the tip of the stone if the ureteral stent cannot be passed because of stone impaction. This can facilitate subsequent double-J ureteral stent insertion after ureterotomy and stone extraction (Fig. 31-4).

After insufflation, the retroperitoneum is first exposed by medial deflection of the colon. Once this has been completed, use a combination of blunt and sharp dissection to expose the ureter where it passes over the psoas muscle or crosses the iliac vessels. The ureter is then isolated, and a vessel loop passed underneath to tent it up and to prevent stone migration. Alternatively, Babcock forceps can be used to grasp the dilated ureter proximal to the uppermost stone for the same purpose. Typically it is easy to identify the stone because it creates a bulge in the ureter or can be palpated with graspers. After stone identification, use a cold knife or nonelectrified

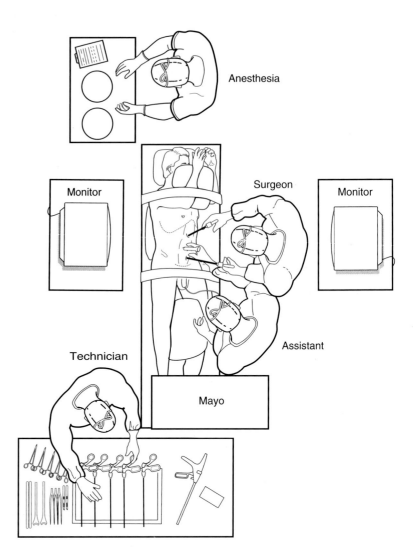

Anesthesia

Monitor

Surgeon

Monitor

Assistant

Technician

Mayo

Figure 31-1. To allow visualization of the procedure by all surgical team members, the surgeon and assistant stand contralateral to the side of the pathologic condition. The scrub nurse or technician stands opposite to help with instrument management.

scissors to incise the ureter over the calculus starting about 0.5 cm proximal to the stone (Fig. 31-5). Loosen the stone and extract it from the ureter with the help of a dissecting instrument (Fig. 31-6). After the stone has been extracted, use spoon forceps or a laparoscopic grasper to remove the stone from the abdomen. Stones too large to pass through the 10-mm port can be placed into a small laparoscopic specimen retrieval bag that can be removed at the end of the procedure. Flush the ureter with saline to remove tiny stone fragments and confirm patency. If necessary, a flexible ureteroscope can be passed through one of the laparoscopic ports and then into the ureter or kidney or both to retrieve any fragments that may have migrated. If less than 1 cm, the ureterotomy may be left open; otherwise, close it with interrupted 3-0, 4-0, or 5-0 absorbable sutures (Fig. 31-7). If a ureteral stent is not already in place, insert one either via laparoscopic manipulation through one of the ports or with the help of flexible cystoscopy. Use of a stent is recommended but not always needed unless the ureteral incision is not sutured. Place a drain in the retroperitoneal space. Fluoroscopy or plain film x-ray examination can then be used intraoperatively to confirm stone-free status and proper stent placement, and ports are removed after CO_2 deflation.

After trocar placement, the steps for retroperitoneal surgery are similar to those for the transperitoneal approach. Postoperative management is also similar.

ROBOTIC PYELOLITHOTOMY (TRANSPERITONEAL)
Operating Room Configuration and Patient Positioning

As is the case with laparoscopic surgery, robotic-assisted surgery requires operating room configuration for ready instrument accessibility and visualization of the procedure. The difference with robotic-assisted surgery is that the surgeon sits at the surgical console separate from the sterile operative field. The patient is placed in the modified flank position with minimal to no flexion of the operating table or elevation of the kidney rest.

Trocar Placement

One option for trocar placement uses three ports, a 12-mm camera port placed at the umbilicus, a 5/8-mm robotic instrument port placed midline supraumbilically, and another 5/8-mm port placed infraumbilically at the midclavicular line (Fig. 31-8). An alternative approach places the 12-mm camera port laterally between the anterior axillary and midclavicular lines, two 8-mm robotic ports triangulated toward the renal pelvis, and two ports for the assistant, 12 mm and 5 mm, placed in the periumbilical midline. This last approach also includes a 5-mm port as needed for liver retraction on the right (Fig. 31-9).

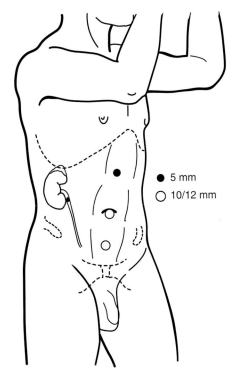

Figure 31-2. Trocar placement in the laparoscopic approach to a proximal ureteral calculus. A 10-mm port is placed at the umbilicus. Then two 5-mm or 10-mm ports are placed under direct vision along the midline, one midway between the umbilicus and the xiphoid process and the other midway between the umbilicus and the pubis.

● 5 mm
○ 10/12 mm

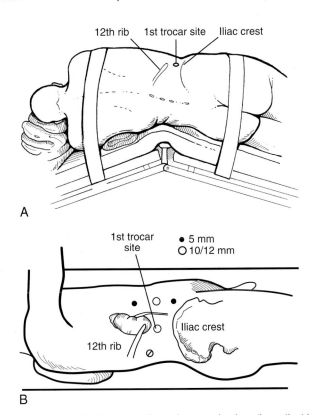

12th rib   1st trocar site   Iliac crest

A

1st trocar site   ● 5 mm
○ 10/12 mm

Iliac crest

12th rib

B

Figure 31-3. A, For the retroperitoneal approach, place the patient in full lateral position. **B,** Trocar placement for right-sided retroperitoneal access. The first trocar is placed approximately two fingerbreadths below the 12th rib. Additional trocars are placed as needed for dissection, retraction, or both.

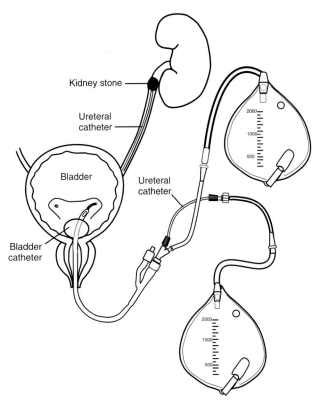

Kidney stone

Ureteral catheter

Bladder

Ureteral catheter

Bladder catheter

Figure 31-4. If a stent or catheter cannot be passed proximal to the stone, an open-ended catheter should be advanced to the stone. A Council-tip bladder catheter can be placed over the open-ended catheter and inflated in the bladder. With a Y-adapter attached to the bladder catheter, urine drainage can be achieved and a wire manipulated through the open-ended catheter once the stone has been removed.

Procedure

After insufflation, expose the renal pelvis through medial dissection and deflection of the colon. Once adequate exposure has been achieved, incise the renal pelvis with nonelectrified scissors. Renal pelvic stones can then be extracted with a robotic grasper or other appropriate instrument. Stones in individual renal calices can be inspected with a flexible nephroscope, and flexible graspers can be deployed as needed to remove calculi. Stones too large to be removed can be fragmented with an energy source such as a holmium laser introduced through the nephroscope or directly through one of the robotic ports. As is the case with ureterolithotomy, it may be prudent to place large or multiple stones in a laparoscopic specimen retrieval bag for later extraction through one of the port sites. Once all stones have been removed, irrigate the renal pelvis. If there is a coexisting UPJO, repair it after all stones have been removed. Use 4-0 or 5-0 absorbable sutures in either a running or interrupted fashion for the pyeloplasty. If no UPJO is present, simply close the pyelotomy with 4-0 or 5-0 absorbable sutures in a running fashion. Before complete closure, place a double-J ureteral stent in an antegrade fashion under vision if one has not already been positioned during an initial cystoscopy. Although not always necessary, it is recommended to place a retroperitoneal drain through one of the port sites at the termination of the procedure. As is the case with laparoscopic surgery, fluoroscopy or plain film x-ray studies can then be used to confirm stone-free status and proper stent placement, and ports are removed after CO_2 deflation.

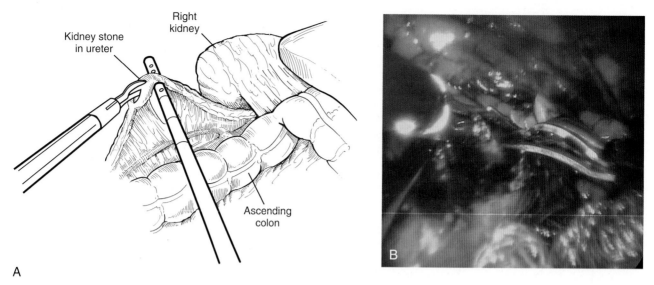

Figure 31-5. A, Once the stone is located within the ureter, the ureter is opened with laparoscopic scissors or a laparoscopic cold knife. **B,** The stone can often be felt with the tip of the scissors.

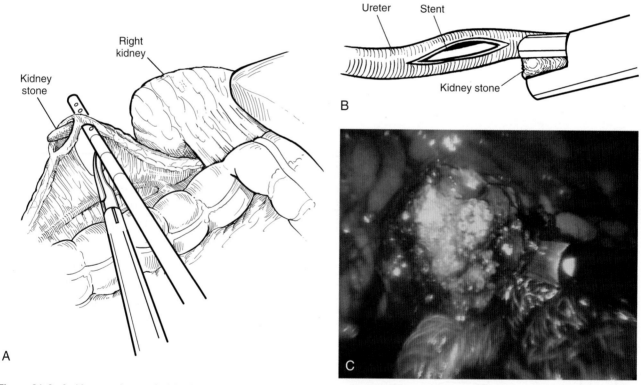

Figure 31-6. A, After an adequate incision has been made, the stone can be manipulated out of the ureter. **B,** Removal from the ureter and from the abdomen can be assisted by the use of spoon forceps. **C,** The incision must be long enough to allow the stone to be removed with minimal trauma to the ureter.

POSTOPERATIVE MANAGEMENT

In most cases, the patient can resume oral food intake on postoperative day 1, and the urethral catheter is then removed on postoperative day 2. The drain can be removed the same afternoon if the output is less than 30 mL. Alternatively, one may wish to check a drain creatinine level before removal to assess for presence of urine leak. The stent is removed 4 to 6 weeks postoperatively, and an intravenous pyelogram or diuretic renal scan is performed 6 weeks later to ensure ureteral patency. Further follow-up varies.

COMPLICATIONS

Minor complications include transient postoperative fever with or without urinary tract infection, postoperative ileus, subcutaneous emphysema, and subcutaneous hematomas. Urine leak is an overall rare event but more common

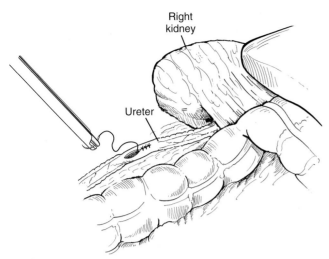

Figure 31-7. Once the stone has been removed, a stent is advanced into the kidney if not already present, and the ureterotomy is closed using freehand suturing or with the help of the Endo Stitch device.

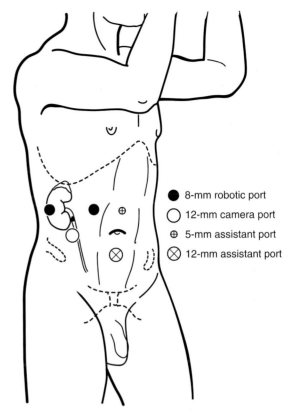

● 8-mm robotic port
○ 12-mm camera port
⊕ 5-mm assistant port
⊗ 12-mm assistant port

Figure 31-9. Alternate trocar placement for robotic-assisted transperitoneal pyelolithotomy. A 12-mm camera port is placed laterally between the anterior axillary and midclavicular lines; two 8-mm robotic ports are triangulated toward the renal pelvis, each one palm breadth from the camera port; and two ports are placed for the assistant, 12 mm and 5 mm, in the periumbilical midline. This approach also includes a 5-mm port as needed for liver retraction on the right.

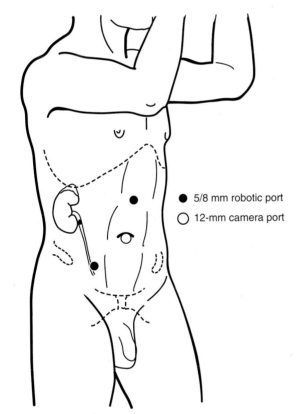

● 5/8 mm robotic port
○ 12-mm camera port

Figure 31-8. Trocar placement for robotic transperitoneal pyelolithotomy. A 12-mm camera port is placed at the umbilicus, followed by placement of a 5/8-mm robotic instrument port midline supraumbilically one palm breadth away. Another 5/8-mm port is placed infraumbilically at the midclavicular line, the same distance away.

along with prolonged urethral catheter drainage. Bowel and vascular injuries, injuries of adjacent organs, venous thromboembolic disease, and incisional hernias are a risk of any laparoscopic or robotic surgery, although they are not more common in ureterolithotomy and pyelolithotomy than in other procedures. There are no long-term results concerning the incidence of postoperative ureteral stricture, nor are there data to suggest that use of electrocautery or laser energy increases stricture rate compared with ureterotomy with a cold knife or nonelectrified scissors. If ureteral stricture develops, management includes a variety of endoscopic and nonendoscopic methods. Residual stones can be managed with ureteroscopy, percutaneous nephrolithotomy, or SWL, as appropriate.

if a ureteral stent is not used; however, it typically is self-limited. If urine leak persists, conservative management is used, first with prolonged urethral catheter drainage, usually in the range of 10 to 14 days. If a urinoma develops, treatment requires percutaneous drainage of the urinoma

TIPS AND TRICKS

- Preoperatively place a double-J ureteral stent to help locate the ureter. If the stone cannot be bypassed because of impaction, leave a guidewire at the tip of the stone. This will facilitate subsequent stent placement after ureterotomy and stone extraction.
- After stone identification, pass a vessel loop underneath the ureter and tent it up to prevent stone migration. Alternatively, a laparoscopic Babcock instrument may be used to grasp the dilated ureter proximal to the uppermost calculus if no vessel loop is available.

32 Robotic-Assisted and Laparoscopic Simple Prostatectomy

Philip T. Zhao, Lee Richstone

Despite technologic advances in endoscopic techniques for management of benign prostatic hyperplasia (BPH) in the past decade, open simple prostatectomy has traditionally been the treatment of choice for patients with giant symptomatic prostatomegaly. Minimally invasive approaches to simple prostatectomy have gained traction in the urologic community since Mariano and colleagues first described laparoscopic simple prostatectomy (LSP) in 2002. The laparoscopic approach demonstrated reduced pain, quicker recovery, and improved cosmesis compared with the open approach, but blood loss remained a major issue, with a tenth of the patients in the initial series requiring blood transfusions. The technique also presented a steep learning curve and challenges for many surgeons not accustomed to the ergonomics of operating in a narrow pelvis and intracorporeal suturing.

More recently, robotic-assisted simple prostatectomy (RASP) has mitigated these challenges and extended the role of robotic-assisted surgery beyond traditional robotic-assisted radical prostatectomy (RARP) for prostate cancer. In 2008, Sotelo and colleagues initially reported RASP in which they used a transperitoneal suprapubic approach similar to that for RARP, applying the same port placement and positioning. Since then, several groups have reported RASP via the retropubic and extraperitoneal approaches. RASP has been established as a safe and effective modality for adenoma excision and is the main technique described in this chapter.

INDICATIONS AND CONTRAINDICATIONS

The indications for minimally invasive simple prostatectomy (MISP) are similar to those for open simple prostatectomy (OSP)—specifically, high-volume (>80 mL), symptomatic BPH refractory to medical therapy or prior endoscopic management. In addition, surgery is generally indicated for men who have renal insufficiency secondary to chronic outlet obstruction, multiple episodes of retention, recurrent urinary tract infections (UTIs), bladder stones, and significant gross hematuria of prostatic origin. Relative indications include the concomitant presence of bladder stones or large bladder diverticula that also require intervention.

Contraindications to MISP include biopsy-proven prostate cancer, elevated prostate-specific antigen (PSA) level, and concerning digital rectal examination (DRE) findings without prior biopsy. The procedure is also contraindicated in men who are poor surgical candidates in general and in those who cannot tolerate extreme Trendelenburg positions for extended periods (e.g., patients with recent neurosurgical procedures who cannot tolerate increased intracranial pressures; those with pulmonary edema associated with congestive heart failure).

PATIENT PREOPERATIVE EVALUATION AND PREPARATION

The diagnostic evaluation of men undergoing MISP consists of a complete physical examination and International Prostate Symptom Score (IPSS) evaluation, PSA level, postvoid residual (PVR) assessment, uroflowmetry, and volumetric imaging of the prostate to determine accurate prostate size. If PSA is elevated or if DRE is concerning, a prostate biopsy should be performed to rule out prostate cancer before proceeding with additional workup of lower urinary tract symptoms (LUTS). Cystoscopy can be helpful to determine the presence of a median lobe, bladder diverticula, and calculi. Formal urodynamic assessment consisting of cystometry and pressure and flow evaluations in patients with more complex conditions and coexisting bladder disease is warranted before prostatectomy.

Urinalysis and urine culture, electrolyte studies, complete blood count (CBC), coagulation studies, and type and screen should all be obtained in patients before proceeding with MISP. Active UTIs should be adequately treated before surgery. Chest x-ray examination and electrocardiography should be part of the presurgical testing for all men older than age 50 and those who have any risk factors for cardiovascular events.

Informed consent should be obtained with the patient having a clear understanding of the surgery and the associated risks, including but not limited to conversion to an open procedure; bleeding; need for transfusions; infections and sepsis; urinary incontinence; and erectile dysfunction or impotence.

OPERATING ROOM CONFIGURATION AND PATIENT POSITIONING

After insertion of an endotracheal tube and induction of general anesthesia, the patient is placed either in a supine position with the legs spread apart on a split table or in the dorsal lithotomy position with all pressure points padded (Fig. 32-1). The arms are tucked at the sides. Sequential compression stockings are placed on both legs, and 5000 units of subcutaneous heparin is given for deep venous thrombosis (DVT) prophylaxis. The patient is then placed into the steep Trendelenburg position (>25%) before preparation and draping to test the configuration and confirm that positioning does not affect anesthetic parameters (e.g., loss of tidal volume and difficulty ventilating), because pneumoperitoneum and CO_2 insufflation can induce hypercapnia and oliguria. After standard preparation and draping, an 18-French Foley catheter is inserted into the bladder with 10 mL of sterile water placed in the balloon.

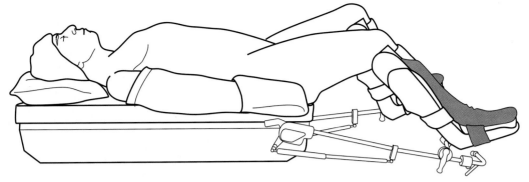

Figure 32-1. The patient's legs are placed apart in stirrups in the low lithotomy position. Both arms should be tucked by the sides and the chest secured with a strap. Shoulder braces are no longer used owing to increased incidence of brachial plexus injury.

TROCAR PLACEMENT

For both transperitoneal laparoscopic and robotic approaches, the pneumoperitoneum is established with a Veress needle inserted at the base of the umbilicus. If the patient has had prior abdominal surgery with incision in the midline or lower abdomen, the Veress needle can be placed at the upper left or right subcostal area. In patients with prior incisions, an additional Veress needle may be used to ascertain if proposed trocar sites are safe by probing the site of placement for escaping gas. After an intra-abdominal pressure of 15 mm Hg has been established, a 12-mm or 8-mm (if using the da Vinci Xi system [Intuitive Surgical, Sunnyvale, Calif.]) camera trocar is then placed in the midline at the umbilicus. The laparoscopic or robotic camera is then inserted through this port and the abdomen is inspected to assess for adhesions or any injuries sustained from Veress needle or port placement. A 12-mm working trocar is placed approximately 15 cm lateral to the camera port on the left, approximately two fingerbreadths superior to the left anterior superior iliac spine. We prefer to place a 12-mm AirSeal System (SurgiQuest, Milford, Conn.) trocar as the working port for both laparoscopy and robotic-assisted surgery because this system allows us to maintain a more stable pneumocavity and prevent sudden loss of insufflation pressure. The valveless trocar system has been demonstrated to improve visualization by decreasing smudging of laparoscopes and evacuating smoke during cauterization, to maintain pneumoperitoneum while suctioning, and to allow easier extraction of specimens and needles.

For RASP, two 8-mm robotic trocars are inserted 8 cm lateral to the camera port on either side of the rectus muscle. A fourth robotic arm trocar is placed 8 cm to the right of the right lateral port above the right anterior superior iliac spine. A 5-mm assistant screw port is placed between the camera port and left robotic trocar and slightly cephalad to them. Some adjustments are needed to ensure that the 5-mm trocar during assistance does not hamper either the robotic or camera arms. The surgeon operates through the three robotic arms and controls the camera while the assistant uses the 12-mm AirSeal port for insertion and retrieval of needles and instruments and the 5-mm port for suctioning and irrigation. See Figure 32-2 for transperitoneal RASP trocar placements.

Initial access for the extraperitoneal approach requires a 2-cm infraumbilical incision to be made to expose the anterior rectus sheath. A midline vertical incision is made in the sheath itself to expose the rectus muscle, which is then split to delineate the posterior sheath. A balloon dilator PDB or Space-maker (Covidien, Dublin, Ireland) is inserted over the posterior sheath and advanced toward the space of Retzius. This allows the robotic or laparoscopic camera to pass through the balloon port and assist in creating extrapneumoperitoneum.

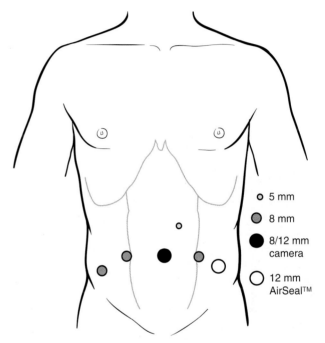

○	5 mm
⬤ (gray)	8 mm
⬤ (black)	8/12 mm camera
○ (large)	12 mm AirSeal™

Figure 32-2. Trocar configuration for transperitoneal robotic-assisted simple prostatectomy. The port placements for the extraperitoneal approach are shifted 2 cm inferiorly.

Care should be taken to preserve the inferior epigastric vessels and not to dissect them off the rectus muscle and also not to inadvertently make a small hole in the peritoneum, which will lead to suboptimal insufflation of the extraperitoneal space.

Once the extraperitoneal space has been developed, the robotic and assistant trocars are placed in similar fashion as for the transperitoneal approach, with emphasis that the ports are not close together to prevent instrument clashing. All trocars are placed slightly below the level of the camera port and under direct endoscopic vision.

The laparoscopic approach also involves establishing pneumoperitoneum with a Veress needle by means of the Hassan technique. A 10-mm camera trocar is placed at the umbilicus. Two 10-mm ports are then placed on each side in the middle of the distance between the anterior iliac spine and the umbilicus. An additional 5-mm port is placed inferior to and lateral to the 10-mm trocar on the surgeon's side. The 12-mm port (AirSeal) is placed on the contralateral side in the same position. See Figure 32-3 for LSP port configuration.

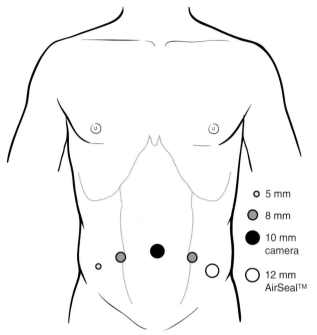

Figure 32-3. Five-trocar configuration for laparoscopic simple prostatectomy.

5 mm
8 mm
10 mm camera
12 mm AirSeal™

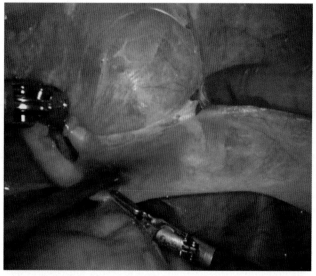

Figure 32-4. The anterior peritoneum is incised lateral to the medial umbilical ligaments to enter the space of Retzius.

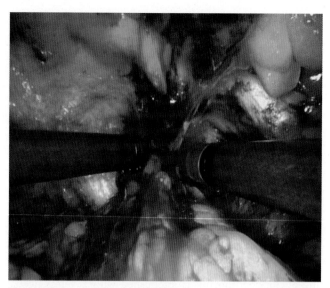

Figure 32-5. Location of the bladder neck is approximated by gently squeezing the distal bladder with both EndoWrist instruments.

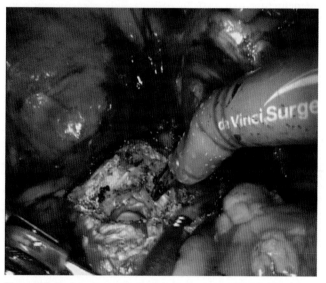

Figure 32-6. A transverse incision is made across the bladder 1 to 2 cm proximal to the vesicoprostatic junction.

PROCEDURE (SEE VIDEO 32-1)
Robotic Simple Prostatectomy: Transperitoneal Approach

Bladder Mobilization

After the pneumoperitoneum is established, the anterior peritoneum is incised lateral to the medial umbilical ligaments bilaterally to the level of the vasa deferentia (Fig. 32-4). The bladder is then dropped to develop the space of Retzius.

Bladder Neck Dissection

Once the retropubic space has been entered, the fat over the vesicoprostatic junction is dissected to expose the bladder neck. The bladder is held taut at the dome with the fourth arm. Approximation of the location of the bladder neck is done by gently squeezing the distal bladder with the wrist of both robotic arms (Fig. 32-5). Some surgeons may prefer to identify the bladder neck by pulling the catheter in and out. In either case, the endopelvic fascia is preserved and the dorsal venous complex (DVC) does not need to be controlled or ligated as is the case with radical prostatectomy. Some superficial dorsal veins may need to be fulgurated if they are present or if any bleeding occurs. The bladder is usually extended by instilling sterile water through the Foley catheter to help define its contours. A transverse incision is made across the bladder approximately 1 to 2 cm proximal to the vesicoprostatic junction (Fig. 32-6). The incision can be extended laterally if a large median lobe, multiple bladder stones, or significant diverticula are present. The Foley balloon is taken down, and irrigation fluid is suctioned out once the cystotomy has been made. The catheter is then withdrawn into the urethra.

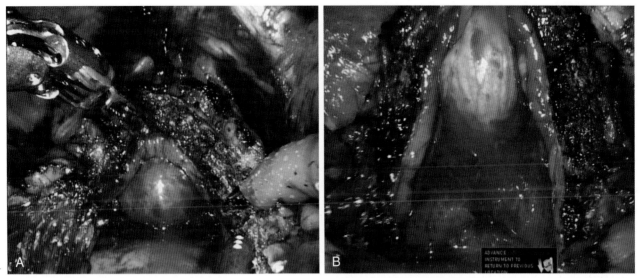

Figure 32-7. A, Through the cystotomy incision, the ureteral orifices must be identified. **B,** Robotic tenacula can be used to lift the prostate or median lobe anteriorly to improve exposure.

Prostatic Adenoma Dissection

Looking into the bladder through the incision, the surgeon must identify and preserve the ureteral orifices (Fig. 32-7). Ureteral catheterization is typically not required; however, it can be performed if the ureteral orifices are particularly close to the bladder neck or median lobe, if there is any suspected cautery or injury to the orifices, or for surgeon comfort early in the learning curve. Monopolar scissors are used to incise the bladder mucosa from the 5 to 7 o'clock positions and identify the correct plane between the full-thickness bladder and the prostate adenoma, ensuring an adequate margin away from the ureteral orifices (Fig. 32-8). The incision is carried circumferentially around the bladder neck. With the assistant holding the bladder flap open and the fourth arm of the robotic system holding the prostate or median lobe anteriorly, posterior dissection is performed with both blunt and sharp dissection. Electrocautery can be applied sparingly to control bleeding. Once the posterior dissection has been completed, anterolateral dissection is performed to mobilize the lateral lobes (Fig. 32-9).

Because the prostate is typically very large in size in patients selected for RASP, sequential dissection may not always be optimal. The fourth arm (with robotic tenaculum) should help to toggle the prostate in any orientation to allow anterior, posterior, and lateral dissections as needed to continue progression of the case (Fig. 32-10). The entire prostatic adenoma should be shelled out between the anatomic and surgical capsules. It may even be helpful to remove parts of the adenoma or the median lobe, if present, early to expose and visualize the deeper parts of the prostate to help with resection (Fig. 32-11). Allow the EndoWrist of the robot to follow the contours of the resection and meticulously and relentlessly cauterize any sources of bleeding. This reduces the time needed to suction out the field and helps with overall hemostasis.

Distal Prostatic Urethral Dissection

Apical dissection is performed underneath the anterior capsule. The distal prostatic urethra is divided after circumferential dissection and the urethra is cut sharply at the apex (Fig. 32-12). Once the adenoma specimen is free, it is placed into a 10-mm or 15-mm Endo Catch bag (Covidien, Dublin,

Ireland) depending on the amount of tissue removed and left in the abdomen until specimen retrieval. Hemostasis is achieved with bipolar or monopolar electrocautery. Any concerning sources of bleeding can be sutured with a 3-0 Monocryl or V-Loc suture (Covidien, Dublin, Ireland). Figure-of-eight sutures with 2-0 V-Loc are applied at the 5 and 7 o'clock positions to control the main prostatic arteries (Fig. 32-13).

Closure of Capsule and Bladder

The empty prostatic fossa is examined to make sure all adenomatous tissue has been resected, and the posterior edge of the bladder neck mucosa is coapted to the posterior edge of the urethra with a 3-0 V-Loc suture (Fig. 32-14). We do not perform a complete vesicourethral anastomosis. A 24-French three-way catheter is inserted into the bladder under direct vision. The transverse cystotomy incision is then closed in a two-layer fashion with separate absorbable V-Loc sutures. One 3-0 suture for the mucosa and one 2-0 suture for the seromuscular layer are run from each end of the cystotomy and tied in the middle (Fig. 32-15). The catheter balloon is then filled with 30 to 50 mL of sterile water (depending on amount of prostatic adenoma that was removed), and the repair is tested by distending the bladder with 120 mL of water (Fig. 32-16). After confirming the repair is intact, a Jackson-Pratt (JP) drain is placed in the pelvis and secured to the skin. A suprapubic tube is not used.

The string to the specimen bag is transferred to the camera port and then extracted after extension of the port incision. Fascia is closed with a 0 Vicryl tie at the 12-mm assistant port, with a suture passer under direct vision. The 8-mm robotic trocar sites and 5-mm assistant port typically do not require fascial closure. The umbilical extraction site fascia is closed with several 0 Vicryl figure-of-eight sutures, and the skin at all port sites is closed with 4-0 Monocryl sutures.

Robotic Simple Prostatectomy: Extraperitoneal Approach

The extraperitoneal approach to RASP is conducted in similar fashion as the transperitoneal approach with creation of the extraperitoneal space. The main advantage of this technique

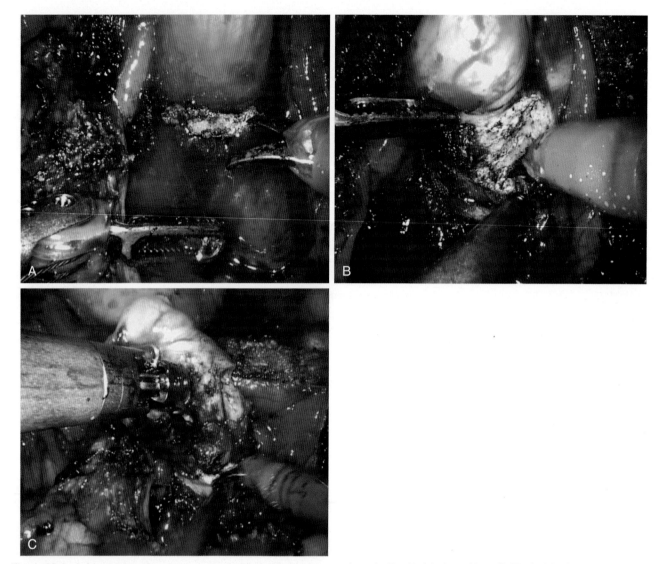

Figure 32-8. A, Monopolar scissors are used to incise the bladder mucosa from the 5 to 7 o'clock positions. **B,** The incision is carried circumferentially around the bladder neck with sharp and blunt dissection. **C,** Removing the median lobe early, if present, helps to expose and visualize the deeper parts of the prostate.

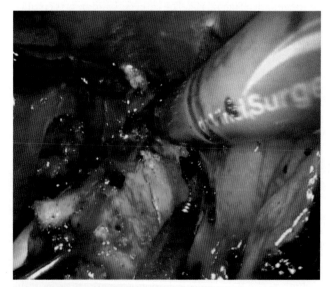

Figure 32-9. Anterolateral dissection is performed to mobilize the lateral lobes.

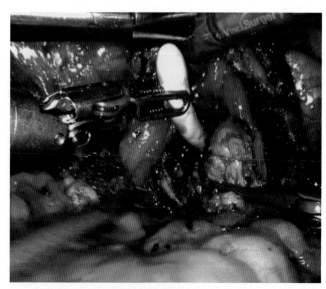

Figure 32-10. The fourth arm can hold the prostate using robotic tenacula and can help to toggle the prostate in any orientation to allow anterior, posterior, and lateral dissections as needed to continue the procedure. The Foley catheter can be held to give countertraction.

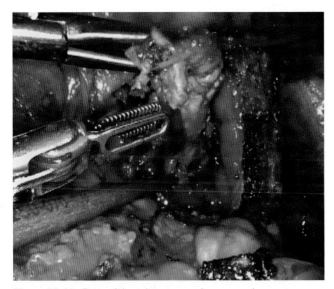

Figure 32-11. Parts of the adenoma can be removed progressively throughout the case to increase surgical space and improve exposure. The assistant can also use laparoscopic tenacula to grasp prostatic adenoma, and the robotic tenaculum can hold the bladder flap, or vice versa.

is that once space has been made, access to the prostate is direct and immediate. This approach also makes minimally invasive excision of prostatic adenoma more feasible in patients with prior abdominal or pelvic surgery and significant adhesions.

Robotic Simple Prostatectomy: Retropubic Approach (Millin Technique)

Retropubic RASP can be performed with either the intraperitoneal or the extraperitoneal approach. Positioning, port placement, and bladder mobilization are all performed in the same way as previously described.

Prostate Capsule Incision

Once the retropubic space has been entered, a transverse incision is made in the prostatic capsule and followed down into the adenoma. The adenoma is bluntly mobilized anteriorly and laterally from the capsule. Robotic tenacula can assist in countertraction of the adenoma to facilitate mobilization. The apex of the prostate is usually dissected sharply after identification of the urethra. The adenoma is placed in an Endo Catch bag and removed at the end of the operation before abdominal port site closures.

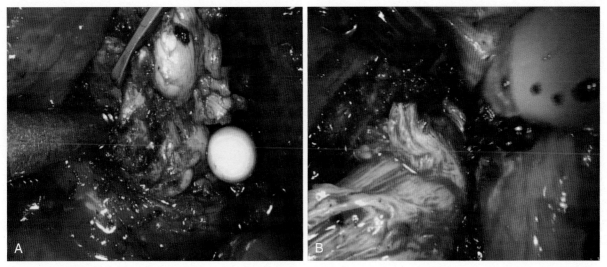

Figure 32-12. A, The Foley catheter is reinserted to identify the urethra. **B,** The distal prostatic urethra is divided after circumferential dissection, and the urethra is cut sharply at the apex.

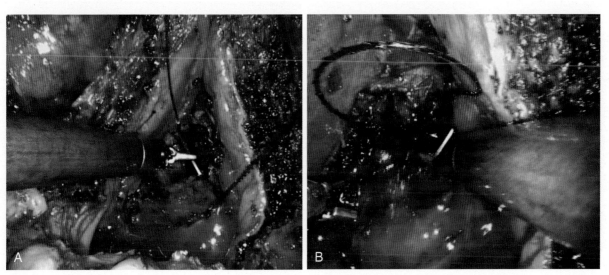

Figure 32-13. A, Figure-of-eight sutures with 2-0 V-Loc (Covidien, Dublin, Ireland) at the 5 and 7 o'clock positions **(B)** to control the main prostatic arteries.

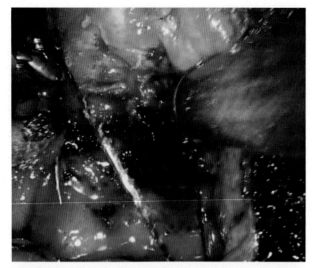

Figure 32-14. The posterior edge of the bladder neck mucosa is co-apted to the posterior edge of the urethra with a 3-0 V-Loc (Covidien, Dublin, Ireland) suture.

Capsular Closure

Once the adenomatous tissues have been removed, bleeding is controlled with bipolar electrocautery or PlasmaKinetic graspers. Several figure-of-eight sutures can be placed at the 5 and 7 o'clock positions at the bladder neck to improve hemostasis. A single dissolvable 3-0 V-Loc suture can be used to reapproximate the posterior plate. A 24-French three-way catheter is then inserted under vision before the anterior capsule being sewn. The catheter balloon is inflated to 30 mL once the capsule is intact, and mild traction of the catheter is applied. The irrigation port in the catheter is usually plugged because continuous bladder irrigation (CBI) is not initiated.

Laparoscopic Simple Prostatectomy

After placement of trocars and establishment of pneumoperitoneum, the space of Retzius is entered and the preprostatic fat is removed. All dissection is performed with an ultrasonic Harmonic Scalpel (Ethicon Endo-Surgery, Somerville, N.J.) and laparoscopic DeBakey forceps. The endopelvic fascia is opened on the lateral sides of the prostate. Several 2-0 Vicryl

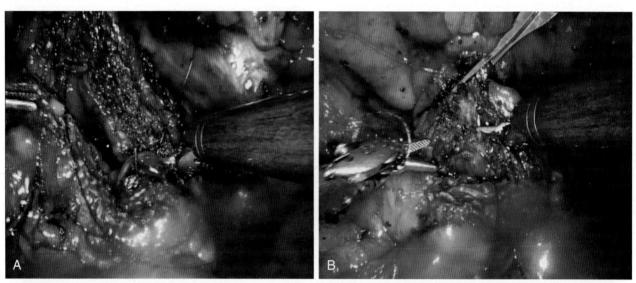

Figure 32-15. A, The transverse cystotomy incision is closed in a two-layer fashion with separate absorbable V-Loc sutures. First, a 3-0 suture is used for the mucosa. **B,** Then, a 2-0 suture is used for the seromuscular layer. Both are run from the ends of the cystotomy and tied together in the middle.

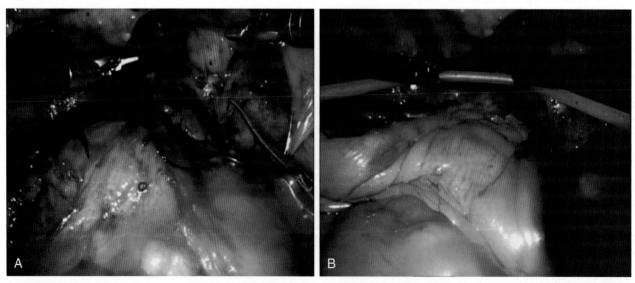

Figure 32-16. A, The repair is tested by distending the bladder with 120 mL of sterile water. **B,** Once closure is confirmed, a Jackson-Pratt drain is placed in the pelvis.

sutures are placed as hemostatic sutures at the DVC and pubo-prostatic ligaments as well as at the lateral prostatic pedicles to control potential bleeding.

The prostatic capsule and bladder neck are opened with a longitudinal midline incision, and the prostatic adenoma is exposed and dissected free with the Harmonic Scalpel and blunt dissection. The isthmus is opened toward the apex so that the prostate can be divided into two lobes. Each lobe is carefully peeled off the urethra until the whole adenoma is freed and then removed and placed in an Endo Catch bag. Bladder neck hemostasis is performed with 3-0 Vicryl sutures at the 5 and 7 o'clock positions, and the bladder neck mucosa is advanced to the prostatic fossa. Running 2-0 Vicryl sutures are used to close the capsule and bladder incision in a two-layer fashion. A 24-French three-way catheter is inserted into the bladder, a JP drain is placed, and the rest of the surgery (specimen extraction and port site closure) proceeds in the same method as for the robotic-assisted approach described earlier.

Robotic-Assisted Laparoscopic Endoscopic Single-Site Surgery

The robotic-assisted laparoendoscopic single-site (R-LESS) approach to simple prostatectomy has been described by Sotelo and colleagues, who used a four-channel r-Port (Advanced Surgical Concepts, Bray, Ireland) placed through a 2.5-cm infraumbilical incision. Aside from the simple port used, the resection technique and principles are largely the same as those applied in RASP. The main challenge in these cases is the loss of instrument triangulation and instrument clashing, especially in an unfavorable setting such as the pelvis.

Robotic-Assisted Simple-Port Suprapubic Transvesical Enucleation of the Prostate

Both Desai and colleagues and Fareed and colleagues have described transvesical robotic single-site techniques for RASP. After initial transurethral incision of the prostatic urethra with a Collin's knife, an r-Port or GelPort (Applied Medical, Santa Margarita, Calif.) was placed directly into the bladder 3 cm above the pubis in the suprapubic crease. Robotic trocars were inserted into the single port, and the da Vinci robot was then docked after adequate pneumovesicum had been achieved. The prostatic adenoma was resected intravesically without the need to enter the peritoneum or extraperitoneum with similar outcomes to RASP.

POSTOPERATIVE MANAGEMENT

There is no need for continuous bladder irritation, as the case with OSP, unless there is significant postoperative hematuria.

The catheter is left to straight drainage without traction, and the JP bulb is left to self-suction. Patients are continued on postoperative antibiotics (usually cefazolin 2 g, every 8 hours) for 24 hours. Subcutaneous heparin and compression stockings are continued until patients are fully ambulatory and usually for the duration of their hospitalization.

Patients are given parenteral analgesics in the postanesthesia care unit and then changed to oral pain medication once they are transferred to the floor. They are started on a clear liquid diet once fully awake from anesthesia and advanced to a regular diet as tolerated the next morning.

Basic metabolic panel and CBC are obtained on postoperative day 1. The JP drain is checked for creatinine, and if the level is similar to the serum level, the JP is removed before discharge. Patients usually are discharged during the first or second postoperative day with the catheter connected to a leg bag (supplies including a large drainage bag are included on discharge to allow adequate urinary drainage at night). Follow-up occurs in a week for catheter removal; routine cystograms are not required unless clinically indicated.

COMPLICATIONS

In the 13 published series of RASP, the complication rates have ranged from 7.7% to 33%, largely related to ileus and UTIs postoperatively. Open conversion is rare. The transfusion rate has ranged from 0 to 33% (overall 3.4%). A systemic review of LSP series shows similar results, including a conversion rate of 0, a reoperation rate of 1.3%, and a transfusion rate of 5.6%. Postoperative ileus can occur after any abdominal surgery but can happen more commonly in the setting of urinary ascites. This highlights the importance of a watertight cystotomy closure and avoidance of prostatic capsular rupture during resection of the adenoma.

TIPS AND TRICKS

- On entering the bladder, make the transverse cystotomy incision as distal and as close to the bladder neck as possible to allow adequate exposure of the adenoma during excision. This is especially important in more obese patients and in those with a narrow pelvis.
- Use robotic tenacula to help hold both the bladder flaps as well as the prostatic adenoma for retraction. Tenacula hold tissue better than fenestrated and other graspers.
- The prostatic adenoma can be resected in multiple parts, not necessarily as a single entity. Removing parts of the adenoma will optimize visualization of the excision bed. This is especially true if there is a large median lobe involved.
- Methylene blue or indigo carmine can be injected intravenously to help identify the ureteral orifices intraoperatively.

33 Transperitoneal Radical Prostatectomy

Akira Yamamoto, Li Ming Su

INDICATIONS AND CONTRAINDICATIONS

Prostate cancer is risk stratified on the basis of prostate-specific antigen (PSA), tumor grade, and clinical stage. Low-risk disease is defined by a PSA level lower than 10 ng/mL, a Gleason score of 6 or less, and clinical stage T1c or T2a. Intermediate-risk patients are those with a PSA level between 10 and 20 ng/mL, a Gleason score of 7, or clinical stage T2b, who otherwise do not qualify as high risk. High-risk patients include those with a PSA level above 20 ng/mL, a Gleason score of 8 to 10, or clinical stage T2c. New evidence suggests that men with low- and intermediate-risk disease may not benefit from definitive management, whereas recurrence rates are high after local control of high-risk prostate cancer.

Considering this, the surgeon should take into account the patient's life expectancy; overall health; tumor characteristics; and urinary, sexual, and bowel functions when counseling the patient about management options. Men with clinically localized prostate cancer should be presented all management options, including active surveillance, radiation therapy, and radical prostatectomy, and the unique risks and benefits of each. Radical prostatectomy is intended to cure patients in whom prostate cancer is truly localized. Patients who have incomplete excision or lymph node–positive disease are at risk for recurrence and progression. To date, it is unclear to what extent pelvic lymph node dissection (PLND) benefits survival.

Radical retropubic prostatectomy has long been the gold standard for definitive surgical therapy, but it has been challenged by less invasive approaches such as laparoscopic radical prostatectomy (LRP) and robotic-assisted laparoscopic prostatectomy (RALP). Today, most prostatectomies are performed via a minimally invasive approach. With greater experience, there are few contraindications to LRP and RALP as compared with open surgery.

Absolute contraindications to LRP or RALP include the inability of the patient to undergo general anesthesia because of severe cardiopulmonary comorbidity and uncorrectable bleeding diatheses. Prior abdominal or pelvic surgery increases technical difficulty for transperitoneal RALP especially, but it is not an absolute contraindication. Salvage surgery after primary treatment failure should be approached with caution and is associated with increased risk of urinary incontinence and rectal injury. Morbid obesity may place the patient at risk for respiratory compromise while positioned in steep Trendelenburg position and for rhabdomyolysis if operative times are long. Finally, neoadjuvant androgen deprivation, multiple prostate biopsies, and the surgical management of benign prostatic hyperplasia (BPH) can increase technical difficulty and alter anatomic landmarks but are not absolute contraindications to surgery.

PATIENT PREOPERATIVE EVALUATION AND PREPARATION

Patients are seen preoperatively for a complete history and physical examination, with special attention paid to medical comorbidities and surgical history. An ECG, a chest x-ray, a complete blood cell count, a basic metabolic panel, a coagulation profile, and a urinalysis specimen, with culture if indicated, are obtained. Informed consent is obtained for both laparoscopic surgery and open conversion. Patients are counseled on the risk of bleeding, transfusion, infection, injury to adjacent organs, incisional hernia, impotence, and incontinence. The risks of general anesthesia must also be discussed because laparoscopic prostatectomy cannot be performed with the patient under regional anesthesia. It is our practice to obtain a baseline assessment of urinary symptoms with the International Prostate Symptom Score and erectile function with the Sexual Health Inventory of Men. This allows for improved counseling regarding a realistic forecast of the return of urinary and erectile function.

Bowel preparation varies by surgeon. Magnesium citrate and clear liquids may be started the day before surgery; however, some surgeons prefer to use only a fleet enema on the morning of the operation. Broad-spectrum antibiotics are administered intravenously within 1 hour of incision in accordance with the American Urology Association guidelines.

OPERATING ROOM CONFIGURATION AND PATIENT POSITIONING

The operating room should be large enough to accommodate the da Vinci Surgical System (Intuitive Surgical, Sunnyvale, Calif.) comfortably with ample room for the surgical team and anesthesia staff in the configuration shown in Figure 33-1. At our institution we use the da Vinci Si HD Surgical System with a four-arm technique.

The bedside surgical assistant should be well versed in laparoscopy and troubleshooting the robotic system. The scrub technician must also be familiar with docking the robot and exchanging robotic instruments. Finally, the anesthesiologist must be aware of the physiologic nuances of laparoscopy and steep Trendelenburg positioning. Adequate communication between team members is essential to a smooth operation.

After induction of general anesthesia, the arm boards are removed, and the patient's arms are tucked to the side with two draw sheets and foam padding as shown in Figure 33-2. The hand and wrists are padded, with the thumb oriented upward in an anatomically neutral position.

A split leg table or stirrups may be used to abduct the patient's legs, allowing access to the perineum during the case. When a split leg table is used, the hips are flexed gently. Be careful not to overflex the hips because this can lead to femoral nerve stretch injuries. Care should also be taken when stirrups are used because pressure injuries can occur at the calf if operative times are long. Sequential compression devices are placed and activated.

The patient's upper body is secured with foam padding and heavy cloth tape across the xyphoid process. This prevents the patient from sliding backward when placed in the steep Trendelenburg position. An orogastric tube is placed to decompress the stomach. The abdomen is shaved, prepped, and draped in the usual sterile fashion. The penis is prepped into the field, and a 16-French urethral catheter is placed.

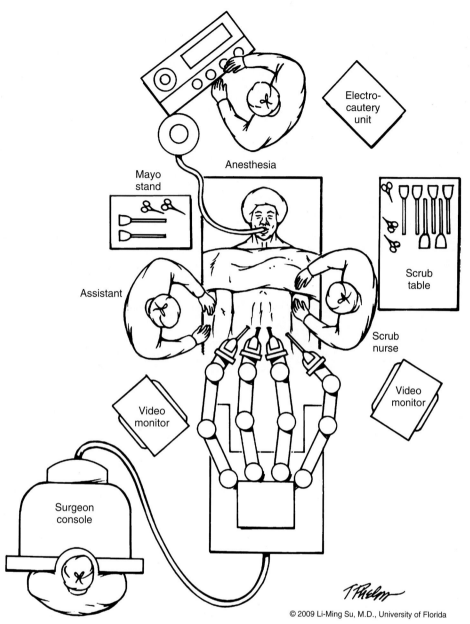

Figure 33-1. Operating room and trocar configuration for laparoscopic radical prostatectomy. The operating room is configured so that the entire team can see the procedure. The assistant stands on the patient's left side.

TROCAR PLACEMENT

A total of six trocars are used for transperitoneal RALP (Figure 33-3). A 12-mm trocar is used for the endoscope and camera. This is placed approximately 15 to 17 cm superior to the pubic symphysis and generally just above the umbilicus. Two 8-mm metal robotic trocars are placed in a pararectus position, approximately 8 cm lateral and slightly caudal to the camera trocar. An additional 8-mm robotic trocar is placed approximately 8 cm lateral to the left robotic trocar to accommodate the fourth robotic arm. The surgical assistant uses a 12-mm trocar in the right lower quadrant just superior medial to the anterior superior iliac spine at the same level as the pararectus trocars that are used for passage of clips and suture. Finally, a 5-mm trocar is placed in the right upper quadrant at the apex of a triangle made between the assistant trocar and the right pararectus trocar that is mainly used for suction and irrigation.

PROCEDURE (SEE VIDEO 33-1)

LRP and RALP can be approached transperitoneally or extra-peritoneally. The transperitoneal approach is presented here with predominant focus on the *posterior* approach. Specific steps salient to the *anterior* approach to robotic prostatectomy are also highlighted.

Step 1: Abdominal Access and Trocar Placement

In a transperitoneal approach, pneumoperitoneum is established with a Veress needle, which is inserted at the base of the umbilicus. Alternatively, an open Hasson technique may be used. The abdomen is insufflated to a pressure of 12 mm Hg. The 12-mm camera trocar is placed first under direct vision with a visual obturator. Once the camera trocar has been placed, the patient is placed in the steep Trendelenburg position, which allows the bowels to fall cephalad and out of the

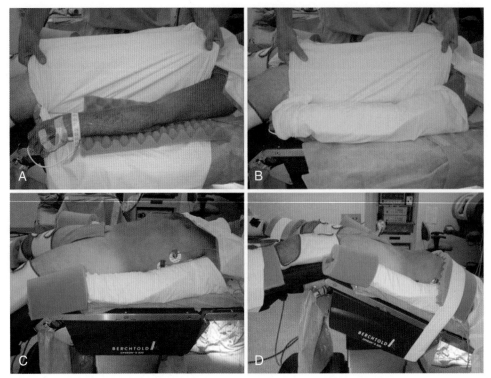

Figure 33-2. Patient positioning for transperitoneal laparoscopic radical prostatectomy. The patient's arms are tucked and padded at the sides **(A-C)** with the operating table placed in the Trendelenburg position **(D)**.

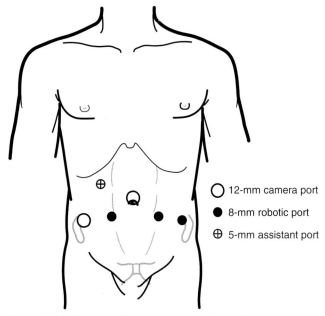

Figure 33-3. Trocar configuration for transperitoneal laparoscopic radical prostatectomy.

○ 12-mm camera port

● 8-mm robotic port

⊕ 5-mm assistant port

pelvic cavity. The 8-mm robotic trocars and the 12-mm and 5-mm assistant trocars are then placed under direct laparoscopic vision. The da Vinci robot is then positioned between the patient's legs, and the robotic arms are docked.

The robotic camera is inserted through the camera trocar. At our institution we exclusively use a 0-degree lens; however, an angled 30-degree lens may be used on the basis of surgeon preference. The robotic instruments are inserted under direct vision. A curved monopoly scissor, Maryland bipolar forceps

(Intuitive Surgical, Sunnyvale, Calif.), and ProGrasp forceps (Intuitive Surgical, Sunnyvale, Calif.) are used in the right, left, and third arms, respectively.

On entry into the abdomen, anatomic landmarks are identified, including the internal inguinal rings, urachus, and medial umbilical ligaments. The peritoneum and bowel are inspected for adhesions, which are taken down sharply (Figure 33-4).

Step 2: Dissection of the Seminal Vesicles and Vas Deferens

The transperitoneal posterior approach begins with dissection of the seminal vesicles (SVs) and vas deferens. The ProGrasp forceps is used to retract the sigmoid colon out of the pelvic cavity. The vas deferens is identified as it courses over the medial umbilical ligaments. The overlying peritoneum is incised, and the vas is traced medially to its coalescence with the ipsilateral SV where it is clipped and divided. The contralateral vas is then dissected. The assistant provides countertraction by lifting the bladder anteriorly in the midline, and the SVs are then dissected. The posterior dissection is carried out first and can be done bluntly. The anterior dissection of the SVs should be performed meticulously because small vessels are frequently encountered entering from the anterior lateral aspect of the SVs. These vessels are clipped with Hem-o-lok clips (Weck Closure Systems, Research Triangle Park, N.C.) and divided sharply with cold scissors to avoid thermal injury to the nearby neurovascular bundle (NVB) (Figure 33-5).

Step 3: Posterior Dissection of the Prostate

The vasa and SVs are lifted anteriorly with the ProGrasp forceps. The assistant provides counter traction by applying downward pressure on the midline rectum with a suction-irrigator. A 2- to 3-cm horizontal incision is made through the

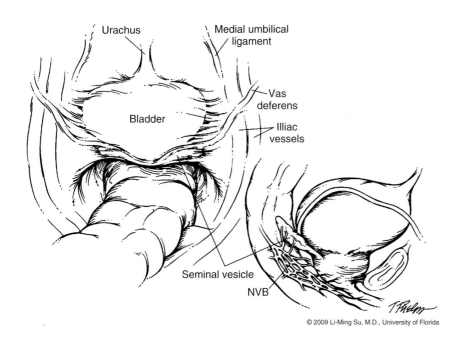

Urachus
Medial umbilical ligament
Vas deferens
Bladder
Illiac vessels
Seminal vesicle
NVB

© 2009 Li-Ming Su, M.D., University of Florida

Figure 33-4. Initial intraperitoneal view detailing the relevant landmarks within the male pelvis during transperitoneal laparoscopic radical prostatectomy. *NVB*, neurovascular bundle.

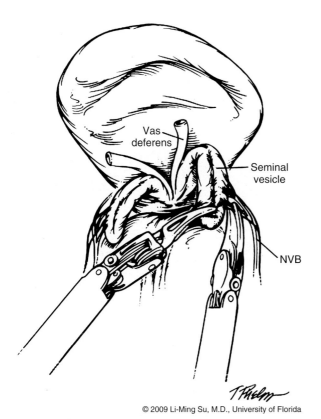

Vas deferens
Seminal vesicle
NVB

© 2009 Li-Ming Su, M.D., University of Florida

Figure 33-5. Seminal vesicle (SV) dissection. In lieu of the use of electrocautery for hemostasis, hemoclips are applied along the lateral aspect and tip of the SV to secure the vascular pedicle and avoid thermal injury to the nearby neurovascular bundles (NVBs). Completed bilateral SV and vas dissection is shown.

cul-de-sac approximately 0.5 cm below the base of the SVs. In patients with low risk, nonpalpable disease, the posterior dissection plane is developed between the prostatic fascia anteriorly and Denonvilliers fascia posteriorly to facilitate later release of the NVB located along the posterolateral surface of

the prostate. In cases of palpable intermediate- or high-risk disease, the posterior dissection is carried one layer deeper, penetrating through Denonvilliers fascia down to the prerectal fat plane. This provides an additional layer of tissue coverage (i.e., Denonvilliers fascia) along the posterior surface of the excised specimen. The plane is developed with gentle sweeping motions, gradually moving toward the prostate apex. Wide dissection of the rectum off the posterior prostate is critical to minimize the risk of rectal injury during later parts of the operation (Fig. 33-6).

Step 4: Developing the Space of Retzius

The transperitoneal *anterior* approach begins with dissection of the bladder and exposure of the space of Retzius. The space of Retzius is entered by incising the peritoneum just lateral to the medial umbilical ligaments. The left hand is used to provide steady traction on the bladder inferiorly to visualize the appropriate plane of dissection. Carry the dissection caudally until the pubic arch is seen. The bladder is then mobilized posterolaterally to the level of the vas deferens as the vas deferens crosses over the medial umbilical ligament, ensuring a tension-free vesicourethral anastomosis (Fig. 33-7).

Step 5: Incision of Endopelvic Fascia and Management of the Deep Dorsal Venous Complex

Once the bladder is dropped, the fat overlying the anterior prostate is removed. The superficial dorsal venous complex (DVC) lies in the midline with branches decussating through the anterior preprostatic fat. The superficial DVC is coagulated with bipolar electrocautery before division, and the preprostatic fat is completely removed. At the completion of this step, visible landmarks include the anterior aspect of the bladder and prostate, puboprostatic ligaments, endopelvic fascia, and pubis (Fig. 33-8).

The endopelvic fascia and puboprostatic ligaments are sharply divided, and this division exposes the levator muscle fibers attached to the lateral and apical portions of the prostate. Once complete, the DVC is clearly seen. The ProGrasp forceps are used to bunch the DVC along the anterior prostatovesical junction while simultaneously applying slight

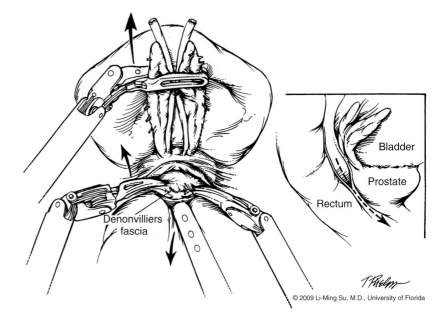

Figure 33-6. Posterior dissection of the prostate. The fourth robotic arm is used to apply upward traction on the seminal vesicles (SVs) and vasa while the assistant provided downward traction on the rectum. A transverse incision is made in Denonvilliers fascia below the SVs, and blunt dissection is used to develop a plane between Denonvilliers fascia and the rectum. Inset demonstrates the direction of posterior dissection toward the prostatic apex.

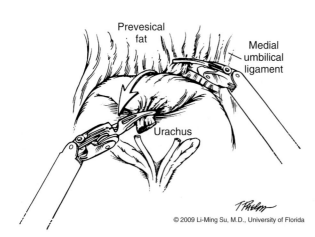

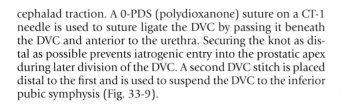

Figure 33-7. Division of urachus and entry into the space of Retzius. Cephalad and posterior traction on the urachus helps to identify the fatty alveolar tissue immediately anterior to the bladder, marking the proper plane of dissection. The medial umbilical ligaments demarcate lateral extent of the bladder dissection.

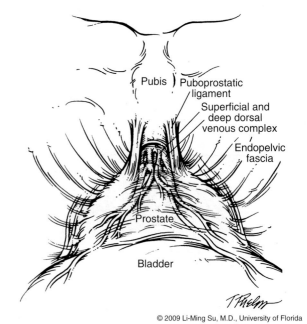

Figure 33-8. Retropubic view of the bladder and prostate following entry into the space of Retzius. The removal of the fatty tissue overlying the anterior aspect of the prostate exposes the puboprostatic ligaments and endopelvic fascia.

cephalad traction. A 0-PDS (polydioxanone) suture on a CT-1 needle is used to suture ligate the DVC by passing it beneath the DVC and anterior to the urethra. Securing the knot as distal as possible prevents iatrogenic entry into the prostatic apex during later division of the DVC. A second DVC stitch is placed distal to the first and is used to suspend the DVC to the inferior pubic symphysis (Fig. 33-9).

Step 6: Anterior Bladder Neck Transection

Several maneuvers are used to help identify the plane of dissection between the bladder and prostate in preparation for transection of the bladder neck. First, visual inspection of the prevesical fat as it transitions to the bare anterior prostate gland can often define the bladder neck. Second, lifting the dome of the bladder cephalad with the ProGrasp forceps creates a tenting effect that defines where

the bladder connects to the base of the prostate. Third, a bimanual "pinch" can be performed by compressing the tissues of the bladder and prostate between the two robotic instruments. Finally, the surgical assistant can provide traction on the urethral catheter, bringing the balloon to the bladder neck. See the associated video for demonstration of all of these techniques. When in doubt, a more proximal plane of dissection is used to avoid inadvertent entry into the base of the prostate, which can result in a positive bladder neck margin. Keep in mind that the bladder neck can always be reconstructed after the prostate has been removed.

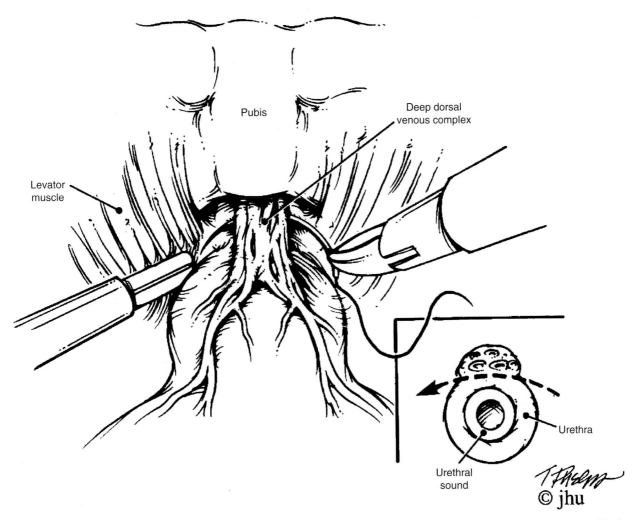

Figure 33-9. Ligation of the deep dorsal venous complex. A suture is passed from right to left, ligating the dorsal vein as distal as possible. Inset demonstrates the proper passage of the needle immediately anterior to the urethra. A urethral sound can be placed to ensure that the urethra is not incorporated in the suture.

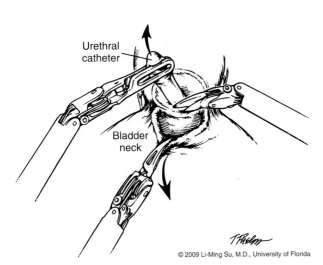

Figure 33-10. Posterior bladder neck division. The third robotic arm is used to lift the catheter tip anteriorly, exposing the posterior bladder neck. Horizontal dissection is carried out through the posterior bladder neck.

The anterior bladder neck is divided transversely, staying close to the midline. Lateral dissection can result in unwanted bleeding from the lateral bladder pedicles. Once the anterior bladder neck is transected, the urethral catheter is exposed. The catheter balloon is deflated, and the catheter tip is advanced through the anterior bladder defect. The ProGrasp is used to lift the catheter tip to the anterior abdominal wall. At the same time, the distal end of the catheter is cinched by the assistant at the penile meatus, effectively suspending the prostate anteriorly (Fig. 33-10).

Step 7: Posterior Bladder Neck Transection

The mucosa of the posterior bladder neck is inspected to identify the presence or absence of a median lobe (i.e., bulge or mass effect) and location of the ureteral orifices. The bladder mucosa is incised transversely, beginning at the midline to avoid bleeding from the lateral bladder pedicles. After the posterior bladder neck is incised through the bladder mucosa, the angle of dissection is oriented 45 degrees downward to avoid inadvertent entry into the prostate base, as well as excessive thinning of the posterior bladder neck. If excessive bleeding occurs, one should be concerned about entry into the prostate gland.

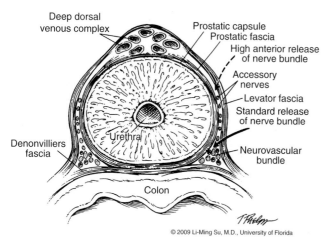

Figure 33-11. Cross section of the prostate demonstrating the periprostatic fascial planes with respect to the location of the neurovascular bundles (NVBs). After anteromedial incision of the levator fascia, the dashed line indicates the direction of interfascial dissection (i.e., between the levator and prostatic fascia) to accomplish release of the NVB from the prostate.

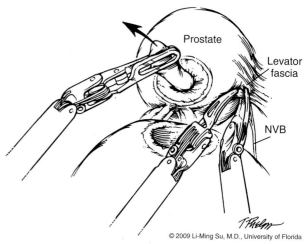

Figure 33-12. Developing the right lateral neurovascular bundle *(NVB)* groove. After the right levator fascia is incised, the monopolar scissors are used to develop the interfascial plane between the elevator and prostatic fascia.

Once the retrovesical space is entered, the SVs and vasa are grasped with the ProGrasp forceps and delivered through the opening between the prostate and bladder. In the *posterior* approach, the SVs and vasa have already been dissected free, and this dissection allows these structures to be identified and lifted easily. Conversely, in the *anterior* approach, the SVs and vasa require dissection with release of the NVBs at this step. Once complete, the remaining lateral attachments between the prostatic base and bladder are divided between Hem-o-lok clips.

Step 8: Lateral Interfascial Dissection of the Neurovascular Bundles

The NVB travels between the levator and prostatic fascia as seen in Figure 33-11. The decision of whether to perform nerve preservation depends on the patient's preoperative sexual function and expectations, as well as clinical grade and stage and site-specific biopsy information (e.g., lateral versus medial, number of positive cores, and percent core involvement). In general, for patients with low-risk disease, a more aggressive nerve-sparing approach may be safely used, beginning with a high anterior release of the levator fascia along the anteromedial border of the prostate. For patients with intermediate- or high-risk disease, a more conservative nerve-sparing approach must be taken to avoid iatrogenic positive margin from dissecting too close to the surface of the prostate. In such cases, a standard release of the NVB is performed through incision of the levator fascia at the 5 o'clock and 7 o'clock positions along the posterolateral surface of the prostate.

For the prostate to be prepared for nerve sparing, the base of the prostate or tip of the urethral catheter is grasped with the ProGrasp forceps and retracted medially to expose the lateral surface of the prostate. This creates a flat surface along the lateral prostate for dissection of the nerve bundles off of the prostate. An opening in the levator fascia is made sharply and carried longitudinally to the apex and base. The interfacial plane between the levator and prostatic fascia is developed bluntly to avoid electrocautery injury to the nerves as they course through this space. The groove between the NVB and the prostate is developed posterolaterally. Insufflation pressure may be temporarily raised to decrease bleeding from periprostatic vessels if necessary (Fig. 33-12).

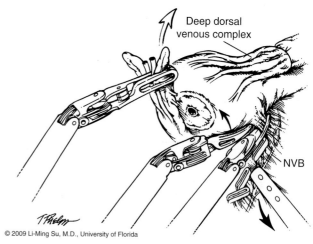

Figure 33-13. Ligation of the right prostatic pedicle and antegrade dissection of the neurovascular bundle *(NVB)*. With countertraction on the seminal vesicles and vasa provided by the fourth robotic arm, the prostatic pedicles are identified, clipped, and divided without electrocautery, staying close to the prostate surface. Direction and course of antegrade NVB dissection are guided by the previously defined lateral NVB groove.

Step 9: Ligation of the Prostatic Pedicles

With the course of the NVBs clearly defined along the lateral aspect of the prostate, the remaining prostatic pedicle is divided by creating tissue packets and clipping them with Hem-o-lok clips, followed by sharp division to minimize thermal injury to the NVBs. The remaining attachments between the NVBs and prostate are gently teased off in an antegrade manner toward the prostate apex. If dense adhesions are encountered between the NVB and the prostate, slightly wider dissection may be carried out to avoid a positive surgical margin, especially in locations at risk for extraprostatic extension. As such, incremental preservation of cavernous nerves can be achieved without sacrificing the entire NVB (Fig. 33-13).

Step 10: Division of the Deep Dorsal Venous Complex

The DVC is divided sharply just proximal to the DVC suture. Care must be taken to avoid inadvertent entry into the apex of the prostate, resulting in a positive margin. Spot electrocautery may be required for small arteries within the DVC. Occasionally, an additional 4-0 polyglactin suture may be needed to oversew the DVC if the original suture is dislodged.

Step 11: Prostatic Apical Dissection and Division of the Urethra

Dissection of the prostatic apex is challenging because of its proximity to the NVBs and DVC, and because of variations in prostatic apical anatomy. The NVBs must be gently swept off the apex without electrocautery. The anterior urethral is divided sharply to avoid injury to the NVB and ensure clear visualization of dissection away from the prostatic apex. After the urethral catheter is exposed, it is withdrawn from the urethra. Before division of the posterior urethra, the contour of the prostatic apex is inspected to ensure that it does not protrude eccentrically beneath the posterior urethra (Fig. 33-14). Once the prostate is free, the pedicles and NVBs are inspected for hemostasis. In case of large venous or arterial bleeding, 4-0 polyglactin figure-of-eight sutures may be used in lieu of thermal energy to secure hemostasis.

Step 12: Pelvic Lymph Node Dissection

In select patients, pelvic lymph node dissection (PLND) is performed before vesicourethral anastomosis. The key initial step is separation of the nodal packet from the external iliac vein by grasping the packet and retracting medially away from the vein. There is a relatively avascular plane between the lymph node packet and the lateral sidewall that can be dissected bluntly with spot electrocautery. Dissection is carried proximally to the iliac bifurcation and distally to the pubis. Retraction of the lymph node packet medially also helps to identify the obturator nerve and vessels. After the distal extent of the lymph node packet is divided with clips, the packet is retracted cranially and then bluntly swept away from the obturator nerve. The proximal extent of the lymph node packet is then clipped and divided at the bifurcation of the iliac vessels. The lymph nodes can typically be removed as a single packet. For identification purposes, a single clip is applied to the left packet to distinguish laterality for the pathologist (Fig. 33-15).

The prostate specimen and pelvic lymph nodes are placed in a 10-mm laparoscopic entrapment bag and stored within the abdomen until the completion of the operation.

Step 13: Vesicoureteral Anastomosis

To reduce tension at the vesicourethral anastomosis and to provide additional support to the bladder neck, we perform a modified posterior reconstruction before proceeding with the vesicourethral anastomosis. A double-armed, 3-0 barbed suture (Quill, Vancouver, British Columbia, Canada) is used. The stitch is begun at the midline through the superficial remnant of Denonvilliers fascia, taken through superficial detrusor of the posterior bladder, and then completed at the posterior rhabdosphincter. Use of the urethral catheter and perineal pressure helps identify the urethral lumen and allows for easier identification of the posterior rhabdosphincter lying just posterior to the urethra. Two complete

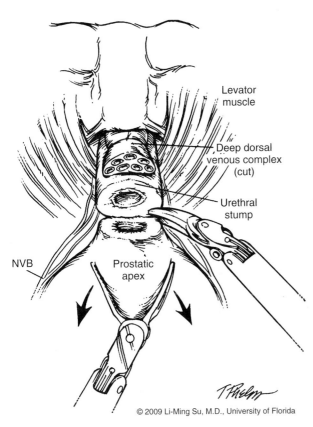

© 2009 Li-Ming Su, M.D., University of Florida

Figure 33-14. Division of the prostatic apex. After transection the of dorsal venous complex, the anterior urethra is divided sharply, taking care to preserve the neurovascular bundles (NVBs) coursing posterolaterally and being mindful of variations in prostatic apical anatomy.

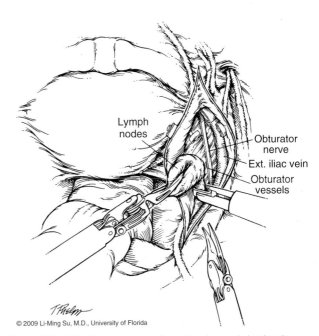

© 2009 Li-Ming Su, M.D., University of Florida

Figure 33-15. Pelvic lymph node dissection. Anatomic landmarks during pelvic lymph node dissection include the external iliac vein and obturator nerve.

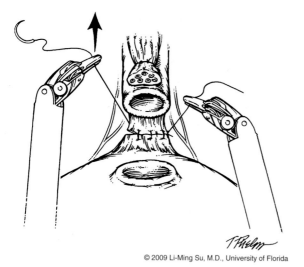

© 2009 Li-Ming Su, M.D., University of Florida

Figure 33-16. Modified Rocco stitch. The remnant Denonvilliers fascia and superficial detrusor from the posterior bladder are reapproximated below the urethra. This additional stitch reduces tension on the vesicourethral anastomosis.

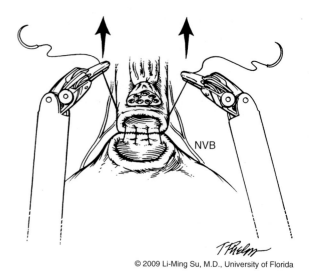

© 2009 Li-Ming Su, M.D., University of Florida

Figure 33-17. Running vesicourethral anastomosis. The vesicourethral anastomosis is performed in a running continuous fashion beginning at the 5 and 7 o'clock positions, outside-in along the posterior bladder neck. The urethral catheter is passed and withdrawn repeatedly to identify the urethral opening during the urethral bites of the anastomosis. *NVB*, neurovascular bundle.

throws are performed on the right and left before pulling up on the suture to reapproximate the bladder neck to the urethra (Fig. 33-16).

The vesicourethral anastomosis is begun as a continuation of the stitch used for the posterior reconstruction. The posterior anastomosis is typically the site of greatest tension and at the highest risk for disruption and subsequent leakage during passage of the urethral catheter if mucosa-to-mucosa apposition is not established. To avoid this, the assistant maintains perineal pressure to expose the posterior urethra during the initial stages of the anastomosis. The anastomosis begins at the 5 o'clock and 7 o'clock positions, outside-in along the posterior bladder neck. Corresponding inside-out bites are taken of the urethra at the 5 o'clock and 7 o'clock positions by the two separate arms of the suture. The urethral catheter may be grasped and lifted anteriorly with the nonthrowing hand to expose the posterior urethral mucosa with each bite. The suture is run anteriorly around the urethral circumference. As the left-sided suture approaches the 11 o'clock position, it is reversed outside-in on the urethral bite and then inside-out on the bladder to allow the final knot to be tied across the anastomosis (Fig. 33-17). In the event of redundancy of the bladder neck, 2-0 polyglactin figure-of-eight sutures may be used to close the anterior bladder. At the completion of the anastomosis, an 18-French urethral catheter is placed by the surgical assistant, and the balloon is inflated to 20 mL of sterile water. The integrity of the anastomoses is tested by filling the bladder with approximately 120 mL of saline through the catheter. Any visible leaks can be oversewn.

If a lymph node dissection is performed, a pelvic drain is placed through the third robotic arm trocar site and secured at the skin with 2-0 nylon suture. The entrapment bag containing the prostate and lymph node packets is delivered via extension of the umbilical incision. The fascia is closed with 0-PDS in a figure-of-eight fashion. The 8-mm and 5-mm trocars generally do not require closure, and the 12-mm assistant trocar also does not need closure if a nonbladed, self-dilating trocar is used.

POSTOPERATIVE MANAGEMENT

Hospital stay is typically 1 to 2 days. Patients receive scheduled acetaminophen and ketorolac as long as the risk of bleeding and renal insufficiency is low to limit narcotic use and avoid associated ileus. Narcotics are available for breakthrough pain. Patients are given clear liquids on the day of surgery, and the liquids are advanced as tolerated. Sequential compression devices are used throughout the hospital stay, and patients are instructed to walk at least 6 times daily to avoid deep vein thrombosis and promote the return of bowel function. Patients are discharged home with the urethral catheter and pelvic drain and return to the clinic for a cystogram on postoperative day 7 to ensure a water-tight vesicoureteral anastomosis before catheter removal.

COMPLICATIONS

Ureteral and rectal injuries are rare events, which are avoided by maintaining good visualization and a sound understanding of surrounding anatomy and orientation. Ureteral injury can occur during three steps. First, during dissection of the vas deferens, it is important to keep dissection close to the adventitia of the vas to prevent inadvertent thermal injury to the ureter, which passes laterally and posterior to the vas. Second, the ureter may be compromised during vesicoureteral anastomosis, especially in cases of a large bladder neck opening, especially in patients with a large median lobe or after TURP [transurethral resection of the prostate]). Imbrication of the bladder at the 5 o'clock and 7 o'clock locations will prevent injury to the ureteral orifices while the vesicourethral anastomosis is completed. Alternatively, a ureteral stent may be passed in a retrograde fashion to protect the ureters. Finally, the ureter may be encountered during PLND as it crosses over the iliac vessels. This is especially true during an extended lymph node dissection. It is important to minimize both thermal and mechanical injury to the ureter by entrapment with hemoclips.

Rectal injuries are rare but devastating complications, and they can be avoided with predominately blunt dissection of the rectum and overlying Denonvilliers fascia and by widely releasing the rectum off of the posterior aspect of the prostate. If a rectal injury does occur, primary laparoscopic closure of the edges in two layers without proximal diversion is acceptable in the absence of a sizable defect or gross fecal contamination. If an injury is suspected but not clearly visualized, a catheter may be placed into the anus with air instilled into the rectum to look for bubbles while filling the pelvic cavity with saline. On completion of the repair, the operative field should be copiously irrigated and drained. Omentum or a peritoneal flap may be used as tissue interposition between the repair and the vesicourethral anastomosis.

Liberal use of hemoclips to secure lymphatics during PLND decreases the risk of postoperative lymphocele. Meticulous hemostasis along the pedicles, NVBs, and DVC during dissection decreases the risk of vesicourethral anastomotic disruption from postoperative pelvic bleeding.

TIPS AND TRICKS

- *Use of a skilled bedside assistant.*
- *Use of insufflation.* Transiently increasing insufflation pressure to 15 to 20 mm Hg may be useful to minimize venous bleeding and optimize visualization.
- *Avoidance of positive margins.* Performance of an oncologically sound operation is paramount to radical prostatectomy because it is well established that the presence of positive surgical margins leads to a higher risk of biochemical recurrence. The following tips can help minimize site-specific positive margins.
  - *Apical margin:* Preparation of DVC is paramount. Make sure to release puboprostatic ligaments and perform a distal ligation of DVC. Also, beware of a posterior-protruding prostatic apex.
  - *Bladder neck margin:* Carefully identify the anterior bladder neck with tips described previously, always erring on the side of more proximal division.
  - *Posterior margin.* The proper plane of posterior dissection can be adjusted according to the presence or absence of palpable, high-volume, or high-risk disease.
  - *Posterolateral margin.* This particular region is perhaps the most challenging for urologists because a decision must be made as to whether nerve sparing should be performed, while an attempt is made to optimize an oncologic cure. The decision as to whether a complete or incremental (i.e., partial) preservation of the NVBs should be performed must be made on the basis of clinical (stage, grade, biopsy findings) and operative (presence or absence of dense adhesions between the prostate and NVBs) findings.

34 Preperitoneal Robotic-Assisted Radical Prostatectomy

Vineet Agrawal, Jean V. Joseph

The preperitoneal (also referred to as an extraperitoneal or retroperitoneal) approach to performing a robotic-assisted radical prostatectomy (RARP) aims to mimic access obtained during an open retropubic radical prostatectomy technique, long considered to be the gold standard surgical management for localized prostate cancer. Maintaining the integrity of the abdominal cavity by performing the entire procedure in the space of Retzius furthers the goal of minimizing the invasiveness of RARP. The preperitoneal approach has unique advantages. However, it is less frequently used worldwide than the transperitoneal approach. Reasons for this can be mainly attributed to training, unfamiliarity with instrumentation during preperitoneal space creation, and a smaller working space. Ability to perform a preperitoneal RARP is a useful skill to acquire. The procedure is particularly beneficial for patients with significant intra-abdominal incisions from prior surgeries; those in whom preservation of the integrity of the peritoneal surface is important, such as patients on peritoneal dialysis who are waiting to be cancer free for transplantation; and patients who cannot tolerate extreme Trendelenburg position.

This chapter describes our step-by-step technique of preperitoneal RARP based on experience with more than 2000 procedures using that approach for over a decade.

INDICATIONS AND CONTRAINDICATIONS

The indications for performing a preperitoneal RARP are no different from those for an open or laparoscopic radical prostatectomy or transperitoneal RARP.

Relative contraindications include previous laparoscopic inguinal mesh hernia repair via a preperitoneal approach. This renders re-creation of the space very difficult. With increasing experience, challenging surgical scenarios such as a large prostate or high body mass index are managed well irrespective of the approach.

PATIENT PREOPERATIVE EVALUATION AND PREPARATION

Fitness to undergo general anesthesia is assessed with a detailed history and examination. Cardiopulmonary conditions that can worsen with hypercarbia are noted.

The patient is maintained on a clear liquid diet after lunch the day before surgery. We perform chemical bowel preparation by administering neomycin and metronidazole the day before surgery. Low-molecular-weight heparin is subcutaneously injected before the procedure. A single dose of intravenous third-generation cephalosporin antibiotic is administered before induction of anesthesia.

OPERATING ROOM CONFIGURATION AND PATIENT POSITIONING

The patient is positioned supine on a split leg bed (Fig. 34-1). We use a beanbag wrapped around the shoulders to secure the patient to the bed to prevent sliding in the Trendelenburg position. After successful induction of general endotracheal anesthesia and placement of an orogastric tube, the abdomen is shaved from the umbilicus to the pubic symphysis. Sequential compression devices are placed on both legs, which are abducted to allow access to the perineum. This allows examination of the prostate as well as docking of the patient cart of the robotic surgical system. Three-inch silk tapes are used to secure the legs to the spreader bars. Arms are placed alongside the torso with padding in egg crate foams. Care is taken to ensure that all pressure points are padded to prevent position-related injuries. The vacuum beanbag is activated after wrapping along the sides and shoulders of the patient.

We place a belladonna and opium rectal suppository at the time of prostate examination under anesthesia. This helps control postoperative bladder spasms. The rectal examination allows more accurate clinical staging before surgery. The abdomen is prepared and draped from the nipples to the upper thighs. A 16-French two-way Foley catheter with a 10-mL balloon is used to drain the bladder before the patient is placed in Trendelenburg position (10 to 15 degrees). Because of the natural retraction of the bowels by the peritoneum in this approach, it is not necessary to place the patient in an exaggerated Trendelenburg position, which is often required in the transperitoneal approach.

EXTRAPERITONEAL SPACE CREATION AND TROCAR PLACEMENT

A 3-cm incision is made adjacent to the umbilicus and deepened to expose the anterior rectus sheath (Fig. 34-2).

A 1-cm transverse cut is made in the anterior rectus sheath. A purse-string suture is placed over the edges of the sheath in preparation for tightening around the camera trocar later to prevent CO_2 leakage. The medial edge of the underlying rectus abdominis muscle belly is pushed laterally to visualize the posterior rectus sheath. The lip of the S-shaped retractor is repositioned into this opening and used for upward retraction (Fig. 34-3).

A 0-degree 10-mm laparoscope (EndoEYE HD II 10 mm; Olympus, Center Valley, N.J.) mounted on an oval balloon dilator (OMS-XB2 Spacemaker Extraview; Covidien, Minneapolis, Minn.) is gently introduced in the plane above the posterior rectus sheath. Its tip is directed upward and medially toward the pubic symphysis. The accompanying pump is used to inflate the balloon, creating the potential preperitoneal space under vision (Fig. 34-4).

The bladder is separated from its attachments to the anterior abdominal wall. The space of Retzius and the retropubic fat are dissected, bringing the pubic symphysis into view (Fig. 34-5).

Too rapid an insufflation can lead to bleeding from tearing of the inferior epigastric vessels. The anatomic landmarks seen at the end of this step are the inferior epigastric vessels bilaterally and pubic symphysis in the midline. After its deflation, the balloon dilator with the laparoscope is withdrawn and replaced by a smooth 12-mm 15-cm-long trocar (Endopath Xcel dilating tip; Ethicon, Somerville, N.J.) (Fig. 34-6).

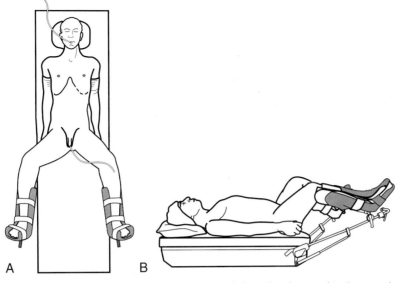

Figure 34-1. Patient positioning. **A** and **B,** The legs are abducted and secured to the spreader bars.

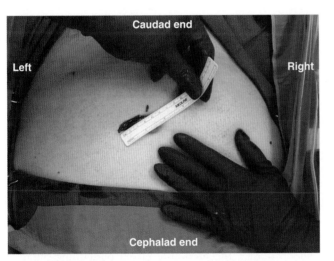

Figure 34-2. A 3-cm left periumbilical skin incision.

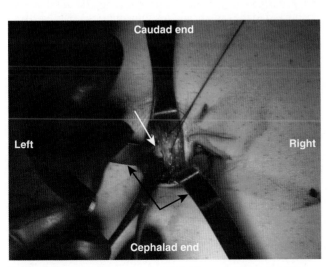

Figure 34-3. Posterior rectus sheath *(white arrow)* seen through a 1-cm incision in the anterior rectus sheath. Two S-shaped retractors *(black arrows)* help with retraction. The purse-string suture can also be seen.

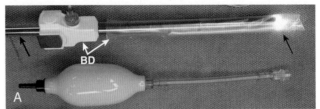

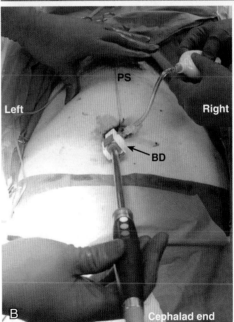

Figure 34-4. A, A 0-degree 10-mm EndoEYE laparoscope (Olympus, Center Valley, N.J.; *black arrow*) placed in a balloon dilator *(BD; top).* The red arrow points to the balloon, which assumes an oval shape after its inflation. Compression pump *(bottom).* **B,** A 0-degree 10-mm EndoEYE laparoscope mounted onto the BD introduced in the plane above the posterior rectus sheath and directed toward the pubic symphysis *(PS).* The compression pump is being used to inflate the balloon.

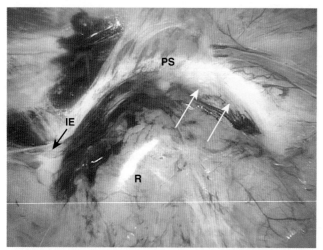

Figure 34-5. View through the balloon. The space of Retzius (R), arch of the pubic bone (white arrows), the pubic symphysis (PS), and the origin of the left inferior epigastric vessels (IE) can be seen.

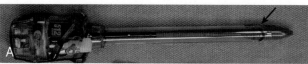

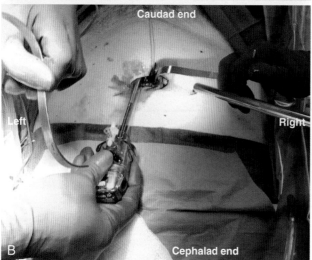

Figure 34-6. A, A smooth 12-mm 15-cm-long trocar with its obturator (arrow points to the beveled edge). **B,** A smooth 12-mm 15-cm-long trocar with beveled edge being inserted on removal of the dilating balloon.

CO_2 is connected to the trocar to insufflate the preperitoneal space created previously. The laparoscope is inserted into the trocar. Under direct vision, the preperitoneal space is further developed laterally to allow placement of the assistant and fourth arm trocars. The beveled edge of the trocar is insinuated under the inferior epigastric vessels and used to sweep the peritoneum cephalad. Following an avascular plane between the transversalis fascia below and rectus abdominis muscle above avoids an inadvertent peritoneal opening. A 12-mm assistant trocar is placed 5 cm cephalad to the right anterior superior iliac spine. During introduction of this trocar, care must be taken to redirect the trocar once it has been visualized to avoid injury to the underlying peritoneum. The left and right 8-mm metallic robotic trocars are inserted about 8 to 10 cm lateral and caudad to the camera trocar. These are

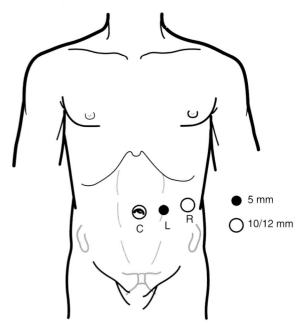

Figure 34-7. Trocar configuration seen prior to docking. C, camera trocar; L, left robotic trocar; R, right robotic trocar.

inserted lateral to the inferior epigastric vessels. We routinely use a hypodermic needle to chart the path of the trocar and prevent inadvertent injury of the vessels. Given that our assistant is left-handed and sits on the patient's right side, we place our fourth arm robotic trocar on the left side of the abdomen. This 8-mm metallic trocar is placed 5 cm cephalad to the left anterior superior iliac spine. Finally, a 5-mm assistant trocar is placed 5 cm lateral to the umbilicus on the right side (Fig. 34-7). Particular care is required to avoid an inadvertent peritoneal opening during sweeping of the peritoneum as the space for this trocar placement is created.

Adequate spacing between the trocars is imperative to avoid external arm collisions. A Xeroform petroleum dressing gauze (DeRoyal, Powell, Tenn.) is wrapped around the camera trocar to prevent CO_2 leakage. (An alternative is to use a double-sleeved balloon trocar.) The previously placed purse-string suture is tightened around this gauze over the camera trocar. The patient cart is moved between the abducted legs and the robotic arms are docked to the camera and instrument trocars (Fig. 34-8).

We use a 0-degree 10-mm da Vinci scope (Intuitive Surgical, Sunnyvale, Calif.) throughout the procedure. The robotic instruments are brought inside the surgical field under vision (Maryland bipolar forceps, scissors, and ProGrasp forceps [Intuitive Surgical, Sunnyvale, Calif.] in the left, right, and fourth arms, respectively). The 12- and 5-mm assistant trocars are used for passage of sutures, clips, and suction and irrigation as necessary.

PROCEDURE (SEE VIDEO 34-1)

The bladder takedown step that has to be performed in a transperitoneal RARP is eliminated in the preperitoneal approach. Similarly, potential adhesiolysis from prior operations or from adhesions between the sigmoid and the anterior abdominal wall is not necessary. All remaining steps are identical to a transperitoneal RARP with slight variation in the specimen extraction and closure steps.

Incision of Endopelvic Fascia

The first step to be performed in a preperitoneal RARP is the incision of the endopelvic fascia (Fig. 34-9). With the use of

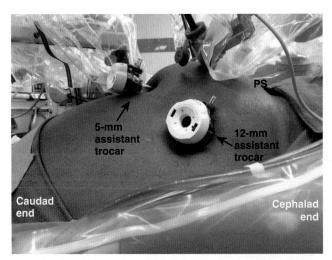

Figure 34-8. Minimal Trendelenburg position used in the extraperitoneal approach as seen in a view from the patient's right side. Selective insufflation of the extraperitoneal cavity can be appreciated. *PS,* pubic symphysis.

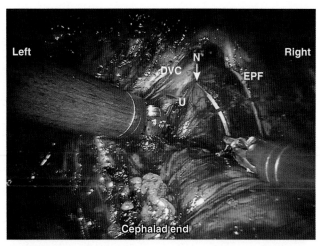

Figure 34-10. Initial throw of the suture in the right "notch" *(N)* between the dorsal vein complex *(DVC)* and the urethra *(U)* visible here on the left side. *EPF,* endopelvic fascia.

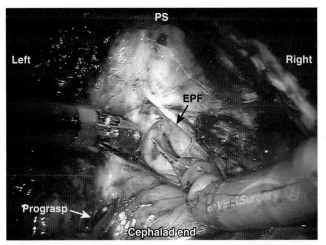

Figure 34-9. Incision of the endopelvic fascia *(EPF),* here visible on the right. The ProGrasp forceps (Intuitive Surgical, Sunnyvale, Calif.) are used to apply cephalad retraction. *PS,* pubic symphysis.

direction into the "notch" between the DVC and the urethra (Fig. 34-10).

After the first and the third throws, the needle is passed through the pubic symphysis to anteriorly suspend the urethra. This has been shown to aid in continence recovery.

Anterior Bladder Neck Transection

The fourth arm retracts the bladder cephalad to expose the plane between the bladder and the prostate. We prefer to begin the anterior bladder neck dissection laterally where the longitudinal bladder fibers can be easily appreciated.

Using a combination of bipolar and monopolar energy, we use a "burn-and-push" technique to develop the plane between the prostate and the bladder neck (Fig. 34-11, *A* and *B*).

Following the funnel of the bladder neck leads to correct anatomic dissection (Fig. 34-11, *B*).

This dissection is carried over to the right side across the midline, with the fourth arm providing optimal countertraction. Once an adequate plane is developed on both sides, the anterior bladder neck is transected sharply in the midline with the catheter coming into view. The catheter is withdrawn.

Posterior Bladder Neck Transection

It is important to identify the location of both ureteral orifices before starting the posterior bladder neck transection. Dissection is carried out in the same plane as for the anterior bladder neck to separate the prostate from the bladder neck (Fig. 34-12).

As the neurovascular bundles (NVBs) course posterolaterally, care should be taken to avoid use of energy in this region. The longitudinal muscle fibers posterior to the bladder are identified in the midline and divided with monopolar cautery to expose the ampullae of the vas deferens (Fig. 34-13).

Dissection of Vas Deferens and Seminal Vesicles

With sweeping motion with the opened jaws of the bipolar forceps, the tissue attachments between the vasa anteriorly and the Denonvilliers fascia posteriorly are separated on both sides. The vasa are followed laterally to the tip of the seminal vesicles (SVs), at which point they are clipped en bloc with the

the fourth arm to retract the prostate medially, the endopelvic fascia is incised on both sides along the lateral aspect of the mid prostate.

Once the initial incision has been made, air entry into the space behind the endopelvic fascia facilitates identification of the correct plane of dissection. We follow the incision toward the apex of the prostate and use a combination of blunt and sharp dissection to separate the levator ani muscle from the lateral prostatic fascia. Energy use should be avoided during this step because this is generally an avascular plane. The dissection is carried out until visualization of the notch between the urethra and dorsal vein. We routinely divide the puboprostatic ligaments to allow better cinching of the dorsal venous complex (DVC).

Securing the Dorsal Venous Complex

We use a 2-0 unidirectional-barbed monofilament suture (V-Loc, Covidien, Minneapolis, Minn.) on an SH needle to secure the DVC using three throws of the suture in a right-to-left

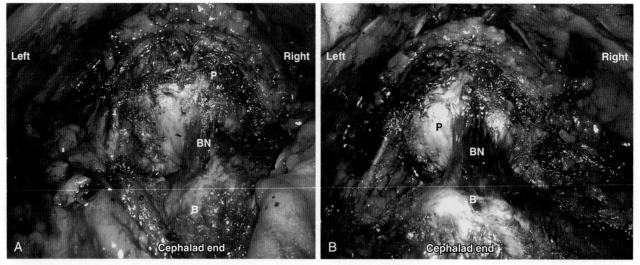

Figure 34-11. A, Use of the "burn-and-push" technique to separate the bladder neck *(BN)* fibers from those of the prostate *(P)*, here visible on the left side. **B,** Following the funnel of the BN leads to the correct anatomic plane for dissection. The left-sided BN dissection has been carried over to the right side across the midline. *B*, bladder.

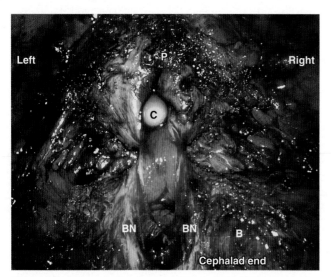

Figure 34-12. View before division of the posterior bladder neck *(BN)*. The anterior BN has been divided. *B*, bladder; *C*, catheter; *P*, prostate.

Figure 34-13. Fibers *(arrow)* posterior to the bladder *(B)* neck that need to be divided to expose the ampullae of the vas and the seminal vesicles. *P*, prostate.

accompanying vessel, located directly between the vas and the adjoining vesicle (Fig. 34-14).

We avoid any use of energy during skeletonization of the SVs, instead preferring to place Hem-o-lok clips (Weck Closure Systems, Research Triangle Park, N.C.) sequentially over vessels entering the SVs laterally. At the end of bilateral vasa and SV dissection, the fourth arm and the assistant grasper pull these structures anteriorly on the left and right sides, respectively (Fig. 34-15).

Posterior Prostate Dissection

A transverse cut is made through the Denonvilliers fascia in midline and extended on both sides (Fig. 34-16).

A combination of blunt and sharp dissection is used to develop the plane between the yellow perirectal fat and posterior prostate. This dissection is carried out toward the apex of the prostate. The assistant provides countertraction by positioning the suction over the Denonvilliers fascia.

Securing the Prostatic Pedicle and Neurovascular Bundle Preservation

We begin this step on the right side with the fourth arm providing countertraction by pulling the prostate to the left side. Vessels entering the prostate base are divided between large Hem-o-lok clips (Fig. 34-17).

The NVB is identified coursing over the posterolateral surface of the prostate. The extent of nerve preservation is determined based on patient and cancer characteristics. Meticulous dissection to gently separate the prostate from the NVB is performed with the aim of joining the plane thus created with the previously performed posterior prostate dissection (Fig. 34-18).

A combination of antegrade and retrograde dissection is now performed to clip the prostatic pedicles, with care taken to avoid injury to the preserved NVB. This dissection is performed from the base to the prostatic apex. A similar dissection is performed on the left side (Fig. 34-19).

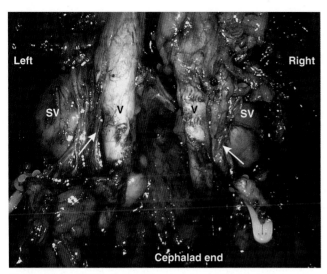

Figure 34-14. Bilateral vasa with artery *(arrows),* and seminal vesicles exposed before their clipping. *SV,* seminal vesicle; *V,* vas.

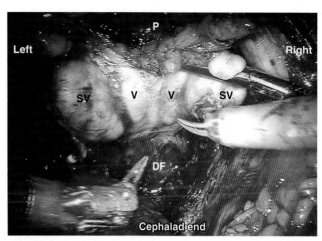

Figure 34-15. The left and right vasa and the seminal vesicles are retracted anteriorly in preparation for posterior dissection. *DF,* Denonvilliers fascia; *P,* prostate; *SV,* seminal vesicle; *V,* vas.

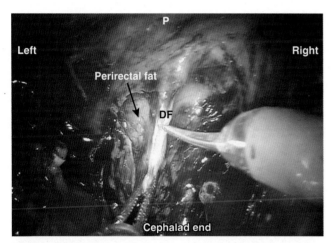

Figure 34-16. Transverse cut in Denonvilliers fascia *(DF)* to expose the yellow perirectal fat. *P,* prostate.

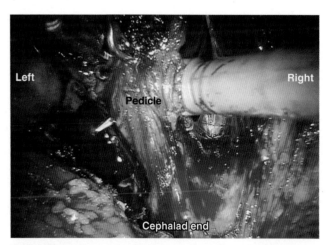

Figure 34-17. Preparation for Hem-o-lok clip (Weck Closure Systems, Research Triangle Park, N.C.) application to the pedicle supplying the right side of the prostate.

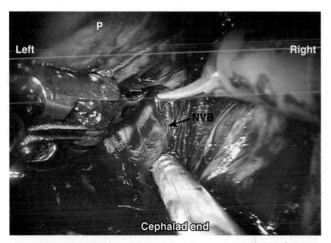

Figure 34-18. Meticulous dissection of the prostate *(P)* off the right neurovascular bundle *(NVB).*

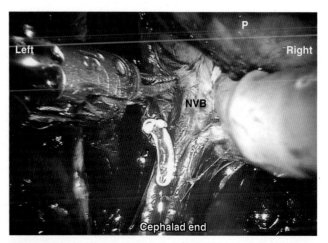

Figure 34-19. Left neurovascular bundle *(NVB)* preservation. *P,* prostate.

Prostatic Apex and Urethral Dissection

The Foley catheter is reintroduced to facilitate visualization of the urethra after DVC transection. We prefer to sharply transect the dorsal vein and urethra. Back bleeding encountered at this stage is of no consequence. Gentle irrigation by the assistant helps clear the field from DVC bleeding, which is generally mild because the DVC was previously ligated. The contour of the prostate apex is followed with the knowledge that this can vary from patient to patient. Care should be taken to avoid transecting the prostatic apex. The dissection should be caudally oriented down to the level of the urethra. Division of the anterior urethral wall leads to exposure of the catheter (Fig. 34-20).

The posterior urethral wall is subsequently divided (Fig. 34-21).

Extreme care is required during final division of the apical fibers to prevent injury to previously preserved NVB fibers coursing close to the apex of the prostate. Occasionally, prostatic tissue in the posterior apex extends caudally behind the urethra. Similar to the anterior dissection, the posterior dissection should follow the contour of the prostate, to ensure that all prostate tissue is resected and avoid a positive surgical margin. The specimen is examined for adequacy of the resection margins, put in a 10-mm specimen bag (Endo Catch, Covidien, Mansfield, Mass.), and moved cephalad out of the surgical field until its extraction at the end of the procedure.

Posterior Reconstruction

The aim is to reconstruct the normal anatomy and reestablish the posterior support of the urethral sphincteric complex. In addition, the posterior reconstruction greatly aids in the next step of vesicourethral anastomosis by bringing the urethra and bladder neck in close approximation, as the urethra is pulled in a more cephalad or intrapelvic location. Two separate 3-0 9-inch V-Lok sutures are used to perform the posterior reconstruction incorporating the posterior median raphe, Denonvillier fascia, and longitudinal fibers posterior to the bladder that were previously covering the SVs (Fig. 34-22).

The sutures are cinched to approximate the bladder neck to the urethra. These sutures are suspended to the Cooper ligament with the aid of Hem-o-Lok clips after vesicourethral anastomosis has been completed. This is a technical modification we have been using with the aim of improving early return of urinary continence. The net effect is to elevate the urethra and bladder neck, as is commonly done with a sling for correction of postprostatectomy incontinence (Fig. 34-23).

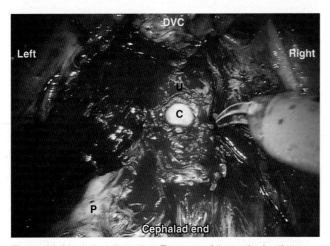

Figure 34-20. Apical dissection. Exposure of the urethral catheter *(C)* on incising the anterior urethra *(U)*. *DVC,* dorsal venous complex; *P,* prostate.

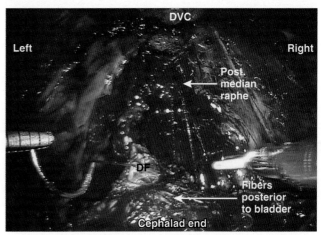

Figure 34-22. Posterior reconstruction. *DF,* Denonvilliers fascia; *DVC,* dorsal venous complex.

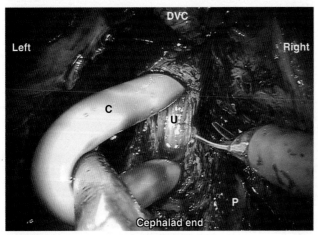

Figure 34-21. Apical dissection. Division of the posterior urethra *(U)*. *C,* catheter; *DVC,* dorsal venous complex; *P,* prostate.

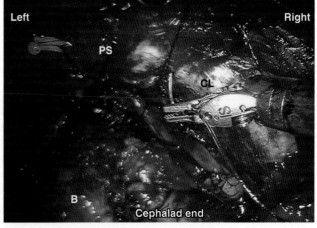

Figure 34-23. Anterior suspension of the posterior reconstruction sutures to Cooper ligament *(CL)*. *B,* bladder; *PS,* pubic symphysis.

Vesicourethral Anastomosis

We use two separate 2-0 9-inch polyglactin (Vicryl) sutures on an RB-1 needle to perform a running anastomosis. The initial throw is placed in an inside-out fashion in the urethra at the 5 o'clock position and then through the bladder in an outside-in fashion (Fig. 34-24).

The suture is then run in a clockwise direction to the 11 o'clock position, ensuring good mucosa-to-mucosa apposition. This completes the posterior layer. For the anterior layer, a second suture is run in a counterclockwise direction from the 4 to 10 o'clock positions. The two sutures are tied separately, providing two distinct suture lines, avoiding reliance on a single knot. A 20-French two-way Foley catheter is inserted with 30 mL of water in the balloon. Filling the bladder with about 180 mL of saline and observing for leakage helps ensure the integrity of the anastomosis.

Drain Placement

The robotic arms of the patient cart are undocked from the camera and instrument trocars. A 19-French Blake drain is inserted and exits via the right-sided 12-mm assistant trocar under vision with the aid of a 0-degree 10-mm laparoscope. The drain is positioned over the pelvis, ensuring it does not lie over the anastomosis, which could result in a falsely high output owing to closed suction drainage. Silk 3-0 sutures are used to anchor the drain to the skin. The 8-mm metallic robotic trocars are removed under vision to ensure there is no bleeding from the epigastric vessels or their tributaries.

Specimen Extraction and Wound Closure

The purse-string suture anchoring the camera trocar is cut. The trocar is removed, taking care to sweep the petroleum jelly from the Xeroform gauze. With the index finger of the left hand inside this wound, the entrapment bag string is transferred from the assistant's 5-mm port to the wound. If the upper abdomen is distended from trapped air, it is useful to make a small opening in the peritoneum to evacuate the air to avoid associated postoperative discomfort. This opening is subsequently closed. The specimen bag is extracted (Fig. 34-25).

We do not routinely close the fascia of the three 8-mm robotic trocar sites. All the skin openings are closed with 4-0 monofilament (Monocryl) sutures. Steri-Strips and dressings are applied over the incisions, and local anesthetic is infiltrated before the reversal of anesthesia.

POSTOPERATIVE CARE

After reversal of anesthesia, the patient is transferred to the postanesthesia care unit and subsequently to the 23-hour stay unit a few hours later. A clear liquid diet is administered, and the diet is advanced as tolerated. Patients are ambulated the same day. Ketorolac or an opiate is used as required for pain relief. Patients are placed on stool softeners as well as proton pump inhibitors. Intravenous third-generation cephalosporin antibiotic prophylaxis is continued for a total of three doses. For thromboembolic prophylaxis, subcutaneous low-molecular-weight heparin and an intermittent pneumatic compression device are used for the duration of the hospitalization. On the morning before discharge, removal of 15 mL of water from the catheter balloon is performed to decrease balloon-related bladder spasms. The drain is removed when the output is below 75 mL in an 8-hour shift. Most patients are discharged home within 24 hours of surgery if they have adequate pain control and are tolerating a regular diet. They are sent home on oral opiate, stool softener, and anticholinergic medications to be used as needed. The Foley catheter is removed in 7 to 10 days in the office. Patients commence performing pelvic floor or Kegel exercises the day after removal of the Foley catheter. Penile rehabilitation with a phosphodiesterase type 5 inhibitor is initiated in preoperatively potent patients who have no contraindications to its use and who underwent a nerve-sparing procedure.

COMPLICATIONS

Complications during a preperitoneal RARP can be intraoperative or postoperative. Many are common irrespective of the approach to performing a radical prostatectomy. In the following text, we focus on the complications associated specifically with the preperitoneal approach.

Intraoperative Complications

Bleeding from Inferior Epigastric Vessels during Preperitoneal Space Creation

Bleeding can occur because of a rapid balloon insufflation or during the 8-mm metallic robotic trocar insertion. A Carter-Thomason needle can be used to pass a suture across the bleeding vessel. Alternatively, the balloon of a Foley catheter inserted via the trocar can be inflated and pulled taut against

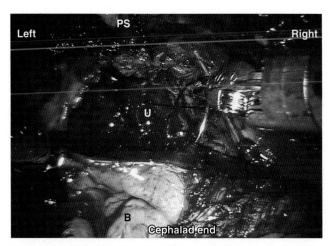

Figure 34-24. Anterior layer of vesicourethral anastomosis. *B*, bladder; *PS*, pubic symphysis; *U*, urethra.

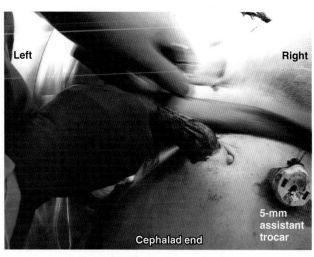

Figure 34-25. Specimen extraction.

the anterior abdominal wall to stop the bleeding. It is for this reason that it is prudent to visualize the removal of the left and right trocars at the end of the procedure; the trocars could be providing a tamponade effect to potentially injured inferior epigastric vessels, which is released on their removal.

Subcutaneous Emphysema

The incidence of subcutaneous emphysema can be relatively higher than with the transperitoneal approach. This may be particularly impressive in the penoscrotal area. It is caused by leakage of CO_2 in the subcutaneous layers of the abdomen around the camera trocar. No treatment is required apart from reassurance because the condition settles down gradually as the patient breathes off the excess CO_2 in the postoperative period.

Inadvertent Peritoneal Opening

It can sometimes be challenging to avoid an inadvertent opening of the peritoneum during the preperitoneal space creation. This is particularly relevant when creating space for the 5-mm assistant trocar insertion near the umbilicus. Making the peritoneal hole larger results in equalization of pressure across the two cavities. The rest of the procedure can mostly be carried out without added difficulties.

Rare intraoperative complications include balloon rupture as a result of its excessive insufflation.

Postoperative Complications

Lymphocele Formation

Lymphocele is occasionally encountered after bilateral pelvic lymph node dissection. It is postulated that unlike with the transperitoneal approach, in which the exposed peritoneal lining absorbs the excessive fluid, with preperitoneal RARP this absorption does not occur. In most cases an expectant approach leads to resolution of this complication, with interventional radiologic drainage used in large lymphoceles or symptomatic patients.

TIPS AND TRICKS

- During preperitoneal space creation, the incision in the anterior rectus sheath is made away from the midline. The tendency to make this cut in the midline should be avoided.
- Application of pressure to the balloon, forcing it across the midline as it is inflated, helps break through the linea alba, allowing the balloon to create the space on both sides of the lower abdomen. Unilateral space creation should be avoided.
- Gentle and coordinated motion of the left and right hand controlling the EndoEYE laparoscope and the long smooth trocar, respectively, helps in cephalad and posterolateral sweeping of the peritoneum off the abdominal wall. This allows the trocars to be placed as far lateral as needed for their adequate spacing to prevent external collision of the robotic arms (10-cm distance between the trocars).
- We use the da Vinci SutureCut needle holder (Intuitive Surgical, Sunnyvale, Calif.) in the left hand. This saves time and gives the operating surgeon control of the suture-cutting process. It improves safety by avoiding passage of scissors for suture cutting by the assistant, which can be associated with inadvertent injuries. However, one has to be careful not to inadvertently cut the sutures as they are being grasped by the SutureCut needle holder.
- Reducing the intensity of the light during the anterior bladder neck dissection helps in taking away the glare and helps in better appreciation of the tissue plane for bladder neck transection.
- Pulling on the Foley catheter before anterior bladder neck transection can help identify a large or irregular median lobe. The catheter balloon tends to be pushed away from the midline in the latter case. In the presence of a large median lobe, extra care has to be taken to avoid injury to the ureteric orifices.
- Reducing the amount of intravenous fluid infusion to less than 1.5 L until the vesicourethral anastomosis (VUA) is complete prevents poor vision caused by excessive urine flooding the operative field.
- Use of perineal pressure and reducing the insufflation by suctioning helps to bring the urethra and the bladder neck together during VUA.

35 Robotic-Assisted Radical Cystectomy

Michael Woods, Raj Pruthi

Radical cystectomy is the standard of care for muscle-invasive and refractory non–muscle-invasive bladder cancer. An open radical cystectomy is the most thoroughly studied approach and remains more frequently used by urologists—although, since the first report of robotic-assisted radical cystectomy (RARC) by Menon and colleagues, we have seen a steady rise in the performance of this minimally invasive approach to radical cystectomy. There has been some controversy surrounding the use of RARC, mainly questioning the true impact on patient morbidity in the setting of unproven oncologic outcomes. However, there continue to emerge numerous reports in the literature suggesting some distinct benefits of the robotic approach, but robust randomized data are lacking. Fortunately, Level I data will be available in the future because the RAZOR (Randomized Open versus Robotic Cystectomy) trial—a large multicenter phase 3 randomized trial comparing open and robotic cystectomy—has recently completed accrual. Despite the current limitations of the available data, RARC is a viable option for radical cystectomy that is being increasingly embraced by both patients and urologists. This chapter outlines a step-by-step approach to RARC and provides some recommendations on preoperative and postoperative management of these patients.

INDICATIONS AND CONTRAINDICATIONS

The indications for RARC are the same as for an open radical cystectomy; in general, RARC will be performed for the treatment of muscle-invasive bladder cancer. An absolute contraindication to RARC is severe pulmonary disease that prohibits adequate ventilation while a patient has a pneumoperitoneum and is placed into steep Trendelenburg position (which is required to perform RARC). Some relative contraindications include extensive prior abdominal surgeries, morbid obesity (positioning and ventilation issues), and bulky or locally advanced tumors. Ultimately, the decision to perform RARC in these situations will come down to surgeon preference and experience.

When a surgeon first starts performing RARC, the procedure can be challenging and lengthy; thus patient selection is extremely important early in one's learning curve. The ideal patient to choose when starting RARC is a nonobese man with no or minimal prior abdominal surgery and a nonbulky primary tumor. It also is advisable to be proficient in robotic-assisted prostatectomy before undertaking RARC.

PATIENT PREOPERATIVE EVALUATION AND PREPARATION

The preoperative evaluation of a patient undergoing RARC is the same as would be performed for open cystectomy. Routine laboratory tests (comprehensive metabolic panel [CMP], complete blood count [CBC], urine culture) should be performed with particular attention paid to renal function because of its impact on choice of urinary diversion. Patients require standard staging studies with computed tomography (CT) of the abdomen and pelvis and chest radiography or chest CT. Additional imaging with a bone scan should be undertaken in the setting of abnormal laboratory findings or symptoms. Although not routinely used, magnetic resonance imaging (MRI) may provide superior soft tissue definition of the primary tumor and aid in patient selection early in one's experience. Patients should be evaluated by an enterostomal nurse preoperatively to choose an appropriate stomal site, and involvement of a dietitian to identify potential nutritional deficiencies should be considered.

When obtaining informed consent for a radical cystectomy, a thorough discussion is required with the patient and any involved family members concerning perioperative morbidity and mortality as well as the impact on quality of life. Radical cystectomy is plagued with high complication and readmission rates; appropriate counseling preoperatively will set realistic expectations for the patient and family. When counseling about RARC, the discussion should include the risk of open conversion and positional injuries, as well as the available data concerning oncologic outcomes and convalescence after RARC versus open radical cystectomy. Regardless of approach used, the oncologic principles of bladder cancer must be followed, and neoadjuvant chemotherapy should be offered to eligible patients.

No bowel preparation is required (if colon is to be used, then we perform a mechanical preparation only). One can consider an enema preoperatively in an attempt to decrease rectal distention, which may improve visualization during the posterior bladder dissection. We routinely use alvimopan (a peripherally acting μ-opioid antagonist) because there is evidence of improved bowel function with its use in the cystectomy population. The first dose is given in the preoperative holding area before surgery. A single dose of antibiotics is given before incision. The choice of antibiotic and timing of readministration, if needed, are based on the Surgical Care Improvement Project (SCIP) guidelines. Venous thromboembolism (VTE) prophylaxis is also initiated in the holding area and typically is continued postoperatively for up to 4 weeks.

OPERATING ROOM CONFIGURATION AND PATIENT POSITIONING

The operating room setup will be very similar to that used for a robotic-assisted prostatectomy. As is the case for prostatectomies, the operating room can be arranged to accommodate either a left- or a right-sided assistant; this is purely a matter of surgeon preference. The following description discusses the operating room configuration for a right-sided assistant.

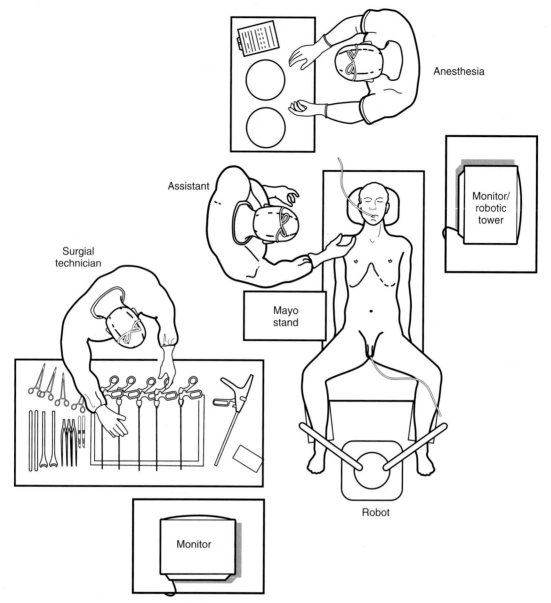

Figure 35-1. Operating room setup for robotic-assisted radical cystectomy with a right-sided assistant. A minimum of two monitors should be used, with one placed across the patient for the bedside assistant. Depending on the particular operating room, the surgical technician and instrument table can be placed on the contralateral side. The robotic console can be placed in various locations depending on the configuration of the given operating room.

We use at least two monitors for the procedure. One should be placed directly across from the bedside assistant, just lateral to the patient's left shoulder; this will be ergonomic for the assistant by preventing rotation of the neck. Of note, this monitor is associated with the robotic tower (i.e., light source, energy sources). The second monitor is located adjacent to the instrument table for use by the surgical technician. The instrument table is located to the right of the patient at the level of the right leg. This allows adequate room for the assistant and surgical technician. The instrument table could also be placed on the left side of the patient based on the configuration of a particular operating room (Fig. 35-1). This arrangement allows the robotic system to be located between the patient's legs, but with the advancements of the da Vinci Xi system (Intuitive Surgical, Sunnyvale Calif.), side docking is possible.

After general anesthesia has been administered, an oro-gastric tube is placed, then a bladder catheter is placed after the patient has been prepared and draped. The patient is positioned in low lithotomy with use of Yellofins stirrups (Allen Medical, Acton, Mass.), and the arms are tucked bilaterally with a draw sheet. Foam is used to protect pressure points, in particular at the calf and elbows. It is our practice to place a strip of 3-inch silk tape over foam at the level of the chest to prevent slippage of the patient while in Trendelenburg position (Fig. 35-2). The use of shoulder blocks should be avoided because of the risk of brachial plexus injury. The use of laparoscopically assisted vaginal hysterectomy (LAVH) drape simplifies the draping of patients undergoing RARC.

TROCAR PLACEMENT

Access to the abdomen and creation of the pneumoperitoneum can be achieved according to the surgeon's preference. Our approach is to use a Veress needle through the site

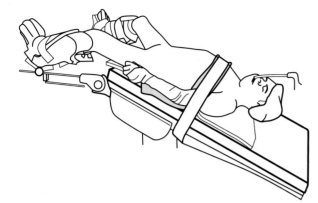

Figure 35-2. Patients are placed in a low lithotomy position for robotic-assisted radical cystectomy. The arms are tucked and all pressure points are carefully padded. The procedure is performed in steep Trendelenburg position. A strip of tape padded by foam placed around the chest is adequate to prevent slippage. Shoulder blocks should be avoided.

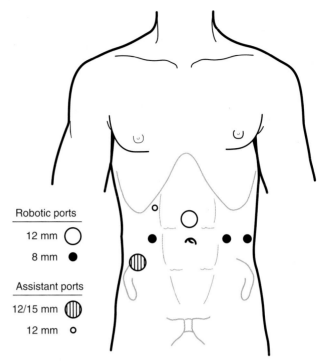

Robotic ports
12 mm ○
8 mm ●

Assistant ports
12/15 mm ◍
12 mm ○

Figure 35-3. Port placement for robotic-assisted radical cystectomy with a right-sided assistant.

where the camera trocar will be placed; this is done before placing the patient in Trendelenburg position. A total of six trocars are used for a RARC: four for the robotic system and two for the assistant. The first trocar, where the camera will be located, is placed 2 to 3 cm cephalad to the umbilicus and is a 12-mm port. The two 8-mm robotic trocars are placed 11 cm lateral to the camera port at the upper edge of the umbilicus. Before placement of any additional ports, the patient should be placed into Trendelenburg position, which will allow additional lateral exposure of the abdominal wall. The last robotic port is placed 11 cm directly lateral to the existing left-side robotic port and will be the site of the fourth robotic arm. Two assistant ports are placed on the right side, 12 mm and 15 mm in size. The 15-mm port is placed approximately halfway between the right robotic port and the right anterior superior iliac spine (ASIS). We prefer a 15-mm port in this location to aid in the extraction of lymph node packets during the pelvic lymph node dissection (PLND) as well as to allow the placement of a 15-mm specimen extraction pouch for the removal of the cystectomy specimen. The remaining 12-mm assistant port is placed directly above (or slightly medial to) the right robotic port just below the costal margin. A 12-mm port in this location allows the placement of a laparoscopic stapler directly onto the vascular pedicles of the bladder. This is discussed in greater detail later in this chapter (Fig. 35-3). A mirror image of this configuration can used to accommodate a left-sided assistant (which is preferred if an intracorporeal urinary diversion is being performed).

PROCEDURE (SEE VIDEO 35-1)

As is the case with an open radical cystectomy, the PLND can be performed either before or after the cystectomy portion of the surgery. This is largely based on surgeon preference. The following section describes the steps for RARC with the PLND being performed first:

1. Right ureteral dissection
2. Right PLND
3. Mobilization of the sigmoid colon, left ureteral dissection, left PLND
4. Transferring left ureter
5. Development of the prerectal space and posterior bladder dissection
6. Division of vascular pedicles to the bladder
7. Anterior bladder dissection
8. Dissection and division of the urethra
9. Specimen extraction and extracorporeal urinary diversion

Right Ureteral Dissection

A 30-degree downward lens should be used at the start of the procedure. This provides a better perspective when working in the pelvis for the ureteral and lymph node dissection. At the outset of the procedure, monopolar scissors are used in the right hand, a fenestrated bipolar instrument is used in the left hand, and ProGrasp forceps (Intuitive Surgical, Sunnyvale, Calif.) are placed in the fourth arm. After releasing any attachment from the cecum and terminal ilium, the pulsations of the right common iliac artery should be identified. In many cases the ureter can be identified at this time. When it cannot be seen, the peritoneum and lymphatic tissue on the proximal common iliac artery should be opened and dissection should be carried distally along the vessel until the ureter is located. The ureter should be dissected away from the posterior structures and freed circumferentially, with care taken to maintain adequate periureteral tissue. The dissection should be carried distally to the insertion of the ureter into the bladder. One needs to be careful not to place too much upward traction on the ureter with the robotic arms, which could result in significant trauma. In female patients, the infundibulopelvic ligament will need to be divided for completion of the distal ureteral dissection.

When the distal dissection is complete, the ureter should be controlled and divided between two locking clips. The proximal clip should have a 10-inch preplaced tie on it. This tie will allow atraumatic manipulation during urinary diversion (Fig. 35-4). If any additional cephalad mobilization of the ureter is required, it should be completed before distal division because this dissection can be challenging once the ureter is free. Proximal dissection should be limited to minimize disruption of the vascular supply and decrease risk of ureteroenteric anastomotic strictures. If desired, a frozen section of the ureter can be sent at this time, although the benefits of its routine use remain uncertain.

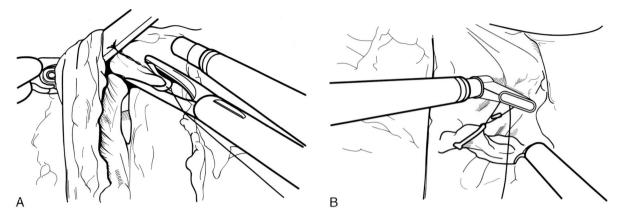

A

B

Figure 35-4. A, The right ureter being controlled with a locking clip with a preplaced tie. **B,** This allows efficient, atraumatic manipulation of the ureter.

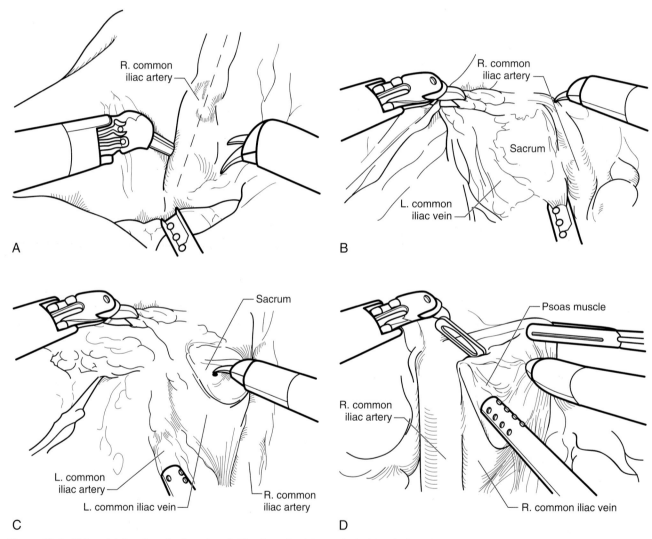

Figure 35-5. Right pelvic lymph node dissection. **A,** The dissection is begun by incising the lymphatic tissue along the full extent of the common iliac vessel in the split-and-roll technique. **B,** Medial deflection of the lymph node packet exposing the left common iliac vein and the sacrum. **C,** Exposure of the left common iliac artery with division of the proximal packet at the aortic bifurcation. **D,** Lateral border of the right common iliac vein.

Right Pelvic Lymphadenectomy

The extent of lymph node dissection in the management of bladder cancer is an area of controversy, but for the purposes of this chapter we describe an "extended" lymph node dissection with the proximal extent being the bifurcation of the aorta.

The lymphadenectomy is performed with the standard split-and-roll technique. We recommend starting the dissection by splitting the lymphatic tissue along the full extent of the right common iliac artery (Fig. 35-5, *A*). The medial packet is then rolled medially, exposing the left common iliac vein and sacral promontory (Fig. 35-5, *B*). At this point the left common iliac

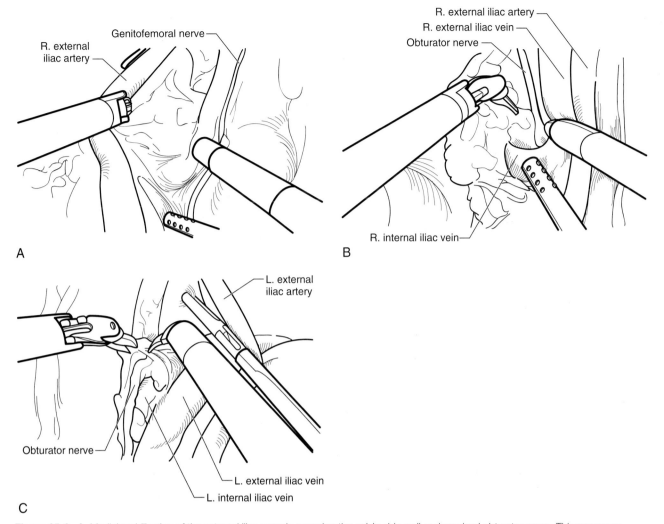

Figure 35-6. A, Medial mobilization of the external iliac vessels exposing the pelvic side wall and proximal obturator nerve. This maneuver simplifies the extraction of the hypogastric and obturator lymph node packets **(B). C,** Lateral exposure of the external iliac vessels provides early identification of the hypogastric vein (shown here during a left-sided dissection).

artery should be exposed. This clearly defines the proximal aspect of the right common iliac packet at the bifurcation of the aorta. It also begins the left PLND and simplifies the completion of this dissection after deflection of the sigmoid colon (Fig. 35-5, C). The dissection is carried distally and completed by dividing the packet at the takeoff of the hypogastric artery. After completion of the medial dissection, the remaining lymphatic tissue is mobilized laterally, exposing the right common iliac vein and distal inferior vena cava (IVC). Once the lateral edges of the venous structures have been defined and the psoas muscle has been exposed, the lymphatic tissue should be separated from the genitofemoral nerve to define the lateral border of the dissection template (Fig. 35-5, D). The packet is divided at the bifurcation of the common iliac, which will allow the completion of the proximal dissection with simple blunt dissection.

The right PLND dissection is continued by splitting the lymphatic tissue along the external iliac artery distally to the level of the circumflex iliac vein. The packet can be rolled medially and laterally, skeletonizing the external iliac vessels. Locking clips should be used to control the distal lymphatics to minimize the risk of lymphocele formation. After completion of the external iliac lymph node dissection, we recommend medial mobilization of the external iliac vessels and all

associated lymphatic tissue, exposing the pelvic side wall and proximal aspect of the obturator nerve (Fig. 35-6, A). This will simplify the removal of the obturator and hypogastric lymph nodes by allowing these packets to be pulled from the underside of the external iliac vein (Fig. 35-6, B). In addition, this lateral approach allows early identification of the hypogastric vein, which can be difficult when approaching solely from the medial aspect of the pelvis, and helps prevent vascular injury (Fig. 35-6, C). We extract all regions of the lymphadenectomy in individual packets using a reusable 10-mm specimen retrieval bag. These should be extracted through the 15-mm assistant port to accommodate the large specimens.

Mobilization of the Sigmoid Colon, Left Ureteral Dissection, Left Pelvic Lymph Node Dissection

The mobilization of the left colon is begun by incising the peritoneum lateral to the bowel. This will allow the colon to be rotated medially, exposing the left common iliac vessels and left ureter. If the ureter is not seen, it may be adherent to the backside of the sigmoid mesentery, which occurs frequently in obese patients. Once the ureter has been identified, it is dissected and controlled in the same manner as described for the right. The left PLND is performed at this

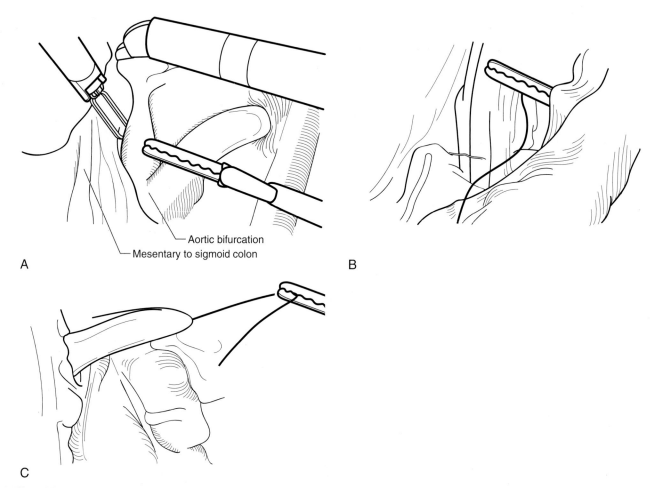

Aortic bifurcation
Mesentery to sigmoid colon

A

B

C

Figure 35-7. Left ureteral transposition. **A,** The bedside assistant passes a blunt-tipped grasper underneath the sigmoid mesentery just anterior to the aorta. **B** and **C,** The ureteral tag is grasped and pulled underneath the left colon and clipped to the right ureteral tag.

point. The dissection begins by splitting the lymphatic tissue over the left common iliac artery. As the dissection is carried proximally toward the aortic bifurcation, the space created by the right-sided PLND is entered and usually the majority of the medial aspect of the left common iliac dissection is complete. This existence of this space simplifies the left PLND. The lateral aspect of the packet is rolled off the common iliac artery until the lateral aspect of the sacrum is encountered, at which point the proximal and distal extent to the packet can be divided. Some caution should be exercised during dissection in this area because there commonly is a lumbar artery present. The remainder of the left PLND is completed in a similar fashion as the right side.

Transferring the Left Ureter

The left ureter can be transferred to the right side under the sigmoid colon with the help of the bedside assistant. A blunt-tipped grasper can be passed from the right under the colon just anterior to the aorta to grasp the tag of the left ureter and transpose it to the right side (Fig. 35-7). This is always straightforward when an extended PLND has been performed, because the overlying sigmoid mesentery has been completely mobilized from the common iliac vessels. When a standard PLND has been performed, some additional dissection separating the back of the sigmoid mesentery from the common iliac lymphatics—generally an avascular plane—can greatly simplify this step. If a left-sided assistant is used, then the

operating surgeon can use the fourth arm and bring it under the colon to transfer the ureter. We recommend transferring the ureter before performing the cystectomy at the completion of the PLND. Clipping the tags of the right and left ureter together at this time can simplify later identification or extraction for urinary diversion.

Development of the Prerectal Space and Posterior Bladder Dissection

We will generally change to a 0-degree lens to optimize visualization during the posterior bladder dissection. In male patients the peritoneum between the bladder and rectum is incised and, with use of blunt and careful cautery, dissection of the prerectal space is developed (Fig. 35-8). Tissue retraction is very important during this portion and is best accomplished by using the fourth robotic arm to elevate the bladder anteriorly and having the assistant depress the posterior peritoneal lip posteriorly. Often the seminal vesicles are seen as this dissection progresses and serve as a landmark confirming the correct plane. The Denonvilliers fascia needs to be incised to carry the dissection as far distally as possible. The dissection should be carried down to the rectourethralis muscle. The degree of posterior dissection should be similar to that routinely performed during a robotic-assisted prostatectomy.

In female patients, a sponge stick should be placed in the vagina to aid the dissection. If a vaginal sparing approach is feasible and desired, the dissection can be performed between

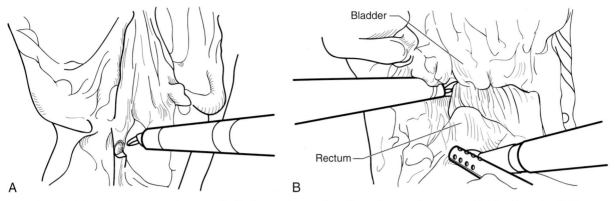

Figure 35-8. A, Incision of the peritoneum between the bladder and rectum is performed to start the posterior bladder dissection. **B,** The posterior dissection continues distally with a combination of blunt dissection and cautery. Posterior retraction by the bedside assistant aids in the development of this plane.

the bladder and vagina with a liberal use of cautery with some blunt dissection. Some benefits of this approach are that no or minimal vaginal reconstruction is required, the chance of vaginal cuff breakdown is minimized, and vaginal length is preserved. The bladder wall can be fairly thin, so one should err toward the vagina during the dissection because vaginotomies are easily repaired. When resection of the anterior vagina is performed with cystectomy, the vaginal cuff is opened onto the sponge stick, and one can divide the lateral vaginal wall and vascular pedicles to the bladder en bloc using a stapler or energy device.

Division of the Vascular Pedicles to the Bladder

After completion of the posterior dissection, the vascular pedicles should be clearly defined bilaterally (Fig. 35-9). If the cystectomy is performed before PLND, then some additional dissection will be required to develop the paravesical space and expose the endopelvic fascia; this will provide the needed definition of the pedicles. It is our preference to divide the pedicles using an endovascular stapler. It is important to note that the stapler should be placed through the 12-mm medial assistant port. This allows the stapler to be applied onto the pedicle in a straight line (Fig. 35-10, *A*). When the stapler is placed through the more lateral assistant port, the angle is usually too acute for division of the ipsilateral pedicle. After the proximal aspect of the pedicle is divided, the endopelvic fascia should be opened bilaterally, if not done already. This allows the stapler to be placed more distally as the remaining pedicle is divided (this will include remaining posterior prostatic attachments). Alternatively, locking clips can be used to control the pedicles and are recommended at the most distal aspect of the pedicle to avoid a rectal injury (Fig. 35-10, *B*).

A few modifications should be made if neurovascular bundle preservation is going to be performed. The neurovascular bundles are located on the posterolateral aspect of the prostate and course from the anterior surface of the colon. The bundles should be mobilized off the prostate by incising the lateral prostatic fascia anterior to the bundles. This should be done before dividing the inferior vesicle pedicles so the bundle can be completely visualized. The lateral dissection is carried medially around the base of the prostate until it is connected to the posterior prerectal dissection. This allows isolation of the inferior vesical and prostatic pedicle, which should be clipped and divided with cold scissors to avoid thermal injury. The nerve sparing should be completed down to the genitourinary diaphragm in a similar fashion to that used during robotic-assisted prostatectomy.

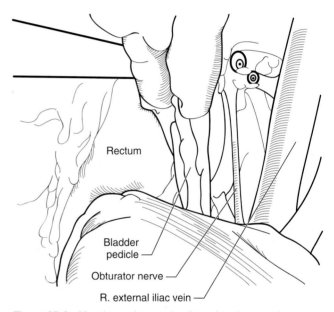

Figure 35-9. After thorough posterior dissection, the vascular pedicles to the bladder are clearly defined and will allow the safe placement of a stapler.

Anterior Bladder Dissection

The medial and median umbilical ligaments should be divided with cautery as far proximally as possible exposing the wispy attachments of the retropubic space. Blunt dissection is used to mobilize the bladder off the anterior abdominal wall, then the remaining peritoneal attachments lateral to medial umbilical ligaments should be divided with cautery. At this point the bladder should be fairly mobile. Any remaining endopelvic fascia and the puboprostatic ligaments should be divided. The dorsal venous complex (DVC) is suture ligated and divided. A stapler can also be used to control the DVC, especially if already used earlier in the surgery.

Dissection and Division of the Urethra

Some effort should be made to dissect out a generous urethral stump. The benefit is obvious when planning a neobladder, but there is still benefit in non-neobladder patients because the additional urethral length will allow placement

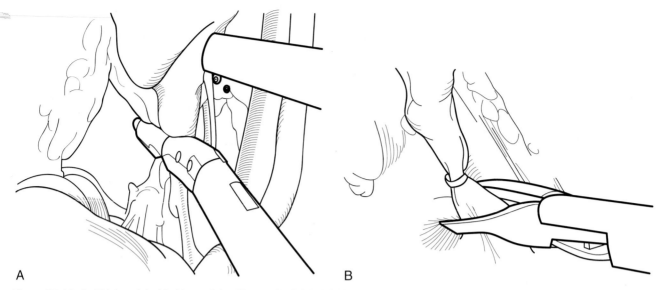

A B

Figure 35-10. A, Division of the bladder pedicle with a stapler. It is helpful for the assistant to lightly depress the rectum to ensure it is not incorporated into the stapler. **B,** Control of the bladder pedicle with a locking clip. This may be necessary at the distal aspect of the posterior dissection owing to limited space between the rectum and prostate.

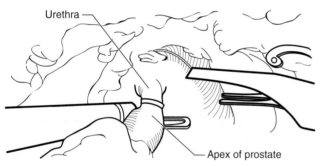

Urethra

Apex of prostate

Figure 35-11. Placement of a locking clip on the urethra to prevent spillage of urine before division.

of a locking clip or suture ligature to prevent tumor spillage during urethral division. If the posterior dissection was adequate, there should be minimal attachments remaining posterior to the urethra, and when the bladder catheter is removed, a locking clip can be placed by the assistant or robotic applier, easily occluding the urethra (Fig. 35-11). The urethra is then divided distal to the clip, and a frozen section can be sent at this time if desired. The specimen is placed into a 15-mm specimen extraction bag and hemostasis is achieved with cautery, suture ligature, or clip placement. If is important to lower the pneumoperitoneum to 5 mm Hg to unmask any venous bleeding being occluded by the increased intra-abdominal pressure.

In most female patients the urethra will be removed unless a neobladder is planned. If compete urethral removal is being performed, it may be beneficial to start the periurethral dissection transvaginally, which will eventually connect to the robotic dissection from above. Alternatively, the bedside assistant can place pressure on the meatus, allowing the operating surgeon to excise the urethra to the level of squamous mucosa of the meatus and avoiding the need for a separate transvaginal dissection. If the anterior vagina has been excised, then the bladder specimen can be extracted through this defect with a blunt-tipped grasper. The vagina should be closed in a

"clamshell" fashion with a large absorbable suture. This closure needs to be meticulous to avoid breakdown and possible herniation of abdominal contents.

Specimen Extraction and Extracorporeal Urinary Diversion

The specimen is entrapped in a 15-mm specimen retrieval bag. This can be extracted though an 8- to 10-cm infraumbilical incision, which can be extended cephalad as needed. Before extraction, the bedside assistant should grasp the ureteral tags with a locking grasper to allow delivery through the extraction incision for the urinary diversion. Another maneuver that can be beneficial is to pretag the terminal ilium with a 10-inch stitch, which can then be clipped to the ureteral tags and be used to rapidly identify the appropriate bowel segment for diversion. This tag can be placed at the outset of the surgery or at the time of controlling DVC, when the robotic needle drivers will already be in use.

The steps for creating an ileal conduit or neobladder through an extraction incision are the same as for a standard open radical cystectomy. A major pitfall that one needs to be aware of is the amount of traction being placed on ureters during extracorporeal reconstruction. The ureteroenteric anastomosis should essentially be performed at the level of the fascia, and any unneeded ureter should be excised. To achieve this, one should make the extraction incision large enough to perform a meticulous anastomosis without placing undue traction on the ureters. A slightly larger extraction incision will not negate the benefits of the robotic approach.

In performing an extracorporeal neobladder, the urethral anastomosis can be completed in either an open or a robotic fashion. If an open anastomosis is used, then the extraction of the specimen should be through a lower midline incision ending near the pubis symphysis to allow placement of the urethral sutures. Preplacement of one or two posterior urethral sutures robotically before extraction can aid in completing the open anastomosis.

If the neobladder–urethral anastomosis is to be completed robotically, then the final urethral catheter is placed

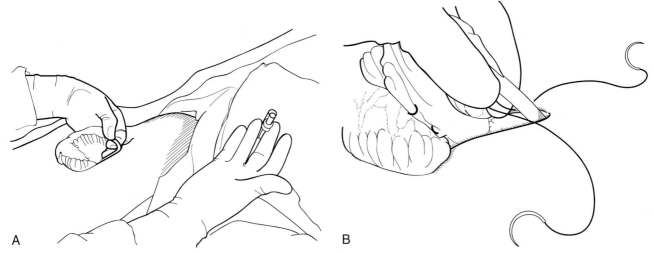

Figure 35-12. Extracorporeal neobladder during robotic-assisted radical cystectomy. **A,** Delivery of the urethral catheter through the extraction incision to allow securing of the diversion stents to the catheter and to aid in bringing the neobladder into the pelvis. **B,** Preplacement of running suture on the bladder neck in anticipation of a robotic-assisted neobladder-urethral anastomosis.

and brought from the pelvis through the extraction incision (Fig. 35-12, *A*). The distal portion of the catheter is placed into the neobladder, and the balloon is inflated. The anastomotic suture is preplaced on the posterior lip of the bladder neck (Fig. 35-12, *B*). We currently use two 2-0 absorbable monofilament sutures on a UR-6 tied together at a length of 7 inches on each side. The urinary diversion stents can be managed in the same fashion as for an open neobladder; we prefer to tie the stents to the final urethral catheter. Gentle traction on the catheter can help deliver the neobladder to the pelvis. The fascia is closed according to surgeon preference, and the robot is re-docked. The patient should be placed in less extreme Trendelenburg positioning than was used during the extirpative portion of the surgery to allow the neobladder to reach the pelvis without tension. The anastomosis is then completed in a running fashion starting at the 6 o'clock position. The urethral catheter balloon should be deflated during the anastomosis to avoid inadvertent puncture. Drains are placed according to surgeon preference.

POSTOPERATIVE MANAGEMENT

Postoperative care pathways are extremely important in the care of patients who have undergone radical cystectomy, whether open or robotic assisted, and have been shown to decrease the length of stay. An effort should be made to create an institution-wide pathway that is followed by all urologists, fellows, residents, and nursing staff. Our postoperative pathway is as follows.

Eligible patients are started on alvimopan in the holding area before surgery; administration is continued until a bowel movement occurs. All patient are given mechanical and medical venous thrombosis prophylaxis preoperatively and postoperatively. A nasogastric tube is not routinely left in place after the procedure. Patients receive scheduled ketorolac (and often intravenous acetaminophen) and a patient-controlled intravenous narcotic for as-needed use. This is typically transitioned to oral narcotic by postoperative day (POD) 2 or when the patient is tolerating a diet. Patients usually sit in a chair or walk on the day of surgery and ambulate in the hallways by POD 1. Patients are given 8 ounces of clear liquids every 8 hours on POD 1 and unrestricted liquids

on POD 2 and are advanced to regular diet on POD 3 or 4 regardless of bowel function as long as no nausea, emesis, or significant abdominal distention is present. Our goal for discharge is POD 4, and we recommend immediate involvement of a caseworker to identify appropriate home resources for patients (e.g., home nursing, physical therapy). Urinary diversion stents are removed on POD 5 to 7 for patients with an ileal conduit, and we perform a cystogram at 2.5 to 3 weeks on neobladders to ensure that no leakage is occurring. As noted earlier, VTE prophylaxis can be continued on an outpatient basis with enoxaparin (Lovenox) 40 mg for up to 4 weeks after surgery.

COMPLICATIONS

The high rate of complications associated with radical cystectomy is well known, and the management of these complications is well established. No particular complications are specific to the robotic-assisted approach, but one may potentially be at a higher risk of having a complication when transitioning from an open to a robotic-assisted approach. We would like to focus on some areas of potential complications so that they may be avoided.

Patient selection is critical when starting to perform RARC. We feel that thin male patients with nonbulky tumors are ideal early in one's experience. Because of the overlap of steps with robotic-assisted prostatectomy, a male patient will provide some additional familiarity in those early cases. Avoid obese patients during the learning curve; exposure during posterior and left ureteral dissection can be challenging because of the large amount of fatty tissue.

Ureteroenteric strictures are a difficult chronic problem to manage. A vast majority of strictures are vascular in nature and arise from poor surgical technique. It is critical to avoid undue tension on the ureter with the robotic instruments. This will result in stripping of periureteral tissue and trauma. One must rely on visual cues to assess tension on the ureter, given the lack of tactile feedback. As mentioned earlier, use of a pretied clip can aid in ureteral manipulation. Finally, to avoid tension on the ureters during extracorporeal urinary diversion, make an adequate extraction incision to allow performance of the anastomosis at the fascial level.

Rectal injuries can be a disaster, resulting in fistula, colostomy, or even death. To avoid such injuries, one must dedicate the appropriate time and effort to a thorough posterior dissection. The dissection needs to be carried distally to completely expose the underside of the prostate, resulting in thin, well-defined vascular pedicles to allow safe application of a stapler, clip, or energy device. If defining the pedicles is difficult because of fibrosis, we recommend proceeding cautiously by isolation of individual tissue pedicles as one progresses distally, using locking clips for vascular control.

The PLND can be a stressful portion of an RARC, especially early in one's experience. To help reduce anxiety and the risk of vascular injury, two maneuvers, which were described earlier, can be used. First, in the case of an extended PLND, start the left PLND from the right side. This allows clear definition of the aortic bifurcation as well as simplifying the access to the left common iliac artery after reflection of the left colon. Second, medial mobilization of the external iliac vessels provides early identification of the hypogastric vein and aids in the extraction of the hypogastric and obturator lymph node packet.

TIPS AND TRICKS

- Careful patient selection should be undertaken early in the surgeon's experience (thin male patient without bulky tumors).
- Avoid excessive tension on the ureters by the robotic instruments.
- Use pretagged locking clips to manipulate ureters after division.
- Perform dissection lateral to the external iliac vessels during PLND to simplify lymph node removal.
- The endovascular stapler can allow for rapid and safe division of the vascular pedicles of the bladder.
- If performing an extracorporeal urinary diversion, make the extraction incision large enough to allow the creation of a meticulous ureteral anastomosis at the level of the fascia and avoid retracting the ureters out of the abdomen.
- Preplace posterior urethral anastomotic sutures robotically before extraction of the specimen when planning a neobladder with an open anastomosis.
- When performing an intracorporeal urinary diversion, use a left-sided assistant.
- Clinical care pathways (also known as enhanced recovery after surgery [ERAS] protocols) provide significant benefits to all cystectomy patients, even those undergoing a robotic-assisted approach.

36 Robotic-Assisted Intracorporeal Ileal Conduit

Johar S. Raza, Tareq Al-Tartir, Ahmed A. Hussein, Khurshid A. Guru

Robotic-assisted radical cystectomy (RARC) has gained substantial acceptance in recent years. This alternate approach is widely practiced because of inherent advantages associated with robotic technology, which have been well documented by randomized and prospective studies. The key benefit of early return of bowel function is pronounced with an intracorporeal approach to urinary diversion. Intracorporeal ileal conduit (ICIC) formation improves outcomes but requires expertise with a stepwise approach and mentored training during the first cases along the learning curve. This chapter reviews the approach to ICIC formation and highlights key points to avoid situations that can potentially make the procedure difficult for surgeons new at adopting it.

INDICATIONS AND CONTRAINDICATIONS

The choice of the diversion method remains a complex issue, which is primarily influenced by patient and disease factors, in addition to the surgeon's training and experience. Ileal conduit (IC) may be considered the most frequently used method of diversion and the most frequent alternative to orthotopic diversion (OD). The main advantage of IC is its ease of performance and acceptance over the last 60 years in addition to the lower incidence of postoperative complications. However, a visible stoma that requires lifelong stoma care may adversely affect personal body image, social relationships, and lifestyle.

Absolute contraindications to continent urinary diversion are renal insufficiency (particularly when serum creatinine exceeds 200 mmol/L), and positive urethral margins at cystectomy or when urethrectomy is required. IC is also preferred in patients with severe hepatic or intestinal dysfunctions. History of pelvic irradiation, urethral stricture, and neurologic disease are other causes to favor IC.

After OD, patients may be unable to void spontaneously and intermittent self-catheterization (ISC) may therefore be necessary. Refusal or inability to perform ISC (as with impaired intellectual ability or the lack of manual dexterity) would favor IC. Other factors that should be considered include advanced age, multiple comorbidities, advanced cancer with poor prognosis, and the possible need for adjuvant therapy.

PATIENT PREOPERATIVE EVALUATION AND PREPARATION

Patients should be fully informed about the risks and benefits of each diversion method, and informed consent should be obtained. A comprehensive preoperative assessment should be done for all patients. This includes assessment of cardiac, renal, and hepatic functions and optimization of modifiable conditions such as hypertension, diabetes, and anemia. A simple cleaning enema the night before surgery has been shown to be sufficient and reliable in patients undergoing IC diversion. A stoma therapist should mark the stoma site before

surgery, and the patient should test and wear the definitive urine collection appliance before surgery. The stoma therapist may play a crucial role in the perioperative management of these patients.

OPERATING ROOM CONFIGURATION AND PATIENT POSITIONING

The operating room configuration and patient positioning are similar to those for RARC (see Chapter 35), in which the procedure is completed in steep Trendelenburg position. An additional short suprapubic port is placed for bowel anastomosis.

TROCAR PLACEMENT

The details of RARC are covered in another section. Port placement is critical for ICIC diversion; it is more cephalad to facilitate bowel maneuvering and performance of extended lymph node dissection. A six-port approach is used, and all ports are placed under direct vision after camera port placement (Fig. 36-1). An additional port is placed in the suprapubic area to facilitate side-to-side bowel anastomosis.

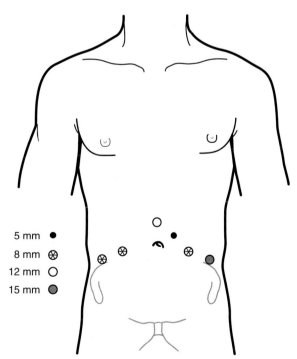

5 mm ●
8 mm ⊗
12 mm ○
15 mm ◉

Figure 36-1. A six-port approach is used, and all ports are placed under direct vision after camera port placement.

PROCEDURE (SEE VIDEO 36-1)
Selection of Bowel Segment and Placement of Marionette Stitch

Once the extirpative part of the procedure has been completed, the bladder and lymph nodes are placed in the retrieval bag and positioned in the empty pelvic cavity. The left ureter is crossed over to the right side and placed alongside the right ureter. The bowel segment is selected by identifying the ileocecal junction (Fig. 36-2) and harvesting a 12- to 15-cm ileal segment approximately 15 cm away from the ileocecal valve (Fig. 36-3). A measuring tape can be used to determine the exact length of the IC. Sometimes the selected bowel segment is taken farther away from the ileocecal valve. The distal ileal segment (close to the ileocecal valve) can be used later if any inadvertent insult happens to the proximal segment (away from the valve). Interbowel adhesions should be released to allow adequate mobilization of the IC. A Keith needle with a 60-cm length of 1-0 silk suture is introduced through the hypogastrium (Fig. 36-4). The suture is passed into the distal end of the conduit (Fig. 36-5) and brought back through the same location in the hypogastrium (Fig. 36-6). This stitch is not tied but controlled with an outside instrument. The extra length of the silk suture allows the distal end of the conduit to be raised and lowered, like a marionette, for easy manipulation of the conduit.

Isolation of Bowel

Isolation of the IC segment starts with creation of two mesenteric windows. This is done by incising the peritoneum of the bowel mesentery with hook cautery. The mesentery is stretched in a fanlike way along three points. The marionette stitch is pulled to hold the bowel segment under tension, close to the abdominal wall. The bowel is stretched on both sides of the marionette with the cobra grasper held in the fourth arm and the assistant grasper. The stretched mesentery is incised by the hook, ensuring adequate width of the mesentery (Fig. 36-7, *A* and *B*). The mesenteric vessels can be controlled in different ways. These include using hook cautery, bipolar grasper, Hem-o-lok clips (Weck Closure Systems, Research

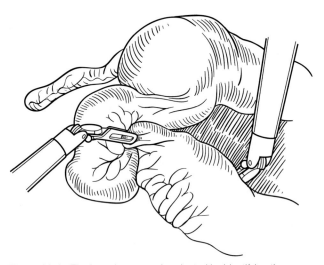

Figure 36-2. The bowel segment is selected by identifying the ileocecal junction.

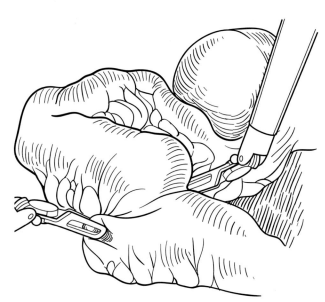

Figure 36-3. A total of 12 to 15 cm of the ileum is harvested approximately 15 cm away from the ileocecal valve.

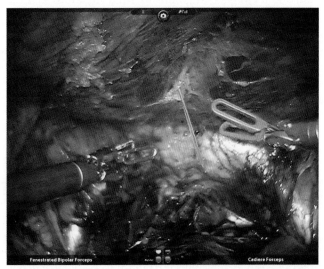

Figure 36-4. A Keith needle with a 60-cm length of 1-0 silk suture is introduced through the hypogastrium.

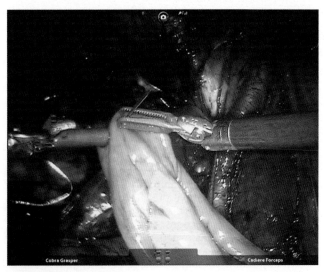

Figure 36-5. The Keith needle is passed into the distal end of the conduit.

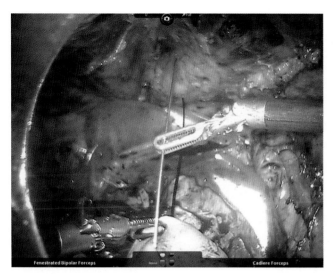

Figure 36-6. The Keith needle is brought back through the entry location in the hypogastrium.

Triangle Park, N.C.), a vascular stapler, or LigaSure (Covidien, Medtronic, Minneapolis, Minn.). Care should be taken when incising the mesentery to avoid inadvertently injuring any structure located posterior to the isolated segment, such as the mesentery of the adjacent bowel. Mesenteric fat layers should be incised in a progressive fashion. A deep cut placed at once may risk injury to the hidden mesenteric vessels, which can be controlled by using Hem-o-lok clips. In addition, care should be taken while manipulating the mesentery because lack of tactile feedback makes mesenteric vessels more susceptible to stretch injury.

After creation of the two mesenteric windows, a 45-mm or 60-mm Endo GIA stapler (Covidien, Medtronic, Minneapolis, Minn.) is passed through the 15-mm assistant port to divide the bowel proximally and distally (Fig. 36-8). Choosing the appropriate length of the Endo GIA stapler is very important when dividing the bowel. It is very crucial to divide the bowel segment with a single Endo GIA throw. If the 45-mm stapler is not enough to encircle the whole bowel diameter, then the 60-mm stapler should be used. Hook cautery is used to create an opening along the distal end of the conduit for introduction of the ureteral stents. Two openings are created along both sides of the

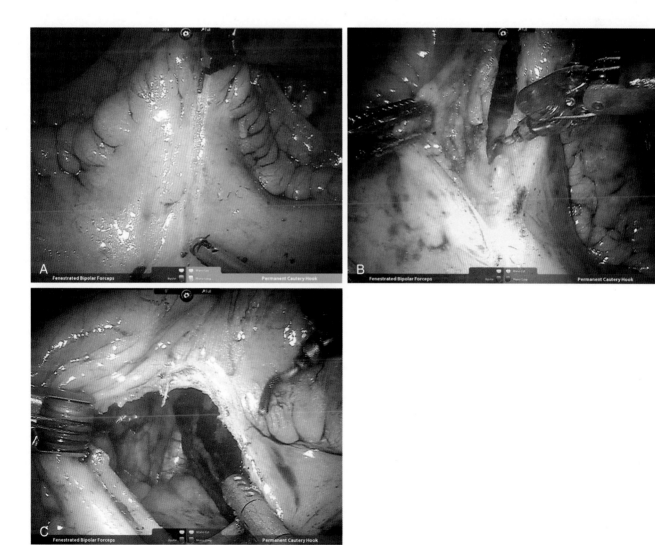

Figure 36-7. A, The stretched mesentery is incised by the hook, ensuring adequate width of the mesentery. **B** and **C,** The mesenteric vessels can be controlled in different ways. These include use of hook cautery, bipolar grasper, Hem-o-lok clips (Weck Closure Systems, Research Triangle Park, N.C.), vascular staple, or LigaSure (Medtronic, Minneapolis, Minn.). Care should be taken when incising the mesentery to avoid inadvertently injuring any structure located posterior to the isolated segment, such as the mesentery of the adjacent bowel.

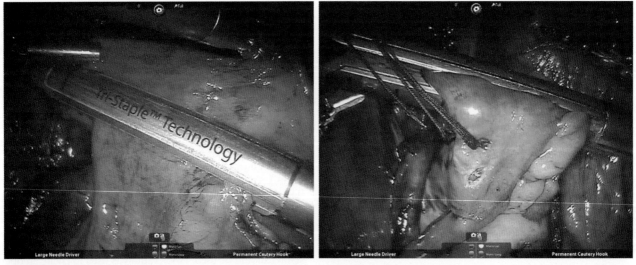

Figure 36-8. After creation of the two mesenteric windows, a 45-mm or 60-mm Endo GIA stapler (Covidien, Minneapolis, Minn.) is passed through the 15-mm assistant port to divide the bowel proximally and distally.

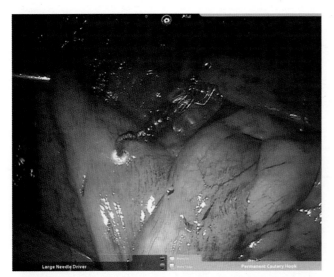

Figure 36-9. Two openings are created along both sides of the proximal end for the ureteroileal anastomoses.

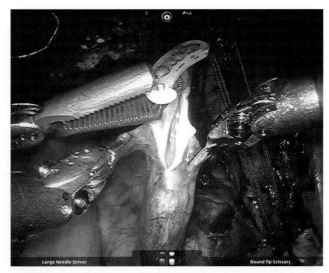

Figure 36-10. The ureter is partially transected and spatulated with robotic scissors for a wide anastomosis.

proximal end for the ureteroileal anastomoses (Fig. 36-9). Bowel continuity is not reestablished at this point; instead, a single No. 0 silk suture is used to bring the two ends of ileum together, preventing malrotation and ensuring proper orientation.

Ureteroileal Anastomosis

Appropriate length of the ureters needs to be confirmed to avoid an anastomosis at tension, or redundant ureter causing difficulty at urine draining in the conduit. Selecting the proper ureteral length can be done by aligning the ureteral end with its respective conduit opening. Any redundant length can be excised, making sure that the ureteral end is viable, and the ischemic end should be excised if any concerns remain.

The left ureteroileal anastomosis is performed first. The fourth arm is used to steadily hold the Hem-o-lok clip placed at the ureteral end. The ureter is partially transected and spatulated with robotic scissors for a wide anastomosis (Fig. 36-10). The marionette stitch is lowered to allow the conduit to lie horizontally for easy manipulation while the ureteroileal anastomosis is performed. If the ureteral length is short, the conduit can be

pulled closer to the ureteral end. A single-armed 4-0 Vicryl suture (5 cm long) is used to create an interrupted anastomosis (or double armed for a continuous anastomosis). In either case, the first anchoring stitch should be placed in an "outside-in" manner on the ureter side at the angle of the spatulation (Fig. 36-11). The suture on the conduit side is placed "inside out," perpendicular to the proximal staple line (Fig. 36-12). After placement of the first stitch, the fourth arm is manipulated to bring the ureteral end close to the conduit opening before the stitch is tied to achieve a tension-free anastomosis. This initial suture ensures proper alignment and placement of the subsequent sutures. Once the first suture has been placed, the remaining anastomosis can be completed in a continuous or interrupted manner. The following tricks can be used to properly identify the mucosal edges for a satisfactory mucosa-to-mucosa anastomosis:

1. Readjustment of the needle position in the right arm and proper use of the grasper held in the left arm; this facilitates exposure of the mucosal edge.
2. Readjustment of the position of the fourth arm.
3. Bowel mucosal eversion.

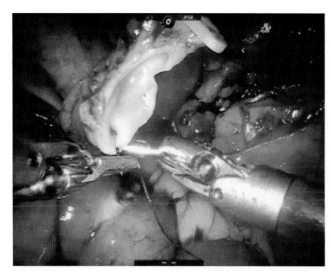

Figure 36-11. The first anchoring stitch should be placed in an "outside-in" manner on the ureter side at the angle of the spatulation.

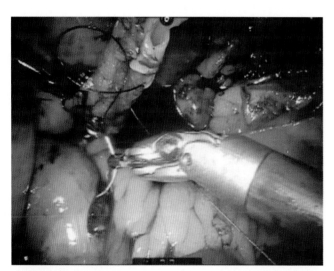

Figure 36-12. The suture on the conduit side is placed "inside out," perpendicular to the proximal staple line.

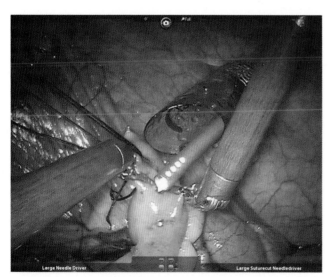

Figure 36-13. A metal laparoscopic suction tube is gently advanced through the 15-mm assistant port, through the distal opening.

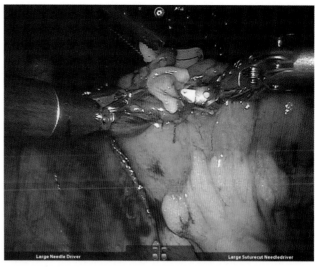

Figure 36-14. The metal suction tip is held in place by the robotic needle driver to allow passage of the stent into the ureter without damaging the anastomosis.

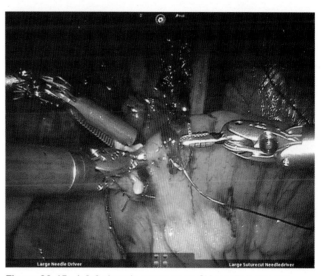

Figure 36-15. A 3-0 chromic suture on an SH needle is used to secure the stent to the conduit to prevent dislodgement.

Improper exposure of the mucosal edges can result in obstruction of the lumen. This is discovered during stent placement, which necessitates the removal of the incorrectly placed stitch, and opening of the ureteral lumen.

Once the posterior wall anastomosis has been completed, the ureteral stent is placed. A metal laparoscopic suction tube is gently advanced through the 15-mm assistant port, through the distal opening (Fig. 36-13), across the conduit. The metal suction tip is held in place by the robotic needle driver to allow passage of the stent into the ureter without damaging the anastomosis (Fig. 36-14). A 90-cm, 8.5-French, single-J ureteral stent with a guidewire is passed through the suction tip and fed into the ureteral opening. It is crucial to not overstretch the ureter when introducing the stent. This can be achieved by adjusting the guidewire tension. Once the stent is pushed all the way, the suction tip is withdrawn while the console surgeon holds the stent. The guidewire is left in the stent to allow easy identification of the stent inside the conduit. A 3-0 chromic suture on short half circle needle (SH) is used to secure the stent to the conduit to prevent dislodgement (Fig. 36-15). The guidewire is

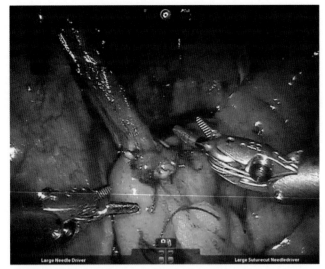

Figure 36-16. The anterior half of the left ureteroileal anastomosis is completed.

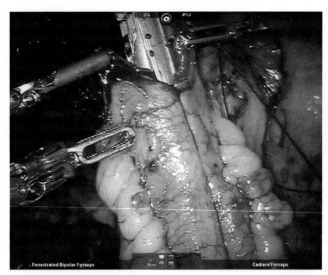

Figure 36-18. Fourth arm Cobra grasper is used to keep the segments aligned while correct orientation is ensured with the right and left robotic instruments.

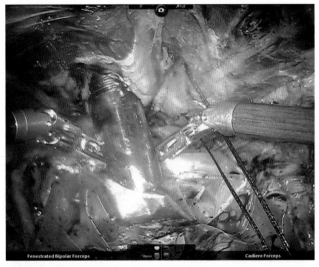

Figure 36-17. Placement of an additional port in the hypogastrium for stapler insertion to restore continuity of the bowel by performing a side-to-side anastomosis.

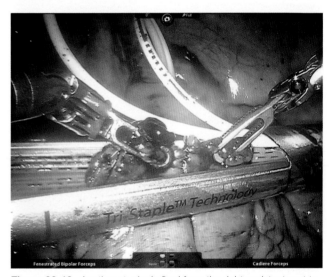

Figure 36-19. Another stapler is fired from the right assistant port to staple the open ends of both bowel segments.

removed after the suture has been placed. The remaining part of the distal ureter is transected and sent for permanent pathologic examination. The anterior half of the left ureteroileal anastomosis is completed (Fig. 36-16). The anastomosis of the right side is performed in similar fashion, keeping in the mind the key step. The marionette can be manipulated to turn the conduit for right ureteroileal anastomosis. After placement of the right stent, the distal ends of both the stents are left in the 15-mm side port; the ex vivo portions of these stents should be left free to prevent accidental dislodgement while maneuvering the conduit inside the abdominal cavity.

Restoration of Bowel

Continuity of the bowel is restored by performing a side-to-side anastomosis. This requires placement of an additional port in the hypogastrium (Fig. 36-17). In male patients, the port is later used to remove the specimen bag via a Pfannenstiel incision around it. The port is placed on the left side just lateral to the midline. The antimesenteric border of the two bowel segments

is incised just below the staple line to allow the jaws of a 60-mm Endo GIA stapler to pass through. The stapler is passed through the hypogastric port, and the bowel segments are slid over the jaws, oriented along the antimesenteric border. A fourth arm Cobra grasper (Intuitive Surgical, Sunnyvale, Calif.) is used to keep the segments aligned, and correct orientation is ensured through use of the right and left robotic instruments (Fig. 36-18). The stapler is fired and removed with care. Another stapler is fired from the right assistant port to staple the open ends of both bowel segments (Fig. 36-19). The distal tip of the staple line is sutured with a single interrupted 3-0 silk suture, and the mesenteric window is closed with interrupted silk sutures.

Creation of Stoma

After completion of the bowel anastomosis, the pelvic cavity is inspected for hemostasis. Specimen bag strings are retrieved from the hypogastric port. A bedside assistant performs the standard approach to creating the stoma. A cruciate incision is made in the anterior rectus sheath, and the rectus muscle is split with a long hemostat. Four stay sutures are placed in the sheath to anchor the conduit once it has been externalized. A vascular clamp is introduced through the stoma opening to grasp the marionette suture and the ends of the ureteral stents, under direct vision. These are pulled out through the stoma along with the conduit, ensuring proper orientation. All robotic ports are removed and the pneumoperitoneum is ended before the stoma is created by a standard open technique.

COMPLICATIONS

The benefits of ICIC urinary diversion are obvious: faster postoperative recovery, early return of bowel function, and reduced analgesia requirements—factors that also affect the overall hospital stay. RARC with intracorporeal urinary diversion (ICUD) has resulted in better outcomes, even when compared with the enhanced recovery pathway. Single-center noncomparative series of RARC with ICUD have reported satisfactory outcomes. Azzouni and colleagues reported outcomes of 100 consecutive ICICs, with a 19% high-grade complication rate at 90 days. Infectious complications were most commonly seen (31%), followed by gastrointestinal complications (22%). There was an appreciable decline in high-grade complications after the first 50 cases. The largest data set for RARC, from the International Robotic Cystectomy Consortium, compared the outcomes between ICUD and extracorporeal urinary diversion (ECUD) after RARC. Complications were comparable between ICUD and ECUD, with a trend favoring ICUD (90-day complication rate: 41% versus 49%, $P = .055$), and significantly fewer readmissions were reported for ICUD (90-day readmission rate: 12% versus 19%, $P = .016$). Gastrointestinal and infectious complications were significantly lower in the ICUD group. The study concluded that ICUD was associated with 32% less likelihood of postoperative complications compared with ECUD. ICIC continues to remain a challenge for surgeons new at adopting this technique. Stepwise, mentored training can help the surgeon attain excellence early, to offer patients the maximum benefits of a completely intracorporeal radical cystectomy.

37 Continent Urinary Diversion

Jason M. Sandberg, Ted B. Manny, Ashok K. Hemal

Urinary diversion is a necessity after cystectomy. For the proper candidate, continent urinary diversion (CUD) may offer significant quality-of-life advantages. Several versions of continent diversion have been described, including the ileal orthotopic neobladder (ONB), Indiana pouch, and ureterosigmoidostomy, among others.

Laparoscopic radical cystectomy (LRC) with extracorporeal urinary diversion was first reported in 1995. LRC with extracorporeal urinary diversion and follow-up has also been reported with satisfactory oncologic and quality-of-life improvement. LRC with a completely intracorporeal ileal neobladder was first reported in two patients in 2002. The first case report of a robotic-assisted, fully intracorporeal procedure was published soon after in 2003. In the same year the first multipatient case series of robotic-assisted radical cystectomy (RARC) with extended pelvic lymph node dissection (ePLND) and urinary diversion was reported in 17 patients. This report detailed three variations of extracorporeal diversion achieved via the 5- to 6-cm incision used to extract the bladder, including the ileal conduit and the W-pouch and double-chimney (or T-pouch) neobladders. The neobladder was constructed extracorporeally through the site of specimen extraction and then was placed back into the pelvis. After the incision was closed, the neobladder-urethral anastomosis was performed robotically. This seminal publication served as the proof of concept for a robotic-assisted operation, which has since evolved.

Since that time, multiple high-volume centers and experienced surgeons have started to perform RARC with completely intracorporeal ONB, the majority of whom use some variation of the Studer pouch. The first multipatient case series was reported in 2010. More recently, a 132-patient series was reported from two institutions, demonstrating improvements in operative times, blood loss, hospital stay, and prevalence of late complications with surgeon experience.

INDICATIONS AND CONTRAINDICATIONS

All patients who are eligible for radical cystectomy should at least be considered as candidates for continent diversion, including ONB reconstruction. However, patients must meet certain criteria, including intact urethral function, absence of stress urinary incontinence, and absence of tumor infiltration into the distal prostatic urethra in men and bladder neck in women. Presence of tumor in the aforementioned areas, either on preoperative biopsy or intraoperative frozen section, contraindicates ONB. In these cases an alternative diversion such as ileal conduit or catheterizable pouch can be pursued. Patients should also be intellectually and physically capable in their understanding of their operation and postoperative care, including voiding behaviors and catheterization if necessary. ONB is also contraindicated in patients with chronic kidney disease and serum creatinine levels above 2 mg/dL (or glomerular filtration rate [GFR] <40 mL/min/1.73 m²), although the procedure can occasionally be offered in the setting of recovered renal function if the condition was caused by obstruction that has since been alleviated.

Reabsorption of ammonia via ileal mucosa in patients with preexisting liver dysfunction can lead to toxic hyperammonemia, thus effectively excluding patients with cirrhosis as candidates.

Furthermore, ONB should not be offered to patients with inflammatory bowel disorders such as Crohn disease. Patients of advanced age or poor functional status or those who have undergone previous radiation therapy should be selected carefully, although these factors do not absolutely contraindicate continent diversion.

PREOPERATIVE EVALUATION AND PREPARATION

The preoperative evaluation of patients undergoing planned RARC followed by ONB is largely similar for most patients as in open surgery but varies slightly depending on the operative indications. All patients should undergo a full and thorough physical examination, including assessment by a preoperative clinic for medical clearance, particularly if the patient is American Society of Anesthesiologists (ASA) class III or greater. Basic laboratory studies to assess for renal function and to rule out metabolic and hematologic abnormalities should be performed. Preoperative urine cultures, review of previous positive cultures, or both are also recommended so that appropriate prophylactic antibiotics can be administered perioperatively. If no positive cultures are available, a third-generation cephalosporin with metronidazole is commonly given on the day of surgery and stopped on postoperative day 2. If malignancy has been diagnosed, standard staging workup including chest radiograph and abdominal computed tomography (CT) are required. Bone scan may be reserved for patients with an elevated alkaline phosphatase level. All patients undergoing radical cystectomy are seen by a medical oncology team to consider neoadjuvant chemotherapy.

A stoma site should be marked in all patients in the event that the procedure is converted to an ileal conduit or catheterizable stoma. Mechanical bowel preparation and preadmission the night before surgery are routinely practiced but are omitted in some series. The patient is allowed clear liquids starting the day before surgery and then nothing by mouth beginning at midnight. During this time, the patient can also be taught clean intermittent catheterization, should the need arise at a later date.

OPERATING ROOM CONFIGURATION AND PATIENT POSITIONING

The patient is placed in the supine position and general endotracheal anesthesia is administered. Intravenous antibiotics are administered. An orogastric or nasogastric tube is placed intraoperatively. A Foley catheter is placed per urethra in preparation for radical cystectomy.

The patient is positioned in the dorsal lithotomy position with the arms tucked, ensuring adequate padding of all extremities to avoid potential compartment syndrome and neurapraxia. The lateral aspects of the patient's knees are appropriately padded. The patient is adequately secured to the table and placed in steep Trendelenburg position (15 to 45 degrees) for RARC (Fig. 37-1). The Trendelenburg position is applied to slide the bowel out of the pelvis and provide adequate exposure. Before proceeding to ONB construction, Trendelenburg should be reduced to 10 to 15 degrees and the robot can be docked traditionally between the patient's

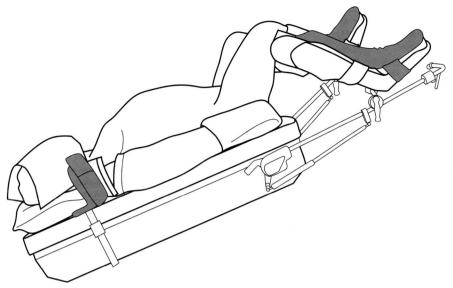

Figure 37-1. The patient is positioned in steep Trendelenburg position (30 to 45 degrees) for robotic-assisted radical cystectomy, which is later reduced to 10 to 15 degrees for the neobladder reconstruction.

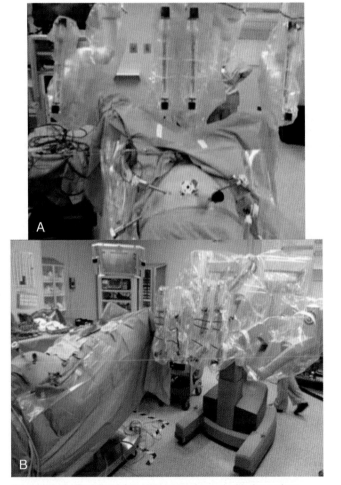

Figure 37-2. The procedure may be performed with the patient in the low Trendelenburg position (30 degrees) to avoid prolonged lithotomy position. The da Vinci Xi robotic system (Intuitive Surgical, Sunnyvale, Calif.) may be docked between the patient's legs **(A)** or optionally side docked **(B).**

legs. Alternatively, the patient can be left supine and the robot can be side docked to avoid prolonged lithotomy position (Fig. 37-2). After induction of general anesthesia, the patient is prepared and draped in the usual sterile fashion. A preparation time-out is performed, and a sterile field is created by preparing the patient's penis or vagina, perineum, and proximal thighs up to the infraxiphoid abdomen after clipper shaving.

All required instrumentation for RARC with intracorporeal ileal neobladder is listed in Box 37-1.

TROCAR PLACEMENT
da Vinci S and Si Robotic Systems

With a Veress needle, the abdomen is insufflated to 15 mm Hg. An Endopath Xcel 12-mm bladeless bariatric trocar (Ethicon, Cincinnati, Ohio) is inserted about 5 cm above the umbilicus. The camera is then inserted and the abdomen and pelvis are inspected for injuries to structures from insertion of the Veress needle, adhesions, and metastatic disease. Under endoscopic guidance, the remaining three 8-mm robotic ports and the two assistant ports are placed (Fig. 37-3, *A*). Two robotic ports are placed on each side of the camera port approximately 7 to 10 cm lateral and above the level of the umbilicus. The additional robotic port is placed in the right lower quadrant of the abdomen approximately 7 to 10 cm lateral to the right-sided robotic port and 5 to 7 cm superior to the iliac crest. This may be inline with or just below the other robotic ports.

An AirSeal trocar (SurgiQuest, Milford, Conn.) is then inserted on the left side 5 to 7 cm superior to the iliac crest. The use of the fourth arm on the right and 12-mm assistant port on the left facilitates bowel manipulation by avoiding acute-angle stapling. A second assistant port can be placed through the premarked stomal site when an ileal conduit is contemplated as an alternative, or it can be placed on the left side, which allows the assistant to have control of both ports from one side. Having an additional 12-mm assistant port close to the midline greatly simplifies pedicle stapling during extirpative cystectomy. The robot is then docked.

We typically use three instruments: Hot Shears (Intuitive Surgical, Sunnyvale, Calif.) in the right robotic arm, PK dissecting forceps (Intuitive Surgical, Sunnyvale, Calif.) in

---

BOX 37-1 Instrumentation for Robotic-Assisted Radical Cystectomy with Intracorporeal Ileal Neobladder

NONDISPOSABLE INSTRUMENTATION

- Four-arm da Vinci Si system (Intuitive Surgical, Sunnyvale, Calif.)
- PlasmaKinetic bipolar generator (Gyrus ACMI PK; Gyrus ACMI, Norwalk, Ohio)
- Laparoscopic grasper
- Laparoscopic scissors
- Laparoscopic KOH Macro Needle Holder (Karl Storz, Tuttlingen, Germany)
- Hot Shears (Monopolar Curved Scissors) (Intuitive Surgical, Sunnyvale, Calif.)
- Maryland (bipolar forceps) (Intuitive Surgical, Sunnyvale, Calif.)
- Atraumatic Cadiere forceps (Intuitive Surgical, Sunnyvale, Calif.)
- Large SutureCut needle driver (Intuitive Surgical, Sunnyvale, Calif.)
- LigaSure (Valleylab, Boulder, Colo.)
- 16-mm stapler (Endo GIA; Covidien, Dublin, Ireland)
- Lapra-Ty absorbable clips (Ethicon, Cincinnati, Ohio)
- Laparoscopic Kelly
- Ligaloop Strings (Braun-Dexon, Spangenberg, Germany)
- 10-mm Stryker suction tip (Stryker, Kalamazoo, Mich.)
- 5-mm-long Stryker suction tip (Stryker, Kalamazoo, Mich.)
- Small, large, and extra-large laparoscopic Hem-o-lok appliers (Weck Closure Systems, Research Triangle Park, N.C.)
- Three 8-mm cannulas with obturator and seals (Intuitive Surgical, Sunnyvale, Calif.)

DISPOSABLE INSTRUMENTATION

- Basic accessory kit and drapes (Intuitive Surgical, Sunnyvale, Calif.)
- Camera head (Intuitive Surgical, Sunnyvale, Calif.)
- 0-degree and 30-degree endoscopes (Intuitive Surgical, Sunnyvale, Calif.)
- StrykeFlow 2 suction/irrigation system (Stryker, Kalamazoo, Mich.)
- Echelon Flex Powered Endopath stapler (Ethicon, Cincinnati, Ohio)

- Weck Hem-o-lok Ligating Clips (Teleflex, Wayne, Penn.)
- Ultra Veress needle (Ethicon, Cincinnati, Ohio)
- One Endopath Xcel 12-mm bladeless bariatric trocar for camera port (Ethicon, Cincinnati, Ohio)
- One Endopath Xcel 12-mm bladeless trocar (Ethicon, Cincinnati, Ohio)
- One Endopath Xcel 15-mm bladeless trocars (Ethicon, Cincinnati, Ohio)
- Endo Catch II 15-mm specimen pouch (Covidien, Dublin, Ireland)
- Two extra-large Hem-o-lok clips prepared with suture attached (Weck Closure Systems, Research Triangle Park, N.C.) for clipping and tagging of the ureters
- AirSeal trocar (Surgiquest, Milford, Conn.)

OPTIONAL INSTRUMENTATION

- ProGrasp forceps (Intuitive Surgical, Sunnyvale, Calif.)
- 0-Vicryl on CT-1 needle (Ethicon, Cincinnati, Ohio)
- Echelon Endopath 45-mm stapler (Ethicon, Cincinnati, Ohio)
- 1-0 V-Loc 90 (glycolic acid–trimethylene carbonate, Covidien, Dublin, Ireland) for vaginal reconstruction
- Harmonic ACE Curved Shears 8-mm (Ultrasonic Energy Instrument, Intuitive Surgical, Sunnyvale, Calif.)
- Large robotic clip applier (Intuitive Surgical, Sunnyvale, Calif.)
- EndoWrist One Suction/Irrigator (Intuitive Surgical, Sunnyvale, Calif.)
- EndoWrist Vessel Sealer (Intuitive Surgical, Sunnyvale, Calif.)
- EndoWrist Stapler (Intuitive Surgical, Sunnyvale, Calif.)
- LigaSure Atlas (Covidien, Dublin, Ireland)
- Enseal Tissue Sealing Device (Ethicon, Cincinnati, Ohio)
- Silicone vessel loops (Aspen Surgical Products, Caledonia, Mich.)
- Endo GIA Ultra Universal stapler (Covidien, Dublin, Ireland)
- Lapro-Clip (Covidien, Dublin, Ireland)
- Firefly near infrared fluorescence visualization system (Novadaq Technologies, Mississauga, Ontario, Canada)

---

the left robotic arm, and Cadiere forceps (Intuitive Surgical, Sunnyvale, Calif.) in the third robotic arm. RARC can be performed entirely with these three instruments to help cut down on operative costs. However, for intracorporeal ONB, two needle drivers inclusive of one suture cut are used. The 0-degree camera lens can be used for a majority of the dissection, but the 30-degree downward lens is helpful for dissecting deep within the pelvis and for the ePLND high up to the aortic bifurcation or inferior mesenteric artery. The 30-degree upward lens may be helpful for dissecting behind the prostate, for retroapical dissection for providing additional urethral length, and for dropping the bladder.

da Vinci Xi Robotic System

As mentioned earlier, a six-port transperitoneal approach is used and all ports are placed about 5 cm cephalad to the umbilicus. On the Xi system the 12-mm camera port is replaced by a da Vinci 8-mm universal camera-robotic port (Fig. 37-3, *B* and *C*). The Xi also lends itself more easily to supine positioning, which may decrease positioning complications.

Laparoscopic Port Placement

A six-port transperitoneal approach is used for LRC with intracorporeal ONB creation (Fig. 37-4). The five previously placed ports for LRC are used as follows: a 10- or 11-mm port above the umbilicus for the camera port; two 12-mm ports, one at the lateral edge of each rectus muscle on the left and right, just inferior to the umbilicus; a 10-mm port in the left iliac fossa; and a 5-mm port on the right at the level of the anterior superior iliac spine. A final 5-mm port is placed midway between the umbilicus and symphysis pubis. While creating the neobladder, instruments can be swapped among the different ports.

PROCEDURE (SEE VIDEO 37-1)

RARC is performed as described in Chapter 35. Attention is then turned to the urinary continent diversion. Several different techniques are available to the urologist.

Completely Intracorporeal Ileal Neobladder

Historically different types of the neobladder can be constructed by using different intestinal segments. We prefer to use ileum whenever possible. We typically place sutures in the urethra in a single pass at the 5 and 7 o'clock positions in an inside-out manner at the start of this portion of the procedure, then pass them through the anterior abdominal wall so they can be retrieved later for the neobladder-urethral anastomosis.

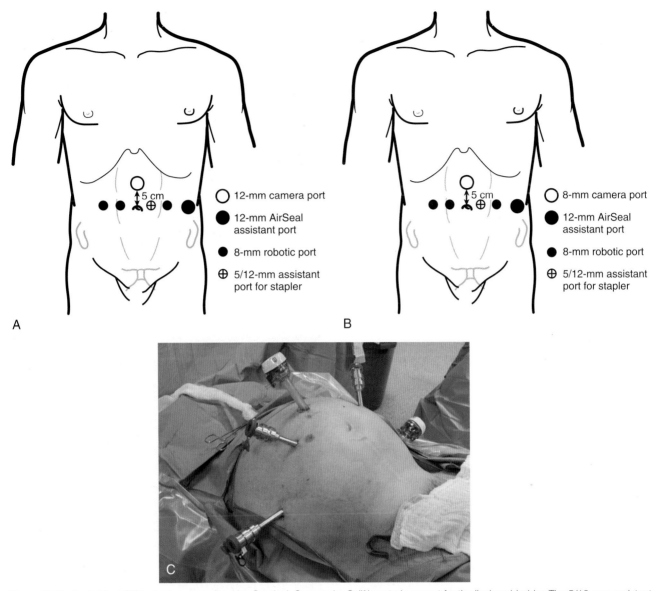

Figure 37-3. A, da Vinci S/Si robotic system (Intuitive Surgical, Sunnyvale, Calif.) port placement for the ileal neobladder. The 5/12-mm assistant port may be placed either on the left (shown) or right. **B,** da Vinci Xi robot port placement for the ileal neobladder. The 5/12-mm assistant port may be placed either on the left *(shown)* or right. **C,** Image showing robotic port placement in an actual patient (Si robot).

Bowel Isolation

To construct the neobladder, we use 60 cm of distal ileum beginning 15 cm proximal to the ileocecal junction. These segments are identified and then marked with the use of two red vessel loops for the distal segment and two blue vessel loops for the proximal segment, placed through the mesentery (Fig. 37-5). A sterile flexible tape measure, premeasured silk suture, or premeasured open-ended ureteral catheter is used to facilitate measurement of bowel segment length (Fig. 37-6). Atraumatic Cadiere forceps are used on the right and fenestrated bipolar forceps on the left robotic arms for bowel manipulation. If needed, double fenestrated forceps or a needle driver can be used to save on cost.

Optionally, before division of the bowel, the anesthesiologist can intravenously administer 2 to 5 mL of 2.5 mg/mL unconjugated indocyanine green (ICG), which enables mesenteric angiography using a Firefly visualization system (Novadaq Technologies, Mississauga, Ontario, Canada) with

the robot. This allows for maximal preservation of blood supply to the ileum used for the neobladder because it is cumbersome to backlight the mesentery intracorporeally. Distal transection of ileum is performed with a 60-mm laparoscopic stapler (Echelon Flex Powered ENDOPATH Stapler; Cincinnati, Ohio) via the 12-mm left assistant AirSeal port and a blue stapler load (3.5-mm thickness) (Fig. 37-7). This distal mesenteric window is further developed with an additional white vascular stapler load (2.5-mm thickness). This is crucial to allow for proper mobilization of reservoir. Preplaced vessel loops help in manipulating bowel.

The transected distal bowel segment (toward the cecum) is marked with a red vessel loop and purple-dyed 3-0 Vicryl suture. With undyed sutures, the ileal segment is marked at approximately 25 cm (denoting the apex of the posterior plate) and 50 cm (denoting the beginning of the afferent limb) from the distal end. After proximal division of the ileal segment, another purple-dyed 3-0 Vicryl suture is placed to mark the proximal transected ileum (Fig. 37-8).

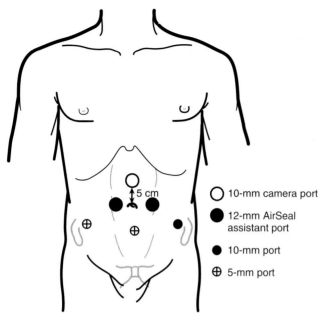

Figure 37-4. Laparoscopic port placement for the laparoscopic intracorporeal ileal neobladder procedure.

○ 10-mm camera port

● 12-mm AirSeal assistant port

● 10-mm port

⊕ 5-mm port

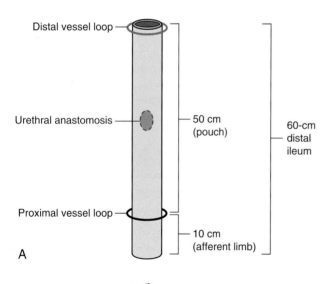

Figure 37-5. Schematic representation of isolated segment of ileum with distal and proximal vessel loops **(A)**. Neobladder configuration after bowel isolation and pouch folding **(B)**.

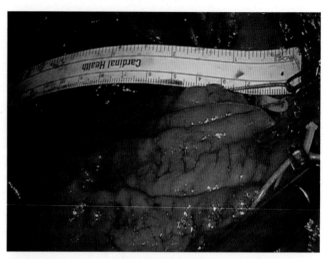

Figure 37-6. For the construction of the Studer neobladder, 60 cm of ileum is isolated. Note the blue and red vessel loops used to not only demarcate the pouch boundaries but also to manipulate the bowel in an atraumatic manner.

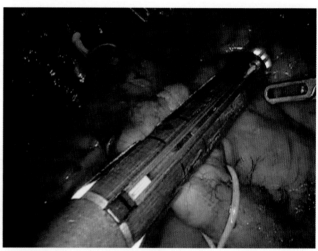

Figure 37-7. The bowel is transected at both the proximal *(blue, shown here)* and distal *(red)* end with a 60-mm laparoscopic stapler. Two vessel loops of the same color are placed on either side of the stapler so that both the residual and isolated ileum holds a color-coded loop. The same stapler is used with vascular load to divide the mesentery.

Restoring Bowel Continuity

With the vessel loops used for traction, the anastomotic bowel segments are brought in apposition, and continuity is reestablished with a standard side-to-side ileoileal anastomosis using two 60-mm laparoscopic tissue stapler loads on the adjacent antimesenteric ileal walls (Fig. 37-9). The open ends of ileum are closed with a tissue stapler load deployed transversely to finish the side-to-side anastomosis (Fig. 37-10). This allows for a single stapler to be used for all bowel stapling. Care is taken to perform the ileoileal anastomosis cephalad to the excluded ileal segment so that the neobladder can be formed in a position caudal to the mesentery and easily moved into the pelvis.

Detubularizing the Bowel

The undyed marking suture at 25 cm from the distal end of excluded ileum is grasped by the fourth robotic arm and

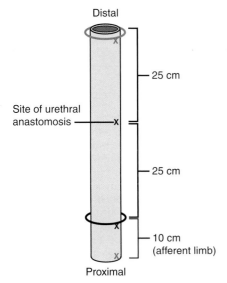

Figure 37-8. The isolated segment of bowel is marked with colored sutures to identify important landmarks including the proximal and distal ends (purple sutures), the site of urethral anastomosis (undyed), and the start of the afferent limb (undyed).

retracted into the pelvis, which helps to symmetrically align two 25-cm ileal segments adjacent to each other. The additional 10 cm of ileum is used for the afferent limb. The 50 cm of ileum is then detubularized with the incision over a 22-French red rubber catheter or chest tube (Fig. 37-11). This may also be completed without any intraluminal tube if desired.

Creation of the Posterior Plate

The apposing edges of the posterior wall of the neobladder are aligned with several 2-0 absorbable interrupted sutures placed at 6- to 8-cm intervals with a 6-cm tag to facilitate manipulation during final suturing (Fig. 37-12). Subsequently, the posterior wall of the neobladder is constructed in a watertight manner with 2-0 running barbed sutures (V-loc; Covidien, Dublin, Ireland) (Fig. 37-13). Once the posterior plate is complete, a 3-0 barbed suture is placed at the midpoint of the right side of the posterior plate at the site of the anticipated urethral-neobladder anastomosis.

Urethral-Neobladder Anastomosis

With the previously placed 3-0 barbed sutures at the 5 and 7 o'clock positions (4, 6, and 8 o'clock positions may be used

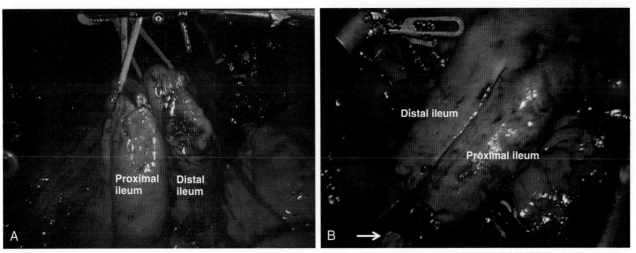

Figure 37-9. A, Bowel continuity is restored after the staple lines are removed; the residual bowel is held in the proper orientation for side-to-side anastomosis. In this image, the staple lines have already been removed with electrocautery. **B,** The 60-mm stapler *(arrow)* is again used to restore bowel continuity with a side-to-side anastomosis.

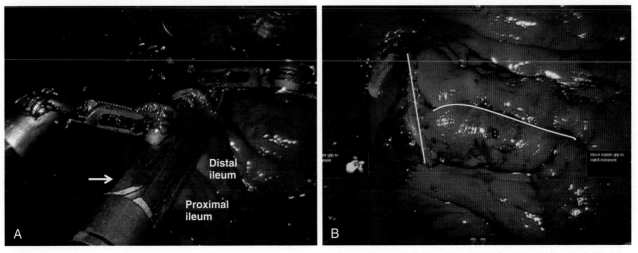

Figure 37-10. A, The open end is then stapled *(arrow)* again to ensure a wide anastomosis. **B,** Completed bowel anastomosis. Staple line is shown in yellow.

if desired) of the urethra, the urethral-neobladder anastomosis is started after rotating the posterior plate counterclockwise 90 degrees with caudal traction. The urethral-neobladder anastomosis is performed in a running fashion with a barbed suture (Figs. 37-14 and 37-24). The posterior portion of the anastomosis is completed over a 24-French hematuria catheter. The anastomosis is completed anteriorly by using interrupted sutures or by continuing to run the previous posterior sutures.

Bilateral Ureteral Anastomosis

Each ureter is then spatulated (Fig. 37-15) and separately anastomosed to the afferent limb with the Bricker technique with interrupted or continuous 5-0 Monocryl sutures. A Vicryl heel stitch may be placed to bolster the anastomosis and to maintain proper orientation (Fig. 37-16). After the posterior wall is sutured and before the anastomosis is completed, each ureter is intubated with completely internalized 6-French 30-cm double-J ureteral stents (Fig. 37-17). These are purposefully long to allow easier cystoscopic retrieval, as was our practice for intracorporeal ileal conduit. The ureteral anastomosis alternatively can

be performed via the Wallace technique in which the medial walls of both spatulated ureters are anastomosed with each other before this newly formed single unit is anastomosed to the afferent limb of the ONB in end-to-side fashion (Fig. 37-18).

Closing the Neobladder

Neobladder closure is started by cross-folding the posterior plate on itself and fixing the midpoint with a horizontal mattress suture. This divides the anterior suture line into two equal halves and aligns the edges for closure. The anterior wall of the neobladder is closed with running 2-0 barbed suture, leaving a small opening for a suprapubic catheter if desired (Fig. 37-19). After placement of the suprapubic catheter into this opening, the anterior closure of the pouch is completed in a running fashion with barbed sutures. This helps in fixation to the anterior abdominal wall, thus preventing some of the small bowel from plastering to the anterior abdominal wall. It may also be helpful for later percutaneous interventions if needed. The neobladder is irrigated via the transurethral Foley catheter to ensure a watertight closure; any leaks are secured with interrupted 2-0 Vicryl sutures. Surgical specimens may be extracted vaginally in women or through extension of the midline camera port incision in men. A closed suction drain is placed in the pelvis through a lateral port site.

Closure of the Abdominal Wall

All 10-mm or larger port sites are reapproximated with 1-0 Vicryl suture at the level of the fascia. The specimen retrieval site is closed at the level of the fascia with figure-of-eight polydioxanone (PDS) followed by reapproximation of the Scarpa fascia with running Vicryl. Monocryl subcuticular sutures are used to close all skin sites, followed by a sterile surgical dressing.

Variations of the aforementioned technique have been described. Wiklund and colleagues perform the neobladder-urethral anastomosis at the beginning of the procedure, immediately after identification of the ileal segment to be used for neobladder construction (Fig. 37-20). After the distal anterior wall is closed in a running fashion, the proximal portion of the neobladder is left open to complete the ureteroileal anastomoses with the Wallace rather than the Bricker technique.

Gill and colleagues have described use of a full 60 cm of ileum for neobladder construction that begins 15 cm proximally to the ileocecal junction. However, they dedicate 44 cm for the reservoir, whereas 16 cm is used for the afferent limb.

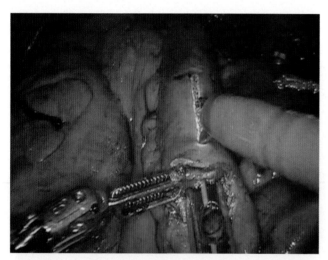

Figure 37-11. After a full-thickness incision is made in the proximal limb of isolated ileum, a 22- to 24-French chest tube is inserted so that the antimesenteric border can be cauterized and incised against a firm backing, effectively detubularizing the proximal limb of the neobladder. The distal limb is similarly incised.

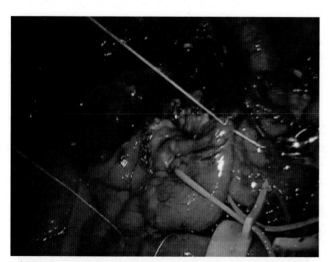

Figure 37-12. Interrupted Vicryl sutures are placed every 5 to 6 cm to approximate the now-detubularized proximal and distal limb when forming the posterior plate.

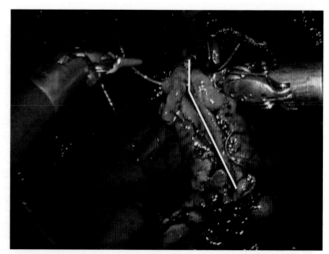

Figure 37-13. The posterior plate is secured with a 2-0 running barbed suture along the approximated proximal and distal limbs *(white line)*.

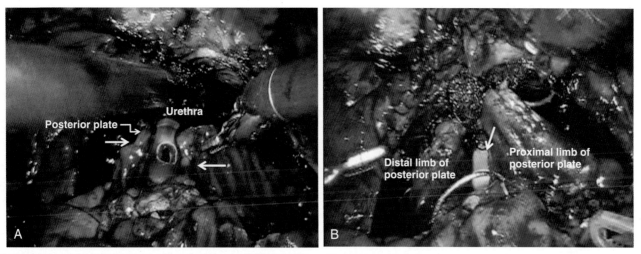

Figure 37-14. A, The previously placed urethral sutures at the 5 o'clock and 7 o'clock positions *(arrows)* are individually brought through the apex of the posterior plate of the neobladder in an inside-out manner. The reconstructed posterior plate can be easily seen. This is done before anterior pouch closure to ensure proper mobilization of the posterior plate without tension on the impending neobladder-urethral anastomosis. Note the transurethral Foley catheter. **B,** The sutures are run toward the 12 o'clock position to complete the urethroileal anastomosis around the Foley catheter *(arrow).*

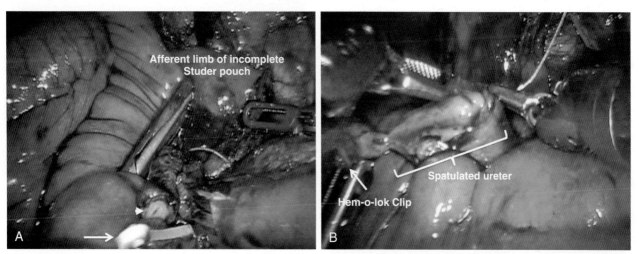

Figure 37-15. A, Both ureters are spatulated in preparation for the ureteroileal anastomoses. The ureter is transected *(arrowhead)* near the Hem-o-lok clip (Weck Closure Systems, Research Triangle Park, N.C.; *arrow*) placed during robotic-assisted radical cystectomy, then spatulated. The ureteral lumen is shown here. **B,** After a small full-thickness segment of bowel is removed from the afferent limb, a Vicryl heel stitch is placed into the spatulated ureter.

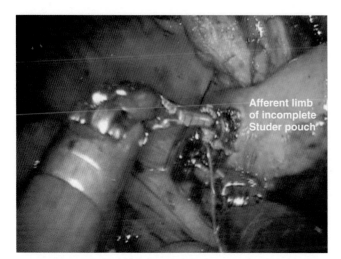

Figure 37-16. The Vicryl heel stitch is then run through the previously made defect in the wall of the afferent limb.

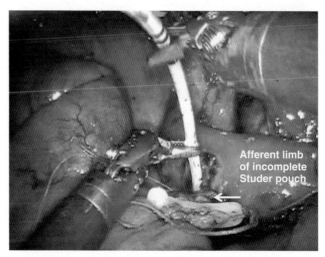

Figure 37-17. A double-J stent is placed over a wire up into the renal pelvis via the ureter *(arrow)* after the heel stitch has been secured. The distal end of the stent is then fed into the ileum so that it will occupy the "inside" of the incomplete Studer pouch.

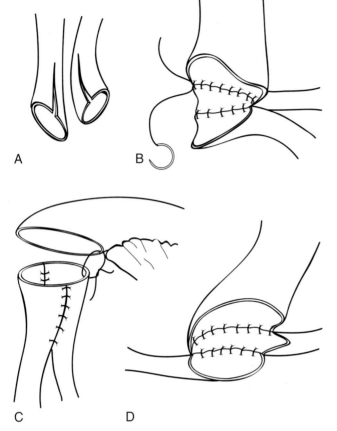

A B

C D

Figure 37-18. The Wallace ureteral anastomosis. **A,** Spatulation of the ureters. **B,** Side-to-side. **C,** Y-type. **D,** Head-to-tail.

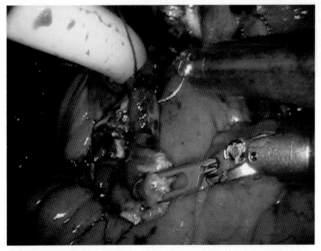

Figure 37-19. Before final pouch closure, a large-bore urinary catheter may be optionally introduced through the abdominal wall and sutured into the pouch to act as a suprapubic tube. Omentum may then be optionally placed over the pouch.

A running urethral anastomosis is completed with a double-armed 3-0 Monocryl suture on an RB-1 needle starting at the 6 o'clock position over a 22-French hematuria catheter. The neobladder is completed in a similar manner to that described earlier in this chapter, including ureteral Bricker anastomoses, internalization of the ureteral stents, and anterior closure of the neobladder. If desired, the sigmoid colon may also be used in constructing the neobladder (Fig. 37-21).

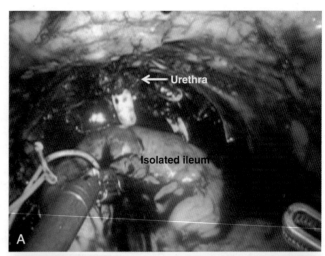

A

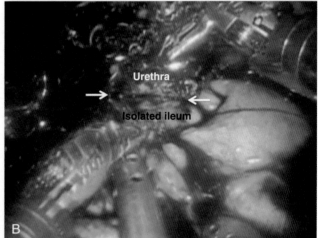

B

Figure 37-20. A, Early urethral anastomosis. The urethroileal anastomosis is performed before creation of the pouch. The Foley catheter may be advanced to the proximal urethra so that it may be readily identified. This ensures that the bowel will reach the urethra, and also provides an anchor point during pouch construction while relieving tension. **B,** Completing the urethroileal anastomosis. The suture line lies between the arrows.

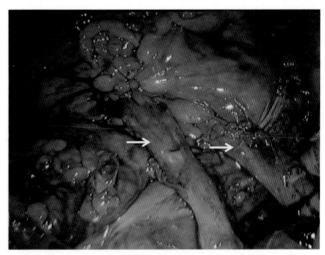

Figure 37-21. Orthotopic sigmoid neobladder. Ureters are marked with arrows.

Extracorporeal (Hybrid) Neobladder Technique

A historically popular method for ONB has been laparoscopic radical cystectomy or RARC, followed by extracorporeal neobladder reconstruction when the surgeon may not feel comfortable with a completely intracorporeal approach. We have found that it is particularly useful to re-dock the robot for ureteral- and urethral-neobladder anastomoses.

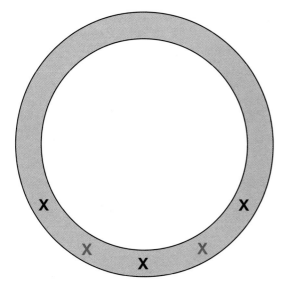

Figure 37-22. Location of early barbed or Vicryl suture placement at the 5 and 7 o'clock positions *(gray)* or alternatively the 4, 6, and 8 o'clock positions *(black)*. These sutures are placed on the urethral side first, which is particularly helpful when performing the extracorporeal (hybrid) neobladder-urethral anastomosis.

Preparing for Extracorporeal Neobladder Construction

After entrapment of the bladder and lymph node specimens in different pouches, several steps are taken before undocking the robot for extracorporeal neobladder construction. Individual Vicryl or barbed sutures are placed on the urethra in a single pass at the 5 and 7 o'clock positions (Fig. 37-22). They may alternatively be placed at 4, 6, and 8 o'clock positions if desired. The right and left ureters are clipped and tagged with dyed and undyed suture, respectively, for later identification. The terminal ileum is marked with a black silk suture, 15 cm from the ileocecal junction. The left ureter is brought beneath the sigmoid mesentery. A 20-French Foley catheter is placed in the urethra. All specimen and anchoring sutures are then secured to a locking grasper brought through the most medial port site to allow for easy retrieval and identification after a midline incision is made.

Specimen Retrieval

After undocking of the robot, a 5- to 6-cm incision extending from the inferior aspect of the midline camera port is made and the specimen is removed (Fig. 37-23). With the previously placed dyed sutures, the ureters are oriented in their correct position. The terminal ileum is identified by the silk suture, and extracorporeal (open) neobladder construction is performed. The neobladder depends on the surgeon's choice; it is created extracorporeally. Common options include the ileal Studer pouch, the ileal W-pouch, and the ileal double-chimney neobladder (or T-pouch), as well as the sigmoid neobladder (Table 37-1).

Ureteral-Neobladder Anastomosis

Ureteral-neobladder anastomosis can be done outside or inside. After creating the neobladder, ureteral positioning is confirmed within the pelvis and checked for proper alignment. Ureteral-neobladder anastomosis can be performed with the Bricker technique using 5-0 Monocryl sutures.

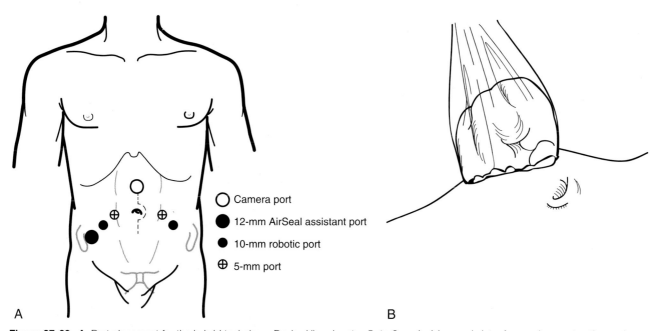

○ Camera port
● 12-mm AirSeal assistant port
● 10-mm robotic port
⊕ 5-mm port

A   B

Figure 37-23. A, Port placement for the hybrid technique. Dashed line denotes 5- to 6-cm incision made later for specimen extraction and delivery of the bowel for extracorporeal neobladder construction. **B,** Extraction of the surgical specimen entrapped in bag. *(**B** reprinted with permission from Menon M, Hemal AK, Tewari A, et al. Nerve-sparing robot-assisted radical cystoprostatectomy and urinary diversion. BJU Int. 2003;92:232-236.)*

Urethral-Neobladder Anastomosis

The urethral-neobladder anastomosis can be performed several ways depending on surgeon preference and patient characteristics. Three popular variations follow.

1. Intracorporeal robotic-assisted anastomosis. After completion of the neobladder, it is placed back in the pelvis and the midline incision is closed. The robotic is re-docked, and the urethral-neobladder anastomosis is performed with the previously placed 4, 6, and 8 o'clock sutures to form a posterior plate. Then, sutures are continued in a running fashion up to the anterior midline (Fig. 37-24, A).

2. Intracorporeal robotic-assisted anastomosis. After re-docking, an intracorporeal hemicircumferential anastomosis is performed. Working from right to left, an initial suture line

TABLE 37-1 Selected Options for Continent Urinary Diversion

Type	Intestinal Segment Used	Continence or Voiding Mechanism	Appearance
Ileal neobladder			
Studer	Ileum	Neobladder, urethral sphincter	
W-pouch	Ileum	Neobladder, urethral sphincter	

TABLE 37-1 Selected Options for Continent Urinary Diversion—cont'd

Type	Intestinal Segment Used	Continence or Voiding Mechanism	Appearance
T-pouch	Ileum	Neobladder, urethral sphincter	
Sigmoid neo-bladder	Sigmoid colon	Neobladder, urethral sphincter	 Arrows indicate ureters.
Indiana (ileocecal) pouch	Ascending (right) colon	Ileocecal valve, catheterizable stoma	

Continued

TABLE 37-1 Selected Options for Continent Urinary Diversion—cont'd

Type	Intestinal Segment Used	Continence or Voiding Mechanism	Appearance
Ureterosigmoidostomy (Mainz II) pouch	Terminal ileum and ascending (right) colon	Anal sphincter	

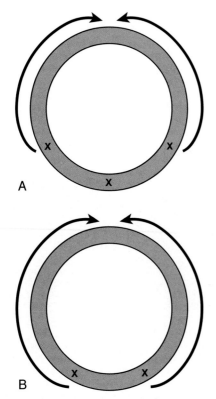

Figure 37-24. The intracorporeal urethral-neobladder anastomosis may be completed with interrupted sutures at the 4, 6, and 8 o'clock positions to form the posterior plate followed by a running suture up toward the 12 o'clock position **(A).** The anastomosis may alternatively be completed with two continuous sutures starting from the 5 and 7 o'clock positions **(B).**

begins by passing the needle outside-in at the 5 o'clock position on the neobladder neck, then inside-out on the urethra and up to the 12 o'clock position to create an adequate posterior plate. The anterior anastomosis consists of a second running suture line starting outside-in on the urethra and then inside-out on the bladder at the 7 o'clock position, and continuing in a counterclockwise fashion up to the point where the other suture is emerging from the neobladder (Fig. 37-24, *B*).

3. Extracorporeal anastomosis. The anastomosis may be performed with the previously placed urethral sutures at the 4, 6, and 8 o'clock positions as in variant 1, earlier.

Laparoscopic Considerations

Performing the ileal neobladder laparoscopically involves many similar steps with major variations owing to differences in equipment, port placement, and ergonomic limitations of traditional laparoscopic tools. This technique was first reported by Gill and colleagues.

Robotic-Assisted Ureterosigmoidostomy

When ONB is contraindicated, particularly in cases of urethral disease or in patients who lack viable ileum owing to previous resection, ureterosigmoidostomy can be offered. However, this procedure has fallen out of favor, especially because of metabolic complications.

POSTOPERATIVE MANAGEMENT

Early mobilization is recommended so that the patients are at least standing at the bedside within the first 24 hours. Diets are advanced via a modified enhanced recovery after surgery (ERAS) protocol. The nasogastric tube is typically discontinued on postoperative day 1, unless clinical status necessitates continuation. Clear liquids are given on postoperative day 1, and patients with ileal neobladders are irrigated gently every 8 hours to prevent mucous formation. The drain is removed on postoperative day 2, or when output is minimal. Pain control is often achieved through the use of patient-controlled analgesia. We do not typically use epidural anesthesia. An incisionally placed anesthetic catheter may be used at surgeon discretion.

Ureteral stents are removed approximately 4 weeks after surgery (Fig. 37-25). Patients are instructed on proper catheter irrigation care so they can continue to prevent mucous plugging at home. Cystoscopy and pouchogram are performed near the time of stent removal, or as far out as 3 to 6 weeks (Fig. 37-26). If no leak is detected, the suprapubic catheter can be removed (if present), followed by removal of the Foley catheter 2 to 3 days later.

Patients need to be monitored for hypochloremic metabolic acidosis and hypovolemia after surgery. The bladder substitute, composed of fully functional healthy ileum, will secrete sodium chloride in response to the initially hypo-osmolar urine in contact with the epithelium. Patients should be instructed to drink 2 to 3 L of fluids per day, or this fluid should be replaced intravenously while the patient is in the hospital, if needed. A high-salt diet is also encouraged to replenish sodium losses from the neobladder. Patients may be managed with oral sodium bicarbonate if base excess exceeds +2.

Rates of severe electrolyte disturbances tend to be much higher in those with colon reconstruction. A higher percentage of these patients require long-term alkali therapy. They are also at higher risk for hypokalemia stemming from total body potassium depletion owing to renal wasting. Symptoms in these individuals may include easy fatigability, anorexia, weight loss, polydipsia, and lethargy.

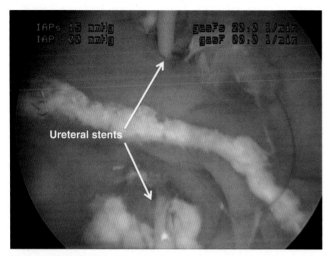

Figure 37-25. Endoscopic view of ureteral anastomosis with ureteral stents in place in the sigmoid neobladder at 3-week follow-up.

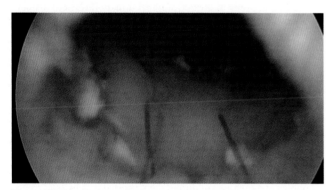

Figure 37-26. Endoscopic view of the neobladder-urethral anastomosis in the sigmoid neobladder 3 weeks after surgery.

Voiding behavior is extremely important after ON creation. Patients are instructed to void every 2 to 3 hours. The voiding interval can then be gradually be increased to every 4 to 5 hours to increase the capacity of the neobladder to an appropriate volume of 0.5 L. If patients exceed reasonable intervals between voids, the neobladder may become overdistended, which results in a floppy pouch with high postvoid residual volumes that does not empty properly. If the patient is not able to void or has high residual urine, he or she should perform clean intermittent catheterization.

COMPLICATIONS

Several single-institution series have been published regarding complications and outcomes after RARC with intracorporeal ONB. One of the largest published series from two institutions analyzed 132 cases and reported a mean hospital stay of 11 days. Early complications (within 30 days) ranging from Clavien-Dindo grade I to IVa were reported in 47% of patients, with 15.2% experiencing grade III or higher. The most common of all early complications were infectious (28.8%). Late complications were observed in 27.3% of patients, with a total of 12.9% graded III or higher. The conversion rate was 2.9%, including 4 out of 136 patients who were ultimately not included in the analysis (Table 37-2).

Sepsis (10%) was the most common early complication (within 30 days), and urinary tract infection (8%) was the most common late complication; 4.5% of patients developed a urine leak, and just over 7% developed a gastrointestinal complication, including four patients with ileus, two patients with a bowel leak, and two patients with neobladder-bowel fistula. Low rates of long-term complications were reported, including reservoir stones (2%), ureteroileal anastomotic stricture (3.8%), and neobladder-vaginal fistula (<1%). Mean operative times as low as 318 minutes have been reported in some small series, and as high as 594 minutes in others.

Overall, complication rates are similar to those of open urinary diversion. A recent single-institution review of 895 patients undergoing open radical cystectomy with some form of urinary diversion reported a hospital stay of 21 days for cases of open orthotopic diversion. Early and late hospital readmission rates for all urinary diversions, including ileal conduit, were 8.6% and 11%, respectively. The most common causes of first-time readmission were upper urinary tract obstruction (13%), pyelonephritis (12.4%), intestinal obstruction (11.9%), and metabolic acidosis (11.3%).

TABLE 37-2 Complications of Significant Published Series of Robotic-Assisted Radical Cystectomy with Intracorporeal Ileal Neobladder

Series	Patients (N)	Operative Time (min)	EBL (mL)	LOS (days)	Clavien I–II Complications	Clavien III–V Complications	Outcomes
Pruthi et al, 2010	3	330	221	5	—	—	—
Goh et al, 2012	8	450	225	8	Early: 63% Late: 0%	Early: 25% Late: 13%	75% daytime continence
Canda et al, 2012*	27	594	429	10.5	Early: 33% Late: 15%	Early: 15% Late: 11%	65% daytime continence; 17.6% nighttime continence
Collins et al, 2014	80	420	475	9	Early: 37% Late: 11%	Early: 27% Late: 19%	87% daytime continence; 80% nighttime continence
Desai et al, 2014†	132	456	430	11	Early: 32% Late: 14%	Early: 15% Late: 14%	84% complete daytime and nighttime continence

*Including two patients with ileal conduit and two patients with extracorporeal Studer neobladder.
†Includes patients from Collins et al, 2014.
EBL, estimated blood loss; LOS, length of stay.

TIPS AND TRICKS

Operating Room Configuration and Patient Positioning

- Move patient into steep Trendelenburg position for RARC and ePLND.
- Shoulder pads should be avoided when positioning the patient because their use poses a greater risk of brachial plexus injury.
- The da Vinci Xi system facilitates side docking in the supine position and may minimize postoperative neuropathy.

Trocar Placement

- Ports are placed supraumbilically, at least 2 inches higher than for robotic prostatectomy.
- The robotic fourth arm (8-mm port) should be placed on the right.
- Assistant ports are placed on the left (best for bowel stapling) and paramedian (best for pedicle stapling and suctioning).

Urinary Diversion After Robotic-Assisted Radical Cystectomy

- Undock, and place the patient into a more shallow Trendelenburg tilt (10 to 15 degrees). Re-dock the robot.

Bowel Isolation

- Accurate measurement of bowel section can be achieved with a premeasured suture or ureteral catheter.
- Color-coded vessel loops are used to indicate relevant ileal landmarks and minimize direct bowel manipulation.
- Use intravenous ICG dye to verify bowel vascularity.

Detubularization of the Bowel

- Incise the ileum over a 24-French lubricated chest tube that keeps the bowel under stretch and safeguards the posterior wall.

Creation of the Posterior Plate

- Use the fourth arm to keep traction via the apical stay suture.
- Use stay sutures placed every 6 to 8 cm to align bowel edges.
- We prefer a hand-sewn approach until robust data are published that demonstrate at least equivalent stone risk and no adverse effect on urodynamic parameters from the use of titanium staples.

Hybrid (Extracorporeal) Neobladder Technique

- The Foley catheter can be advanced through the urethra into the neobladder after it has been created. The neobladder is then dropped into the pelvis and the robot can be re-docked for the urethroileal anastomosis.

Urethroileal Anastomosis

- After the bladder and prostate have been resected en bloc, stitches are applied with barb sutures on the urethral stump, and the sutures are then pulled through the port when the hybrid technique is being performed. Later, these can be used to anastomose with the neobladder neck under direct vision.
- Use a Penrose drain around the isolated ileal mesentery to provide downward traction via the fourth arm.
- A barbed suture between the seromuscular layer of the ileal loop and the rectourethralis can be used to keep the ileal plate close to the urethra.

Ureteral Anastomosis

- Short (3-inch) suture on a cutting needle and continuous sutures are used.
- A 30-cm-long stent allows easier later cystoscopic retrieval from the afferent limb.

Closing

- Fill the neobladder with 50 mL of saline via the Foley catheter under direct vision to check for leakage.

SUGGESTED READINGS

Beecken WD, Wolfram M, Engl T, Bentas W, Probst M, Blaheta R, Oertl A, Jonas D, Binder J. Robotic-assisted laparoscopic radical cystectomy and intra-abdominal formation of an orthotopic ileal neobladder. *Eur Urol.* 2003;44:337–339.

Canda AE, Atmaca AF, Altinova S, et al. Robot-assisted nerve-sparing radical cystectomy with bilateral extended pelvic lymph node dissection (PLND) and intracorporeal urinary diversion for bladder cancer: initial experience in 27 cases. *BJU Int.* 2012;110:434–444.

Collins JW, Sooriakumaran P, Sanchez-Salas R, Ahonen R, Nyberg T, Wiklund NP, Hosseini A. Robot-assisted radical cystectomy with intracorporeal neobladder diversion: the Karolinska experience. *Indian J Urol.* 2014;30:307–313.

Desai MM, de Abreu AL, Goh AC, Fairey A, Berger A, Leslie S, Xie HW, Gill KS, Miranda G, Aron M, Sotelo RJ, Sun Y, Xu Z, Gill IS. Robotic intracorporeal urinary diversion: technical details to improve time efficiency. *J Endourol.* 2014;28:1320–1327.

Desai MM, Gill IS, de Castro Abreu AL, Hosseini A, Nyberg T, Adding C, Laurin O, Collins J, Miranda G, Goh AC, Aron M, Wiklund P. Robotic intracorporeal orthotopic neobladder during radical cystectomy in 132 patients. *J Urol.* 2014;192:1734–1740.

Gill IS, Kaouk JH, Meraney AM, Desai MM, Ulchaker JC, Klein EA, Savage SJ, Sung GT. Laparoscopic radical cystectomy and continent orthotopic ileal neobladder performed completely intracorporeally: the initial experience. *J Urol.* 2002;168:13–18.

Goh AC, Gill IS, Lee DJ, de Castro Abreu AL, Fairey AS, Leslie S, Berger AK, Daneshmand S, Sotelo R, Gill KS, Xie HW, Chu LY, Aron M, Desai MM. Robotic intracorporeal orthotopic ileal neobladder: replicating open surgical principles. *Eur Urol.* 2012;62:891–901.

Harraz AM, Osman Y, El-Halwagy S, Laymon M, Mosbah A, Abol-Enein H, Shaaban AA. Risk factors of hospital readmission after radical cystectomy and urinary diversion: analysis of a large contemporary series. *BJU Int.* 2015;115:94–100.

Hemal AK, Kolla SB, Wadhwa P, Dogra PN, Gupta NP. Laparoscopic radical cystectomy and extracorporeal urinary diversion: a single center experience of 48 cases with three years of follow-up. *Urology.* 2008;71:41–46.

Manny TB, Gorbachinsky I, Hemal AK. Lower extremity neuropathy after robot assisted laparoscopic radical prostatectomy and radical cystectomy. *Can J Urol.* 2010;17:5390–5393.

Manny TB, Hemal AK. Fluorescence-enhanced robotic radical cystectomy using unconjugated indocyanine green for pelvic lymphangiography, tumor marking, and mesenteric angiography: the initial clinical experience. *Urology.* 2014;83:824–829.

Menon M, Hemal AK, Tewari A, Shrivastava A, Shoma AM, El-Tabey NA, Shaaban A, Abol-Enein H, Ghoneim MA. Nerve-sparing robot-assisted radical cystoprostatectomy and urinary diversion. *BJU Int.* 2003;92:232–236.

Mufarrij PW, Rajamahanty S, Krane LS, Hemal AK. Intracorporeal double-J stent placement during robot-assisted urinary tract reconstruction: technical considerations. *J Endourol.* 2012;26:1121–1124.

Pruthi RS, Nix J, McRackan D, Hickerson A, Nielsen ME, Raynor M, Wallen EM. Robotic-assisted laparoscopic intracorporeal urinary diversion. *Eur Urol.* 2010;57:1013–1021.

Sanchez de Badajoz E, Gallego Perales JL, Reche Rosado A, Gutierrez de la Cruz JM, Jimenez Garrido A. Laparoscopic cystectomy and ileal conduit: case report. *J Endourol.* 1995;9:59–62.

38 Robotic-Assisted Laparoscopic Partial Cystectomy

Manish A. Vira, Paras H. Shah

Partial cystectomy has been used in the extirpative management of muscle-invasive bladder cancer since the mid-20th century. However, poor disease-free and disease-specific survival has largely precluded its use in this patient cohort. Improvements in surgical technique, the development of multimodal treatment strategies, and maturation in our understanding of the disease have allowed partial cystectomy to re-emerge as a treatment option for muscle-invasive bladder cancer in carefully selected patients.

Although no prospective trials evaluating efficacy exist, large retrospective series demonstrating acceptable oncologic outcomes and improved sexual function encourage use of this technique to minimize postoperative morbidity and significant quality-of-life changes associated with radical cystectomy. Unlike with other bladder-sparing therapies, partial cystectomy is potentially superior because of accurate staging with full thickness pathologic evaluation of the tumor and concomitant pelvic lymph node dissection. The minimally invasive approach to partial cystectomy offers opportunity to enhance perioperative outcomes, including decreased operative blood loss, decreased postoperative pain, and shorter length of stay. Of course, careful patient selection is required to achieve equivalent oncologic efficacy; it is currently estimated that only 5% to 10% of all patients with muscle-invasive bladder cancer are eligible for partial cystectomy.

INDICATIONS AND CONTRAINDICATIONS

Critical review of patient pathology and disease history is of paramount importance when determining eligibility for partial cystectomy. In general, surgery is reserved for patients with pathologic stage T2 disease on initial staging specimen who demonstrate invasion of the muscularis propria without imaging evidence of more locally advanced disease. Within this cohort, optimal disease features include the presence of a solitary tumor situated in the anterior bladder wall or bladder dome, away from the trigone. Resection should be performed with intent to achieve a histologically negative margin of 2 cm; inability to obtain an adequate disease-free perimeter would preclude partial extirpative therapy. Intraoperative frozen sections of the bladder wall taken from the edge of the resection bed should be used to ensure the absence of residual disease. Positive margins may be indicative of a more infiltrative process for which radical cystectomy would be better suited.

Tumor multifocality and the concomitant presence of carcinoma in situ (CIS) are both highly predictive of disease recurrence, with the latter particularly associated with the development of advanced disease. Accordingly, pathologic evidence of these entities during initial staging is a contraindication to partial cystectomy. Before planned partial cystectomy, the patient should undergo thorough examination of the remaining bladder, ideally with random bladder biopsy to confirm the absence of tumor multifocality or CIS. Although partial cystectomy is typically performed on tumors in the anterior wall and bladder dome, the location is not inherently associated with oncologic outcomes. Rather, the oncologic efficacy of the operation is determined by the ability to achieve an adequate negative surgical margin. Tumors in the posterior or lateral wall are potentially amenable to an organ-sparing approach when combined with concomitant ipsilateral ureteral reimplant. However, tumors at the trigone or bladder neck are generally not amenable to a partial approach, given the technical challenge of achieving an adequate surgical margin. Although no specific size restrictions exist, the patient should be counseled on the direct correlation between increasing size and risk for local recurrence. Finally, patients with severe bladder dysfunction or markedly reduced bladder capacity should be counseled against partial cystectomy for bladder cancer treatment.

PATIENT PREOPERATIVE EVALUATION AND PREPARATION

Optimal patient selection is critical before initiation of treatment. The nature and extent of disease must be accurately defined to ensure patients are not placed at increased risk for tumor recurrence or progression. Preoperative assessment of patients should begin with history and physical examination. Diagnosis is made most often during evaluation for either microscopic or macroscopic hematuria. Flank pain may occasionally be reported and may occur secondary to ipsilateral ureteral obstruction at the level of the bladder. Although bladder cancer does not lend itself to many positive findings on physical examination, a fixed bladder on bimanual examination or the presence of palpable lymphadenopathy may indicate an advanced disease process.

Relevant laboratory studies include urinalysis, basic metabolic profile, complete blood count, liver function tests, urine culture, and urine cytology. Microscopic hematuria may be the initial presentation leading to a diagnosis of bladder cancer. The presence of atypical or malignant cells on urine cytology may be suggestive of high-grade disease and warrants a thorough evaluation, particularly to rule out CIS. Because partial cystectomy is often performed as part of a multimodal treatment approach, optimization of serum creatinine may be necessary before administration of neoadjuvant or adjuvant chemotherapy. For the risk of infection to be minimized, a negative urology culture should be documented before surgical intervention.

Cross-sectional imaging of the abdomen and pelvis is indicated during the initial workup for both microscopic and macroscopic hematuria. Computed tomography (CT) with contrast is the study of choice to help determine a potential genitourinary source. Intraluminal areas in the upper urinary tract or bladder devoid of contrast (i.e., filling defects) on delayed, excretory phase images should raise suspicion for a neoplastic process. Alternatively, a more infiltrative process in the bladder may appear as asymmetric thickening of the bladder wall. If a patient cannot undergo contrast-enhanced cross-sectional imaging, retrograde pyelography and ureteroscopy can be performed at the time of cystoscopy to evaluate for upper-tract disease. More recently, dynamic contrast and diffusion-weighted magnetic resonance imaging is being used to develop more accurate clinical staging models for bladder cancers.

Cystoscopy is central to the workup because it allows direct visualization of the tumor as well as mapping of the bladder.

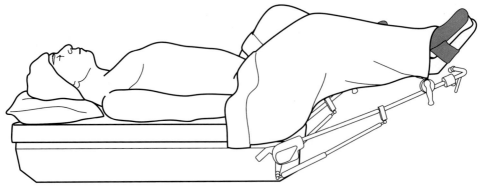

Figure 38-1. Dorsal lithotomy positioning.

Tumors most amenable to partial cystectomy are solitary and situated in the anterior wall or dome. Transurethral resection of the tumor should be performed with the intent to resect to completion. The concomitant presence of CIS must be ruled out. Random bladder biopsies may be performed at the time of primary tumor resection or during second-look cystoscopy. Prostatic urethral involvement would also preclude partial cystectomy; debate exists regarding when prostatic urethral biopsy should be performed, but in general it is performed if urethral abnormalities are observed, if positive cytology findings are present in the absence of gross tumor in the bladder, if CIS is identified, or if tumor is situated in the bladder neck.

Once invasion of the muscularis propria has been established during primary transurethral resection, restaging resection, as is often done in the setting of noninvasive high-risk disease, is not necessary unless there remains question regarding the presence of synchronous lesions, particularly CIS, or if complete resection of the tumor was not achieved during initial resection.

Staging workup for muscle-invasive disease is completed with cross-sectional imaging of the chest, abdomen, and pelvis to evaluate for systemic disease. Imaging of the bone and brain is reserved for symptomatic presentation or abnormal laboratory values.

Patients should be counseled before surgery about the possible need to convert to radical cystectomy at the time of surgery (if more extensive disease or positive frozen section is discovered), and appropriate bowel preparation should be given to the patient.

OPERATING ROOM CONFIGURATION AND PATIENT POSITIONING

All anesthetic preparations are made with the patient supine, after which the patient is placed in a dorsal lithotomy position with the hips abducted (Fig. 38-1). It is critical that the patient be secured to the operating table and appropriately padded in anticipation of placement into steep Trendelenburg position. Such positioning permits the small bowel to fall out of the pelvis and enhances visualization during the transperitoneal approach. The arms are padded and tucked at the patient's side. Gel pads are placed on the patient's shoulders, and the thorax is taped in a crisscross manner over the shoulders and across the chest just above the costal margin; care should be taken to not restrict respiratory excursion. The groin and perineum are prepared in a sterile manner along with the abdomen and pelvis. An 18-French Foley catheter is placed.

The da Vinci system robotic tower (Intuitive Surgical, Sunnyvale, Calif.) is situated between the patient's legs, after

which the patient is placed in low lithotomy to enable steep Trendelenburg positioning. The robotic arms are subsequently docked to the trocars (Fig. 38-2).

TROCAR PLACEMENT

A Veress needle is first placed through the umbilicus to establish a pneumoperitoneum of 15 mm Hg (Fig. 38-3). Six ports are subsequently placed in a configuration similar to that for robotic-assisted laparoscopic prostatectomy. A 12-mm camera port is placed approximately 2 cm superior to the umbilicus (20 to 25 cm above the pubic symphysis). Alternatively, the 12-mm camera port can be placed under direct vision by the Hasson technique. Two 8-mm robotic ports are placed 8 cm lateral to the midline on each side at the level of the umbilicus. A third 8-mm robotic port and a 12-mm assistant port are placed 8 cm lateral to the previously placed trocars on the right and left sides, respectively, again at the level of the umbilicus. A 5-mm port is placed left of the midline approximately 8 cm away from both camera port and the second robotic trocar (Fig. 38-4). In general, we prefer to use the AirSeal insufflation system (SurgiQuest, Milford, Conn.) to maintain the pneumoperitoneum.

PROCEDURE (SEE VIDEO 38-1)

The procedure begins by performing a bilateral extended pelvic lymph node dissection (see Section II of this book). After lymph node dissection, mobilization of the bladder is undertaken. The anterior peritoneum is incised immediately lateral to each medial umbilical ligament with monopolar electocautery (Fig. 38-5). The incision is carried superiorly toward the umbilicus to allow transection of the urachus. Although division of the medial umbilical ligaments can be performed with impunity, care must be taken to avoid lateral encroachment onto the lateral umbilical folds that overlie the inferior epigastric arteries.

The space of Retzius is accessed with a combination of blunt and sharp dissection through loose alveolar connective tissue in a lateral-to-medial fashion from the medial umbilical folds and a superior-to-inferior manner from the urachus toward the pubic bone. Development of the space of Retzius allows complete mobilization of the bladder off the anterior abdominal wall (Fig. 38-6).

Approximately 150 mL of normal saline is instilled into the bladder, after which a longitudinal cystotomy is made at the dome with electrocautery (Fig. 38-7). Alternatively, transillumination through the bladder with intraoperative flexible cystoscopy may help better delineate the site of initial incision so as to not cut into the tumor site. As the bladder is entered, urine and fluid should be aspirated with a suction device to

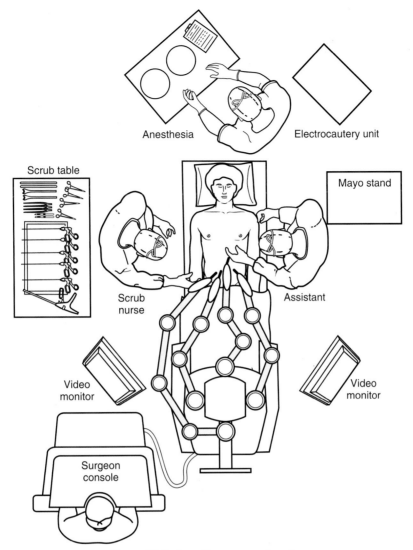

Figure 38-2. Operating room configuration.

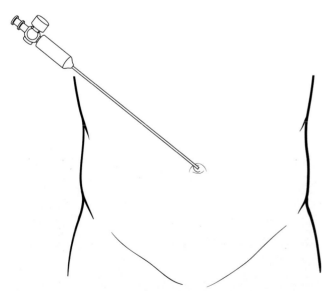

Figure 38-3. Veress needle is placed through the umbilicus to establish pneumoperitoneum of 15 mm Hg.

minimize risk for tumor seeding. The Foley balloon is taken down to facilitate inspection of the bladder mucosa. It is critical that the bladder tumor site be visualized in its entirety to assess the feasibility of a 2-cm tumor-free resection margin as well as to exclude the presence of metachronous lesions. In addition, the location of the tumor relative to the ureteral orifices should be noted (Fig. 38-8).

Full-thickness resection of the bladder wall and periad-ventitial tissue is performed in a circumferential manner around the tumor site (Fig. 38-9). The bladder mucosa may be scored with electrocautery before resection to help facilitate a 2-cm tumor-free margin. The surgical specimen is placed in a 10-mm Endo Catch bag (Medtronic, Minneapolis, Minn.) (Fig. 38-10). Mucosal and detrusor tissue is sampled from four quadrants at the edge of the resection bed and sent for frozen section analysis (Fig. 38-11). The absence of tumor must be demonstrated on all frozen section specimens before completing the cystorrhaphy.

The bladder wall is reapproximated in an appositional pattern and closed in a two-layer running fashion with 2-0 V-Loc sutures (Medtronic, Minneapolis, Minn.); alternatively, 2-0 polyglactin suture may be used. The primary layer should capture the mucosa and submucosa, and the secondary layer should incorporate the seromuscular layer

(Fig. 38-12). The bladder is subsequently filled with 150 mL of sterile saline to evaluate for the presence of urinary leak. Full-thickness buttressing sutures may be used to close bladder wall defects.

The initial Foley catheter is exchanged for a 20-French Foley catheter which is placed to gravity drainage. A 19-French Blake drain is situated anterior to the bladder closure and brought out through the right lateral robotic trocar site (Fig. 38-13). A 2-0 nylon suture is used to secure the drain to the skin. After hemostasis is confirmed, gas insufflation is stopped, the robot is undocked, and trocars are removed. Specimens are extracted through extension of the upper midline trocar site. After the specimens are delivered, the fascia is reapproximated with interrupted figure-of-eight 0-polyglactin sutures. The 12-mm left lateral assistant port is also closed with a 0-polyglactin suture. The wounds are irrigated and the skin is closed with 4-0 monofilament sutures.

POSTOPERATIVE MANAGEMENT

The patient may be started on a clear liquid diet and advanced on return of flatus. Patient-controlled anesthesia, either intravenous or via an epidural catheter placed preoperatively, can be offered. A 20-French Foley catheter is left in the bladder and placed to gravity drainage to facilitate healing of the cystotomy healing suture line. A pelvic drain situated anterior to the bladder wall closure is placed to self-suction and can be used to evaluate for urine leak. Although drain outputs are an important metric to monitor, fluid creatinine may be more indicative of the integrity of the bladder closure because it is less likely to be confounded by fluid shifts related to third-spacing. In the setting of adequate drainage from the Foley catheter and decreasing outputs from the pelvic drain, a fluid creatinine measurement mirroring that of serum suggests appropriate healing of the bladder closure. The drain is discontinued the day before discharge unless the drain fluid creatinine is elevated relative to serum, in which case the drain is continued for a longer duration. The Foley catheter is removed 10 to 14 days postprocedure after cystography demonstrates the absence of contrast extravasation.

Postoperative surveillance of patients who undergo partial cystectomy for muscle-invasive disease is imperative, given the relatively high risk of recurrence and progression. Voided urine cytology and cystoscopy should be performed every 3 months for at least the first 2 years after surgery. Frequent cross-sectional imaging, preferably CT urography, allows for evaluation of recurrence in the upper tract.

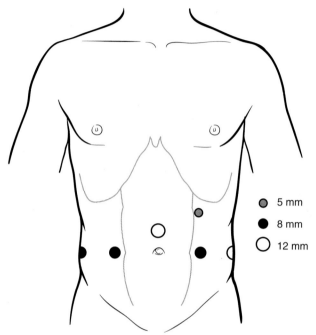

Figure 38-4. Placement of robotic ports. A 12-mm camera port is placed 2 cm superior to the umbilicus or, alternatively, 20 to 25 cm above the pubic bone. Two 8-mm ports are placed 8 cm lateral to the midline on each side at the level of the umbilicus. A third 8-mm port is placed on the right at the level of the umbilicus 8 cm lateral to the second port; a 12-mm AirSeal port (SurgiQuest, Milford, Conn.) is placed at the corresponding location on the left. A 5-mm port is placed 8 cm away from both the camera port and the left robotic port to the left of the midline.

- 5 mm
- 8 mm
- 12 mm

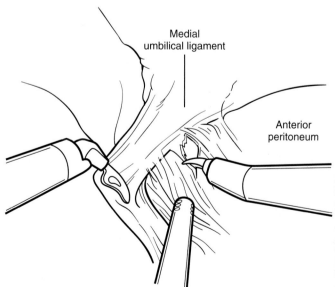
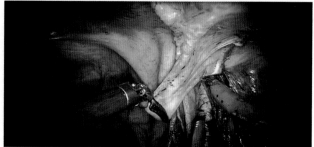

Figure 38-5. The medial umbilical ligament is placed on medial traction to allow incision along its lateral border with monopolar electrocautery.

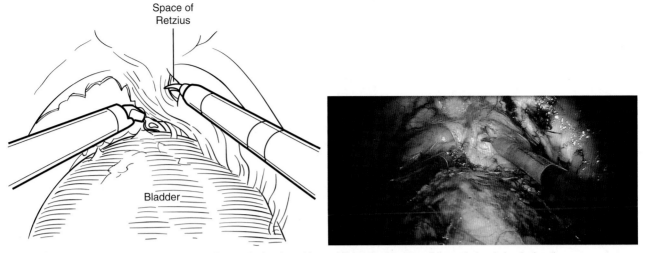

Figure 38-6. The space of Retzius is developed by mobilizing the bladder off the anterior abdominal wall.

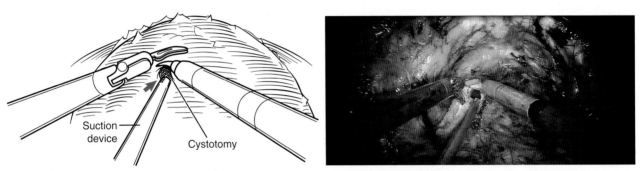

Figure 38-7. A cystotomy is made away from the tumor site after instillation of 150 mL of normal saline into bladder. A suction device is used to aspirate urine and irrigant fluid as the bladder is entered.

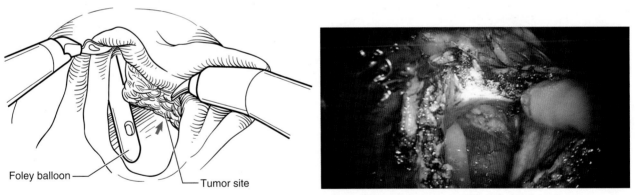

Figure 38-8. After extension of the cystotomy, the tumor site is visualized in its entirety to assess the feasibility of achieving a 2-cm tumor-free margin. The Foley balloon is deflated to facilitate inspection of the bladder mucosa and to rule out the presence of satellite disease.

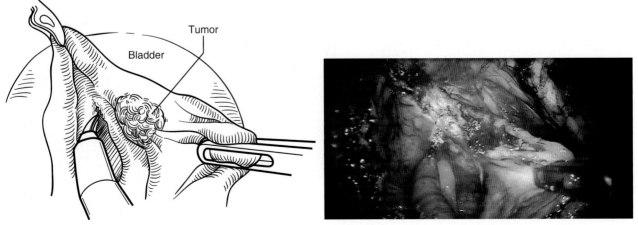

Figure 38-9. The tumor site is excised circumferentially, maintaining a 2-cm tumor-free margin.

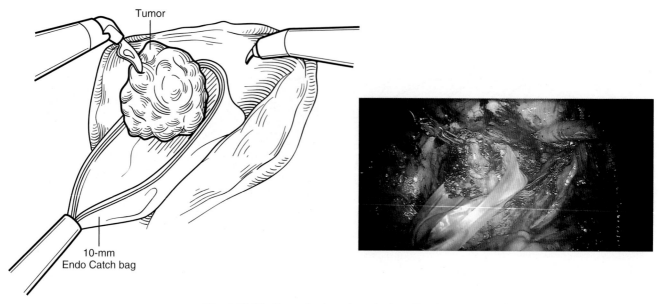

Tumor

10-mm
Endo Catch bag

Figure 38-10. The excised specimen is placed in a bag.

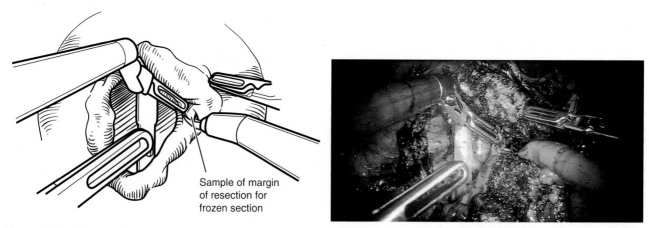

Sample of margin
of resection for
frozen section

Figure 38-11. Mucosal and detrusor tissue is sampled from four quadrants at the margin of the resection bed and sent for frozen section analysis to rule out the presence of residual disease.

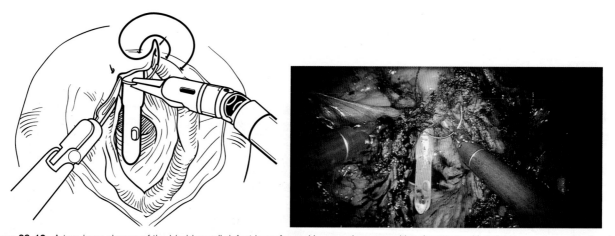

Figure 38-12. A two-layer closure of the bladder wall defect is performed in a running, appositional manner with 2-0 V-Loc sutures (Medtronic, Minneapolis, Minn.). The bladder is subsequently filled with 150 mL of normal saline to assess integrity of the cystorrhaphy.

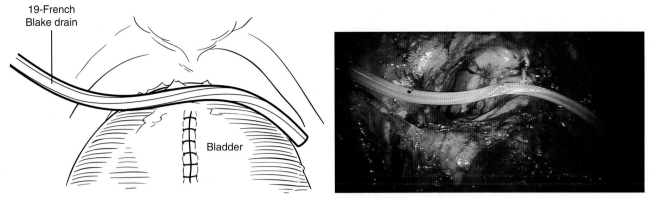

19-French
Blake drain

Bladder

Figure 38-13. A pelvic drain is placed anterior to the suture lines to aid in the diagnosis and management of a potential urinary leak across the wall closure.

COMPLICATIONS

Urine leak is a recognized complication after partial cystectomy. A high index of clinical suspicion should exist with the development of fever and leukocytosis in the early postoperative period. In addition, high output and elevated fluid creatinine from a pelvic drain placed anterior to the bladder wall closure may herald urinary extravasation across the suture lines. Conservative measures should be used initially in the event a leak is suspected. Continued drainage of the bladder with a Foley catheter is critical in helping facilitate healing. The drain should not be removed until outputs diminish and equivalence between drain fluid and serum creatinine is demonstrated. A cystogram should be obtained before removal of the Foley catheter. Imaging is not necessary for diagnosis of urinary leak unless there exists concern for an infected urinoma, which may be amenable to percutaneous drainage. Failure of conservative measures may necessitate urinary diversion, generally with bilateral percutaneous nephrostomy tube placement.

Iatrogenic injury to the ureter during resection around the tumor site may manifest as ipsilateral flank pain, varying degree of acute kidney injury, or the development of a urinoma. It is important to remain cognizant of where the ureteral orifices lie relative to the tumor site, given efforts to obtain a wide margin of resection. If injury to the ureter is suspected intraoperatively, an attempt can be made to place a ureteral stent in a retrograde manner; inability to do so would require reimplantation of the ureter at the time of surgery.

Injury suspected in the postoperative setting can be confirmed with CT of the abdomen and pelvis, which may demonstrate new-onset hydronephrosis. If renal function is amenable, delayed-phase images after administration of intravenous contrast will allow for integrity of the ureter to be assessed. Disruption of the ureter would necessitate insertion of an ipsilateral percutaneous nephrostomy tube. An antegrade attempt at placement of a nephroureteral tube can be made; however, if the attempt is unsuccessful, delayed ureteral reimplantation should be performed.

TIPS AND TRICKS

- Proper patient selection is key to achieving good surgical and oncologic outcomes.
- Pay special attention to the positioning, padding, and securing of the patient on the operating room table to avoid position-related injury during steep Trendelenburg.
- Cystoscopic placement of ureteral catheters may help to prevent ureteral orifice injury during excision for lateral wall tumor.
- Posterior tumors may be approached without mobilization of the bladder off the anterior abdominal wall. The peritoneum is dissected off the posterior wall, and the cystotomy is made.
- Optimize the patient's voiding function before the procedure with use of α-blockers, such as tamsulosin or alfuzosin, to avoid high-pressure voiding after Foley catheter removal.
- Consider adjuvant chemotherapy for patients with tumor invasion into the perivesical fat or lymph node involvement.

39 NOTES-Assisted Laparoscopic Transvesical Bladder Diverticulectomy

Ahmed Magdy, Günter Janetschek

Several techniques have been described for bladder diverticulectomy. These include open, endoscopic fulguration, and laparoscopic transperitoneal or retroperitoneal and robotic-assisted approaches. Pansadoro and co-workers first described the transvesical approach in 2009. Then Stolzenburg and co-workers described a series of laparoscopic endoscopic single-site (LESS) procedures via a transperitoneal approach through the umbilicus. Roslan and co-workers in 2012 published a small case series of transvesical laparoscopic endoscopic single-site (T-LESS) procedures. We introduce here our modification, which uses the natural orifice of the urethra as an extra port for diverticular wall traction and bladder wall suturing (Natural Orifice Transluminal Endoscopic Surgery—hence the term *NOTES-assisted*).

INDICATIONS AND CONTRAINDICATIONS

Indications

Indications include secondary "acquired" bladder wall diverticula with one or more of the following criteria:

- Retentive bladder diverticula with postvoid residual (PVR) volume of 80 mL or more
- Recurrent urinary tract infections
- Significant compression of the nearby structures

To date, we have not applied this approach to cases of primary diverticula.

Contraindications

Contraindications include the following:

- Patients with unresolved bladder outlet obstruction
- Invasive bladder diverticular tumors in candidate patients for partial cystectomy

Roslan and co-workers have applied the T-LESS technique for extraction of bladder diverticula with noninvasive bladder tumors; however, this was a small case series with no data about subsequent follow-up.

PREOPERATIVE EVALUATION AND PREPARATION

Routine evaluation includes the following:

- Routine preoperative blood tests
- Urine analysis
- Urine culture to ensure sterile urine before the operation
- Anteroposterior and lateral retrograde cystogram with postvoid films (see Fig. 39-10)

Optional, case-specific evaluation includes the following:

- Ultrasound to evaluate to PVR volume
- Computed tomography with intravenous contrast, including delayed films of the urinary tract, to evaluate for possible diverticular masses and their extension
- Magnetic resonance imaging
- Neurogenic evaluation
- Flowmetry

OPERATING ROOM SETUP AND PATIENT POSITIONING

Under general anesthesia, the patient is placed in lithotomy position. The surgeon stands between the patient's extended legs as in the performance of normal cystoscopic procedures. The assistant "holding" the camera stands to the right of the surgeon, and the scrub nurse stands with the instruments table to the left of the surgeon. The cystoscopy-laparoscopy tower faces the surgeon at the patient's head (Fig. 39-1).

TROCAR PLACEMENT

Before trocar placement, diagnostic cystoscopy is performed. Diagnostic cystoscopy is used to assess the diverticular site; inspect the diverticular wall from inside for suspicious masses or carcinoma in situ; place a ureteral catheter to secure the ureter in cases of paraureteral diverticulum; assess the ideal position for transvesical trocar placement with a needle; and fill the bladder with saline (NaCl 0.9%) to facilitate insertion of the transvesical ports, to avoid transperitoneal fixation and consequent intestinal injury.

We normally use three trocars for this procedure. One 11-mm trocar is inserted two fingerbreadths above the symphysis pubis. Under cystoscopic guidance, we insert another two 5-mm trocars in a flat triangular pattern into the bladder (Fig. 39-2).

We use special trocars with an internal fixation balloon that are self-retentive with less likelihood of dislodging from the bladder.

PROCEDURE (SEE VIDEO 39-1)

- Diagnostic cystoscopy is performed as mentioned earlier in the discussion of trocar placement, with or without ureteric catheter insertion according to the site of the diverticulum (Fig. 39-3).
- Self-retentive trocar placement is performed in the full bladder in a flat triangular pattern (Fig. 39-4).
- The bladder is insufflated with CO_2 until a pressure of 12 mm Hg is attained.
- We use a 30-degree laparoscope for the whole procedure.
- The diverticulum is inspected.
- A circumferential incision of the bladder mucosa is made at the mouth of the diverticulum (Fig. 39-5).
- The diverticular mucosa is grasped with a grasper, followed by blunt and sharp peeling of the diverticular mucosa from the detrusor muscle attachments (Fig. 39-6).
- When the diverticulum is large, traction can be applied to the diverticular mucosa through a grasper inserted through the urethra.

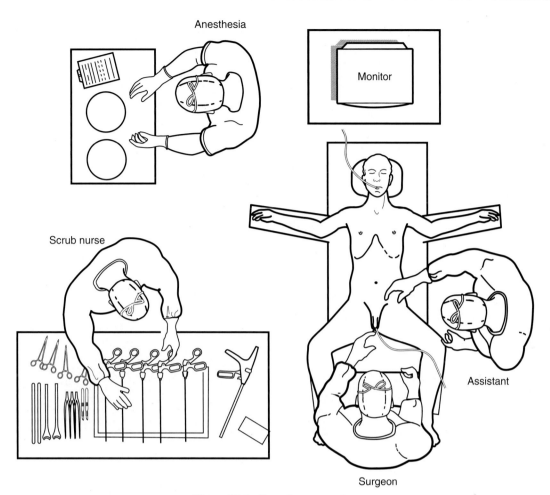

Anesthesia

Monitor

Scrub nurse

Assistant

Surgeon

Figure 39-1. Operating room setup.

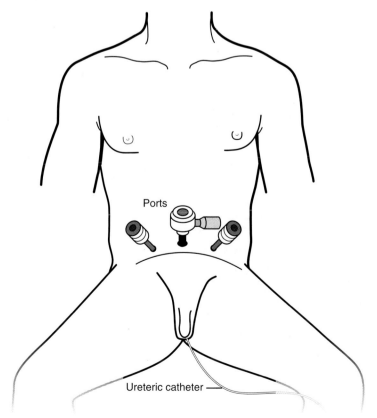

Ports

Ureteric catheter

Figure 39-2. Port configuration.

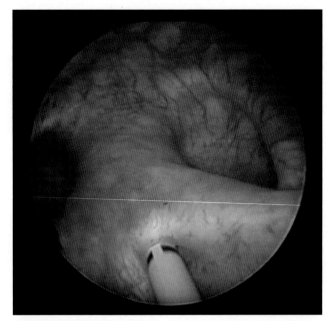

Figure 39-3. Insertion of ureteric catheter with cystoscopy in case of paraureteral diverticulum.

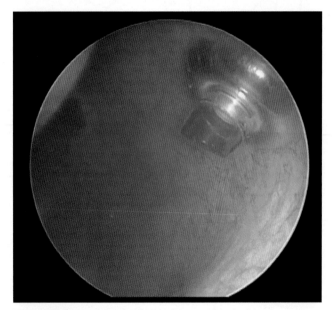

Figure 39-4. Insertion of self-retentive trocars in the bladder under cystoscopic guidance.

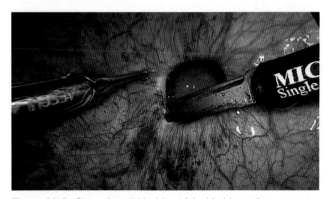

Figure 39-5. Circumferential incision of the bladder wall mucosa at the mouth of the diverticulum.

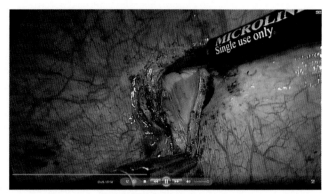

Figure 39-6. Stripping of the diverticular mucosa from the detrusor muscle attachments with blunt and sharp dissection.

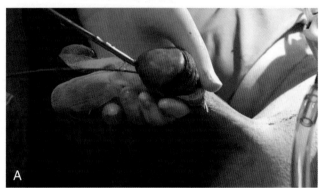

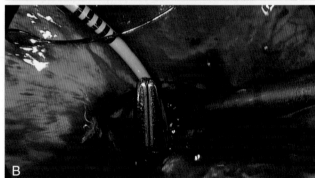

Figure 39-7. Insertion of the needle holder through the urethra. **A,** External view. **B,** Laparoscopic view.

- After the mucosa has been totally separated from the detrusor, it is then extracted through the laparoscopic ports or via cystoscopy under laparoscopic guidance.
- Good hemostasis at the excision bed is ensured, with or without drain insertion into the dead space, according to the surgeon's own preference and the operative situation.
- The 2-0 V-Loc sutures (Covidien, Dublin, Ireland) are inserted through the camera port.
- The needle holder is inserted through the urethra. Depending on whether most of the diverticula are located at a paraureteral or posterolateral wall position, suturing with a needle holder inserted through the urethra is much better with regard to ergonomics than using the transvesical ports to close the bladder wall (Fig. 39-7).
- The detrusor muscle and bladder mucosa are sutured in one layer (Figs. 39-8 and 39-9).

- Depending on the surgeon's preference, a Lapra-Ty device (Ethicon, Cincinnati, Ohio) may be used after suturing of the bladder wall through the camera port to secure the sutures.
- A urethral catheter is placed.
- Closure of the port sites is performed in layers—sheath, subcutaneous tissue, and skin.

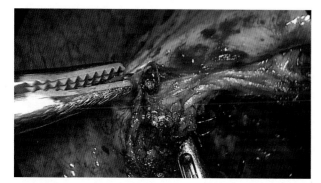

Figure 39-8. Closing the bladder wall mucosa and muscle in one layer.

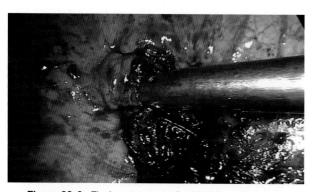

Figure 39-9. Final appearance after bladder wall closure.

POSTOPERATIVE CONSIDERATIONS

The urethral catheter is monitored for gross hematuria postoperatively, with the possible insertion of a three-way catheter with irrigation when needed.

For paraureteral diverticula, we recommend leaving the ureteric catheter in place for 2 to 3 days postoperatively to keep the ureter patent and prevent ureteric obstruction caused by postoperative edema at the vesicoureteral junction.

The urethral catheter is left for 10 days postoperatively. Then a retrograde cystogram is performed at postoperative day 10 to evaluate for any extravasation (Fig. 39-10).

TIPS AND TRICKS

- Under cystoscopic guidance, insert a needle into the bladder to locate the optimum placement site for the camera and working trocars.
- Insert the special self-retentive transvesical trocars after filling the bladder with saline under cystoscopic guidance.
- Strip the diverticular mucosa with both blunt and sharp dissection.
- Use the urethra to insert a grasper to retract the diverticular mucosa; this especially helps in dissection of large diverticula.
- Use the urethra as an extra port to insert the needle holder and suture the bladder.
- Leave the ureteric catheter in cases of paraureteral diverticula for 2 to 3 days, until the edema at the ureteric ostium resolves, to avoid ureteral obstruction and the need for auxiliary procedures (e.g., nephrostomy).
- Ensure good hemostasis.
- Leave a drain in the dead space whenever needed.
- There is no need to close the bladder wall. Just leave a urethral catheter.
- Perform retrograde cystoscopy before removing the urethral catheter.

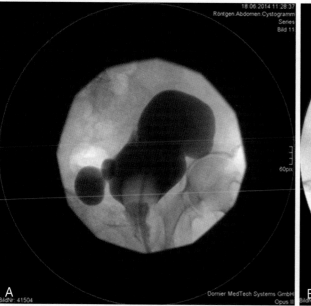
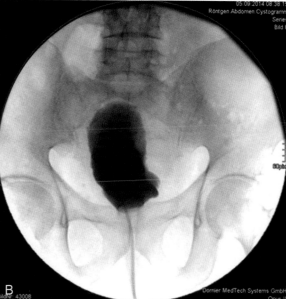

Figure 39-10. A, Retrograde cystogram showing three retentive bladder diverticula. **B,** Retrograde cystogram at postoperative day 10 showing no extravasation and complete resolution of the bladder diverticula.

SUGGESTED READINGS

Pansadoro V, Pansadoro A, Emiliozzi P. Laparoscopic transvesical diverticulectomy. *BJU Int.* 2009;103:412–424.

Roslan M, Markuszewski MM, Kłącz J, Krajka K. Laparoendoscopic single-site transvesical ureteroneocystostomy for vesicoureteral reflux in an adult: a one-year follow-up. *Urology.* 2012;80:719–723.

Stolzenburg JU, Do M, Kallidonis P, et al. Laparoendoscopic single-site bladder diverticulectomy: technique and initial experience. *J Endourol.* 2011;25:85–90.

40 Laparoscopic Adrenalectomy

Mary E. Westerman, George K. Chow

Since the introduction of laparoscopic adrenalectomy in 1992, it has rapidly become the gold standard for surgical management of adrenal pathology. In this chapter, we describe current indications and techniques for laparoscopic adrenalectomy and discuss perioperative management and potential complications.

INDICATIONS AND CONTRAINDICATIONS

The indications for adrenalectomy are summarized in Box 40-1. Adrenal masses 1 cm and larger require metabolic evaluation and imaging for appropriate classification, the details of which are beyond the scope of this chapter. Benign lesions can be either functional (metabolically active) or nonfunctional (inert). Metabolically active lesions should be removed in appropriate surgical candidates, with very careful attention to their perioperative management. Inert adenomas larger than 6 cm (some argue 4 cm) or with more than 1 cm of growth on follow-up imaging are to be considered malignant until proven otherwise and should be removed. Solitary metastatic lesions from a nonadrenal primary cancer (commonly lung, breast, kidney, and melanoma) can be removed laparoscopically, although the long-term benefits for the patient should be carefully considered.

Relative contraindications to laparoscopic adrenalectomy include prior abdominal surgery, obesity, and tumor size. Extensive scarring and adhesions from prior abdominal surgery may increase the difficulty of a transperitoneal approach, but a retroperitoneal or transthoracic approach may be feasible. Similarly a flank approach may be more appropriate in obese patients. Body habitus may increase the technical difficulty, but the less invasive laparoscopic approach may be more beneficial for these patients because of their already compromised functional status. Currently, tumors up to 10 to 12 cm are generally considered resectable by experienced laparoscopic surgeons. However, patients must be carefully selected because tumors larger than 5 cm are significantly more likely to be malignant and are technically more difficult.

Resection of adrenal cortical carcinoma (ACC) should not be attempted laparoscopically if it will compromise cancer control. ACC is aggressive, with locoregional recurrence rates of more than 60%, and any degree of spillage or residual tumor may be harmful to the patient. These tumors are usually large and infiltrative, and the surgeon must be prepared for en bloc resection. ACC with evidence of extra-adrenal tumor invasion or adrenal vein thrombus extending into the inferior vena cava (IVC) is considered the only absolute contraindication to laparoscopic resection.

There are few indications for partial adrenalectomy. Patients with inherited disorders who have an increased propensity for recurrent adrenal lesions, such as multiple endocrine neoplasia (MEN) or von Hippel-Lindau (VHL) disease, are candidates for partial adrenalectomy. It may be considered for patients with a solitary adrenal gland as well.

PATIENT PREOPERATIVE EVALUATION AND PREPARATION

All patients should be counseled about standard surgical risks including infection, bleeding, damage to surrounding structures (spleen, liver, kidney, major vascular structures), and possible conversion to an open procedure, which occurs in 2% to 5% of cases. If ACC is suspected, patients should be counseled and should give informed consent for adjacent organ removal.

Specific considerations for pheochromocytoma include initiation of an α-blocker (typically phenoxybenzamine) at least 2 weeks before surgery and addition of a β-blocker if necessary. Give anesthesia advance notice, even for inert masses, because 5% of patients with pheochromocytomas have normal blood studies. Patients with glucocorticoid-producing tumors need adequate blood glucose control, and in some cases may benefit from adrenolytic agents such as mitotane, aminoglutethimide, or metyrapone. Perioperatively, hydrocortisone should be given. For aldosterone-secreting tumors, hypertension should be adequately controlled weeks before surgery and hypokalemia should be corrected, either by replacement or use of a potassium-sparing diuretic.

In the operating room, place sequential compression devices (SCDs) and a Foley catheter. For transperitoneal cases, a nasogastric or orogastric tube and preoperative bowel preparation may be helpful. Ensure that pressure points are properly padded, and administer perioperative antibiotics. If there

---

BOX 40-1 Indications for Adrenalectomy

BENIGN

Functional

Catecholamine
Mineralocorticoid
Aldosterone

Nonfunctional

Size >4-6 cm
Enlarging (>1 cm)

MALIGNANT

Adrenal cortical carcinoma
Solitary lesion from nonadrenal primary

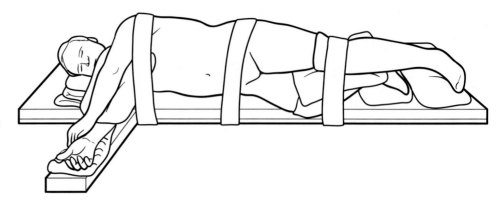

Figure 40-1. Modified flank position (transperitoneal approach). The flank is placed directly over the break in the table so that the table can be flexed. The arms are carefully padded and secured. Wide cloth tape is used to secure the hips and chest.

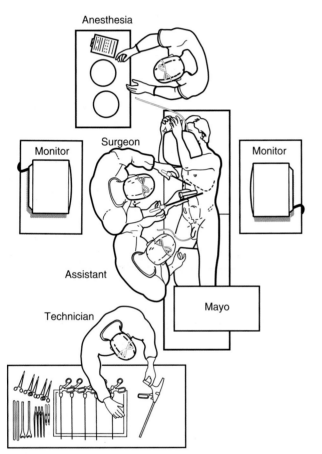

Figure 40-2. Operating room setup for the transperitoneal approach. Both the surgeon and the assistant stand on the patient's ventral side; the technician stands at the feet or on the dorsal side.

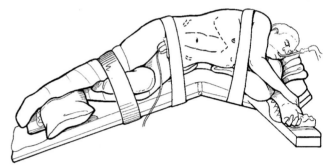

Figure 40-3. Full flank position (retroperitoneal approach). Again the flank is directly over the table break. Flexion of the table is recommended when the space between the twelfth rib and the iliac crest is narrow. With the table flexed, the head is lowered to create a level operating surface. Both arms are extended in front of the patient as previously described, and an axillary roll is carefully placed.

is concern for rapid hemodynamic changes, close monitoring via an arterial line or pulmonary artery catheter may be warranted.

OPERATING ROOM CONFIGURATION AND PATIENT POSITIONING

Transperitoneal Approach

Place the patient in a modified flank position, 20 to 30 degrees back from vertical, using a beanbag device or a padded roll if needed to keep the patient in position. The table should

be flexed only during conversion to open surgery. Extend the lower arm on a standard arm board and place an axillary roll just caudad to the axilla. Bring the upper arm across the body and support it with a Krause (sling) rest, double arm board, or several pillows (Fig. 40-1). To avoid undue strain on the upper shoulder joint, ensure the upper arm is adequately extended. Pad both arms under the elbows and wrists. SCDs should be placed on the calves. Then gently flex the legs and place a pillow between them and foam beneath the feet and ankles. Secure the patient to the table with wide tape strips across the hips and chest. Both surgeon and assistant stand on the patient's ventral side (Fig. 40-2) while the technician stands at the feet or on the dorsal side. Two monitors are positioned to ensure all members of the surgical team can view the procedure.

Retroperitoneal Approach

For the retroperitoneal approach, place the patient in full flank position (Fig. 40-3). The flank should be positioned directly over the table break with the patient on a beanbag. Flex the table to adequately open the space between the 12th rib and the iliac crest. With the table flexed, adjust the bed to create a level operating surface (usually by raising the head). Arm extension and leg positioning are the same as for the transperitoneal approach. For the retroperitoneal approach, the surgeon and assistant stand on the patient's dorsal side. Again, the configuration in the operating room allows for visualization of the procedure by the entire surgical team (Fig. 40-4).

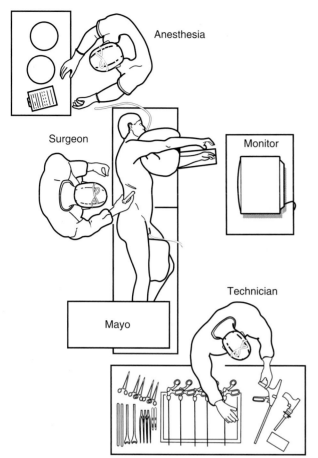

Figure 40-4. Operating room setup for the retroperitoneal approach. The surgeon stands at the patient's back.

TROCAR PLACEMENT

Transperitoneal Approach

Left-Sided Adrenalectomy

A left-sided adrenalectomy requires three ports along the costal margin with an optional fourth port if additional retraction is needed. The primary site is a 10-mm port two fingerbreadths below the costal margin in the midclavicular line. Note that in the lateral position, most patients have a slight hollow at this site. Two 5-mm secondary ports are placed just below the costal margin. The first is placed medially and cephalad, just lateral to the rectus abdominis muscle, and is used primarily for retraction and irrigation-aspiration. The second 5-mm port is placed lateral and caudad to the primary site to accommodate scissors, dissectors, and a clip applier (Fig. 40-5). Finally, if difficult anatomy or dissection requires the use of a fourth port, place it laterally. Some flexibility in port use allows exposure of the adrenal to be optimized by shifting the laparoscope according to anatomy and body habitus. This setup is considered a lateral transperitoneal approach.

Right-Sided Adrenalectomy

A right-sided transperitoneal adrenalectomy always requires four ports to allow for continuous liver retraction during the procedure. As with the left side, place the primary 10-mm port

in the midclavicular line. Access this site in a caudad direction to avoid injuring the liver on initial entry. Subsequent 5-mm ports should be placed along the costal margin as shown in Figure 40-6. Alternate between these ports as needed to access the short adrenal vein during the procedure.

Retroperitoneal Approach

For the retroperitoneal approach, port placement is the same for both right- and left-sided adrenalectomy. Three ports are routinely used and a fourth port is optional. First, place the primary site using a 2-cm incision placed between the tip of the 12th rib and the iliac crest. Develop the retroperitoneal space using finger dissection, and place a Hasson port. Under direct visualization, place the second port posterior to the primary site, just below the angle formed by the 12th rib and the vertically oriented paraspinous muscles (Fig. 40-7). Note that this port must not be too close to the paraspinous muscles because this may limit the range of motion. Finally, place the third port 3 to 4 cm medial and slightly superior to the primary site in the anterior axillary line, taking care to avoid the peritoneal reflection. This arrangement allows the camera to sit between the two working ports, optimizing orientation. These ports may be 5 mm or 12 mm, depending on preference and availability of instruments. If a fourth port is desired for retraction, it is placed in the anterior axillary line, 5 to 7 cm inferior to the working port. Alternatively, the two anterior axillary ports can be used, omitting the posterior port site.

PROCEDURE

Transperitoneal Approach

Left-Sided Adrenalectomy

Create pneumoperitoneum with CO_2 according to preference. Inspect the peritoneal cavity and trocar sites first for evidence of access-related injury. Anatomic landmarks are identified and orientation is achieved.

First, mobilize the colon. On the left, divide the lienophrenic attachments of the splenic flexure to the abdominal wall using a curved grasper and cautery scissors. Then incise the line of Toldt along the descending colon and sweep the colon medially. Next, mobilize the spleen by extending the lateral incision cranially along the splenic border. This releases the spleen and allows it to fall away from the suprarenal fossa by gravity. Keep this incision close to the spleen to avoid injuring the diaphragm (Fig. 40-8). Using electrocautery, make a transverse incision through the lienocolic ligaments (superficial attachments of spleen to the transverse colon) overlaying the left kidney. Incise these attachments to allow both the colon and the spleen to fall away from the upper pole of the kidney. Sufficient mobilization has been accomplished when the renal hilum is exposed (Fig. 40-9).

Next, identify the adrenal gland. The characteristic golden-orange hue of the adrenal gland can be confused with the surrounding yellow fatty tissue; therefore, careful dissection is paramount. The left adrenal sits within the perinephric fat at the superior pole of the left kidney. The left adrenal vein generally descends from the inferomedial aspect of the gland to the left renal vein (see Fig. 40-9). The adrenal vein may be divided close to the adrenal gland; therefore, complete exposure of the renal vessels is typically not needed. However, in the event of a difficult dissection or pheochromocytoma, it is helpful to identify the adrenal vein early at its confluence with

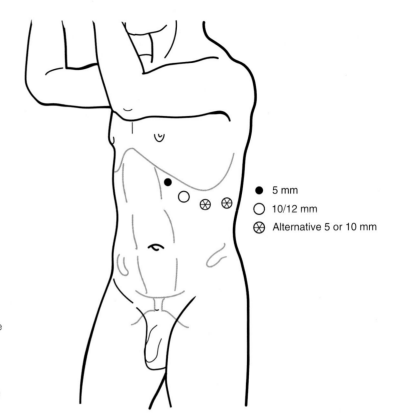

Figure 40-5. For transperitoneal left-sided adrenalectomy, three ports are placed along the costal margin initially, with an optional fourth port if additional retraction is needed. The primary site is located two fingerbreadths below the costal margin in the midclavicular line. A 10-mm port is used for the primary laparoscopic port. Secondary ports are also placed just below the costal margin. A 5-mm port is medial and cephalad, just lateral to the rectus abdominis muscle. This port is primarily used for retraction and irrigation-aspiration. A 5-mm port is placed lateral and caudad to the primary site to accommodate scissors, dissectors, and a clip applier.

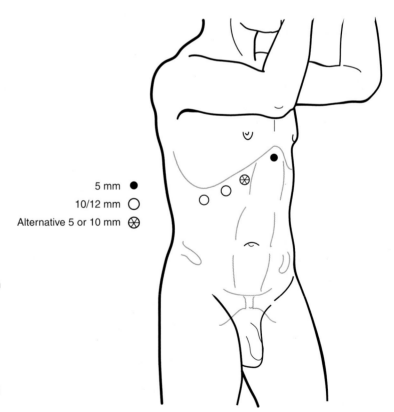

Figure 40-6. For transperitoneal right-sided adrenalectomy, four ports are always used because the liver requires active retraction. Similar to the left side, the primary 10-mm port is placed in the midclavicular line. The superomedial port is usually a 10-mm port to accommodate a large fan retractor, although a 5-mm retractor could also be used. The third port is 10 mm and is commonly used for the laparoscope, and the fourth (medial) port can be 5 mm, placed just under the xiphoid process in the midline. The surgeon may alternate between ports 1 and 3 for initial dissection, and ports 2 and 4 when the medial port is used for retraction of the liver.

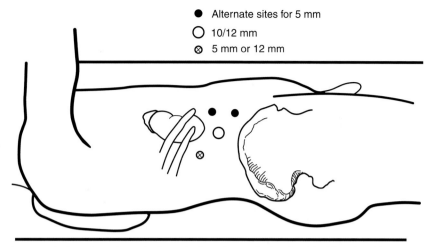

- ● Alternate sites for 5 mm
- ○ 10/12 mm
- ⊗ 5 mm or 12 mm

Figure 40-7. For trocar placement in the retroperitoneal approach, the primary site is a 2-cm incision placed between the tip of the 12th rib and the iliac crest. After finger dissection to develop the retroperitoneal space, a Hasson port is used here. Two additional ports are routinely used, and a fourth port is optional. The port placement is similar on the right and left sides. The laparoscope is placed at the primary port. The second port is placed 3 to 4 cm medial and slightly superior to the primary site in the anterior axillary line. The third port is placed posterior to the primary site, just below the angle formed by the twelfth rib and the vertically oriented paraspinous muscles. This allows the camera to sit between the two working ports to optimize orientation. The posterior port must not be too close to the psoas muscle, which could limit the range of motion. These ports may be 5 mm or 12 mm depending on the surgeon's preference and availability of instruments. The optional fourth port may be used for retraction and is placed in the anterior axillary line, about 5 to 7 cm inferior to the working port.

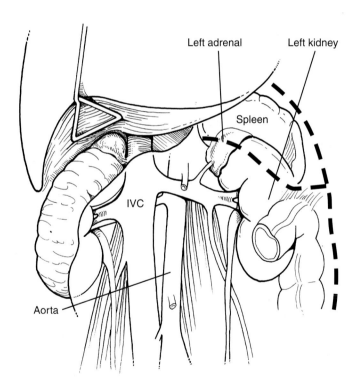

Figure 40-8. The lateral incision is extended high up along the spleen so that the spleen is released and allowed to fall away from the suprarenal fossa. The incision is made close to the spleen to avoid injury to the diaphragm. *IVC,* inferior vena cava.

the left renal vein (Fig. 40-10). The splenic vessels course near the left adrenal, but there is a clear plane between the splenic vessels and tail of the pancreas and the anteromedial surface of the adrenal gland. The splenic artery pulsations are a recognizable landmark, and dissection should not be carried out medial to this artery. Once the adrenal vein has been identified, perform careful vascular dissection with a right-angle dissector to expose a sufficient length of vein. Place standard laparoscopic clips—two proximally, one distally—and divide the vein (Fig. 40-11).

With the adrenal borders clearly identified, carry out a complete dissection. The adrenal is fragile and will bleed easily if mishandled. To minimize bleeding, dissect by lifting or pushing the adrenal rather than grasping it. Use electrocautery to effectively divide the many small feeding vessels. There are generally no specific arteries that need to be identified. Rather, the arterial supply consists of an extensive array of small arteries around the medial side of the adrenal that can be easily handled with electrocautery or other dissecting energy (Fig. 40-12). The remainder of the dissection consists

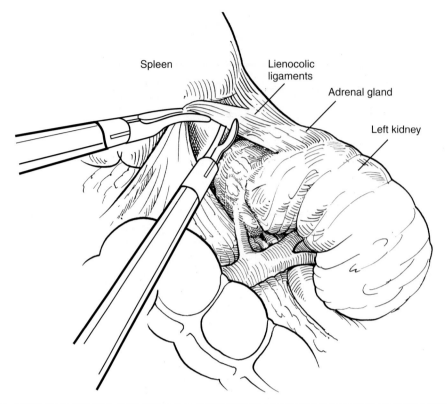

Figure 40-9. Additional mobilization of the spleen is accomplished by a transverse incision through the lienocolic ligaments.

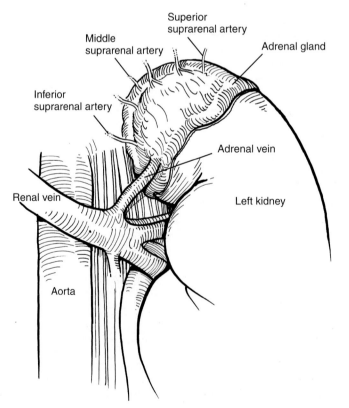

Figure 40-10. Anatomy of the left adrenal gland. The left adrenal vein is usually found medial to the level of insertion of the gonadal vein on the renal vein and at the lateral edge of the aorta. Practically speaking, the adrenal vein is usually more medial than expected.

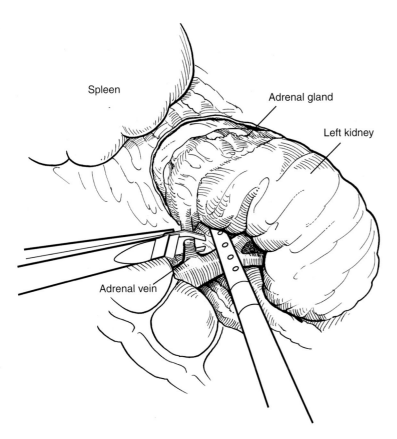

Figure 40-11. After the vein has been ligated and divided, complete dissection is performed. This can be done by lifting or pushing the adrenal rather than grasping it. Electrocautery effectively divides the many small feeding vessels. The remainder of the dissection consists of freeing the adrenal from its bed. Infrequently, additional variant veins may require clips and should be identified.

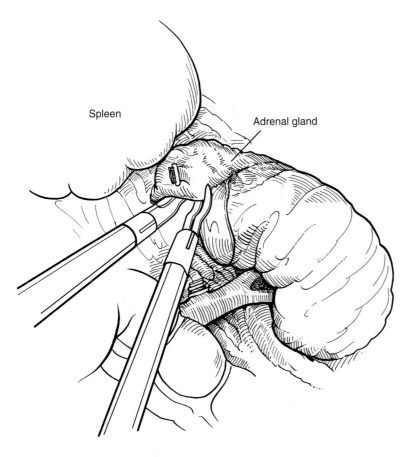

Figure 40-12. Once the adrenal vein is divided, the adrenal gland is separated from the upper pole of the kidney and freed posteriorly, leaving the superior attachments, which are then divided with electrocautery or other energy.

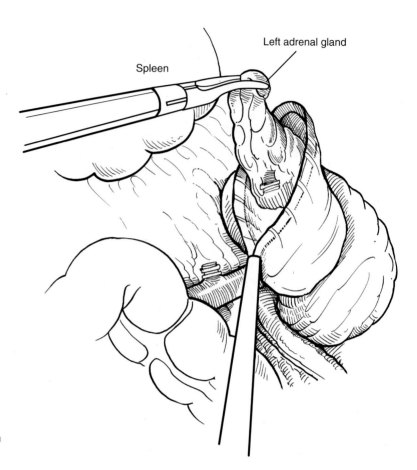

Spleen

Left adrenal gland

Figure 40-13. The dissected adrenal gland is placed into a commercial retrieval pouch and removed through the largest port site.

of freeing the adrenal from its bed. Infrequently, additional variant veins may require clips and need to be identified. Once the adrenal has been dissected entirely, place it into a retrieval bag and remove it through the largest port site (Fig. 40-13). Close the port sites in standard fashion (see Chapter 12).

TIPS AND TRICKS: LEFT TRANSPERITONEAL ADRENALECTOMY

- Aggressively mobilize the spleen to expose the suprarenal fossa.
- Keep dissection lateral to the splenic vessels.
- Use laparoscopic sonography to help localize the adrenal within the perinephric fat.
- The left adrenal vein is found at the inferomedial border of the adrenal; once divided, this makes a better "handle" than the fragile adrenal parenchyma for lifting up the adrenal.
- If the adrenal is buried in fatty tissue, find the splenic vessels medially and the renal capsule laterally; the adrenal vein lies between the two at the upper edge of the renal vein.

Right-Sided Adrenalectomy (See Video 40-1)

Dissect down along the ascending colon and medially just below the liver until the colon falls away, exposing the kidney. There is often minimal or even no mobilization of the colon if the suprarenal fossa is easily exposed by lifting up the liver. Mobilize the liver from its abdominal wall attachments high up along its lateral aspect (Fig. 40-14). Retraction of the liver, which is necessary to sufficiently uncover the adrenal gland and complete the dissection, can be achieved with a retractor through either the most medial or most lateral port (Fig. 40-15).

The right adrenal gland is closer to the IVC than the left adrenal is to the aorta, which makes this side more challenging. The right adrenal vein usually arises from the posterolateral

aspect of the IVC (Fig. 40-16). If the adrenal gland is readily identified, dissect right along the edge of the gland. Expose the IVC directly and extend this dissection up to the top of the adrenal gland. Just above the junction of the IVC and renal vein, use a blunt retractor to push the adrenal gland laterally, away from the IVC, creating a working space.

Divide the vessels along the medial edge of the adrenal with electrocautery until the short adrenal vein is identified. At this point, expose the short adrenal vein with a right-angle dissector and divide it between clips or with an endovascular GIA stapler (Fig. 40-17). If using the vascular stapler, ensure that there is adequate space between the vena cava and the edge of the adrenal gland to prevent avulsion of the adrenal vein during insertion and activation of the stapler. In addition, venous variations may exist, with additional venous branches arising from the right renal vein or hepatic veins. As on the left side, simply divide the array of adrenal arteries with cautery (Fig. 40-18).

With the main adrenal vein divided, the remainder of the dissection is less worrisome. When the adrenal gland is completely free, place it in a retrieval bag and remove it through a port site. Close the incisions in standard fashion.

TIPS AND TRICKS: RIGHT TRANSPERITONEAL ADRENALECTOMY

- The adrenal lies close to the IVC; create space between the two structures to facilitate the critical dissection of the adrenal vein.
- The short right adrenal vein usually runs transverse to the IVC.
- Close dissection right on the IVC may prevent inadvertent injury.
- Aggressively mobilize the liver from its lateral attachments and actively lift with a retractor.
- If the adrenal gland seems to lie more posterior to the IVC, shift the laparoscope to work through the lateral ports while retracting the liver through the most medial port.

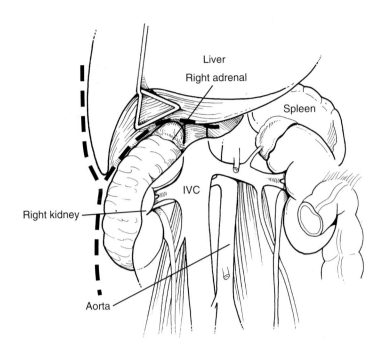

Figure 40-14. During a right-sided, transperitoneal adrenal dissection, the peritoneum is opened along the ascending colon and medially just below the liver until the colon falls away sufficiently from the kidney. As with the spleen, the liver is mobilized from its abdominal wall attachments high up along its lateral aspect, staying close to the liver to avoid diaphragmatic injury. *IVC,* inferior vena cava.

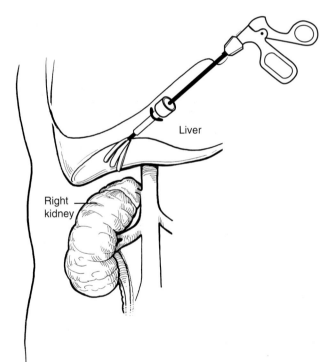

Figure 40-15. Retraction of the liver is necessary to sufficiently uncover the adrenal gland and complete the dissection. This can be achieved with a fan retractor through the most medial port.

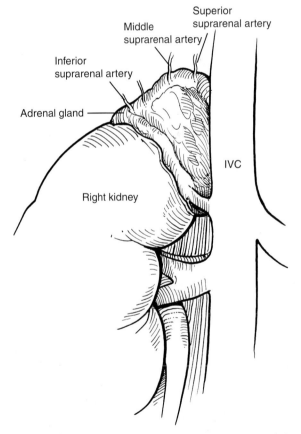

Figure 40-16. Anatomy of the right adrenal gland. The adrenal gland on the right side lies close to the inferior vena cava (IVC), and the right adrenal vein usually arises from the posterolateral aspect of the IVC.

Retroperitoneal Approach
Techniques for Both Sides

The key to the retroperitoneal approach lies in understanding the orientation, which is distinctly different from the transperitoneal approach. We prefer to use the center trocar for the camera, giving a slightly inferior and lateral perspective toward the hilum. The retroperitoneal approach is less frequently used but offers some flexibility in patient selection. Patients with extensive prior abdominal surgery may benefit from this approach because the retroperitoneum may be easier to access than a scarred and adhesion-ridden peritoneum.

Through the primary incision, perform a muscle-splitting dissection with exposure created by S-retractors. Confirm access to the retroperitoneal space by inserting one finger and

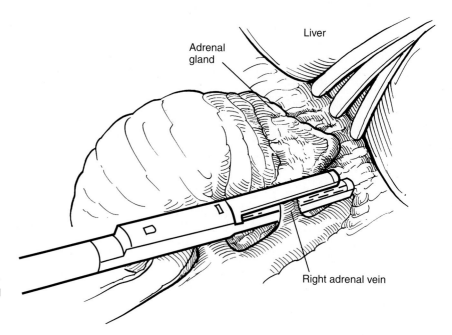

Figure 40-17. At the medial aspect of the adrenal, the short adrenal vein is identified, exposed with a right-angle dissector, and divided between clips or, if there is adequate room, divided with the endovascular stapler.

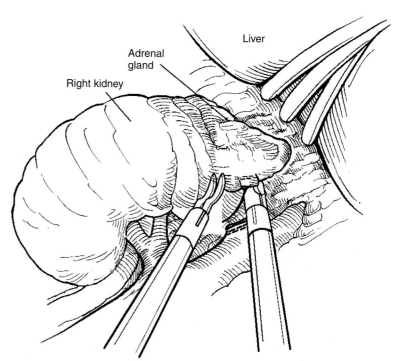

Figure 40-18. With the main adrenal vein divided, the remainder of the dissection is performed with cauterization of small vessels feeding the adrenal. After division of the adrenal vein, the adrenal is dissected from the edge of the vena cava. The inferior attachments to the upper pole of the kidney are then released.

palpating the inner surface of the 12th rib above and the iliac crest below. Also use this finger to identify the psoas muscle and begin to sweep the kidney anteriorly. Create the retroperitoneal working space with a commercial balloon dilator or Gaur balloon using the finger from a size 9 glove and a 20-French red rubber catheter (Fig. 40-19). Place the trocar-mounted balloon posteriorly along the abdominal wall and cephalad from the incision. This mobilizes the kidney and perinephric fat away from the back wall. Then secure the Hasson port. The pneumoretroperitoneum is generated. Place and secure additional ports.

Positioning the balloon dissector more cephalad facilitates access to the adrenal gland. It may be useful to reposition the balloon a second time and reinflate it. Typically, we inflate initially in a more cephalad direction and then a second time in

a more caudal direction. The initial view is usually somewhat tattered, but key landmarks can be identified. The psoas muscle is easily identified and serves as a guide for longitudinal orientation. Many random veils of tissue near the psoas can be swept aside or divided to clarify the view.

Dissecting medially, the great vessels can be identified by their pulsations as they run parallel to the psoas fibers. The renal vessels are found by identifying the pulsations of the posteriorly situated renal artery, although exposure of these vessels is not always necessary. The kidney may be relatively difficult to identify if there is an abundance of perinephric fat. If the patient is thin and the adrenal mass prominent, locating the area of interest may be straightforward. However, a small mass in the midst of abundant fat can present a challenge. For these patients, intraoperative sonography is helpful.

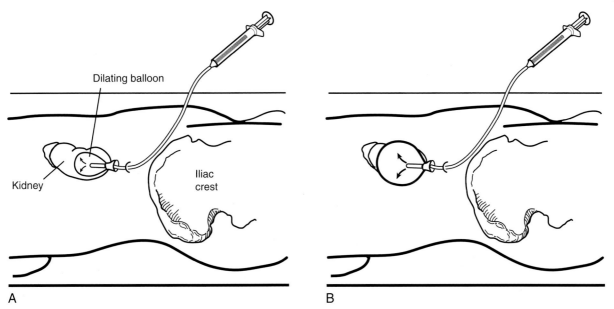

Figure 40-19. Access into the retroperitoneal space is confirmed by inserting one finger and palpating the inner surface of the 12th rib above and the iliac crest below. This finger can also identify the psoas muscle and begin to sweep all anterior structures away. One may also create the retroperitoneal working space with a constructed catheter balloon device or a commercial dilating balloon (Origin Medsystems, Menlo Park, Calif.). **A,** The trocar-mounted balloon is placed posteriorly along the abdominal wall and cephalad from the incision. **B,** This mobilizes the kidney and perinephric fat away from the back wall.

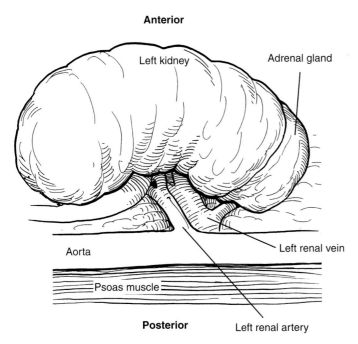

Figure 40-20. Once the initial dissection is complete and the landmarks and orientation have been identified, the adrenal mass must be located. Because there is often scant fatty tissue posterior to the adrenal, the golden hue may be quickly noted. The dissection should be carried cephalad along the psoas to the upper pole of the kidney. We tend to approach the adrenal from a lateral angle and then find the adrenal vein along the inferomedial border, where it can be exposed, clipped, and divided. If locating the adrenal is difficult, or if the mass is a pheochromocytoma, the adrenal vein can be found first by identifying the left renal vessels and locating the junction of the adrenal vein with the left renal vein.

Left-Sided Adrenalectomy

Once the initial dissection is complete and the landmarks and orientation have been identified, locate the adrenal mass. Because there is often scant fatty tissue posterior to the adrenal gland, the gland's golden hue is quickly noted. Carry the dissection cephalad along the psoas to the upper pole of the kidney.

If locating the adrenal is difficult, or if the mass is a pheochromocytoma, find the adrenal vein via identification of the left renal vessels and subsequently identify the confluence of the adrenal and left renal vein (Fig. 40-20). Because the adrenal vein tends to course along the medial aspect of the kidney, keep the dissection strictly posterior. This prevents the kidney and adrenal gland from falling down into the field of view. After dividing the adrenal vein, detach the remainder of the gland, remembering to lift and push, rather than grasp, the adrenal gland tissue.

Once the adrenal is completely mobilized, place a laparoscope through one of the secondary ports so that the gland may be removed through the largest incision (the primary site). Place the gland in a retrieval bag and remove it. Close the port sites in standard fashion.

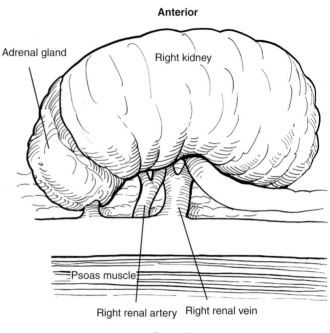

Figure 40-21. The right side is somewhat more difficult with a retroperitoneal approach because of the position of the adrenal and the length of the adrenal vein in relation to the inferior vena cava (IVC). The same principles of retroperitoneal laparoscopy apply. Dissection moves cephalad along the psoas muscle with careful attention to orientation, so that the renal vein is not mistaken for the adrenal vein. The kidney is held anteriorly by its own attachments or by an optional retractor. The adrenal gland must be located before the adrenal vein can be approached. Identification and dissection of the IVC above the renal vessels may be helpful but may also be difficult. The right adrenal rests somewhat more medial to the kidney than the left adrenal, and the upper pole of the kidney may interfere with exposure of the adrenal.

Right-Sided Adrenalectomy

Again, the right side is generally more difficult because of the position of the adrenal gland and the length of the adrenal vein in relation to the IVC (Fig. 40-21). As with the left-sided adrenalectomy, move the dissection cephalad along the psoas muscle, paying careful attention to orientation. The kidney is held anteriorly by its own attachments or with an optional retractor. Locate the adrenal gland before approaching the adrenal vein. Identify and dissect the IVC above the renal vessels, if needed. The right adrenal gland rests somewhat more medial to the kidney than the left gland, and the upper pole of the kidney may interfere with exposure of the gland. Once the adrenal gland is located, mobilize and lift it anteriorly to expose the adrenal vein, which can then be clipped and divided. As with the other approaches, mobilize the remainder of the adrenal gland with electrocautery and remove it in a retrieval bag. Close the port sites as previously described.

TIPS AND TRICKS: RETROPERITONEAL ADRENALECTOMY
Identify the key landmarks: psoas muscle, kidney (and hilar vessels), IVC, and aorta.

- Locate the adrenal gland by knowing its position relative to the landmarks.
- Use laparoscopic sonography to help localize the adrenal gland within the perinephric fat.
- Keep the line of dissection posterior along the psoas muscle so that the kidney maintains its anterior attachments.
- The left adrenal vein is found at the inferomedial border of the adrenal gland.
- The right adrenal vein is short, transverse, and medial to the adrenal gland.

Additional Tips and Variations

Other energy sources, such as Harmonic Scalpel (Ethicon Endo-Surgery, Cincinnati, Ohio) or plasma kinetic energy, can be used for much of the dissection in place of electrocautery. Intraoperative laparoscopic sonography is particularly helpful when the tumor is small or is buried in a large amount of adipose tissue. Watch for accessory or aberrant veins, even after securing the main adrenal vein. The medial dissection is always the most critical, because this is where the risk of aberrant vessels is greatest. In general, no significant arteries are identified. Because the dissection circumscribes the gland, use electrocautery to divide arterial feeders in the case of smaller vessels and between clips for larger vessels.

The introduction of robotics into laparoscopy has led some to investigate the potential benefit of robotic-assisted laparoscopy for adrenalectomy. Although robotic assistance has been helpful for procedures that require extensive suturing, there has not been a significant benefit for adrenalectomy. This is an expected outcome because laparoscopic adrenalectomy has been mastered early by the community of laparoscopic surgeons.

There may be a role for adrenal-sparing procedures if both adrenal glands are pathologically involved, as with bilateral adenomas or VHL disease. Typically, partial adrenalectomy is considered when these tumors are smaller and more laterally situated, although some authors have even divided the main adrenal vein, removed the tumor, and left a remnant of the adrenal with function confirmed by scintigraphy. However, because the incidence of multifocal lesions is not known, partial adrenalectomy should be done only in select situations.

POSTOPERATIVE MANAGEMENT

At the conclusion of the surgery, remove the Foley catheter and orogastric tube, leaving the SCDs in place. For routine operations, no drains are necessary. Continue antibiotics for 24 hours. A diet can be resumed on postoperative day 1, and early ambulation should be encouraged. Check a complete blood count and electrolytes postoperatively and again the morning after surgery.

Consultation with an endocrinologist may be helpful for the postoperative management of patients with functional adenomas. Some patients with pheochromocytoma require intensive care unit monitoring because the abrupt catecholamine withdrawal results in hypotension. Patients with glucocorticoid-producing tumors should be monitored for acute adrenal insufficiency, which can develop even after a unilateral or partial adrenalectomy. Typically, some degree of mineralocorticoid replacement is required for these patients. Removal of aldosterone-producing tumors can result in potassium abnormalities—usually hypokalemia, but occasionally hyperkalemia, results from salt wasting from long-term suppression. Patients left without adrenal tissue postoperatively require replacement with fludrocortisone.

COMPLICATIONS

Complications can arise from obtaining access, intraoperatively, and postoperatively. Access-related complications are the same as for other laparoscopic procedures. Abdominal wall hemorrhage can occur from port placement. Because of the smaller incisions, cutaneous nerve injury is much less likely than with open procedures, although possible. Finally, visceral injury is a concern when a Veress needle is used, although in our experience is uncommon.

Bleeding is the most common intraoperative complication and accounts for approximately 30% of open conversions (Box 40-2). Thermal injury risk can be minimized by keeping the cautery tips in view and minimizing use around viscera. Place and hold retractors on organs such as the liver and spleen carefully because they are often out of the field and can be injured. Because of the glands' anatomic location and proximity to major vasculature, correct identification of structures is vital to avoid injury. The great vessels and renal and splenic vessels are most commonly injured. If bleeding is encountered, it can be controlled by clamping with an Allis clamp and suturing the defect closed. For an IVC injury, a vascular clamp may be needed. Keep in mind that an accessory adrenal vein may be present in up to 10% of the population. The right adrenal vein is significantly shorter than the left and empties into the IVC, leaving a small space in which to control the vessel. Injury to a segmental renal artery may require a revascularization attempt or result in ischemic damage. The superior mesenteric vein can be injured if there is significant anatomic distortion present. Injury can be fatal, so a high degree of suspicion should be maintained. Adrenal tissue is fragile and prone to bleeding. Surrounding tissue should be retracted or dissected away for exposure. Never directly grasp the adrenal, because this results in persistent oozing, making the remaining dissection impossible.

Visceral injuries can also occur during laparoscopic adrenalectomy. The pancreas can be injured during a right or left adrenalectomy. The tail of the pancreas is more susceptible during a left-sided procedure and the head (pancreatic ducts) during a right-sided procedure. A distal pancreatectomy can be done if there is damage to the tail, whereas damage to the head should be repaired. In either case, drains should be left

BOX 40-2 Intraoperative Complications
VISCERAL INJURY
Tail of pancreas
Head of pancreas
Spleen
Liver
Colon
Renal ischemia or infarct
VASCULAR INJURY
Inferior vena cava or aorta
Renal vessels
Splenic vessels
Superior mesenteric vein

BOX 40-3 Postoperative Complications
Ileus
Fever
Wound infection
Port site hernia or hematoma
Neuromuscular pain or weakness
Bowel injury
Delayed hemorrhage
Pancreatitis
Hiccups

in place. High triglyceride output from the drains is indicative of an ongoing pancreatic leak and should be managed with bowel rest and total parenteral nutrition. Splenic injury is more common with left-sided adrenalectomy and can be managed with an argon beam coagulator, methyl cellulose, or splenorrhaphy. If these methods fail, a splenectomy can be done, and splenic vaccinations should be given postoperatively. Liver injuries are more common on the right side and can be managed with an argon beam coagulator and methyl cellulose. Larger injuries should be sutured with a blunt-tipped liver needle. Very rarely, a colonic injury may occur. Serosal injuries can be repaired primarily; however, if there is gross spillage of fecal material, a formal repair should be done by a general or colorectal surgeon.

Postoperative complications are listed in Box 40-3 and include infection, ileus, and port site problems similar to those in most laparoscopic abdominal operations. Of note, patients with severe Cushing disease are particularly at risk for developing wound-related complications as well as systemic infections and are at long-term risk for osteoporosis and fractures.

41 Partial Adrenalectomy

Daniela Colleselli, Ahmed Magdy, Günter Janetschek

Laparoscopic partial adrenalectomy can be performed via a transperitoneal, a posterior, or a retroperitoneal approach. In this chapter we highlight the most often applied transperitoneal approach.

INDICATIONS AND CONTRAINDICATIONS

Partial adrenalectomy has become the therapy of choice for patients at highest risk of developing adrenal insufficiency after surgery, because the demand for lifelong steroid replacement is associated with a decreased health-related quality of life. Patients with certain hereditary syndromes including von Hippel-Lindau (VHL) disease and multiple endocrine neoplasia type 2 (MEN2) are at highest risk of developing bilateral disease. Pheochromocytomas, for example, occur bilaterally in 3% to 11% of all patients and in up to 60% of patients with those hereditary syndromes. Partial adrenalectomy is also gaining acceptance as a treatment option in patients with a sporadic hormonally active mass such as aldosterone-producing adenoma because there is evidence that patients who have undergone only unilateral adrenalectomy may demonstrate an impaired response to stress states. Moreover, similar surgical outcomes and perioperative complications were observed in comparison to total adrenalectomy, which makes partial adrenalectomy a more surgically challenging but safe and feasible procedure.

But not every lesion might be suitable for partial adrenalectomy because of its possible malignant potential. Therefore size plays a critical role as an indicator of potential malignancy. A cutoff of 4 cm has been described to differentiate adrenal carcinomas from other histologic features. Small non–hormonally active adrenal masses are considered benign and do not require surgical intervention.

The ideal indication for partial laparoscopic adrenalectomy, therefore, is a small (<4 cm) hormonally active mass in a patient with either a solitary adrenal gland or adenomas related to a hereditary syndrome.

PATIENT PREOPERATIVE EVALUATION AND PREPARATION

The preoperative evaluation of a patient with a suspected hormonally active tumor consists of imaging techniques and laboratory studies. Radiologic evaluation includes an abdominal computed tomography (CT) scan. A three-dimensional reconstruction of the abdominal spiral CT provides reliable images of the arterial and venous anatomy and thus gives information about the spatial relationship of the tumor to the adjacent vessels. If there are contraindications to CT contrast media (e.g., patients with allergy to CT contrast media; patients in whom radiation exposure should be limited, such as children or pregnant women), magnetic resonance imaging (MRI) should be performed. The use of iodine 123 (^{123}I)-metaiodobenzylguanidine (MIBG) scintigraphy as a functional imaging modality is recommended in patients with metastatic pheochromocytoma or patients at increased risk of metastatic disease owing to the large size of the primary tumor.

In addition to laboratory testing for blood count and coagulation, specific laboratory measurements for the diagnosis of pheochromocytoma and Conn adenoma are indicated. Initial biochemical testing for pheochromocytoma should include measurements of plasma free metanephrines or urinary fractionated metanephrines. When a pheochromocytoma is diagnosed by clinical appearance and laboratory findings, a preoperative medical blockade must be performed to prevent perioperative cardiovascular complications. Preoperative treatment for about 14 days with α-adrenergic receptor blockers should lead to normalized blood pressure and heart rate. The additional use of a β-antagonist may be required.

If a cortisol-producing adenoma is suspected, serum cortisol and plasma adrenocorticotropic hormone (ACTH) levels and urinary free cortisol level should be obtained, and a 1-mg overnight or high-dose dexamethasone suppression test (DST) should be performed. Preoperative treatment of hypertension, diabetes, or electrolyte aberrations should be conducted.

When Conn adenoma is suspected, testing for serum aldosterone, 24-hour urine aldosterone, and serum potassium levels should be performed, and treatment with aldosterone antagonists should be started.

Before starting any intervention, informed consent must be obtained. Always inform the patient that there is a small chance of conversion to an open procedure and of postoperative adrenal insufficiency. Although one third of adrenal remnant might be sufficient, the risk of lifelong steroid dependence cannot be ruled out preoperatively. Patients undergo blood typing and screening, although blood transfusion is rarely necessary. A broad-spectrum antibiotic should be administered perioperatively. Bowel preparation is not mandatory, but many surgeons choose to order a bowel regimen to help decompress the colon during the transperitoneal approach.

OPERATING ROOM CONFIGURATION AND PATIENT POSITIONING

The operating room configuration is identical to that for laparoscopic nephrectomy. The surgeon and the camera holder stand on the contralateral side, facing the patient's abdomen (Fig. 41-1). The scrub nurse and any other assistant, if needed, stand facing the patient's back. The primary monitor should be across the table from the surgeon at the level of the patient's chest. After induction of general anesthesia, a bladder catheter is inserted.

For a transperitoneal approach, the patient is positioned in a modified flank position with the operative side elevated 30 degrees to 45 degrees. The ipsilateral arm is folded across the chest, the contralateral arm secured to an arm board (Fig. 41-2). Care should be taken to pad all pressure points including the contralateral elbow and both legs and ankles. An axillary roll may be needed to protect the brachial plexus of the contralateral arm. The patient must be secured properly to the table with wide tape over the legs, hips, and shoulders to rotate the patient safely during the procedure as necessary. The skin should be prepared from the nipples to the pubis and from the contralateral rectus muscle to the paraspinal muscles. Images should be present in the operating room to verify the side of the surgery.

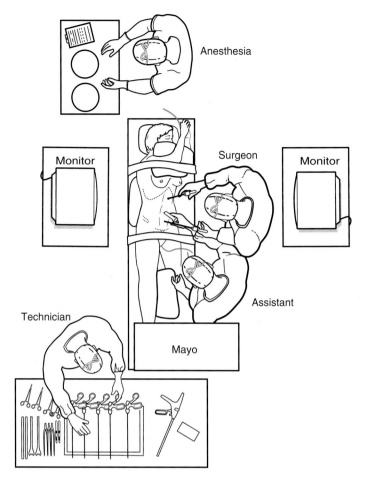

Figure 41-1. The operating room configuration includes two monitors so that all members of the surgical team can follow the procedure. The surgeon and the camera holder stand on opposite sides facing the abdomen of the patient. The scrub nurse stands at the patient's feet. If a second assistant is needed, he or she stands at the patient's back.

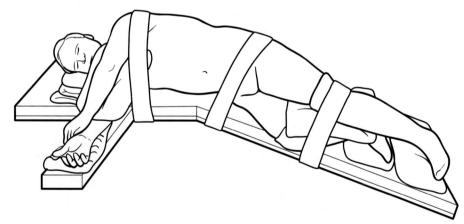

Figure 41-2. The patient is positioned in a modified Trendelenburg position. Care should be taken to pad all pressure points. The patient must be safely secured to the operating table so that rotation is possible without any risk.

TROCAR PLACEMENT

After the table is rotated backward in the right position, the Veress needle is inserted lateral to the rectus muscle between the xiphoid and the umbilicus. CO_2 insufflation is used to maintain a pressure of 20 mm Hg and to generate a sufficient pneumoperitoneum during port placement. For dissection, three ports might be sufficient, but in most cases, especially during partial adrenalectomy on the right sight, a fourth trocar for retraction is of benefit.

The first 10/12-mm trocar for the camera is inserted through an incision at the level of the Veress needle position. Then a second 10/12-mm trocar is placed at the same line, right under the costal margin. The third, 5-mm, port is placed

in the midclavicular line under the costal margin. For a right-sided partial adrenalectomy, a fourth port of 5 mm is useful to assist with specimen retraction, liver elevation, or organ entrapment (Fig. 41-3). Place this port, after all adhesions have been mobilized, in the midline between the two 10/12-mm trocars. Trocar placement for left-sided partial adrenalectomy is identical to that for a right-sided procedure except for the placement of the fourth trocar. In case of left-sided partial adrenalectomy, the fourth trocar is optional. When placed, it should be positioned lateral and caudal to the 5-mm trocar (Fig. 41-3).

During insertion, the trocars all should be placed in the direction of the adrenal gland. Operate through the ports under the costal margin while the assistant holds the laparoscope in

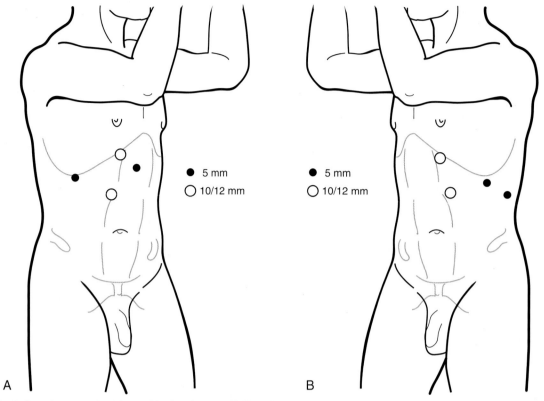

Figure 41-3. A, Port placement for right partial adrenalectomy. **B,** Port placement for left-sided adrenalectomy. The fourth trocar on the left side is optional.

the lower pararectal port. The port for lateral retraction is also manipulated by an assistant.

PROCEDURE (SEE VIDEO 41-1)

After placement of the laparoscopic ports, a partial adrenalectomy involves the following steps:

- Exposure of the right adrenal gland
- Exposure of the left adrenal gland
- Identification of the adrenal mass
- Dissection of the adrenal mass
- Control of hemostasis
- Entrapment and removal of the intact specimen through a small incision
- Closure of the incision and trocar sites

For partial adrenalectomy, the surrounding heathy tissue should be as unaffected as possible. Therefore proper exposure of the adrenal gland is mandatory. The first steps are the same as for total adrenalectomy. After safe laparoscopic access and port placement, diagnostic laparoscopy is performed to rule out other pathologic abnormalities or injuries from port placement. Preparation of the right and left adrenal gland involves some major differences.

Exposure of the Right Adrenal Gland

When performing right-sided partial adrenalectomy, retraction of the liver is a crucial step for better exposure. At the beginning, the liver is mobilized anteriorly and medially by incising the retroperitoneal attachments medially. Then the triangular ligament is divided, and the liver is carefully retracted cranially with a locking grasper, which is inserted through the 5-mm midline port. The grasper is fixed to the lateral abdominal wall and retracts the liver.

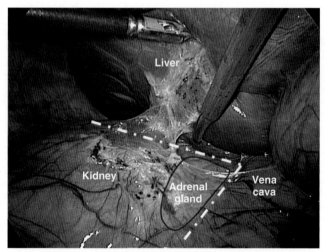

Figure 41-4. Location at which the peritoneum must be incised for right-sided partial adrenalectomy. First the liver is mobilized anteriorly and medially by incision of the retroperitoneal attachments. Then the triangular ligament is divided and the liver is carefully retracted cranially by different retractors through the 5-mm midline port.

Alternatively, a blunt grasper, fan retractor, or snake-type retractor may be used for retraction (Fig. 41-4). Mobilizing the liver is mandatory for proper exposure, which is often complicated in obese patients, especially those with Cushing syndrome.

In contrast to left-sided partial adrenalectomy, the colon rarely has to be mobilized. In some cases, however, it has to be mobilized for better visualization. Therefore the hepatic flexure can be mobilized inferiorly and medially with sharp dissection. On the right side, the adrenal gland should be

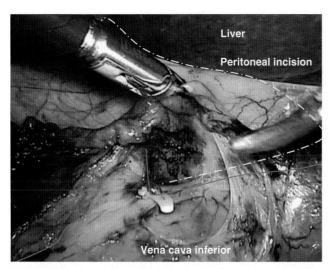

Figure 41-5. The peritoneum is incised along the vena cava to better visualize the medial margin of the adrenal gland.

identified at this time because it is located directly under the peritoneum. The next step for better visualization is the preparation of the infrahepatic vena cava. The peritoneum is incised laterally off the vena cava (Fig. 41-5). Sometimes the duodenum has to be mobilized for better preparation of the lateral aspect of the vena cava. At this time the adrenal vein should also be identified. Injuries and subsequent ligation of the adrenal vein should be avoided, but sometimes ligation of smaller branches is inevitable for further preparation.

Exposure of the Left Adrenal Gland

The left adrenal gland is covered by the left colonic flexure, the spleen, and sometimes the pancreatic tail. For exposure on the left side, the peritoneum is incised along the line of Toldt from the sigmoid to the splenic flexure, and the incision is then continued up to the diaphragm (Fig. 41-6). In addition, the splenocolic ligament may be incised (Fig. 41-7, *A*). The spleen and the pancreatic tail have to be mobilized until the spleen can be rotated medially about 180 degrees (Fig. 41-7, *B*). It should then fall out of the field of view by itself.

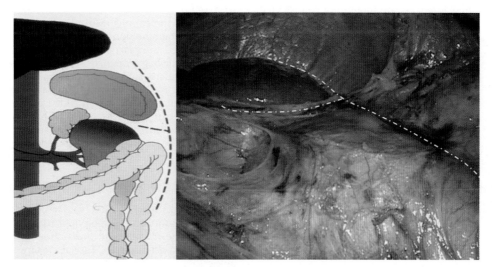

Figure 41-6. Peritoneal incision for left-sided partial adrenalectomy. The peritoneum has to be widely incised along the line of Toldt from the sigmoid to the diaphragm.

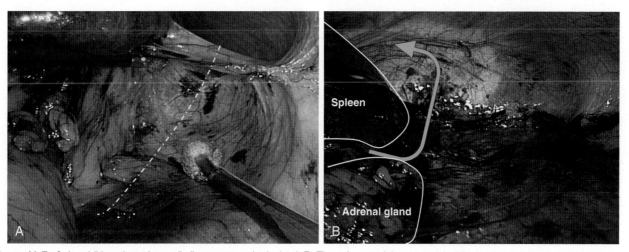

Figure 41-7. A, In addition, the splenocolic ligament may be incised. **B,** The spleen and the pancreatic tail must be mobilized until the spleen can be rotated medially about 180 degrees.

Identification of the Adrenal Mass

In most cases the identification of the adrenal mass is quite simple. The adenoma can often be seen as a prominent tumor right after the exposure of the adrenal gland (Fig. 41-8). In some cases, however—especially in smaller masses—the identification might be more challenging because there is no possibility for palpation. In these circumstances the use of a laparoscopic ultrasound device can be recommended. The adenoma is seen as a hyperechogenic lesion. The application of the fluorescent dye indocyanine green can also help to better distinguish the adenoma from the surrounding tissue. Therefore, in addition to a white light camera, a special camera is needed to detect fluorescence. After intravenous application of the dye, the adenomas are seen as hypofluorescent masses in the adrenal tissue under fluorescent light.

Dissection of the Adrenal Mass

After identification of the adrenal mass, dissection can be performed. For dissection, UltraCision Harmonic Scalpel (Ethicon, Cincinnati, Ohio) or monopolar scissors can be used. Dissection should be done within safe surgical margins (Fig. 41-9). The surrounding adrenal tissue should not be dissected

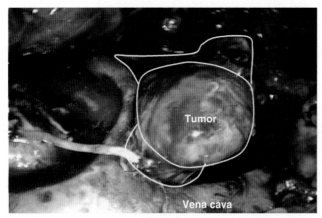

Figure 41-8. Usually the adenoma is seen as a prominent tumor in the adrenal gland.

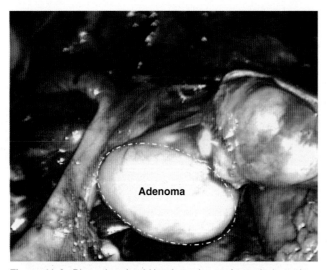

Figure 41-9. Dissection should be done along safe surgical margins with monopolar scissors or UltraCision Harmonic Scalpel (Ethicon, Cincinnati, Ohio).

and should be left as unaffected as possible. Smaller branches of the adrenal vein may have to be cut to reach the tumor. The vessels are divided between double 5-mm locking polymer clips. Smaller branches can be dissected either with UltraCision or after bipolar coagulation. While the specimen is being freed from all sides, forceps or suction can be used for retraction.

Controlling Hemostasis

After the specimen has been completely freed in the abdominal cavity, graspers are used to move it from the adrenal remnant and place it over the liver or spleen, where it can be easily found again. Closely observe the entire operative field and address any unrecognized bleeding or injury at this time. For hemostasis, bipolar forceps are usually used in smaller vessels; alternatively, clips have to be set. Sometimes it is advisable to use a hemostatic sealant to further control hemostasis.

Entrapping and Removing the Intact Specimen

As soon as complete hemostasis is achieved, the specimen can be removed. Small adenomas can be removed directly through the 10/12-mm port. Lager specimens have to be entrapped in a self-opening specimen retrieval bag (e.g., Endo Catch [Covidien, Minneapolis, Minn.]). The bag is usually passed directly through the skin after the caudal 10/12-mm trocar has been removed and placed in the caudal quadrant of the abdomen. Then the bag is opened and a grasper is used to place the specimen under vision on the bottom of the bag (Fig. 41-10). Then the bag is closed by pulling under direct vision to ensure that vital structures are not included in the device. Once the specimen is entrapped, the bag is withdrawn through the trocar site. Sometimes there is need for an incision to extract the specimen. The size depends on the specimen so that the bag can be easily retracted with the application of light force.

Closure of the Incision and Trocar Sites

After the intact specimen has been removed, inspect the bowel and retroperitoneum for potential bleeding or injury before removing the trocars. The ports should be removed under laparoscopic visualization. Fascial closure sutures are placed at the 10/12-mm trocar sites. The skin is closed at all port sites in standard fashion.

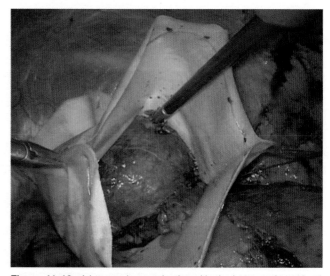

Figure 41-10. A larger adenoma is placed in the bottom of a retrieval bag for removal.

POSTOPERATIVE MANAGEMENT

The patient starts on a clear liquid diet after surgery and is advanced to a regular diet as tolerated. The urethral catheter is usually removed on the first day if the patient is fully mobilized. Immediate postoperative pain control is achieved with a patient-controlled analgesia device administering narcotics. By the second postoperative day, oral analgesics consisting of nonsteroidal antiphlogistics are usually sufficient. Postoperative antibiotic prophylaxis is usually not needed. Hydrocortisone administration should start intraoperatively and must be continued postoperatively with continuous reduction of intake. Up-titration is necessary when signs of hydrocortisolism are occurring. In case of pheochromocytoma, blood pressure, heart rate, and plasma glucose levels should be closely monitored for 24 to 48 hours to discover postoperative hypertension, hypotension, and hypoglycemia. To document successful tumor removal, biochemical testing for metanephrines in plasma and urine should be performed 4 weeks after surgery. Patients can be discharged depending on age, physical status, and comorbidities from the second postoperative day onward.

COMPLICATIONS

Complications can occur at all steps of the procedure. Potential access-related complications include trocar site bowel herniation, abdominal wall hematoma, and bowel or solid organ injury. Intraoperatively, liver, spleen, bowel, pancreatic, and vascular injuries, especially vena cava trauma, can occur. Small caval injuries may be compressed and coagulant agents applied with good success. If bleeding continues, laparoscopic suturing is required. The surgical team must be prepared for emergent conversion to an open procedure secondary to such injuries. A general laparotomy set with vascular clamps must be readily available for each procedure. Potential postoperative complications include urinary tract infection, prolonged ileus, bleeding, thrombosis, and adrenal insufficiency.

TIPS AND TRICKS

- Expose the margins of the whole gland and the tumor completely before beginning the partial resection.
- The unaffected portion of the gland should not be dissected to preserve vascular supply to the remaining gland.
- Avoid the use of vascular staplers for partial resection because these staplers allow only a straight cut and are too wide. You might risk losing an unnecessary amount of normal tissue by compromising vascular supply with this technique.
- Intraoperative ultrasound or the application of the fluorescent dye indocyanine green may be helpful to identify the adrenal mass.

42 Laparoscopic Orchiopexy

Arun Srinivasan, Mazyar Ghanaat

In the era of minimally invasive surgery, there is a growing amount of evidence and support for the role of laparoscopy in the management of cryptorchidism. There has been a tremendous improvement in technology and laparoscopic technique over the past few years. Laparoscopy has been proven to be a safe and effective alternative to open exploration for the nonpalpable testis in experienced hands. This chapter outlines indications, preoperative considerations, and description of our laparoscopic approach to the nonpalpable testis, and postoperative results and potential complications.

INDICATIONS AND CONTRAINDICATIONS

Cryptorchism or undescended testis (UDT) is a commonly encountered pediatric disorder, especially in preterm infants. The latest American Urological Association (AUA) guidelines recommend referral to a pediatric urologist for surgical management of UDT at 6 months of age (corrected for gestational age). The rational for waiting is twofold. First, spontaneous descent may occur as a result of gonadotropin surge within 2 to 3 months of life. Second, anesthetic risks are increased in younger infants. Indications for correction of UDT include risk of progressive infertility, testicular malignancy, testicular torsion, associated inguinal hernia, and potential social implications for both the child and family. Orchiopexy is preferably done at 6 months and before 12 months because of potentially unfavorable histologic changes after that time period.

UDT is further classified as palpable or nonpalpable, which requires a through history and physical examination. The palpable inguinal or high scrotal testis is traditionally approached via a small inguinal incision or occasionally through a scrotal approach (Bianchi technique). In the case of a nonpalpable testis, diagnostic laparoscopy is indicated if examination under anesthesia reveals a truly nonpalpable testis. Further surgical management is dictated by intraoperative findings and the surgeon's preference and expertise. In this chapter we focus on the therapeutic laparoscopic management of UDT of a nonpalpable testis.

It should be noted that in a patient with bilateral nonpalpable testes, evaluation for disorder of sexual development (DSD) should be performed before any surgical management.

Absolute and relative contraindications to laparoscopic surgery should be considered, including but not limited to insufficient expertise of the surgeon, peritonitis or abdominal wall infection, extensive previous abdominal or pelvic surgery, significant cardiopulmonary disease, coagulopathy, and risk associated with anesthesia.

PATIENT PREOPERATIVE EVALUATION AND PREPARATION

The clinical finding of a unilateral nonpalpable testis will ultimately reveal one of four scenarios:

1. Intra-abdominal testis

2. Atrophic ("vanishing") testis
3. High canalicular ("peeping") testis
4. Agenesis of the testis

A common physical examination finding that may suggest vanishing testis or agenesis, although not predictive or definitive, is hypertrophy of the normally descended contralateral testis. Hormonal therapy is no longer recommended owing to low response rates and lack of evidence for long-term efficacy and will not be discussed. We do not recommend ultrasound or other imaging modalities in the management of unilateral nonpalpable testis because imaging will not affect decision making or patient management owing to low sensitivity and specificity. To date, only laparoscopy can unequivocally diagnose the presence or absence of a unilateral intra-abdominal testis.

Informed Consent

Parents are advised of the standard laparoscopic operative risks of bleeding, infection, general anesthesia, hernia, air embolus, and injury to intra-abdominal or retroperitoneal viscera or vessels. Informed consent for orchiopexy specifically includes the risks of testicular atrophy and injury to the vas deferens or gonadal vessels. The potential for conversion to an open procedure, the need for orchiectomy, the need for a staged procedure, and the potential finding of agenesis or vanishing testis are also discussed.

OPERATING ROOM CONFIGURATION AND PATIENT POSITIONING

The operating room configuration traditionally includes one monitor at the foot of the bed to allow adequate visualization of the pelvis by all members of the surgical team (Fig. 42-1). In a modern operating room equipped for laparoscopic and robotic-assisted surgery, multiple monitors may be positioned as desired by the surgical team. The surgeon stands on the side contralateral to the affected testis.

After induction of general endotracheal anesthesia, administer prophylactic broad-spectrum antibiotics before making any incisions. Place a grounding pad. Secure the child to the operating room table in supine position with the legs parted moderately or frog-legged. Repeat examination of the groin under anesthesia may identify a testis and obviate the need for laparoscopic evaluation. Pad all pressure points without elevating the extremities to an extent that will compromise exposure to the scrotum or pelvis.

Prepare and drape the child from the xiphoid to the upper thighs including the scrotum. Placement of an orogastric tube for decompression may be considered. Place a small urethral catheter after the sterile preparation to decompress the bladder. The catheter may be removed once the bladder is emptied.

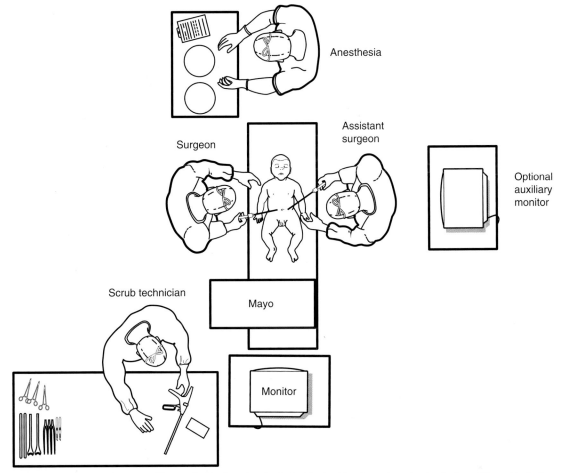

Figure 42-1. Operating room configuration. The monitor is placed at the foot of the bed to allow adequate visualization of the pelvis for the entire surgical team. The surgeon stands contralateral to the affected testis with an optional auxiliary monitor placed across the table for the primary surgeon.

TROCAR PLACEMENT

In the standard technique, three ports are usually sufficient to complete the procedure. Place the first 5-mm trocar in an immediate supraumbilical or infraumbilical position, as described later in the chapter. Increase the peritoneal pressure temporarily to 15 mm Hg for insertion of additional trocars under direct visualization, if desired. Diagnosis is made regarding the type of nonpalpable testis, and for patients with abdominal testis, additional ports are placed. Place the second and third ports, each 3 to 5 mm in size, at the level of the umbilicus in the midclavicular line (Fig. 42-2). The vector of each trocar is toward the affected groin. Care should be taken to avoid the epigastric vessels. Placement of these ports just above the level of the umbilicus instead allows additional room for movement of instruments in the smaller infant. This configuration affords freedom for the surgeon and camera without compromising the triangulation needed for the laparoscopist to work efficiently.

Trendelenburg positioning with table rotation to the unaffected side will facilitate displacement of the bowel for safe visualization of the anatomy.

Single-Site Port Placement

Depending on availability and the surgeon's expertise, a laparoscopic endoscopic single-site (LESS) technique can be used and performed with a single infraumbilical incision. After confirmation of the nonpalpable abdominal testis by diagnostic laparoscopy (as described later), the camera is removed and the skin and fascial incisions are extended to allow insertion of the GelPoint (Applied Medical, Rancho Santa Margarita, Calif.). The inner ring is placed into the peritoneal cavity and secured in place. The port is then prepared by placing three trocars in a triangular fashion, and the post is secured in place on the ring in a standard fashion. The three ports can then be used to complete the operation as described later, identical to the classic technique (Fig. 42-3).

PROCEDURE (SEE VIDEO 42-1)
Diagnostic Laparoscopy

Achieve peritoneal insufflation in children via a small semilunar incision in the infraumbilical or supraumbilical rim or by a transumbilical approach; excellent cosmesis results in each case. Dissect through the subcutaneous fascia to approach the rectus fascia. Place two hemostats on the fascia to facilitate lifting up and provide back pressure when placing a Veress needle. Obtain access to the peritoneum via direct blind puncture (Veress needle technique) or open insertion (Hasson trocar technique). Insert the trocar at a 45-degree angle toward the pelvis to minimize the risk of visceral injury. These techniques and respective precautions are described in detail elsewhere in the text, and the approach largely depends on the training and preference of the surgeon. After insertion of a 5-mm umbilical port, perform CO_2 insufflation at low flow to achieve a pressure of 12 mm Hg in infants and 15 mm Hg in older children. Use disposable or reusable blunt trocars. Defer placement of additional ports until the gonad has been identified and plans for therapeutic laparoscopy are in place.

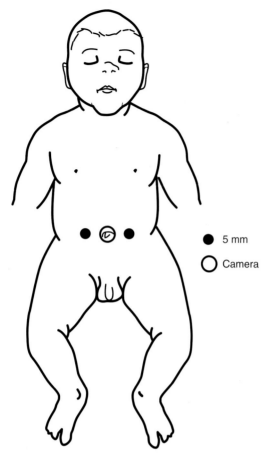

Figure 42-2. Trocar placement. A periumbilical port is initially placed, with second and third ports placed at the level of the umbilicus in the midclavicular line.

● 5 mm

○ Camera

After safely entering the peritoneal cavity, briefly inspect the abdominal and pelvic contents to rule out injury or obvious coincident disease. Rare adhesions are carefully dissected to facilitate exposure.

The inguinal ring may be more difficult to see in the child with a high abdominal testis because the anatomic landscape is less populated. The contralateral ring is a useful reference in that situation. The normal inguinal ring is marked by the confluence of the vas deferens (medial) and spermatic vessels (lateral) (Fig. 42-4). Their relationship with the iliacs and ureter, as well as the obliterated umbilical artery and inferior epigastric vessels, is also noteworthy for the progression of the case.

The vas deferens travels in the retroperitoneum in the deep pelvis, crossing the obliterated umbilical artery laterally and the distal ureter medially after exiting the deep inguinal ring. The spermatic vessels come into view from just beneath the ipsilateral colonic peritoneal deflection and follow a retroperitoneal course toward the internal inguinal ring. The vessels guide the surgeon to the testis, which can be anywhere along the course of normal testicular descent from the renal hilum to the pelvis. Uncommonly, the testis may be found near the liver or spleen, in the deep pelvis behind the bladder, or ectopic in the contralateral hemipelvis. The vas deferens, gonadal vessels, and testis compose a triangle, with the testis at the apex (Fig. 42-5). This triangle serves as the platform for the posterior peritoneal dissection and pedicle mobilization.

Intraoperative Decisions

The next phase of surgical intervention depends on the findings of laparoscopic exploration; potential scenarios are as follows:

1. An intra-abdominal testis is identified. If the testis is located near the internal ring or below the level of the iliac vessels, one-stage laparoscopic orchiopexy is appropriate. However, for a very high testis with a short vascular leash, consider a

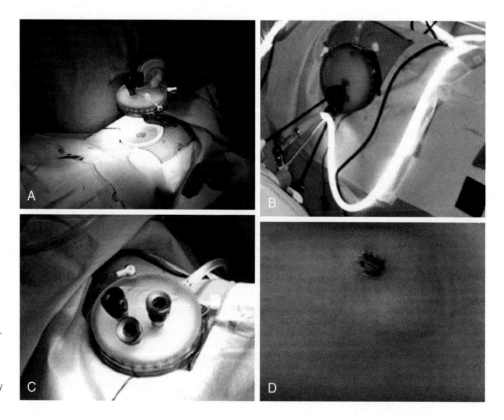

Figure 42-3. A to **C,** Single-site laparoscopy with GelPoint port (Applied Medical, Rancho Santa Margarita, Calif.). Placement and use of the port. **D,** The appearance of the wound after surgery, completely hidden inside the umbilicus.

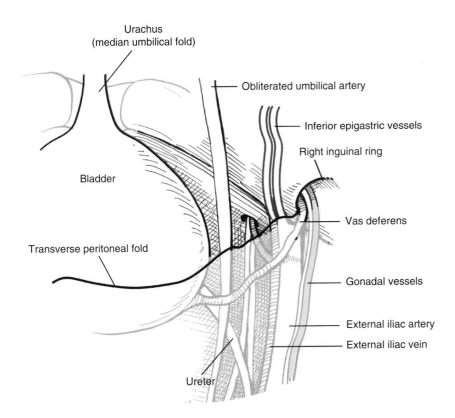

Urachus
(median umbilical fold)

Obliterated umbilical artery

Inferior epigastric vessels

Right inguinal ring

Bladder

Vas deferens

Transverse peritoneal fold

Gonadal vessels

External iliac artery

External iliac vein

Ureter

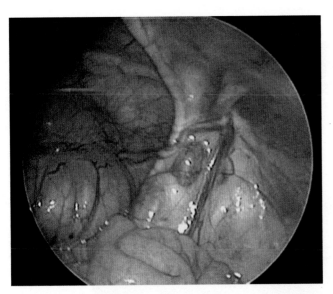

Figure 42-4. Normal right inguinal ring. Note the confluence of the vas deferens and vessels at the internal ring. The inferior epigastric vessels and obliterated umbilical artery are clearly visualized.

two-stage procedure before extensive dissection (see discussion of two-stage laparoscopic Fowler-Stephens procedure).

2. A normal vas deferens and spermatic vessels exit the inguinal ring. If the inguinal ring is closed, explore the groin for a probable vanishing testis. The need for excision of these remnants is controversial, but it is recommended because the "nubbin" contains viable germ cell elements in 10% of patients. If the inguinal ring is open, a peeping testis may be located just inside the canal and may be milked into the abdomen for laparoscopic mobilization. Otherwise, perform inguinal exploration.

3. Blind-ending vas and vessels are identified. This is the only scenario in which no further exploration is required.

4. Blind-ending vas is identified. Further laparoscopic exploration is required to identify the gonadal vessels. Dysjunc-

tion can occur between the testis and wolffian structures; if a testis is present, it will be related to the vessels. Blind-ending vessels are required to terminate exploration.

Components of Laparoscopic Orchiopexy

After peritoneal insufflation and identification of a low intra-abdominal or a peeping testis at the internal ring, laparoscopic orchiopexy is completed with the following basic steps:

1. Place trocars (see earlier).
2. Dissect the testis and vascular pedicle.
3. Create the dartos pouch.
4. Perform the laparoscopic Prentiss maneuver.
5. Deliver the testis with orchiopexy.

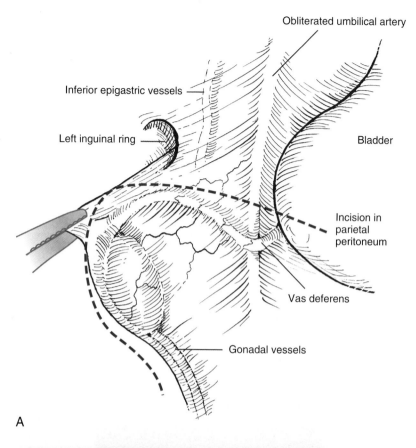

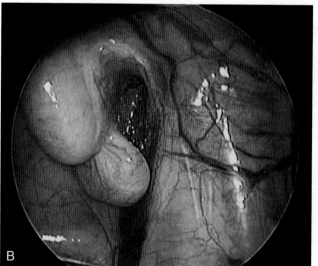

Figure 42-5. A, The vas deferens, gonadal vessels, and testis compose a triangle covered by peritoneum, with the testis at the apex of the triangle. This peritoneal triangle is scored for dissection of the testis, vas, and gonadal vessels. **B,** Left abdominal testis at the internal ring. Note the prominent vascular leash in the retroperitoneum.

Dissection of the Testis and Vascular Pedicle

The triangle of the vas deferens, testis, and gonadal vessels provides guidance for the dissection of the parietal peritoneum off the pelvic floor and side wall. Using a fine laparoscopic grasper, elevate a fold of peritoneum lateral to the gonadal vessels. Incise the peritoneum with the dominant hand using Endo Shears (Covidien, North Haven, Conn.), parallel to the gonadal vessels toward the ipsilateral internal inguinal ring. Grasp the peritoneum just distal to the testis and retract it cranially to expose the gubernaculum and processus vaginalis. Thin these tissues

before dividing them in order to avoid injury to a long-looping vas. Use electrocautery to divide the vascular gubernaculum (Fig. 42-6). Incise the peritoneum medial and parallel to the vas deferens as well, and bluntly mobilize the peritoneal triangle from the underlying iliac vessels, ureter, and obliterated umbilical artery. Preserve the peritoneal triangle between the vas deferens and the spermatic vessels as much as possible because this maximizes the blood supply to the mobilized testis but may have to be divided to maximize testicular mobilization.

Assess adequacy of pedicle mobility and length by guiding the mobilized gubernacular remnant and testis toward

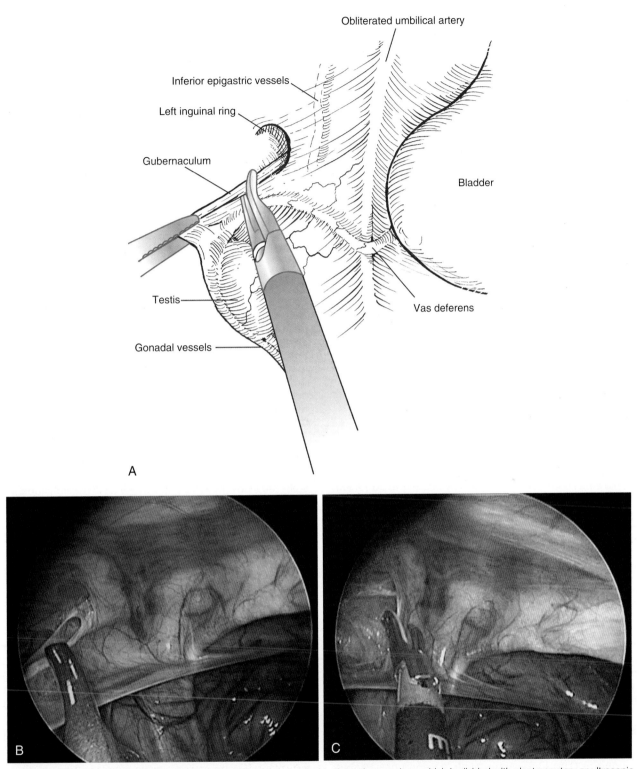

Figure 42-6. A and **B,** Division of the gubernaculum. Traction is applied to the gubernaculum, which is divided with electrocautery or ultrasonic coagulation. **C,** Incise the peritoneum medially parallel to the course of the vas deferens. The peritoneal triangle is developed and mobilized from the underlying iliac vessels, ureter, and obliterated umbilical artery.

the contralateral inguinal ring (Fig. 42-7). If the testis can safely reach this landmark, typically it can be placed in the scrotum without tension. If the testis cannot reach the contralateral ring, further proximal dissection is required. Continue the peritoneal incision lateral and parallel to the gonadal vessels, at times requiring deflection of the ipsilateral colon. High transverse incision of the peritoneum over the gonadal vessels (perpendicular to the axis of the vessels) may relax the pedicle for further length. Again, take care to minimize incision of the peritoneum distally between the vas and vessels, but this can be done if mobility is suboptimal.

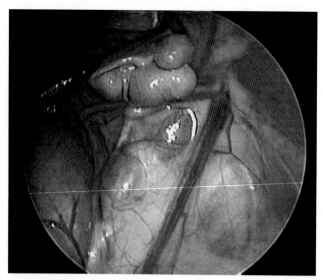

Figure 42-7. Verify that mobilized testis can reach the contralateral ring.

Creation of the Dartos Pouch

Create the dartos pouch through a 1-cm ipsilateral mid to low scrotal incision along natural skinfolds. Create this subcutaneous pouch with fine scissors or a fine hemostat, taking care to avoid dissection into the true hemiscrotum.

Laparoscopic Prentiss Maneuver

Once the dartos pouch is adequate, deliver the testis anterior to the pubic tubercle and into the scrotal incision. This is performed either with or without a radially dilating 10- to 12-mm trocar. We prefer placement of a trocar because this aids nontraumatic delivery of the testis into the scrotum. Alternatively, a grasper can be placed under laparoscopic guidance to grab the testis and deliver it into the scrotum.

We place a Veress needle with sheath through the scrotal incision, over the pubic tubercle, and enter the peritoneal cavity under laparoscopic guidance medial to the inferior epigastric vessels but lateral to the medial umbilical ligament (Prentiss maneuver), taking care to avoid the lateral wall of the bladder (Fig. 42-8). A 10- to 12-mm radially dilating trocar is then placed through the sheath, and this effectively creates a new inguinal tract for surgical descent of the testis, decreasing the length of pedicle needed to reach the scrotum. Verify adequacy of urethral catheter drainage before performing this maneuver in order to avoid bladder injury.

Delivery of the Testis with Orchiopexy

Advance a locking grasper through the scrotal trocar into the peritoneum (Fig. 42-9). Apply gentle traction on the gubernaculum to guide the testis over the pubis and through the scrotal incision while removing the trocar. If a 10-mm port is selected for scrotal access, the testis can typically be drawn safely into the trocar for smooth delivery into the scrotum. Endoscopically monitor descent of the testis into the scrotum from above to ensure delivery without torsion of the pedicle. Fix the testis within the dartos pouch according to surgeon preference for open orchiopexy.

Decrease the insufflation pressure and examine the field for active bleeding. Close the fascial port sites to avoid hernia, and inject the incisions with bupivacaine.

Two-Stage Fowler-Stephens Laparoscopic Orchiopexy (See Video 42-2)
First Stage

When an intra-abdominal testis is too high to bring down into the scrotum without excessive tension, perform a Fowler-Stephens orchiopexy. In the first stage, advance a 5-mm laparoscopic clip applier to ligate the gonadal vessels en bloc. A limited peritoneotomy medial to the vessels allows ligation without extensive dissection (Fig. 42-10). We do not divide the vessels in the first stage, but this can be done with electrocautery. We do not move the testis in the first stage, keeping the dissection to a minimum. Alternatively, one can place the fully mobilized testis and its divided vessels deep in the pelvis in the vicinity of the inferior epigastric vessels. In this case, although the testis is well positioned for the second stage, the secondary adhesions may complicate the second-stage dissection.

Second Stage

Final mobilization and delivery of the testis occur 6 months after the first stage. This waiting period is intended to maximize the quality of the vasal circulation through collateral flow. Minimal adhesion formation is typical after simple ligation during the first stage. Advise the parents that atrophy may have occurred and could result in orchiectomy during the second stage. Divide the clipped vessels, and proceed with peritoneal mobilization as described earlier for standard laparoscopic orchiopexy. Take great care to preserve the peritoneal triangle and all perivasal tissues.

One-Stage Fowler-Stephens Laparoscopic Orchiopexy

Some surgeons prefer to perform gonadal vessel ligation and transscrotal delivery of the testis in the same setting, possibly increasing the risk of acute testicular atrophy. Once it is clear that the mobilized testis and pedicle have insufficient length to reach the scrotum, clip and divide the vessels. The remainder of the procedure is as described earlier for standard laparoscopic orchiopexy. Outcomes equivalent to those of two-stage procedures have been reported if no prior testicular mobilization has been performed.

POSTOPERATIVE MANAGEMENT

Laparoscopic orchiopexy is an outpatient day surgery. Diet is advanced as tolerated. The child may shower or bathe 24 to 48 hours after the surgery. It is generally recommended to abstain from straddle toys and rough play for 2 to 3 weeks. We do not routinely prescribe narcotic pain medication owing to potential side effects. It is our experience that patients usually do well with acetaminophen and ibuprofen as needed. Follow-up in 3 months for the first postoperative visit is recommended.

With any history of cryptorchid testis, monthly bilateral testicular self-examination is recommended after puberty.

SURGICAL RESULTS

Validation of therapeutic laparoscopy in management of the intra-abdominal testis requires comparison with the gold standard of open surgical exploration. The desired technical outcome is a well-positioned scrotal testis without acute atrophy. Techniques must be stratified according to preservation or division of the gonadal vessels and whether a staged procedure is performed. There continues to be growing evidence that laparoscopic orchiopexy techniques for intra-abdominal testis are

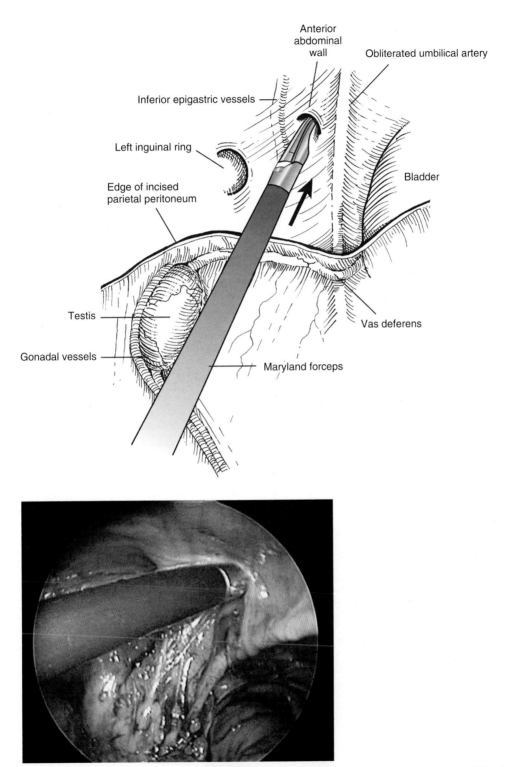

Figure 42-8. Laparoscopic Prentiss maneuver. Maryland forceps facilitate gentle penetration of the anterior abdominal wall fascia, medial to the inferior epigastric vessels but lateral to the obliterated umbilical artery.

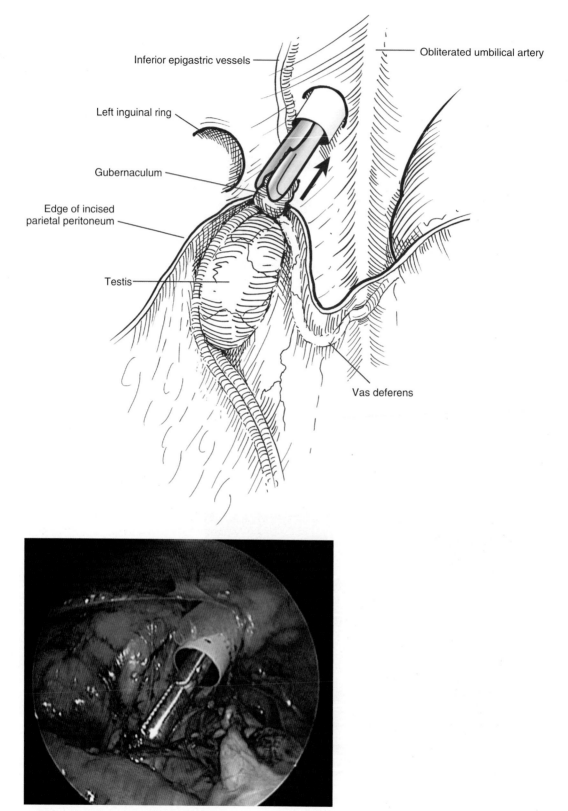

Figure 42-9. Delivery of the testis. A locking grasper is introduced through a scrotal trocar to deliver the testis to the scrotum. Descent is monitored laparoscopically to ensure delivery without pedicle torsion.

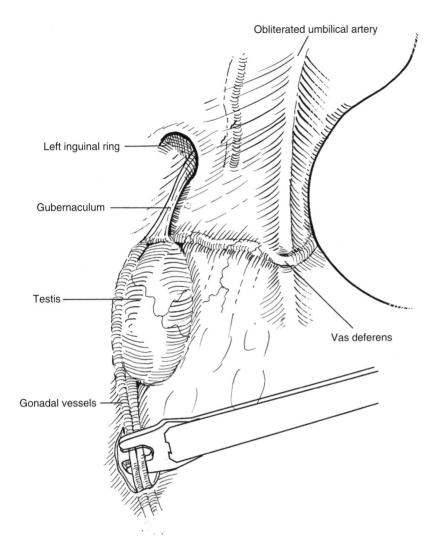

Figure 42-10. Fowler-Stephens maneuver. A 5-mm laparoscopic clip applier is advanced to ligate the gonadal vessels en bloc.

Obliterated umbilical artery

Left inguinal ring

Gubernaculum

Testis

Gonadal vessels

Vas deferens

TABLE 42-1 Success Rate as Defined by Intrascrotal Testis with No Testicular Atrophy

	Open FSO	Lap FSO One-Stage Procedure	Lap FSO Two-Stage Procedure
Success rate	81.7%	80%	85%

Data from Elyas R, Guerra LA, Pike J, et al. Is staging beneficial for Fowler-Stephens orchiopexy? A systematic review. *J Urol.* 2010;183:2012-2019.
FSO, Fowler-Stephens orchiopexy; *Lap FSO*, laparoscopic Fowler-Stephens orchiopexy.

safe and effective with the benefits of minimally invasive surgery. See Table 42-1 for success rates as defined by intrascrotal testis with no testicular atrophy.

COMPLICATIONS

Testicular atrophy and recurrent cryptorchidism are seen in both open and laparoscopic orchiopexy; however, operative complications are fortunately uncommon. Injury to abdominal viscera is more likely with blind insertion of a trocar after Veress needle insufflation than with open insertion of the initial trocar, particularly given the short distance between the anterior wall and the retroperitoneum in children. Injury to the bowel, bladder, great vessels, vas deferens, and gonadal vessels occurs infrequently.

TIPS AND TRICKS

- In young children it is difficult to dissect proximally because there is limited intracorporeal space to provide traction to aid dissection. We have found that delivering the testis into the scrotum and applying slight traction through the scrotum enables more proximal dissection and helps with visualization and further mobilization.
- In spite of maximal mobilization, if the testis reaches only to the upper scrotum, we can fix the testis to that position and plan for a second procedure a few months later for further mobilization. Alternatively, a traction button can be used to fix the testis to the lower scrotum and removed 2 weeks later.
- Children with prune belly syndrome are particularly at risk for bladder injury during scrotal port placement. Special care needs to be taken to be sure that the entry point is lateral to the median umbilical ligament.
- Challenges arise with LESS surgery. Surgeon preference and expertise are critical for a successful single-site procedure. Obvious challenges are loss of triangulation and overlying instruments. The advantage is that the incision is completely within the umbilicus, thus providing the patient with arguably better esthesis. An articulating laparoscope may also obviate some of the difficulties with single-site laparoscopy.

43 Laparoscopic Orchiectomy

Casey A. Seideman, Lane S. Palmer

INDICATIONS AND CONTRAINDICATIONS

The necessity for surgical removal of an intra-abdominal testicle or gonad is a rare event limited to gonadectomy in patients with gonadal dysgenesis and other forms of disorders of sexual differentiation, older patients with undescended testicles, or patients with inadequate testicular volume, and those in whom orchiopexy is not feasible.

Often, laparoscopic orchiectomy is a potential surgical decision made at the time of surgery for an undescended testicle. The ability to adequately mobilize the testicle and the size and quality of the testicle differ in each individual case. There are current recommendations to remove the intra-abdominal testicle in postpubertal patients up until age 50, when the risk of neoplasm is negligible. In addition, laparoscopic orchiectomy is indicated if an intra-abdominal nubbin is found on diagnostic laparoscopy for an undescended testicle.

PATIENT PREOPERATIVE EVALUATION AND PREPARATION

The preoperative evaluation of a child who will undergo a laparoscopic orchiectomy consists essentially of physical examination, with imaging and serum studies performed in selected cases. The physical examination is aimed at determining whether the testes are palpable and their location distal to the external inguinal ring. In the case of a nonpalpable testis, the presence of a descended contralateral testis measuring more than 2 cm in length may be a harbinger of an absent or a small intra-abdominal testis that will be removed laparoscopically. In general, the finding of a nonpalpable testicle in a young child does not warrant preoperative imaging because diagnostic laparoscopy offers the most definitive assessment. A scrotal and groin ultrasound may be useful in obese boys, in whom the identification of a testis may be difficult. A pelvic ultrasound is useful in boys with a disorder of sexual development (DSD) to assess for müllerian structures or the presence of an intra-abdominal gonad.

No routine laboratory studies are required before surgery, unless the patient has a predisposing medical condition or a DSD is being evaluated. In addition, we do not advocate preoperative bowel preparation before laparoscopic surgery in children unless they have a long-standing history of constipation.

OPERATING ROOM CONFIGURATION AND PATIENT POSITIONING

After the induction of general anesthesia, physical examination is repeated to confirm the absence of a palpable testis. A Foley catheter or feeding tube may be placed to empty a distended bladder, but this may be deferred until the bladder distention is assessed laparoscopically. Similarly, an orogastric tube may be placed for gastrointestinal decompression, at the surgeon's discretion. A dose of perioperative antibiotics may also be useful.

The patient is placed in the supine position with the arms tucked at the side and then is prepared from the xiphoid down to the mid thighs, including the scrotum (Fig. 43-1).

TROCAR PLACEMENT

The camera port is placed through the umbilicus. In the small child the umbilicus can be opened directly in the vertical midline; in the larger child, two towel clamps placed on lateral sides of the umbilicus can be used to invert the umbilicus, and the vertical incision is made. In younger children, a naturally occurring umbilical hernia may be present, into which a 5-mm trocar can be placed. In older children or adults the Hassan procedure can be used to gain abdominal access and reduce the risk of injury to an intra-abdominal organ.

The abdomen is insufflated at a low rate (3 to 5 L/min) to a low intra-abdominal pressure (8 to 12 cm H_2O), and a 0-degree or 30-degree laparoscope is introduced for diagnostic laparoscopy. When an intra-abdominal testicle is visualized, additional working trocars (3 mm, 5 mm, or 10 mm for removal of a large testis) are placed under direct visualization at or just below the level of the umbilicus at the lateral rectus margin (Fig. 43-2).

The patient is placed in moderate Trendelenburg position to allow the bowel to fall back and the surgeon to better visualize the working area in the pelvis.

PROCEDURE

After insertion of the laparoscope, a diligent and systematic inspection is performed (Fig. 43-3). This includes assessment for any injury during port placement and inspection of both internal inguinal rings to assess whether they are open or closed. If DSD is present or suspected, then müllerian structures and then the gonads are assessed. In the case of a possible intra-abdominal testis, the ipsilateral side of interest is inspected, first looking for the presence, course, and thickness of the internal spermatic vessels; the presence of a testis at the end of the vessels; and then the presence and course of the vas deferens.

If the testis (gonad) is to be removed laparoscopically, laparoscopic Maryland dissectors and laparoscopic scissors are used to grasp and incise the peritoneum overlying or just adjacent to the gonadal vessels. The vessels are carefully dissected off the posterior abdominal wall and isolated for about 2 cm distance (Fig. 43-4). Transection of the cord can be performed with the scissors between laparoscopic clips or with thermal energy devices, according to the surgeon's preference (Fig. 43-5). The testicle is now attached by the vas medially and the gubernaculum caudally. These attachments are divided with cautery via the laparoscopic scissors, and hemostasis is achieved with electrocautery.

The specimen is extracted through a working trocar. If the specimen is too large to remove from the trocar, it can be placed in a small Endo Catch bag (Medtronic Minimally Invasive Therapies, Minneapolis, Minn.), one of the lateral 5-mm port sites

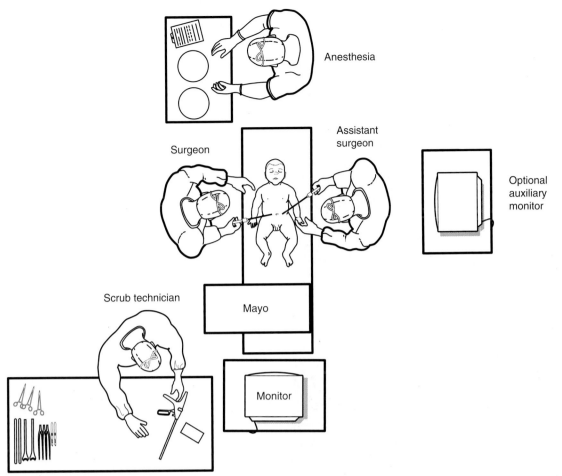

Figure 43-1. Operating room configuration. The monitor is placed at the foot of the bed to allow adequate visualization of the pelvis for the entire surgical team. The surgeon stands contralateral to the affected testis with an optional auxiliary monitor placed across the table for the primary surgeon.

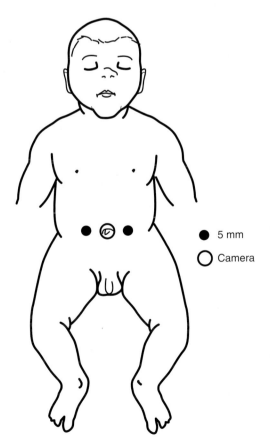

Figure 43-2. Trocar placement. A periumbilical port is initially placed, with second and third ports placed at the level of the umbilicus in the midclavicular line.

● 5 mm

○ Camera

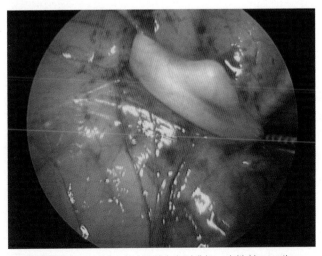

Figure 43-3. Intra-abdominal testicle is visible on initial inspection at the level of the internal ring. The testicle is small with atrophic vasculature.

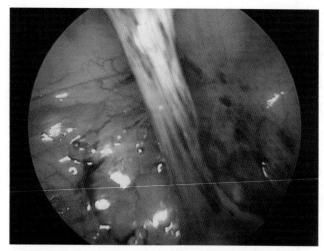

Figure 43-4. The vessels are dissected off the peritoneum and isolated for about a 2-cm segment, in preparation for clipping and transection.

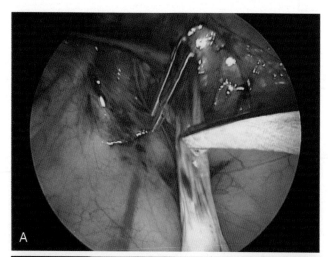

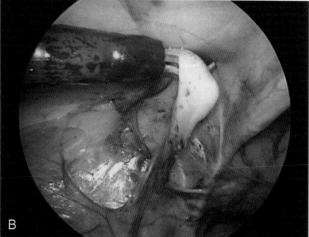

Figure 43-5. The vessels are isolated and clipped **(A)** and then transected with monopolar scissors **(B)**.

can be enlarged, and the specimen can be removed. If the port site is enlarged, the fascia is closed with 3-0 polyglactin suture. The remaining ports are removed under visual guidance, and the surgical site is again inspected for hemostasis. The skin is closed with a running subcuticular poliglecaprone stitch or with 2-octyl cyanoacrylate.

POSTOPERATIVE MANAGEMENT

The patient is discharged from day surgery. Typically, patients are sent home with a prescription for oral narcotics for pain control. Diet can be advanced as tolerated.

COMPLICATIONS

Complications secondary to laparoscopic orchiectomy are rare and similar to those related to any pediatric laparoscopic pelvic surgery. There is a small risk of injury to surrounding structures, including the bladder, which should be decompressed before port placement. Injuries to the bowel and vessels are also uncommon but are a serious complication risk. In addition, there is a risk of incisional hernia if the ports are not closed adequately. Currently, we advocate the fascial closure of all ports in small children.

TIPS AND TRICKS

- At the surgeon's discretion, one should consider scrotal fixation of solitary testis to avert later torsion and risk of anorchia.
- Always assess the size and quality of the contralateral testicle before orchiectomy.
- Bowel preparation can be considered in patients with chronic constipation.

44 Laparoscopic Varicocelectomy

Haris S. Ahmed, David A. Leavitt

Scrotal varicoceles can be found in approximately 15% of the adolescent population, with the prevalence ranging anywhere from 3% to 43% in adults. Although varicoceles are a common finding in males, the natural history is poorly understood and the true impact on future fertility potential is unknown. There is, however, ample evidence of the effects of varicocele on testicular size, growth, and spermatogenesis. The goal of treatment in children and adolescents is preservation or improvement of potential fertility and resolution of pain in those with symptomatic varicoceles. Varicocelectomy has been performed successfully via several techniques including the retroperitoneal Palomo approach, the Ivanissevich inguinal approach, microsurgical repair, retrograde embolization, antegrade sclerotherapy, and retroperitoneoscopic and transperitoneal laparoscopic procedures.

Laparoscopic varicocele ligation was first described in 1988 by de Badajoz, following the principles detailed by Palomo in 1949 for the open varicocelectomy, and has since become the most popular technique for the treatment of varicoceles in children. Over the last decade several modifications have been described, including two trocar approaches, single-incision approaches, and retroperitoneoscopic and needlescopic techniques. Improvements in lighting and instrumentation have allowed laparoscopic varicocele ligation to evolve into a highly safe and efficacious modality for the treatment of clinically significant varicoceles. This chapter describes a transperitoneal laparoscopic lymphatic- and artery-sparing varicocelectomy.

INDICATIONS AND CONTRAINDICATIONS

Varicocelectomy is indicated in patients with significant (20% or more) size discrepancy with left testicular hypotrophy, bilateral testicular hypotrophy, pain attributable to the varicocele, and abnormal semen parameters, which usually manifest as low sperm counts, poor motility, or both. Laparoscopic varicocelectomy may be of particular benefit in those with prior groin surgery, such as hernia repair, wherein adhesions and scar tissue may complicate traditional open or subinguinal microscopic approaches. With appropriate presurgical planning to avoid additional incisions, the laparoscopic approach can also be of benefit in treating bilateral varicoceles. There is some evidence to suggest that prophylactic ligation of varicoceles in prepubertal boys may allow for improved potential fertility and testicular catch-up growth, although this remains debatable.

There are few contraindications to performing laparoscopic varicocele ligation. Instances in which an alternate approach may be prudent include patients with extensive prior abdominal or retroperitoneal surgery, infections such as those of the abdominal wall or peritonitis predisposing to dense adhesions, large abdominal wall hernias, respiratory or cardiac compromise precluding sufficient pneumoperitoneum, and uncorrected coagulopathy. Prior surgery in the area of concern, specifically prior suprainguinal varix ligation by any approach or inguinal hernia repair with mesh, can lead to dense adhesions, making identification and mobilization of structures considerably more challenging, and complications more likely. If the artery is not to be spared, prior surgery that may have potentially compromised collateral blood supply to the testes also becomes a contraindication. Finally, although not a contraindication per se, obesity can increase the technical difficulty of the procedure and increase the possibility for complications.

PATIENT PREOPERATIVE EVALUATION AND PREPARATION

The preoperative evaluation of the adolescent with a clinically significant varicocele is the same whether an open, microscopic, or laparoscopic approach is planned. A thorough history should elucidate details regarding discomfort (pain, heaviness, visible and palpable varices) along with exacerbating and alleviating factors, such as varicocele reduction during recumbency. Physical examination should focus on a complete genital examination with palpation of the cord in both the upright and supine positions, and with the patient performing the Valsalva maneuver. Size discrepancy between the testes is of particular importance and should be documented clearly. Abdominal examination is performed to exclude abdominal masses.

Routine laboratory studies can be performed before laparoscopic surgery. In the adult patient, baseline semen parameters can be obtained; however, this is generally considered unnecessary in the adolescent patient. Imaging of the abdomen or scrotum is not routinely necessary. An exception is the isolated right-sided varicocele, which merits evaluation of the retroperitoneum, abdomen, and pelvis with cross-sectional imaging to rule out an underlying malignant process. On occasion, ultrasonography of the scrotum and spermatic cord for other indications may detect subclinical varicosities, for which treatment is customarily not recommended.

In obtaining informed consent, the patient should always be counseled on the possibility of conversion to open surgery if it becomes unsafe to proceed laparoscopically. No bowel preparation is required for laparoscopic varicocele ligation, nor is there a need to make blood available. However, some surgeons may choose to type and screen blood because there is a small risk of bleeding. A single perioperative dose of a broad-spectrum antibiotic, such as cefazolin, should be administered before the start of the procedure.

OPERATING ROOM CONFIGURATION AND PATIENT POSITIONING

The operating room configuration consists of a single monitor positioned at the foot of the bed, and an optional second monitor positioned for use by and across the operating table from the assistant and/or scrub nurse. The surgeon and assistant are positioned opposite one another, with the surgeon on the right side of the patient, facing the foot of the bed. The scrub nurse and any additional assistants are positioned behind the surgeon (Fig. 44-1).

The patient should void before entering the operating room to avoid the need for urinary bladder catheterization at the time of operation. Place the patient in the supine position and take care to pad all potential pressure points. The patient's arms can either be abducted on arm boards, making sure to leave enough room for the surgeon to work comfortably, or adducted and tucked. Securing the patient with wide tape over the legs, hips, and shoulders is not routinely done

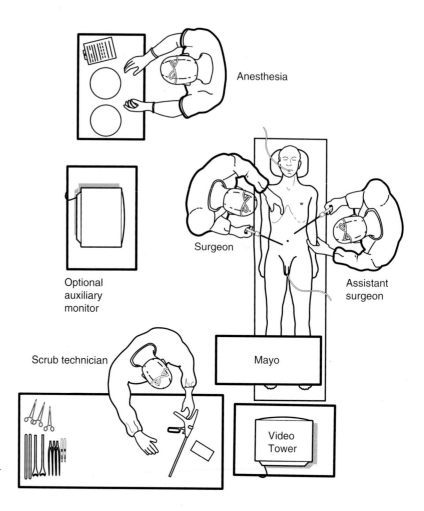

Figure 44-1. Operating room configuration. The surgeon stands on the right side and faces the monitor at the foot of the bed.

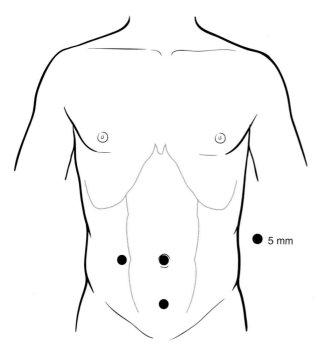

Figure 44-2. Port placement for a left-sided varicocelectomy. The periumbilical port is placed initially. One additional port is placed in the midline midway between the pubis and umbilicus, and the other is placed lateral to the rectus belly at the level of the umbilicus.

but does allow for safe rotation of the bed and steep Trendelenburg positioning should this become necessary during the procedure. After establishment of the pneumoperitoneum, the patient is situated in a slight Trendelenburg position and usually remains there throughout the duration of the procedure. Surgically prepare the skin from the level of the xiphoid down to the upper thighs, and laterally to the anterior superior iliac spines. The penis and scrotum should be included in the surgical field, which will allow for traction on the testicle to aid in identification of the ipsilateral spermatic vessels.

TROCAR PLACEMENT

Trocar placement can be achieved with either the Veress needle technique or a modified Hassan technique. Our preferred method of access involves making an umbilical incision and carrying this down to the level of the fascia. The fascia is then tented up (with a Kocher or Edna clamp), and the Veress needle is used to enter the abdomen and insufflate the peritoneal cavity. Pneumoperitoneum is maintained at a pressure of 10 to 15 mm Hg depending on the size of the patient, with the higher pressures reserved for larger adolescents.

Three ports are usually sufficient for completion of laparoscopic varicocele ligation, although two-port and single-port techniques have been reported with good success (Fig. 44-2). Trocar location may vary according to surgeon preference, but we find the herein described three-port configuration to be ergonomic and helpful for minimizing surgeon fatigue. Step trocars can be placed when smaller instruments are being used, although contemporary instrumentation and laparoscope optics are such that the entire procedure can frequently be accomplished with only 5-mm, or smaller, ports.

The first trocar is placed at the umbilicus through the same puncture site as the Veress needle. A 5-mm camera can then be used to inspect the abdomen and guide remaining trocar placement under direct vision. The second port is placed in the midline approximately halfway between the pubis and the umbilicus. This port can be placed more cephalad in taller or older patients, making sure that the gonadal vessels remain easily within reach of the working ports. The final port is placed lateral to the rectus muscle at the level of the umbilicus on the ipsilateral side of the varicocele. The operation is carried out through the umbilical and lateral ports; the laparoscope is held in the lower midline port. In cases of bilateral varicocelectomy, the umbilical trocar is repositioned laterally such that a single trocar is situated on the lateral abdomen on each side of the rectus abdominis muscle. The lower midline trocar remains the same, allowing a bilateral varicocelectomy to be performed through three port sites as well.

PROCEDURE (SEE VIDEO 44-1)

After placement of the laparoscopic ports, varicocelectomy is performed via the following steps:

1. Identify the spermatic vessels.
2. Create a lateral peritoneotomy and extend it medially.
3. Identify and isolate the largest varix.
4. Preserve the testicular artery.
5. Dissect the adventitia away from the isolated varix.
6. Preserve the lymphatics running within the adventitia.
7. Clip and ligate the isolated vein.
8. Inspect for additional varices. Then isolate, secure, and divide them.
9. Reduce pneumoperitoneal pressure and inspect for bleeding.
10. Close the trocar sites and skin incisions.

Through the lateral port, 5-mm curved scissors are introduced, and a curved grasper (Maryland) through the umbilical port. After initial peritoneal inspection, the spermatic vessels are identified as they course toward the ipsilateral internal inguinal ring and join the vas deferens (Fig. 44-3). Traction on the ipsilateral testicle will aid in identifying the lateral and medial margins of the spermatic cord structures when the anatomy is unclear. Occasionally, lysis of adhesions and even mobilization of the descending or sigmoid colon may be necessary to gain exposure to the internal ring and spermatic vessels. Maintaining the patient in slight Trendelenburg position will also aid in exposure by allowing the intestines to fall away with gravity.

Once the spermatic vessels have been adequately exposed, the peritoneum superolateral to the spermatic vessels is

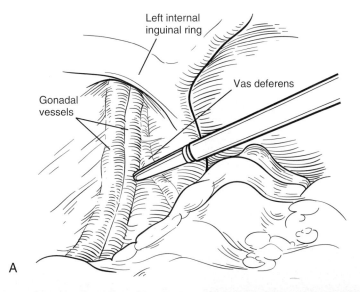

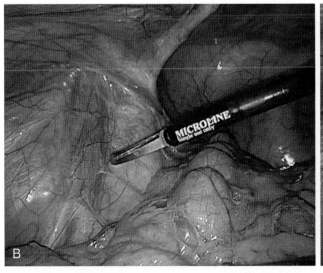

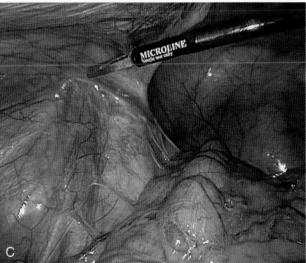

Figure 44-3. **A** to **C,** Anatomic landmarks including the gonadal vessels **(B)** and the internal inguinal ring **(C).**

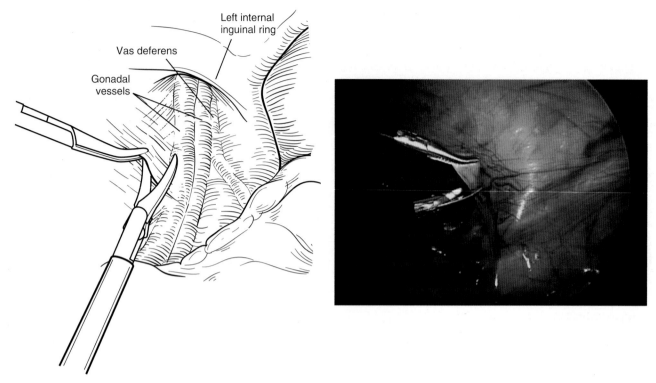

Figure 44-4. The peritoneum is tensioned and incised lateral to the gonadal vessels and superior to the internal inguinal ring in a direction parallel to the vessels.

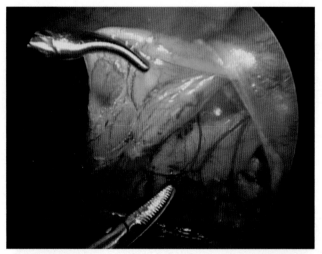

Figure 44-5. Identification and traction of the main varicose vein. Gentle traction on the testicle can help to reveal the medial and lateral limits of the vessels.

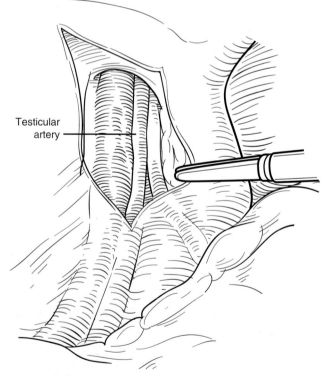

Figure 44-6. The testicular artery can be seen coursing adjacent to the main varix.

grasped and tensioned away from the retroperitoneum, and a peritoneotomy is created with the monopolar scissors (Fig. 44-4). The peritoneotomy can be extended in a craniocaudal direction for a few centimeters, parallel to the vessels, with the distal limit at least a few centimeters above the internal ring. The incised peritoneal edge is regrasped and elevated anteromedially. With this exposure, the scissors are used to extend the peritoneotomy medially past the medial aspect of the spermatic vessels, to the edge of the iliac vessels.

Once the peritoneum has been adequately dissected from the spermatic vessels, the varicocele(s) is easily identifiable, as often is the artery (Fig. 44-5). If the testicular artery is to be spared, laparoscopic Doppler can be helpful in confirming the artery's position, which often courses adjacent to the largest varix (Fig. 44-6). With the spermatic vessels exposed, the largest spermatic vein can then be identified and isolated.

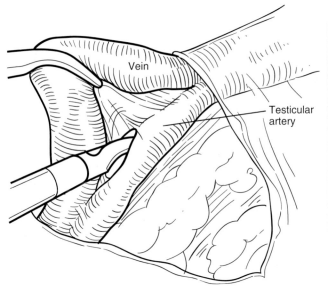

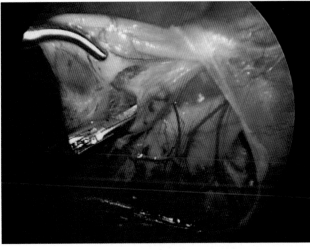

Figure 44-7. A combination of gentle blunt and sharp dissection can free the main vein from associated adventitia, the lymphatics, and the testicular artery.

This is best achieved by using the grasper to pick up the varix of interest and using the tip of the curved scissors to separate the vessel from the surrounding adventitia; a combination of blunt and sharp dissection may be required (Fig. 44-7). This also isolates the vessel into a packet sufficiently small for safe clipping. Careful separation of this adventitia is key during a lymphatic-sparing procedure, because this is where the bulk of the lymphatics are found and can thus be preserved (Fig. 44-8).

With the adventitia dissected off of the vessel, the curved tip scissor can be passed medially under the vessel to hold it up for clipping. The vessel can also be held with a grasper. Most commonly, either titanium clips or 5-mm Hem-o-lok clips (Teleflex, Morrisville, N.C.) are used to double-ligate the vessel both proximally and distally (Fig. 44-9). Clipping the vessel close to the edge of the peritoneotomy will help bury the clips in the retroperitoneum once the vessel is cut and the clipped ends retract. The clip applier can then be used to tension the vessel while it is transected with the scissors (Fig. 44-10). The same procedure is carried out for any remaining veins isolated from the adventitia and lymphatics (Fig. 44-11). Alternatively, silk ties or a vascular sealing device can also be used to control the spermatic veins (Fig. 44-12).

The peritoneum is not routinely reapproximated. After careful inspection for bleeding, the working trocars are removed under direct vision. The camera port can be used to assist in deflating the abdomen, after which it is removed. Some prefer to reinspect the surgical bed at low insufflation pressure (5 mm Hg), which may expose venous bleeding not appreciated under full pneumoperitoneum. After removal of all trocars, the port sites are then closed.

POSTOPERATIVE MANAGEMENT

Postoperative management for laparoscopic varicocelectomy is no different than for open varicocele ligation. The surgery is performed on an outpatient basis, with patients discharged home from the recovery room the same day. Limitations on activity are surgeon dependent, but in general, normal activity can be resumed on the first postoperative day and strenuous activity after the first week. The patient is able to return to a regular diet postoperatively, and excellent pain control is usually achieved with minimal narcotic requirement.

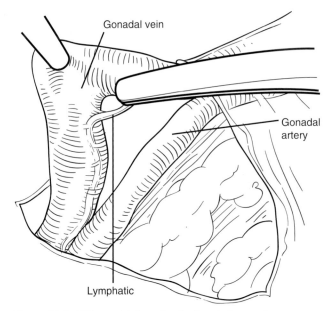

Figure 44-8. With careful dissection the lymphatics can be separated from the vein and preserved. One such large lymphatic channel is illustrated here.

Follow-up after laparoscopic varicocele ligation takes place within 1 to 2 weeks postoperatively, and then at 3 months, 6 months, and 1 year.

COMPLICATIONS

There are several important complications to be aware of that may result from laparoscopic varicocele ligation. In addition to the many well-described complications associated with laparoscopy in general (e.g., visceral organ injury, abdominal wall hernias, bowel obstruction secondary to adhesion formation, hypercapnia, infection, bleeding), a few complications specific to varicocele ligation include hydrocele formation, atrophy of the testicle, and nerve injury. Hydrocele represents the most common postoperative complication after varicocelectomy,

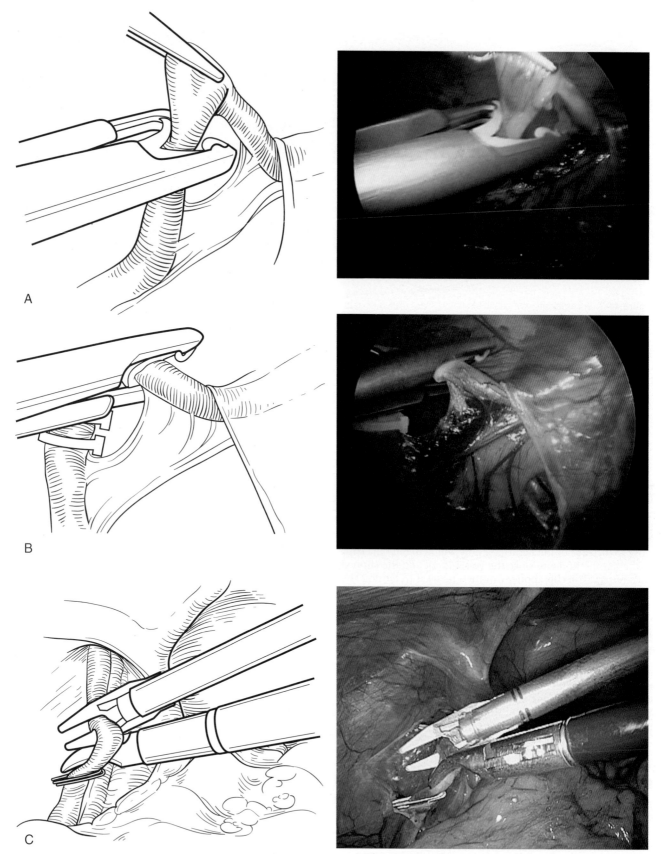

Figure 44-9. The varices can be controlled by a number of different measures, and are most commonly secured with Hem-o-Lok clips (Teleflex, Morrisville, N.C.) (**A** and **B**) or metal clips (**C**).

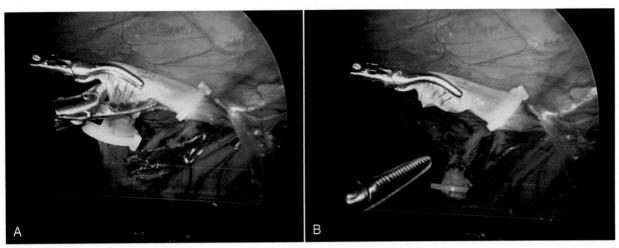

Figure 44-10. After proximal and distal ligation of the varix, it is transected **(A)**. In this case, cold scissors are used. Retraction of the proximal end of the vessel occurs after transection **(B)**.

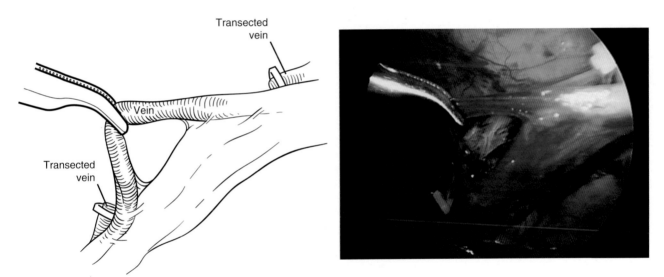

Figure 44-11. Additional veins are isolated and controlled in a similar manner.

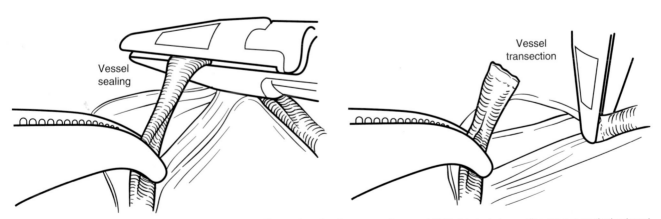

Figure 44-12. A vascular sealing device is shown controlling and cutting the spermatic vessel. With this technique, clips are not routinely placed across the vessel(s).

with a significantly decreased incidence after lymphatic- and artery-sparing procedures (30% versus 0% to 4%). Testicular atrophy and nerve injury occur infrequently. Testicular atrophy is most often seen when prior inguinal surgery has been performed, compromising collateral blood supply, and may be mitigated by artery-sparing approaches. Injury to the genitofemoral nerve is usually signaled by postoperative numbness or paresthesia along the groin and inner thigh. These symptoms most often resolve within 3 to 6 months with observation alone. Finally, both recurrence and persistence of the varicocele can occur. These are rare but more commonly encountered in artery- and lymphatic-sparing approaches in which there is a greater likelihood of missing a clinically significant varix.

TIPS AND TRICKS

- Have the patient void before he enters the operating room.
- Surgically preparing the genitalia in the operative field will allow for traction on the testicle to aid with identification of the spermatic vessels.
- Using slight Trendelenburg position facilitates exposure of the internal inguinal ring and spermatic vessels.
- Sparing of the lymphatics is best achieved by carefully dissecting the adventitia away from the vessels.
- Ensure that vessel packets are not too large for clipping and that clips are lying down securely across the entire vessel.
- At the end of the operation, inspect the surgical site under low insufflation pressure to elucidate any potential bleeding.

45 Laparoscopic Denervation for Chronic Testicular Pain

Salvatore Micali, Giacomo Maria Pirola, Angelo Territo, Giampaolo Bianchi

INDICATIONS AND CONTRAINDICATIONS

Chronic testicular pain (CTP) is a rare condition that for some patients can be severely debilitating and is a special challenge for the urologist. CTP is defined as unilateral or bilateral, intermittent or continuous testicular discomfort of at least 3 months' duration that interferes with the patient's daily activities.

Often the cause is difficult to assess, although the specific factors that mostly relate to chronic pain include urinary tract infections (e.g., prostatitis), testis tumor, inguinal hernia, hydrocele, spermatocele, varicocele, and prior surgery (e.g., vasectomy).

Pain is the major symptom, referred in 2% to 10% of patients with varicocele. Pain is described as heaviness or a dull ache, typically occurring after prolonged ambulation and worsening with physical activity and straining. In many cases, the clinical examination findings are normal; investigations such as scrotal ultrasonography and microbiologic urine analysis can yield unremarkable results.

Diagnosis and treatment of CTP have been difficult and an often unrewarding clinical situation; CTP is challenging to treat and might need a multidisciplinary approach.

First-line treatment should be restricted to a pharmacologic approach, such as antibiotics, nonsteroidal anti-inflammatory drugs, and antidepressants. If these options fail, surgery should be considered. Because testis pain has many different causes, caution should be used before recommending surgery for treatment of testicular pain. A cord block with a long-lasting anesthetic should be considered before recommending surgical denervation. If the patient has complete relief from the cord block, he is likely to benefit from surgical cord denervation.

Among surgical procedures, testicle-sparing epididymectomy, vasectomy reversal, hydrocelectomy, and inguinal testicular denervation have been considered and proposed. It is important to consider that inguinal denervation requires microsurgical skills and can compromise testicular blood supply, particularly in patients with a history of scrotal surgery.

Few reports have examined varicocelectomy as a suitable option for the treatment of chronic scrotal pain. The optimal technique is still a matter of controversy, but the following criteria for the optimal procedure have been stated: preservation and improvement of testicular function, elimination of the varicocele with a low recurrence rate, minimal intraoperative and postoperative complications and morbidity, and cost-effectiveness.

Surgical approaches include open surgical ligation of the spermatic vein, retrograde or anterograde sclerotherapy, microsurgery, and laparoscopy. Of course, each technique has its own advantages and disadvantages, with different results reported in the scientific literature.

A laparoscopic approach should be proposed depending on the experience of the surgeon with this procedure, advising the patient about the possibility of an open conversion if necessary.

Testicular denervation requires a precise knowledge of scrotal neuroanatomy. The innervation of the testis and epididymis is both autonomic and somatic, with fibers coursing in the spermatic cord. Cremasteric and layers (parietal and visceral) of the tunica vaginalis are innervated by the genital branch of the genitofemoral nerve; nociceptive fibers from the testis, vas deferens, and epididymis course within the sympathetic supply of each organ. Therefore, testicular nociceptive fibers course in the sympathetic plexus (T10 to T12), close to the testicular artery and vein, whereas the deferential and epididymal pelvic plexus (T10 to L1) is situated along the vas deferens.

Contraindications to surgical treatment are the finding of testicular tumor, chronic infection of the testis or epididymis, indirect inguinal hernia, spermatocele, or hydrocele.

PATIENT PREOPERATIVE EVALUATION AND PREPARATION

Preoperative evaluation of the patient is the same whether an open or a laparoscopic approach is planned. Laboratory studies should be performed as indicated; semen analysis is performed in all patients to investigate male infertility.

Transabdominal sonography is necessary to exclude abdominal masses and aortic aneurysms.

Patient preparation begins with informed consent. The patient undergoing laparoscopic surgery must always be informed of the potential necessity of conversion to an open procedure.

Antibiotic prophylaxis, such as with cefazolin, is administered before the patient is taken to the operating room. Antithrombotic prophylaxis is performed with anticoagulants (heparin) and with the use of elastic stockings.

There are no specific contraindications; only previous abdominal surgery is a relative contraindication.

PATIENT POSITIONING AND OPERATING ROOM CONFIGURATION

Under general anesthesia the patient is positioned on the operating table in supine position on a mattress with silicone to prevent slipping during Trendelenburg positioning. A Foley catheter is placed in the bladder.

The video monitor and the columns are positioned at the foot of the patient, in front of the operators (Fig. 45-1).

TROCAR PLACEMENT

The abdomen is insufflated to 15 mm Hg, and a 10-mm umbilical port is placed under direct vision. The table is tilted to elevate the operative side, and a second infraumbilical 5-mm port is placed in the midline. If necessary, an additional 3- or 5-mm port is placed lateral to the umbilicus on the ipsilateral midclavicular line to assist with dissection. The overlying peritoneum is incised and the gonadal vessels are isolated circumferentially proximal to the internal inguinal ring and vas deferens. The gonadal artery and vein with all perivascular tissue are divided between sutures or multiple clips. Care is taken to ensure that the vas deferens and its vasculature are well preserved. Trocar sites are closed in a standard fashion.

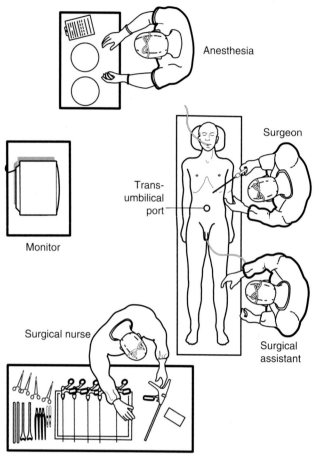

Figure 45-1. Surgical setting for right spermatic cord ligation. The umbilicus is the site for the laparoscopic endoscopic single-site surgery port.

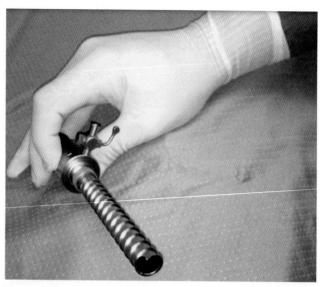

Figure 45-2. Ternamian EndoTIP 10-mm optical trocar. (Karl Storz Endoscopy-America Inc., El Segundo, Calif.) *(From Micali S, Ghaith A, Martorana E, et al: Bilateral spermatic cord en bloc ligation by laparoendoscopic single-site surgery: preliminary experience compared to conventional laparoscopy. BMC Urol. 2014;14:83.)*

PROCEDURE (SEE VIDEO 45-1)

Laparoscopic testicular denervation as a testis-sparing procedure is a minimally invasive technique. By complete division of the gonadal artery, vein, and perivascular tissue, interruption of the autonomic and nociceptive innervations of the testis is guaranteed. However, because fibers to the tunica vaginalis, vas deferens, and epididymis are spared, one would not expect complete scrotal denervation or universal success, despite a successful preoperative cord block.

Laparoscopic testicular denervation provides another advantage compared with inguinal denervation in patients with a history of testicular surgery (vasectomy) and is a less technically challenging way of preserving arterial flow to the testis. In these patients, unlike with the inguinal approach, when preserving the integrity of the testicular artery is essential for testis viability, laparoscopic testicular denervation allows for simple division of artery and vein. This division is possible because it occurs proximal to vessel confluence with the vas deferens.

Ultimately, in laparoscopic testicular denervation, distal gonadal artery flow can be provided via collaterals from the proximal deferential artery, even in patients with prior vasectomy.

Conventional Laparoscopic Varicocelectomy

The abdomen is insufflated to 15 mm Hg, and a 12-mm transumbilical optical trocar is used for the 0-degree lens. A second 5-mm port and an additional 10-mm port are placed in the midline between the umbilicus and the symphysis pubis and used for dissection with standard 5- and 10-mm laparoscopic instruments. The overlying peritoneum is incised, and the spermatic cord is isolated circumferentially proximal to the internal inguinal ring and the vas deferens. The gonadal vein is identified and adjacent tissue with lymphatics is swept away, and the vein is then ligated using titanium clips. Alternatively, en bloc ligation of the spermatic cord and surrounding tissue is performed with Hem-o-lok clips (Weck Closure Systems, Research Triangle Park, N.C.).

Recovery time after laparoscopic varicocelectomy is shorter than with the standard open inguinal approach (microsurgical subinguinal varicocelectomy), especially in bilateral cases. Patients are treated with a 1-day regimen and are able to return to normal activities after 3 or 4 days.

Laparoscopic Endoscopic Single-Site Surgery

The abdomen is insufflated with carbon dioxide at 15 mm Hg. To start, an incision of 2 cm is made on the lower margin of the umbilicus. Transperitoneal access is created with a 10-mm optical laparoscopic visual reusable trocar (EndoTIP 10 mm; Karl Storz, Tuttlingen, Germany) (Fig. 45-2). This trocar allows dissection of each tissue layer under direct vision, with complete control of blood vessels by the surgeon.

It is possible to replace the optical trocar with a disposable multiport trocar (GelPoint; Applied Medical, Rancho Santa Margarita, Calif.) (Fig. 45-3), performing an open technique to access the abdominal cavity and to position the port.

Transumbilical access has two advantages: obtaining better cosmetic results through use of a preexisting scar, and quick identification of the spermatic cord and vas deferens bilaterally by the same incision (Fig. 45-4). We introduce through the GelPoint a 5-mm flexible laparoscope Endo-EYE camera system (Olympus America, Melville, N.Y.) that minimizes the internal and external clashing of the instruments. Standard 5- and 10-mm laparoscopic instruments are used to perform the procedure. A 3- to 4-cm T incision of

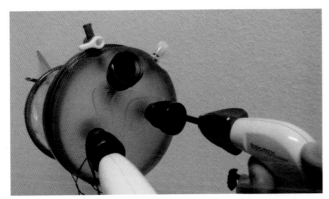

Figure 45-3. GelPoint laparoscopic endoscopic single-site surgery (LESS) port (Applied Medical, Rancho Santa Margarita, Calif.). *(Courtesy Ethicon Endo-Surgery, Cincinnati, Ohio.)*

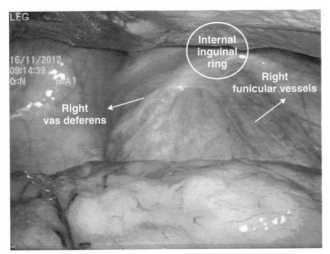

Figure 45-4. Right internal inguinal ring identification, with a view of the spermatic vessels and, medial to them, the vas deferens.

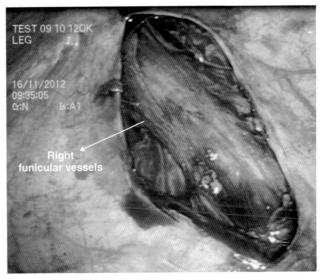

Figure 45-5. T incision of peritoneum and right spermatic cord exposure.

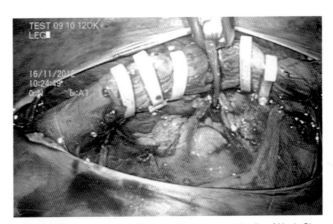

Figure 45-6. Left gonadal clamping with Hem-o-lok clips (Weck Closure Systems, Research Triangle Park, N.C.) and following transection with cold scissors.

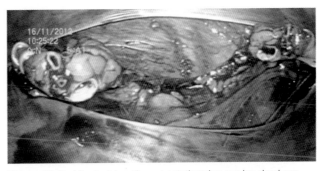

Figure 45-7. After incision, the cut ectatic veins can be clearly appreciated.

peritoneum is performed lateral to the spermatic cord and proximal to the internal ring and vas deferens (Fig. 45-5). The spermatic cord is isolated en bloc and Hem-o-lok clips are placed for hemostasis (Figs. 45-6 and 45-7). It is important to ensure vas deferens preservation with its artery to ensure blood supply to the ipsilateral testis. Finally, the abdominal cavity is slowly deflated for accurate hemostasis control.

POSTOPERATIVE MANAGEMENT

The bladder catheter is left in place for 8 to 10 hours to enable careful monitoring of urine output. Patients are started on liquids the morning after the surgery and advance to regular diet as tolerated. On average, patients are ready for discharge by postoperative day 1 and are allowed to gradually increase their activity with no restrictions after 3 to 4 days.

COMPLICATIONS

Bleeding caused by vascular injury is the most significant complication and is the most common cause for conversion to an open procedure. Bleeding can occur from the gonadic vessels but more commonly arises from injury to the iliac veins and arteries.

Unrecognized injury to the bowel is a possible complication of any laparoscopic procedure and may occur in an atypical fashion. The patient who has pain at one trocar site, low-grade fever, leukopenia, abdominal distention, and diarrhea even in the absence of peritoneal signs and ileus may have an unrecognized bowel injury.

Prompt diagnosis is important because mortality and significant morbidity can result from delayed recognition. Prompt imaging of the abdomen and pelvis with a CT scan is valuable in establishing the diagnosis of the type of injury. When a bowel injury has been identified, immediate exploration is required.

TIPS AND TRICKS

- Deflate the bladder and place a Foley catheter.
- The first key point is correct identification of the internal inguinal ring, with clear exposure of the gonadal vessels and, medial to them, the vas deferens. This will minimize the risk of vas deferens damage.
- The only therapy for chronic testicular pain is total denervation, which can be achieved with a funicular clamp en bloc. Many authors are skeptical about this technique because it includes the clamping of a gonadal artery; however, the deferential artery is sufficient for a complete testicular blood supply. This surgical technique can also be applied as a therapy for varicocele because it ensures a complete spermatic venous clamp.
- On the left side, it is important to mobilize the sigmoid colon, which is often located over funicular vessels. As in all laparoscopic procedures, take care to avoid bowel injury and, most important, to identify and not injure the internal iliac artery.

Index

Page numbers followed by *f* indicate figures; *t*, tables; *b*, boxes.